Hamilton Bailey's
Demonstrations of
PHYSICAL SIGNS
in Clinical Surgery

Hamilton Bailey's
Demonstrations of

PHYSICAL SIGNS

in Clinical Surgery

EDITED BY

Allan Clain MB (Cape) FRCS (Eng)

Consultant Surgeon and Surgical Tutor,
Dudley Road Hospital, Birmingham,
Senior Clinical Lecturer, Medical School, Birmingham

SIXTEENTH EDITION

Four hundred and five thousand

With 957 illustrations, of which 65 are unnumbered

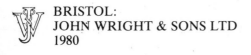
BRISTOL:
JOHN WRIGHT & SONS LTD
1980

First Edition, 1927
Second Edition, 1930
Third Edition, 1931
Fourth Edition, 1933
Fifth Edition, 1935
Sixth Edition, 1937
Seventh Edition, 1940
Eighth Edition, 1942
Ninth Edition, 1944
Tenth Edition, 1946

Eleventh Edition, 1949
Twelfth Edition, 1954   Assistant Editor: Allan Clain
Thirteenth Edition, 1960

Fourteenth Edition, 1967
Fifteenth Edition, 1973
Reprinted 1976   } Edited by Allan Clain
Reprinted 1978
Sixteenth Edition, 1980

German First Edition, 1939
German Second Edition, 1956
German Third Edition, 1959
German Fourth Edition, 1965
German Fifth Edition, 1967
German Sixth Edition, 1974
German Seventh Edition in preparation
Turkish Edition, 1953

Spanish First Edition, 1963
Spanish Second Edition, 1971
Spanish Third Edition, 1979
Spanish Fourth Edition in preparation
Bulgarian Edition, 1948
Jugoslav Edition, 1953
Italian Edition, 1965
Greek Edition, 1969

Four hundred and fifth thousand excluding foreign editions.

CIP Data

Bailey, Hamilton
  Hamilton Bailey's demonstrations of physical
  signs in clinical surgery. – 16th ed.
  1. Diagnosis, Surgical
  I. Clain, Allan   II. Demonstrations of physical
  signs in clinical surgery
  617'.075'4   RD35

ISBN 0 7236 0518 1

E.L.B.S. Edition first published 1967
E.L.B.S. Edition of Fifteenth Edition 1973
E.L.B.S. Edition of Sixteenth Edition 1980

PRINTED AND BOUND IN ENGLAND BY
HAZELL WATSON AND VINEY LTD, AYLESBURY, BUCKS

'If it is a question of doubt in diagnosis, you may often observe that one man solves the doubt when the others could not, and the way in which one man happened to solve it is this: he applied to the diagnosis of the case some method of examination which the others had not applied.' (Lockwood)

★ ★ ★

'Clinical diagnosis is an art, and the mastery of an art has no end; you can always be a better diagnostician.' (Clendening)

★ ★ ★

'The wards are the greatest of all research laboratories.' (Wade)

★ ★ ★

'There can be no substitute for detailed appraisal of the history and clinical signs.' (Ellis)

★ ★ ★

CHARLES BARRETT LOCKWOOD, 1856–1914, *Surgeon, St. Bartholomew's Hospital, London.*
LOGAN CLENDENING, 1884–1945, *Professor of Clinical Medicine, University of Kansas.*
SIR HENRY WADE, 1877–1955, *Surgeon-in-ordinary, Royal Infirmary, Edinburgh.*
HAROLD ELLIS, *Contemporary Professor of Surgery, Westminster Hospital Medical School, London.*

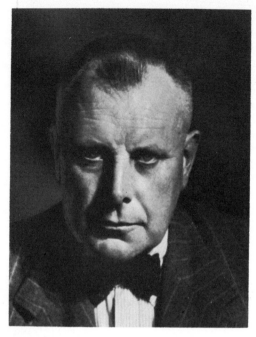

Hamilton Bailey 1894–1961

Born in Bishopstoke, Hampshire, where his father was a general practitioner, Henry Hamilton Bailey grew up in Southport, Eastbourne, and Brighton, where his father was successively in practice. His mother was a nurse, so not surprisingly he became a medical student at the London Hospital at the early age of sixteen, after schooling at St. Lawrence College, Ramsgate.

At the outbreak of the First World War he was a fourth-year medical student, and volunteered for the Red Cross, being dispatched with the British Expeditionary Force to Belgium. Almost inevitably he was taken prisoner-of-war and set to work on the German railways. A troop train was wrecked and Bailey, with two Frenchmen, was held on a suspicion of sabotage. One of the latter was actually executed but Bailey was reprieved (apparently by the good offices of the American Ambassador in Berlin) and repatriated via Denmark, where he continued his medical studies temporarily.

In 1916 he joined the Royal Navy as a Surgeon-Probationer, serving in H.M.S. *Iron Duke* at the battle of Jutland. During the battle he helped with casualties in near darkness, the electricity supply being damaged for most of the action. While in the Navy he qualified, and later returned to the London Hospital, where he gained the FRCS (Eng) in 1920. During his period as surgical registrar at the London Hospital he pricked his left index finger, and tendon-sheath infection, a common sequel in those days, ensued. The end-result was an amputation of the stiff finger (this can be seen in several illustrations in this book), but he soon overcame the disability.

Appointments as Assistant Surgeon at Liverpool Royal Infirmary, Surgeon to Dudley Road Hospital, Birmingham (1925), and finally as Surgeon to the Royal Northern Hospital, London (1931), followed:

In a quarter of a century Bailey produced this work, his *Emergency Surgery*, and *Short Practice of Surgery* (jointly with R. J. McNeill Love (1891–1974), contemporary as a surgical registrar at the London Hospital and as a Surgeon at the Royal Northern Hospital), edited *Surgery of Modern Warfare* during the Second World War, and revitalized *Pye's Surgical Handicraft*. These were his most successful works; all rapidly attained a wide circulation with many editions, and it has been said '. . . it will readily be conceded that the present excellence of illustrations in medical text-books owes much to his inspiration and striving for perfection'. In addition to these major contributions, he wrote over 130 original papers and 9 other books.

All this, together with a busy practice, particularly in surgical emergencies, was too much even for Hamilton Bailey's massive frame, and in 1948 he suffered a breakdown in health, aggravated, no doubt, by the death of his only child, a son, in a railway accident in 1943. He retired to Deal, Kent, and later to Malaga, Spain, but continued his literary work. He died of carcinoma of the colon, and is buried in the peaceful little English cemetery in Malaga. His missionary zeal for teaching medical students has been perpetuated by the use of the royalties from his books to expand medical school libraries in developing countries.

Preface to the sixteenth edition

Over fifty years have passed since the gestation of this work at Dudley Road Hospital, then, as now, one of the largest hospitals in the British Isles with a tremendous wealth of clinical material. I have been fortunate recently in obtaining a copy of the first edition of the book and it is interesting to note that, although a good deal of effort has gone into producing new illustrations for this edition (totalling approximately two hundred), there are still some twenty of the original photographs, taken by Mrs Hamilton Bailey, which have never been improved upon.

If seven foreign editions are taken into account (quite apart from a pirate Chinese edition) over half a million copies have been published and the last English edition ran to nearly 100,000 copies which seems to indicate that my policy of adhering to Hamilton Bailey's original aims as set out on p. xi still meets the requirements of surgical trainees. *Demonstrations of Physical Signs* is intended primarily for the medical student commencing clinical studies, and for him it is sufficient to read the sections in ordinary type. Small-print sections are intended for postgraduates but for the medical student in the tropics some of the small-print sections are basic. The number of Medical Schools and students in the tropical world is constantly increasing and the English Language Book Society Edition of this work is distributed widely in the tropics. Further efforts have been made in this edition to increase the conditions listed in the Appendix on Tropical Diseases.

Some believe that the zenith of clinical surgical diagnosis has been attained. To refute this new material and illustrations demonstrating diagnostic signs in the following conditions have been added: acute epiglottitis, oro-antral fistula, bronchial tear, pseudomyxoma peritonei, ischaemic colitis, pseudo-intestinal obstruction, yersinia enteritis, seat belt injury, intermittent claudication in a young person, crescent sign in calf haematoma, common peroneal nerve entrapment, recurrent dislocation of the shoulder, glomus tumour, lower limb shortening and battered baby. Rigorous pruning of obsolete material and illustrations has led to a slight reduction in size.

Grateful acknowledgement is given on pp. xiii–xiv to surgeons the world over for borrowed illustrations without which the book could not have reached its foremost position. Professor J. K. A. Clezy of the University of Papua New Guinea has kindly revised the section on leprosy and Mr Ernest Robin of Birmingham has given helpful advice on his specialty of Ear Nose and Throat Surgery. Other colleagues at Dudley Road Hospital have been generous in allowing me the use of their clinical illustrations, all of which (together with my own) have been skilfully produced by the hospital's Medical Photographic Department. My medical artist, Mrs June Clain, has replaced almost all the art work in the course of the three editions which I have edited. I am particularly grateful to Professor Ronald A. Malt of Harvard Medical School who offered, entirely unsolicited, to bring the biographical footnotes relating to American Surgeons up to date.

For this new sixteenth edition the Publishers have re-set the book completely in a new format. I am most appreciative of Mr A. H. B. Symons' care in applying John Wright & Sons' meticulous standards of technical skill with which many readers will be familiar.

Edgbaston,   ALLAN CLAIN
Birmingham

From the prefaces to the first to thirteenth editions

There is a growing tendency to rely upon laboratory and other auxiliary reports for a diagnosis. A former chief was wont to picture the modern graduate of medicine, when summoned to an urgent call, driving up to the patient's house followed by a pantechnicon containing a fully equipped X-ray installation, and a laboratory with a staff of assistants. Without these aids the future doctor would be unable to formulate a diagnosis. The history, and physical methods of examination, must always remain the main channels by which a diagnosis is made.

Written originally for the student commencing clinical work in the surgical wards and the out-patient department, it is to him or her that this book is still principally addressed. Couched in language that should be understood easily by anyone who has been trained in anatomy and physiology, when a term with which the beginner is unlikely to be familiar is introduced, its meaning and derivation are explained.

When I have felt not fully competent to speak from personal experience, I have studied the relative literature and sought advice from those who are better able to assess the value of particular physical signs than myself.

Individual physical signs are often known by the name of the person who first described them. In many respects this is an advantage, for an anatomico-pathological label is often cumbersome. On the other hand, an array of proper names is apt to bore the reader, especially if they do not conjure up personalities. By adding historical footnotes, not only is this objection overcome without lengthening the text, but due credit is given to whom we owe so much. If the reader is not interested, the footnotes can be disregarded.

The book has never presumed to be a complete treatise on clinical surgery; its scope is clearly set out in Chapter I. I have always intended it to be what its name implies—demonstrations—hence the pictures.

HAMILTON BAILEY

Acknowledgements

FOR READING THE PROOFS
Frank W. Wallis, *Stratford-upon-Avon*

FOR PRESENTING ILLUSTRATIONS
Girdharlal D. Adhia, *Bombay*. Fig. 853.
Lewis Aldridge, *Birmingham.Fig*. 406.
Cecil D. Alergant, *Liverpool*. Fig. 620.
Alan J. Alldred, *Dunedin, New Zealand*. Fig. 704.
Richard S. Allison, *Belfast*. Fig. 426.
'A.M.A. Archives of Surgery'. Fig. 518.
Stephen T. Anning, *Leeds*. Fig. 851.
Alan G. Apley, *Pyrford, Surrey*. Figs. 818, 826.
John Apley, *Bristol*. Fig. 229.
John Atkins, *Shrewsbury*. Fig. 243.
Stanley O. Aylett, *London*. Fig. 141.
Francis Bauer, *Liverpool*. Figs. 119, 159, 167, 249, 252, 659.
Edward A. Benson, *Leeds*. Fig. 772.
Peter G. Bevan, *Birmingham*. Figs. 73, 155, 310, 594, 632, 643.
C. Allan Birch, *Hastings*. Fig. 166.
Peter M. F. Bishop, *London*. Fig. 169.
Theodor Blum, *New York*. Figs. 230, 237.
'British Journal of Radiology'. Fig. 292.
'British Journal of Surgery'. Figs. 218, 523, 726, 772.
Ian Buchanan, *Birmingham*. Figs. 12, 13, 19.
Harold J. Burrows, *London*. Figs. 725, 832.
William H. P. Cant, *Birmingham*. Fig. 521.
Kenneth Clezy, *Papua New Guinea*. Figs. 621, 677–9, 875.
John H. Cobb, *Guildford*. Fig. 275.
Sean Corkery, *Birmingham*. Figs. 297, 498.
Mark B. Coventry, *Rochester, Minnesota*. Figs. 869, 879.
Vic Delal, *Birmingham*. Fig. 306.
Clyde L. Deming, *New Haven, Connecticut*. Fig. 612.
Edinburgh University Collection. Fig. 857.
Wray Ellis, *Stockton-on-Tees*. Fig. 361.
Keith Eltringham, *Bristol*. Figs. 654, 656.
Charles Engel, *London*. Fig. 216.
Philip R. Evans, *London*. Figs. 163, 811.
Maurice Feldman, *Birmingham*. Fig. 90.
Frederick P. Fitzgerald, *London*. Fig. 699.
Louis Forman, *London*. Fig. 873.
William Fowler, *Birmingham*. Fig. 581.
Paul F. Fox, *Chicago*. Fig. 518.
Thomas R. C. Fraser, *London*. Fig. 137.
Eric Freeman, *Lincoln*. Fig. 59.
Shyam Garg, *Zaria, Nigeria*. Fig. 87.
Durga D. Gaur, *Bombay*. Fig. 458.
Karl-Ove Gedda, *Göteborg, Sweden*. Fig. 796.

David L. Griffiths, *Manchester*. Figs. 779, 786.
Peter Hansell, *London*. Figs. 127, 130, 131.
Herbert E. Harding, *London*. Fig. 670
Francis D. Hart, *London*. Fig. 391.
D. St. Clair L. Henderson, *Birmingham*. Fig.34.
John H. Hicks, *Birmingham*. Fig. 702.
Maynard K. Hine, *Indianapolis, Indiana*. Fig. 236.
Harvey Jackson, *London*. Fig. 140.
James B. Jones, *Lynchburg, Virginia*. Fig. 814.
Allan E. Kark, *London*. Figs. 104, 343, 360, 496, 550, 854.
Weston M. Kelsey, *Winston-Salem, North Carolina*. Fig. 165.
James Kirby, *Birmingham*. Fig. 179.
Ivor R. H. Kramer, *London*. Fig. 217.
Sydney M. Laird, *Manchester*. *Fig*. 617.
Frank W. Law, *London*. Figs. 125, 128.
John F. Lipscomb, *Farnborough, Kent*. Fig. 298.
Arthur Lister, *London*. Fig. 124.
George C. Lloyd-Roberts, *London*. Fig. 703.
George R. W. N. Luntz, *Birmingham*. Fig. 794.
Ronald C. MacKeith, *London*. Fig. 101.
Brian McConkey, *Birmingham*. Figs. 152, 791, 792, 793.
John McKinnon, *Birmingham*. Fig. 335.
Thomas J. McNair, *Edinburgh*. Figs. 714, 765, 855.
Cecil P. Malley, *London*. Figs. 250, 255.
John Masterton, *Melbourne*. Figs. 175, 344, 693.
David N. Matthews, *London*. Fig. 579.
Colin Melnick, *Birmingham*. Figs. 219, 630, 631.
Samuel Movsas, *New York*. Fig. 522.
Philip H. Newman, *London*. Fig. 392.
Karl I. Nissen, *Sherborne, Dorset*. Fig. 816.
Keith Norcross, *Birmingham*. Fig. 887.
Archibald P. Norman, *London*. Figs. 411, 696.
Wilfred G. Oakley, *London*. Fig. 676.
Magdi Obeid, *Birmingham*. Fig. 480.
John S. Oldham, *Birmingham*. Figs. 149, 368.
Robert G. W. Ollerenshaw, *Manchester*. Figs. 380, 735, 748, 827.
'Oral Surgery, Medicine and Pathology'. Fig. 236.
Messrs. Parke, Davis & Co. Ltd. Fig. 241.
Alexander Paton, *Birmingham*. Figs. 94, 354, 680.

Max Pemberton, *Enfield, Middlesex. Figs.* 370, 592.

Harry Piggott, *Birmingham. Figs.* 710–13.

'Practitioner'. *Fig.* 137.

The 'Proceedings of Royal Society of Medicine'. *Fig.* 720.

Clive Quinnell, *Bath. Figs.* 690, 744-5.

'Radiology'. *Fig.* 890.

Anthony J. H. Rains, *London. Fig.* 432.

Frederick H. Robarts, *Edinburgh. Figs.* 287, 662.

Ernest Robin, *Birmingham. Fig.* 242.

Helmut Röckl, *Munich. Figs.* 771, 773.

Gordon K. Rose, *Oswestry. Figs.* 698, 843, 868.

Tristram A. S. Samuel, *London. Figs.* 281–4.

Eugene W. Scheldrup, *Iowa City. Fig.* 742.

Charles G. Scorer, *London. Fig.* 601.

Edmund Shephard, *Maidstone, Kent. Fig.* 720.

Samuel L. Simpson, *London. Figs.* 95, 167.

Michael M. L. Sutcliffe, *London. Fig.* 523.

Michael N. Tempest, *Chepstow, Mon. Fig.* 218.

David Trevor, *London. Fig.* 740.

'U.S. Armed Forces Journal'. *Fig.* 612.

George Vas, *Budapest. Figs.* 653, 848.

Robert F. Whitley, *London. Figs.* 800, 844, 884.

Alistair Wilson, *Birmingham. Figs.* 325, 425, 497.

Brian W. Windeyer, *London. Fig.* 292. .

Roy G. Yarwood, *Birmingham. Figs.* 53, 309, 468.

David Young, *Birmingham. Fig.* 707.

Contents

Chapter 1

INTRODUCTION

The making of a surgical diagnosis resolves itself into seven stages—often not more than three or four of these should be necessary.

1. A history is taken and a general observation of the patient is made.

2. Physical signs are elicited.

3. A mental process takes place on the part of the surgeon, whereby (1) and (2) are sifted and correlated, and a logical conclusion is drawn. Some would invoke the aid of a computer: no computer is as efficient as the *trained* human mind.

4. A differential diagnosis is entertained: this is also a mental process—largely one of exclusion, but reinforced, when possible, by further physical signs.

5. The more accessible parts of the interior are rendered visible by ingeniously constructed instruments, such as the cystoscope, sigmoidoscope, bronchoscope, oesophagoscope, gastroduodenoscope and colonoscope.

6. Confirmatory investigations are carried out. These may be relatively simple biochemical, bacteriological or radiological examinations, or, in obscure conditions, complicated technological procedures involving the use of radio-isotopes, ultrasound or computer tomography.

7. A biopsy or an exploratory operation is performed.

If a diagnosis is still found wanting after the seven stages have been exploited two possibilities remain: Nature cures the patient of his disease, and the diagnosis is for ever one of surmise; or he dies, and a post-mortem, the final court of appeal, if performed, reveals the exact pathology.

The seven stages may be termed the 'surgical crescendo'. *It is mainly with the second stage and the latter part of the fourth that this book is concerned.*

' "Data, Data, Data!" cried Sherlock Holmes. "I can't make bricks without clay." '* In the following demonstrations an earnest endeavour has been made to train the student to elicit and assemble facts upon which to formulate a reasoned diagnosis.

Another important objective is to bring before the reader selected patients with surgical conditions for demonstration, so that not only can a physical sign or signs be sought, but in a number of instances attention can be drawn to some characteristic feature or syndrome† helpful in arriving at a diagnosis.

Not all the patients presented suffer from conditions that will be encountered frequently. Whereas a particular disease is rare in one part of the world, sometimes it is not uncommon in another. Also possibly, the reader, having seen

---

* *The Copper Beeches*, Sir Arthur Conan Doyle.

† *Syndrome.* Greek, συνδρομή = concurrence: an aggregation of symptoms and physical signs that collectively constitute a clinical entity. With three leading criteria, the term 'triad' is employed (e.g. Hutchinson's triad, p. 89).

an illustration and read the corresponding text, sometimes will be enabled to make a correct diagnosis having never before encountered the condition.

Armamentarium. A few simple instruments are necessary; their cost is small. Practically all the apparatus employed in the tests described is shown in *Fig.* 1.

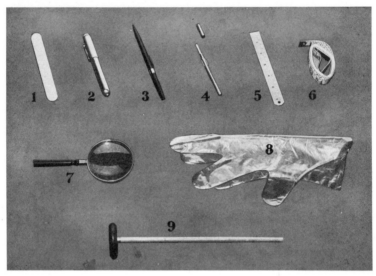

Fig. 1. Apparatus used for diagnostic purposes in this book. 1, Wooden tongue depressor; 2, Electric pocket torch; 3, Skin marking pen; 4, Clinical thermometer; 5, Metal ruler; 6, Linen tape-measure; 7, Magnifying glass; 8, Disposable glove; 9, Tendon hammer.

To become a competent clinician, the student and the practitioner must become familiar with the use of rectal, vaginal and nasal specula, together with the auroscope, ophthalmoscope and laryngeal mirror. In spite of requests to do so, no attempt to demonstrate the use of these important aids to diagnosis has been made because: (1) it is considered beyond the scope of physical signs; (2) an adequate description would greatly increase the size of the book.

Note-taking. Accurate records are essential, not least for medicolegal reasons. The history, which may be all-important in suggesting the diagnosis, should be noted. For the artistically inclined a sketch is a good method of documenting the physical signs. For the inartistic rubber stamps (*Fig.* 2) are useful.

The Boundaries of Surgical Diagnosis. The expanding frontiers of surgical treatment dictate that specialist surgeons require an understanding of the intricacies of medical diagnosis *in their particular domains*. Thus the neurosurgeon must be able to confirm the physical signs of, say, a cerebral tumour. The chest surgeon should recognize the signs of a heart lesion amenable to surgical treatment. However, the patient is examined initially by the relevant medical specialist who correlates the (sometimes complex) specific investigations necessary.

It is felt that physical diagnosis falling within such spheres is beyond the compass of this work, which is intended for the medical student and the trainee surgeon. The former will be instructed by those responsible for imparting the elements of medical diagnosis; the latter, if intending to specialize, should acquire the requisite knowledge during his training by surgeons in the specialty. Attention will thus be confined to the territory of what is usually regarded as general surgery *in the wider sense*. Gynaecological diagnosis is thus excluded, but genito-urinary and orthopaedic surgery are included.

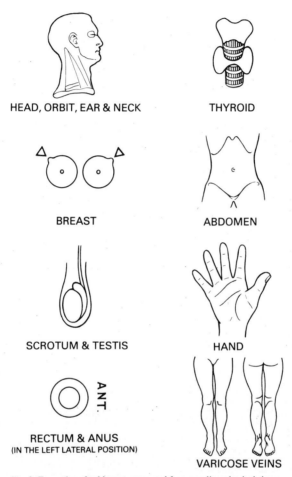

HEAD, ORBIT, EAR & NECK   THYROID

BREAST   ABDOMEN

SCROTUM & TESTIS   HAND

RECTUM & ANUS
(IN THE LEFT LATERAL POSITION)

VARICOSE VEINS

Fig. 2. Examples of rubber-stamps used for recording physical signs.

Communication. Finally, the diagnosis being reached, the doctor's next duty is to take the trouble to explain to the patient or a relative in simple terms, understandable to the layman, what is wrong and the steps necessary to correct it.

Chapter 2

BASIC PHYSICAL SIGNS

Before commencing to describe individual physical signs, let us tune up by harping for a moment on a fundamental principle of clinical surgery—*comparison*. When it is possible to compare an injured or diseased member or side with its opposite number (*Figs.* 3–6), the opportunity should be seized greedily. Observe this principle studiously.

THE VALUE OF COMPARISON

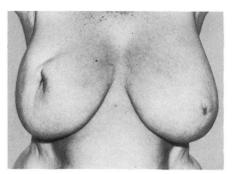

Fig. 3. Comparison of the nipples. This case of carcinoma of the right breast shows that the nipple is both raised and retracted (*see* p. 165).

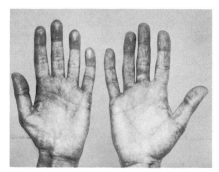

Fig. 4. Left cervical rib (*see* p. 146). Note the thenar wasting.

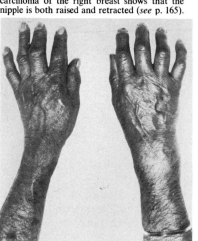

Fig. 5. Tuberculosis of the right wrist (*see* p. 461) in an Indian.

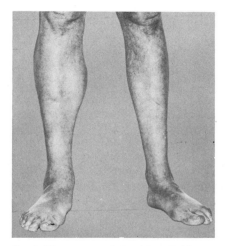

Fig. 6. Fibrosarcoma of the right calf. The swelling is not attached to the skin and can be moved freely on the tibia. With the calf muscles contracted the mobility of the swelling decreases.

Another fundamental principle is, after concluding the examination of a local inflammatory or neoplastic lesion, *remember the regional lymphatic field*. This should become so inculcated that it comes, not as an afterthought, but as a reflex. Conversely, when a lymph node (or group of lymph nodes) is found to be enlarged, the primary focus must be sought. Such omissions lead to failure in examinations and are a cause of embarrassing mistakes in practice.

INCIDENTAL OBSERVATION OF THE FACE AND HANDS

'You are looking better'; even a layman can discern signs in the face that portray improvement in a patient's condition. There is no doubt that the experienced clinician subconsciously makes more use of observing the facies than he realizes.

A glance at the face of a patient previously seen will often indicate (without other methods of examination) whether the condition from which he is suffering is responding to treatment. Important as is this relative assessment, we are concerned here particularly with the first glance at the face of a patient. The general diagnostic importance of the facies is enormous, but unfortunately much that can be learned from it cannot be put into words.

The eyes—those windows of the mind*—tell much, but not as much as once was thought (*Fig.* 7). Even the way the patient looks at you while he recounts his history may reveal sincerity or shiftiness. Slight bulging of the eyeballs, especially if combined with a nervous manner, should foretell the necessity of excluding hyperthyroidism in due course. Pin-point pupils, or at least small pupils (*Fig.* 8), suggest tabes dorsalis or narcotic drug addiction.

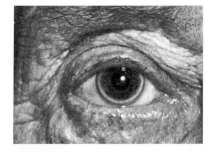

Fig. 7. So-called arcus senilis. While this undoubtedly becomes commoner with advancing age, it is not unduly associated with atherosclerosis, hypertension, myocardial infarction, stroke, or diabetes. It is relatively common in those of African descent.

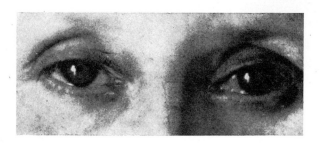

Fig. 8. 'Pin-point', slightly irregular pupils were noticed as this patient was giving her history of 'being unable to hold her water'. The pupils gave the Argyll Robertson reaction.† Knee jerks were absent. Diagnosis—incontinence of urine due to tabes dorsalis.

---

* 'Mistress, look on me; Behold the window of my heart, mine eye.' Shakespeare, *Love's Labour's Lost*, V. 2. 848.

† Absence or diminution of the pupillary reflex to light but an active contraction to near vision.

D. ARGYLL ROBERTSON, 1837–1909, *Ophthalmic Surgeon, Royal Infirmary, Edinburgh.*

A faint yellow tinge of the sclerae, unnoticed by others, may be apparent in good daylight to a trained observer. *In electric light even moderate jaundice may be missed.*

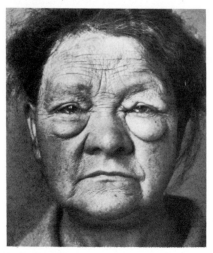

Fig. 9. In addition to bagginess under her eyes this patient had very dry skin and a sallow complexion. Case of myxoedema (*see* p. 159).

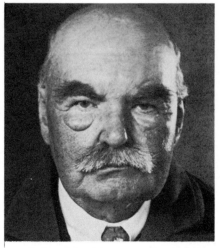

Fig. 10. Complains of frequency and nocturia. Bagginess under the eyes suggested nephritis. Urine loaded with albumin with microscopic casts but no pus cells.

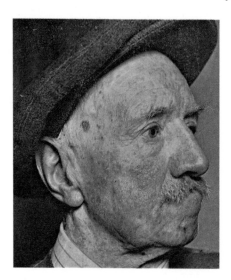

Fig. 11. Polycythaemia rubra vera. The florid plum-coloured complexion is accompanied by similar coloration of the tongue and mucous membranes.

In the heyday of life there is some foundation for the popular idea that bagginess under the eyes is a sign of debauchery; more often it is of ominous clinical significance (*Figs.* 9, 10).

Persons with acne rosacea or with polycythaemia rubra vera (*Fig.* 11) are liable to go through life branded as secret drinkers, an unwarranted assumption.

'Is he weather-beaten, or is it a faint cyanotic tinge?' We look at the nail-beds to determine this point. The patient has a bulldog jaw and heavy features, suggesting acromegaly (*Fig.* 12). He is requested to hold up his hands; spade-like hands (*Fig.* 13) confirm the suspicion. Regarding the hands 'one does not need the mysteries of palmistry to read in them something of the past, a great deal of the present, and even a little of the future. In them is written the record of age and sex; of occupation and habits; of skill or ineptitude; of hard work or indolence' (Cutler). A number of references to the hands in relation to general disease will be found in the pages of this book.

So much for a superficial introduction to an important and fascinating study of the first impression concerning the patient, in which the aspiring clinician should strive to acquire experience and proficiency.

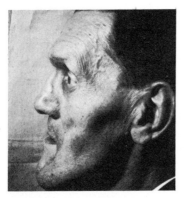

Fig. 12. 'Lantern jaw' acromegaly.

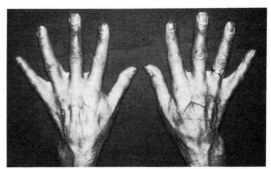

Fig. 13. Spade-like hands belonging to patient shown in *Fig.* 12.

THE PULSE

Details of examination of the pulse are dealt with in medical works. A few points of surgical importance are noted here.

1. Always regard with suspicion the pulse reading of a patient *immediately* after he has entered hospital, when he is likely to be excited and nervous. A reading after 20 minutes bed-rest is more likely to be accurate.

2. The *normal* pulse rate varies with age, especially with children. In the first few months of life the pulse rate normally may increase to 170 beats per minute during periods of crying and activity.

Age in years	Normal pulse rate per minute
Fetus	140–160
0– 1	135
1– 2	120
3– 4	110
5– 9	90
9–11	85
12–17	80
Adult	72

CONDICT W. CUTLER, 1888–1958, *Surgeon, Goldwater Memorial Hospital, New York City.*

3. A few perfectly healthy individuals have a much slower pulse rate (bradycardia*) than is set out in the standard table.

4. Frequent pulse readings are of considerable assistance in the diagnosis of internal haemorrhage. By 'frequent' is meant not a 4-hourly chart, but an hourly, or even quarter-hourly, record. This can be tabulated on a separate piece of paper, or it can be charted in red ink above the temperature chart. Usually temperature, pulse, and respirations are recorded graphically (preferably in different colours) so that any change in the patient's condition is apparent instantly.

5. Oft-repeated pulse readings are of paramount importance in the management of cases of head injury. A gradual slowing of, or a rise in, the rate is of such diagnostic importance in early cases that it is advisable to make a routine practice of recording it every quarter-hour.

6. If the pulse cannot be felt, try the other wrist; occasionally the radial artery is absent. If unsuccessful in feeling the pulse at either wrist, try the femoral arteries (*see* p. 380).

THE TONGUE IN RELATION TO THE GENERAL CONDITION

Because of its particularly rich blood supply with a capillary network close to the surface, the colour of the tongue is dark red. Normally it is covered by a slight greyish coating. It has been said that the tongue will tell the clinician many things, not only by what he hears, but by what he sees upon it. First, the very way in which the patient responds to the request 'Put out your tongue' may give some valuable information. There is no mistaking the agility, the extent and the willingness to display as much of the tongue as possible that comes of long practice before a mirror by a hypochondriacal patient.

Regarding coating on the tongue a myth should be dispelled; evidence collected from large series has proved that there is no relationship between a tongue more heavily coated than usual and constipation (Loudon).

Excessive Furring will be found to result from:

1. *Local Infection* arising from the mouth itself (as in stomatitis), from the nose or throat (as in tonsillitis, colds and sinusitis), or from the lungs (as in bronchitis and pneumonia).

2. *Dehydration of the Mouth* resulting from general dehydration, from pyrexia, from blocked nose (mouth-breathing), or from tobacco smoking.

Discoloration of the Tongue can result from chewing or sucking coloured foodstuffs, etc., the leading examples of which are betel nut (bright red), liquorice and iron-containing medicine (black), black cherries and blackberries (purple), and oral antibiotics which exterminate the normal flora of the buccal cavity with consequent growth of fungi, especially *Monilia*.

The Significance of a Dry Tongue. In surgical practice it is the relative dryness of its dorsum that makes the tongue a most valuable indicator. In late intestinal obstruction, renal failure and dehydration from any cause, the tongue is dry, brown and often encrusted, the dryness being due to diminished secretion of the salivary glands. However, a similar appearance can be caused by mouth breathing by an ill but not dehydrated patient.

(For examination of the diseased tongue *see* p. 119.)

---

* *Bradycardia*. Greek, βραδύς = slow.

IRVINE S. L. LOUDON, *Contemporary General Practitioner, Wantage, Berkshire.*

THE LOCATION OF PAIN

When pain is a feature instruct the patient to *point to the site of the pain*. More often than not he will indicate an area vaguely, or commence to rub the part. Ask him to place *one finger* on the spot where the pain is felt most (*see Fig.* 505, p. 289). In order to ascertain if there is a tender place it is often advisable to go further and to insist upon the patient palpating the area himself; only after the patient has concluded *his* examination do you commence *yours*.

The possibility of pain being *referred* should be to the fore in the clinician's mind. Notable examples are shown in *Fig.* 14.

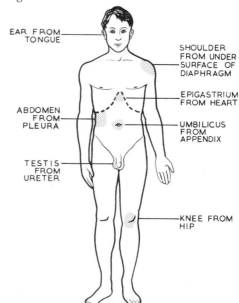

EAR FROM TONGUE

SHOULDER FROM UNDER SURFACE OF DIAPHRAGM

EPIGASTRIUM FROM HEART

ABDOMEN FROM PLEURA

UMBILICUS FROM APPENDIX

Fig. 14. Leading examples of referred pain.

TESTIS FROM URETER

KNEE FROM HIP

LOCAL TEMPERATURE

A sign of great value in early cases of inflammation is increased heat of the affected part. A good method of testing for this, but one that requires a little practice, is to pass the hand rapidly from the non-affected to the affected area, and back again (*Fig.* 15). This, and other signs of inflammation, later tend to be

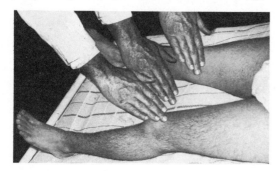

Fig. 15. Testing local temperature in the case of the knee joint. The hand is passed rapidly from the non-affected side, and back again.

masked by antibiotic therapy. As a result cold abscesses, formerly almost always tuberculous, are now frequently encountered following pyogenic infections.

PITTING ON PRESSURE

In order to confirm a suspicion of oedema, pressure is exerted by the thumb or a finger in the case of a massive infiltration (e.g. of the legs) (*Fig.* 16). With a comparatively circumscribed swelling the index finger should always be employed. Pressure is maintained for 10–15 seconds. Should the sign be positive, a pit will be produced and will remain where the pressure was exerted (*Fig.* 17) for upwards of half a minute. When the area is tender (e.g. inflammatory oedema) the index finger is employed and increasing pressure is exerted very slowly. Should a visible depression be doubtful, the palmar surfaces of the fingers are passed over the area, for minor degrees are sometimes better felt than seen.

'Oedema gives rise to a soft pitting, while if pus be present, induration can always be felt. If this fact is borne in mine, many embarrassing mistakes will be avoided' (Kanavel).

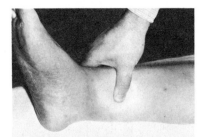

Fig. 16. Pitting on pressure. Case of oedema due to a failing heart. Pressure being exerted by the thumb.

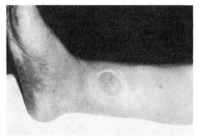

Fig. 17. A deep pit remains after removing the thumb. Same case as *Fig.* 16.

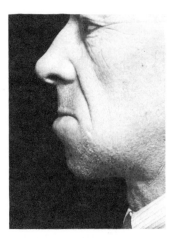

Fig. 18. Angioneurotic oedema of the lower lip.

Oedema of subcutaneous tissues can be due to a number of causes, examples of which are outpouring of lymph into the tissue spaces associated with

ALLEN B. KANAVEL, 1874–1938, *Professor of Surgery, Northwestern University, Chicago.*

inflammation, blocking of lymphatic vessels by carcinoma cells or by filarial nematodes, a defective peripheral circulation (e.g. a failing heart), nephritis, excessive intravenous fluid, extravasation of urine, and vitamin B_1 deficiency (e.g. that associated with beri-beri: it also occurs following starvation resulting from a duodenal fistula). Perhaps the most astonishing form is *angioneurotic oedema* (*Fig.* 18), due to allergy. Swelling of the affected part can take place before one's very eyes, and abate with such rapidity that it has gone, or almost gone, before the students can be summoned from a nearby refectory to observe it.

Oedema of the Ankle or Ankles, see p. 534.

Local Oedema confined to a limb, usually to a lower limb, can be due to venous thrombosis, compression of large veins by a tumour or enlarged lymph nodes. When the cause is obscure, always perform a rectal examination to exclude a carcinoma of the rectum, or other pelvic tumour. In residents in the tropics (at present or previously), when no other cause is apparent, lymphatic obstruction due to filariasis should be suspected. Finally, bear in mind oedema of one or both lower limbs due to maldevelopment of the lymphatics. (*See* p. 399.)

Oedema due to Endocrine Disorders. Myxoedema is sometimes accompanied by slight pitting oedema. Occasionally the oedema is considerable, and is accompanied by effusion into serous cavities, especially the pericardium.

Pretibial Myxoedema (*Fig.* 19) occurs only in persons suffering from, or, much more frequently, those who have suffered from thyrotoxicosis and who, as a result of treatment, are now otherwise symptom-free apart, sometimes, from persistent exophthalmos (*see* p. 73).

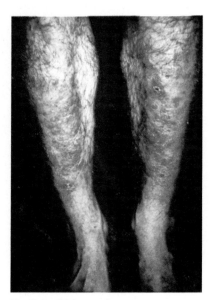

Fig. 19. Pretibial myxoedema.

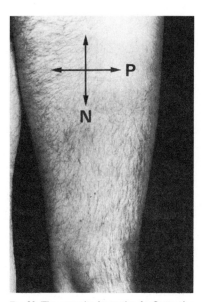

Fig. 20. The necessity for testing for fluctuation in two planes. P, Positive fluid impulse transversely, N, Negative impulse vertically.

FLUCTUATION AND TRANSMITTED IMPULSE

Fluctuation is the most elementary, and probably the oldest, physical sign in surgery. Yet how frequently one sees this test attempted in such a manner as to render the result absolutely valueless! The technique was described by Marsh thus:

'Fingers straight, a little flexed upon the metacarpals; the number of fingers depends upon the size of the swelling—usually the index finger of each hand is sufficient.'

Fluctuation implies transmitted impulse in two planes at right-angles to each other. To illustrate the necessity of this basic principle, the familiar experiment of transmitted fluid impulse across the normal thigh may be undertaken. An impulse through the quadriceps can be elicited in a transverse direction; if, however, the experiment is repeated in the longitudinal axis of the limb, the sign will be absent (*Fig.* 20).

Proceed to examine a swelling of moderate size for fluctuation. The pulp of the tip of the right forefinger is placed halfway between the centre and the periphery of the swelling. This is the 'watching finger', *and it is kept motionless throughout the procedure* (*Fig.* 21). The left forefinger is now placed upon a point at an equal distance from the centre, diagonally opposite the first. This is the 'displacing finger'. If the 'watching finger' is displaced by the pressure exerted by the 'displacing finger' *in both axes of the swelling*, then fluctuation is present, and we know that the swelling in question contains fluid.

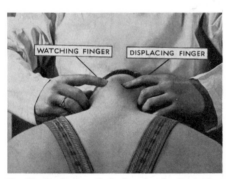

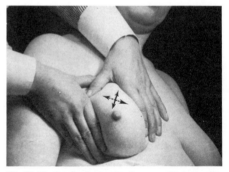

Fig. 21. Standard method of testing for fluctuation. Case of tuberculous abscess connected with the third cervical vertebra.

Fig. 22. Testing for fluctuation in a movable lump. The lump must first be fixed by an assistant. When this has been done, fluctuation can be sought in the usual way.

A second method of eliciting the sign is suited particularly to small swellings. The two fingers of the left hand are the 'watching fingers' and should be kept motionless. The right index finger is the 'displacing finger' (**A**) ⟶ This also must be tried in two planes at right-angles to one another before the sign is pronounced positive.

When a swelling is mobile in a soft surrounding medium (e.g. a cyst of the breast), it is necessary, before testing for fluctuation, to have the lump 'fixed' by an assistant or other onlooker (*Fig.* 22).

FREDERICK H. MARSH, 1839–1915, *Surgeon, St. Bartholomew's Hospital, London.*

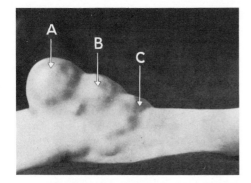

Fig. 23. Transmitted impulse could be demonstrated from A to B but not from B to C. This proved that the swelling A–B was a distended prepatellar bursa and the swelling C a distended infrapatellar bursa, which, as is well known, has no communication with the former.

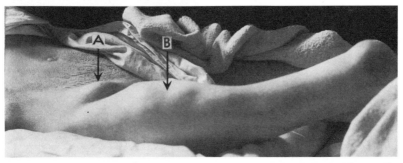

Fig. 24. Transmitted impulse could be demonstrated from above to below the inguinal ligament (A–B) in this case of psoas abscess.

Examples of *transmitted fluid impulse* are shown in *Figs*. 23 and 24.

Fallacies of Fluctuation. 1. *Does a lipoma fluctuate?* This is a vexed question, and one that puzzles the student considerably. Some lipomata appear to fluctuate. Fluctuation spells fluid; fat is semi-fluid at body temperature.

2. *In swellings of less than 2 cm in diameter* the sign of fluctuation is unreliable.

The reason for this is that in eliciting fluctuation the displacing finger (A), instead of merely increasing tension within a cystic swelling, displaces the swelling (irrespective of whether it is cystic or solid) and so imparts movement to the watching finger (B), viz. ⟶

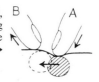

BALLOTTEMENT *

This sign, used for the confirmation of pregnancy (of more than 3 months' standing), has several non-obstetric applications:

Renal Ballottement. In the case of an intra-abdominal swelling suspected of being an enlarged kidney, with the patient supine, one hand is laid flat upon the abdomen, so that the greater part of the flexor surfaces of the fingers overlies the swelling, while the pulps of the slightly flexed fingers of the other hand are insinuated behind the loin so that they contact the area lateral to the sacrospinalis

---

* French, *ballottement* = a tossing about.

muscle. Short, quick, forward thrusts are made by the fingers of the posterior (displacing) hand, and if these movements impart a bouncing sensation (due to impacts of the swelling against the anterior abdominal wall) to the anteriorly placed (watching) hand, the sign is positive (*Figs*. 25, 26).

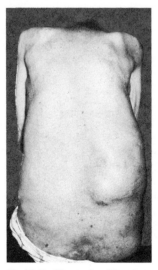

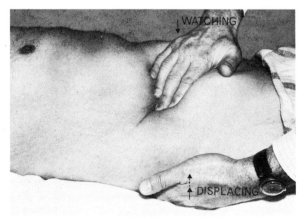

Fig. 25. Swelling produced by a large right-sided hydronephrosis.

Fig. 26. Showing the method of eliciting ballottement in the same patient as in *Fig.* 25.

Ballottement of Intraperitoneal Swellings can sometimes be elicited in great enlargements of the spleen when the organ is untethered by adhesions. It is not infrequently present with other swellings, particularly those at least fairly mobile, and especially when filled with fluid, e.g. ovarian cysts. However, ballottement is particularly helpful when a mass is present within a peritoneal cavity filled with fluid (ascites) when there is doubt whether an intraperitoneal swelling is present.

Ballottement of a Swelling rising out of the Pelvis. The left (watching) hand is laid over the hypogastrium, while the displacing finger of the right hand is inserted into the vagina, in contact with the cervix uteri if the uterus is thought to be the swelling. In *virgo intacta*, and in males with a large swelling occupying the true pelvis, it can be attempted by the displacing finger in the rectum.

TRANSLUCENCY

The routine application of this very useful sign often sheds light upon the nature of a swelling. There is one trap which must be borne in mind constantly, and that is '*normal skin illumination*' (*Fig.* 27). Unfortunately, it is not possible always to work with a torch of exactly the same power. Therefore always try out the 'normal skin illumination'. If this precaution is neglected, this sign becomes unreliable. In a strong light, especially in the summer sunlight, it should be elicited in the shade of a screen. In doubtful cases the room must be darkened.

Brilliantly translucent swellings are a vaginal hydrocele (*Fig.* 28), an encysted hydrocele of the cord, a cyst of the canal of Nuck (*see Fig.* 451, p. 259), a cystic hygroma, and a spinal meningocele. Two fallacies of transillumination are:

1. In a baby or a young child an inguinal hernia containing small intestine is translucent.

2. A vaginal hydrocele of many years' standing (owing to the deposition of fibrin and often blood pigment on its walls) is usually opaque.

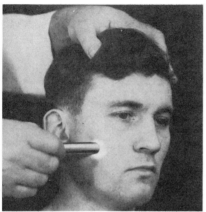

Fig. 27. Normal skin illumination.

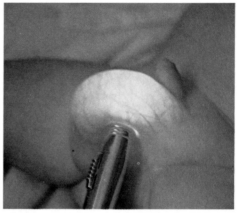

Fig. 28. A brilliantly translucent vaginal hydrocele in an infant.

CREPITUS

There are several varieties of crepitus, each being of fundamental importance.

Bone Crepitus. An attempt to elicit this sign of a fracture should be made only rarely when facilities for X-ray examination are not available. Great circumspection and gentleness are required. On movement of the part, coarse grating is so characteristic as to make the diagnosis of a fracture unmistakable.

Joint Crepitus. The joint is moved with one hand while the other hand is laid upon the joint (*Fig.* 29).

When present, joint crepitations are unmistakable. They comprise:

1. Fine, evenly spaced, crepitations, which are present in many subacute and chronic joint affections ⟶

2. Coarse, irregular, crepitations, which usually signify osteoarthrosis ⟶

3. A 'click' that can be re-elicited often proves a significant sign of a displaced cartilage or a loose body ⟶

Crepitus of Tenosynovitis is found over an inflamed tendon sheath when the inflammation is mild and allows of movement. An excellent example is de Quervain's disease (*see* p. 462). The hand is laid upon the arm above the wrist, and the patient is instructed to open and close his hand (*Fig.* 30). At the point where the extensor pollicis brevis and abductor pollicis longus cross the extensores carpi radialis longus et brevis (*Fig.* 30, inset) crepitus may be felt in cases of obscure pain near the wrist.

Crepitus of Subcutaneous * Emphysema. In four conditions gas is present in the subcutaneous tissues. In all a peculiar crackling sensation is imparted to the examining fingers. When one places the fingers fanwise on the affected area and exerts light pressure, a sensation similar to that of likewise palpating a horsehair mattress is experienced (Dooley). A stethoscope exerting steady pressure over the suspected area will enable crackling to be heard even though the crepitus is indefinite.

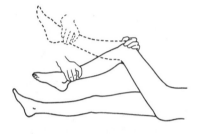

Fig. 29. Method of examining the knee joint for crepitus.

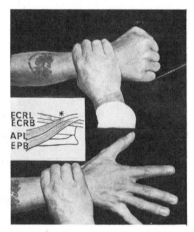

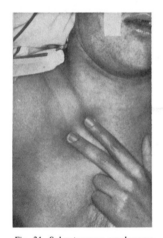

Fig. 30. Testing for crepitus in suspected de Quervain's disease. The site of tenosynovitis is depicted below the asterisk of the inset.

ECRL—Extensor carpi radialis longus. ECRB—Extensor carpi radialis brevis. APL—Abductor pollicis longus. EPB—Extensor pollicis brevis.

Fig. 31. Subcutaneous emphysema following multiple rib fractures.

1. *Traumatic* (*Fig.* 31). Most commonly complicates a fractured rib which penetrates the lung, and air extravasates into the subcutaneous tissues (*see* p. 182). Emphysema may extend widely, sometimes from the angle of the jaw to the scrotum. Inquire where the swelling commenced. If it began on one side of the face probably there is a fracture of a nasal air sinus, and air has been forced into the subcutaneous tissues by the patient blowing his nose. Similar facial

---

* The older term 'surgical emphysema' is still in use.

DENIS DOOLEY, *Contemporary, Her Majesty's Inspector of Anatomy, Ministry of Health, London.*

involvement has followed dental treatment when compressed air has perforated thin bone at the apex of a tooth root allowing air to escape into the soft tissues. Other sources of traumatic air extravasation into the subcutaneous tissues are a breach of continuity of the larynx (sometimes due to an accident, but usually due to tracheostomy) or bronchus (*see* p. 184) and a fractured skull implicating an air sinus such as the frontal (*see* p. 60).

2. *Infective*. Crepitus similar to the above is found in gas gangrene, but the patient always exhibits other signs of that condition (*see* p. 388).

3. *Extraneous*. Subcutaneous effusions of blood are wont to produce crepitus. A common source of perplexity to the uninitiated is when air becomes imprisoned during the closure of an operation wound or as a result of trauma to a limb. The house-surgeon may elicit subcutaneous crepitus and think that gas gangrene has developed in the wound which, except for crepitus, shows nothing amiss and the patient's condition gives rise to no anxiety.

4. *Subcutaneous Emphysema complicating Rupture of the Oesophagus* (*see* p. 196).

OBSERVING NORMAL AND ABNORMAL SUPERFICIAL VEINS

To assess the venous pressure, and thereby reap a harvest of highly important clinical data, it is only necessary to retract the garment that hides the root of the patient's neck (*Fig.* 32).

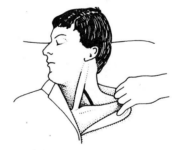

Fig. 32. Retracting the night attire in order to display the external jugular vein should become a clinical habit. In patients who are undergoing continuous intravenous therapy the external jugular vein should be kept uncovered for all to see.

The External Jugular Vein. When the venous pressure is within normal limits, with the head resting upon a pillow, the external jugular vein is either invisible, or visible only for a short distance above the clavicle (Lewis). If the venous pressure is raised, as in myocardial failure, the external jugular vein will indicate it. From a surgical point of view, by far the most important cause of this phenomenon is over-hydration; *engorgement of the external jugular vein is the earliest and best clinical sign that a patient is receiving too much fluid intravenously.*

Bilateral enlargement of the external jugular vein is seen in singers, due to continued endeavour to reach the top note. If the enlargement is unilateral it may be due to the vein being partially occluded in the supraclavicular fossa by enlarged lymph nodes, a neoplasm, or a subclavian aneurysm.

Enlarged Veins over the Superior Thoracic Aperture are sometimes the key to the diagnosis of a retrosternal goitre (*see* p. 157) and also of obstruction to the superior vena cava (*see* p. 191).

Sir Thomas Lewis, 1881–1945, *Physician-in-Charge of Clinical Research, University College Hospital, London.*

Unilateral Enlargement of Veins over the Upper Part of the Thorax usually is due to pressure on the subclavian vein.

A Series of Superficial Venules over the Costal Margin (*Fig.* 33,*A*) is often seen. They are without any clinical significance.

The Caput Medusae (*Fig.* 33,*B*). Radiating veins issuing from the umbilicus can be taken as positive evidence of obstruction to the portal venous system. Often the caput is incomplete, only enlarged epigastric veins being seen.

Inguino-axillary Veins (*Figs.* 33,*C*, 34). Obvious superficial communication between the veins of the axilla and those of the femoral triangle on both sides (*Fig.* 34) is evidence that the inferior vena cava is obstructed. When one side is affected, it signifies blockage of the common or external iliac vein of that side. For **Varicose Veins** *see* p. 395.

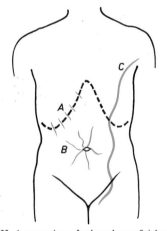

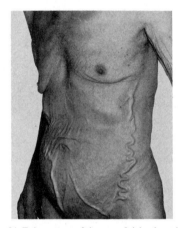

Fig. 33. A symposium of enlarged superficial veins of the trunk. *A*, Superficial venules over the costal margin; *B*, Caput Medusae; *C*, Inguino-axillary.

Fig. 34. Enlargement of the superficial epigastric and inguino-axillary veins due to obstruction of the inferior vena cava.

HICCUP

Hiccup, which is caused by spasmodic contractions of the diaphragm, is sometimes of considerable surgical significance. Occurring in the course of peritonitis, repeated hiccup often indicates that the diaphragmatic peritoneum has become implicated by upward extension of the inflammatory process. Hiccup is a fairly regular accompaniment of advanced renal insufficiency—even one diaphragmatic explosive contracture may give a lead. Ask the patient to protrude his tongue. If it looks less moist than normal it is likely that investigation will show that the urinary output is inadequate and the level of the blood urea is high.

As a rule, hiccup occurring in the early postoperative period signifies pressure on the under-surface of the diaphragm by a dilated stomach or coils of small intestine resulting from paralytic ileus or intestinal obstruction. At this time, so ominous is the sound of hiccup—perchance one muffled hiccup—that this should be a signal to pass a gastric aspiration tube and empty the stomach forthwith.

MEDUSA, *one of the three Gorgons whose fine hair was turned into snakes (Greek mythology).*

VOMIT

It is possible to recognize only:

1. The vomit of ingested material which has not had time to be altered by the digestive processes. Such vomit is acid in reaction.

2. Vomit containing blood which may be red or partly clotted or old ('coffee-grounds').

3. Vomit containing gastric juice when the patient has not eaten recently, i.e. a clear watery fluid, also acid in reaction.

4. Vomit containing bile, i.e. yellow in colour.

5. Vomit containing upper small bowel contents, i.e. green in colour.

6. 'Faeculent' vomit, i.e. lower small bowel contents, brown and smelly.

7. Vomit containing faeces.

8. A peculiar vomit associated with acute dilatation of the stomach (*see* p. 312).

The value of inspecting the vomitus should not be underestimated, but it is necessary to emphasize that it is asking too much to expect to formulate a diagnosis by its aid alone. Other data must be taken into account.

Sometimes there is a doubt whether the specimen contains blood or dark bile. Dilute it with water. If it is bile a green tinge will become apparent.

Vomit containing disintegrated old blood clot has aptly been called 'coffee-grounds' vomit. Unfortunately the term is much abused, and every dark vomit tends to be reported as 'coffee-grounds'. Red wine or medicine containing iron may give rise to a 'coffee-grounds' appearance.

Faeculent vomiting is found in late intestinal obstruction. It is distinguished not so much by its appearance as by its odour. Vomited tea may *look* like it.

Vomit containing formed faeces is rare, and signifies that there is a communication between the colon and the stomach, unless the patient is a coprophagist.*

The witnessing of the act of vomiting is valuable, it may be noted that the vomitus is ejected forcibly, as in the projectile vomiting of infantile pyloric stenosis, or that it is effortless and comes up in mouthfuls, as in established peritonitis.

Information regarding the progress of a case of intestinal obstruction may be obtained by the passage of a gastric aspiration tube, and aspiration of the stomach contents from time to time. If untreated, as the obstruction proceeds the character of the aspirations will change from clear gastric juice to greenish bile-stained fluid, and then to typical faeculent material. In the event of spontaneous relief of the obstruction, e.g. in paralytic ileus, this sequence will be reversed.

FAECES

Inspection of the faeces often provides an important clue to the diagnosis. Typical stools of surgical importance are shown in *Figs*. 35–38.

The Stools in Early Life. *Meconium*† is the scanty, semi-liquid, sticky, greenish-

---

* *Coprophagist.* Greek, κόπρος = dung.

† *Meconium.* Greek, μήκων = a poppy. The physicians of Ancient Greece believed that meconium was the substance responsible for keeping the fetus asleep in utero.

black, odourless excreta passed by the neonate during the first two or three days of life. It gradually gives place to slightly sour-smelling faeces, which by the end of the first week are a thin golden-yellow paste in a breast-fed baby, but paler and putty-like in a bottle-fed baby. As the infant takes more solid food the stools become less frequent, less smelly, darker, and better formed.

Blood in the Stools

*Melaena.** Blood arising from haemorrhage high in the alimentary canal, e.g. from a duodenal ulcer, is partly digested before it it passed. Usually it is evacuated by frequent actions of the bowels as black, tarry (sticky) stools (*Fig.* 37). The black stools passed by patients taking iron, bismuth, or charcoal are well formed, small and not sticky.

CHARACTERISTIC STOOLS

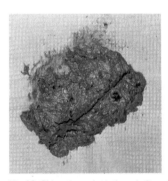

Fig. 35. China clay-coloured stool. Complete obstruction of the common bile duct by carcinoma of the pancreas.

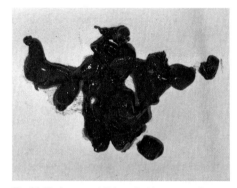

Fig. 36. 'Red-currant jelly' stool of intussusception.

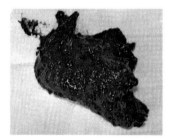

Fig. 37. Melaena stool. Bleeding duodenal ulcer.

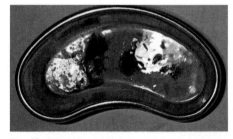

Fig. 38. Ulcerative colitis. Note the bloodstained mucus clinging to the bed-pan.

Stools with Dark Red Fragmented Clots suggest that the bleeding is coming from the small intestine, e.g. peptic ulcer within, or in the vicinity of, a Meckel's

---

* *Melaena.* Greek, μέλαινα, fem. of μέλας = black.

JOHANN F. MECKEL, the Younger, 1781–1833, *Professor of Anatomy and Surgery, Halle.*

diverticulum, but this assumption is unreliable, for massive gastroduodenal haemorrhage passing rapidly through the intestinal tract frequently results in red, as opposed to melaena, stools.

Bleeding from the Large Intestine gives rise to dark red jelly-like material streakily intermingled with the motion.

Blood arising from the Rectum or in the Anal Canal is characteristically bright red, and is either passed separately or as an incomplete coating on the surface of the faeces. One streak of bright red blood on the motion should alert the clinician to the possible presence of a fissure-in-ano or internal haemorrhoids or a more serious lesion.

Steatorrhoea. A severe degree of pancreatic insufficiency causes diarrhoea, characterized by malodorous and voluminous stools which float on the water in the lavatory pan. Pancreatic insufficiency is practically certain if the patient passes quantities of fat or oil that separates from the non-fatty portion of the faecal matter; such fat resembles butter that has melted and then becomes solid again (Bright).

Pipe-stem Stool. Totally unreliable is the pipe-stem stool supposed to occur in stenosis, particularly carcinomatous stricture of the rectum.

Toothpaste Stool of Hirschsprung's disease (*see* p. 241) is an unusual finding. The faeces are expressed as toothpaste is from a tube; spurious diarrhoea or absolute constipation is much commoner.

THE URINE

The macroscopic examination of the urine is considered on p. 335.

Chapter 3

LOCALIZED SWELLINGS

Deformity. Medical students often have difficulty in defining this term. The dictionary definition is 'that which mars or spoils the beauty of a thing' or 'marked deviation from the normal in size or shape of the body or of a part'. Thus a fair majority of surgical diseases, including all those discussed in this chapter, exhibit deformity as do such common conditions as external herniae. Generally speaking, however, the term is reserved to describe an abnormality of bone or joint, notably in disorders of a limb or of the spine. If a bone is out of its anatomical alignment it is deformed; if a joint cannot be placed in its neutral anatomical position it is deformed. 'Fixed deformity' denotes the angle between the neutral position of the normal joint and the position the deformed joint will reach (*see* Thomas's test, p. 490).

In elucidating the cause of deformity in a limb the student should consider the following categories:
Skin contracture across a joint.
Fascial contracture, e.g. Dupuytren's contracture, p. 486.
Muscle or *Tendon* contracture, e.g. Volkmann's ischaemia, p. 486.
Joint ankylosis.* The joint cannot be put through its normal range of movements.
Bone angulation, i.e. due to a fracture, recent or old.

THE DIAGNOSIS OF A LUMP

Step 1. The first essential is to leave no stone unturned in the endeavour to ascertain the *anatomical plane* in which the lump is situated. Ask yourself, 'Is it in the skin (*Figs.* 39 and 50), subcutaneous tissue (*Fig.* 87), muscle (*Fig.* 52), tendon, nerve, or bone (*Fig.* 45); or is it attached to some particular organ?'
Step 2. Determine the physical characteristics of the lump. Is it tender or non-tender? If not acutely tender determine its:
Size: Express as a measurement preferably in metric units.† Comparison with common objects is to be deprecated; even hen's eggs vary in size.
Shape: Round or flattened; regular or irregular.
Consistency: Five convenient gradations of consistency have proved tolerably satisfactory: very soft (like jelly), soft (as relaxed muscle), firm (like a contracted muscle), hard (as a contracted biceps of a boxer), and stony or bone hard.
Step 3. Having completed the examination, if the diagnosis is still uncertain run through the following little catechism to yourself:
  1. Is the lump congenital? If not—
  2. Is it traumatic?
  3. Is it inflammatory? If so, is it acute or chronic?
  4. Is it neoplastic? If so, is it benign or malignant? If malignant, is it primary or secondary?

---

* *Ankylosis.* Greek, ἀγκύλος = crooked. Stiffness or fixation of a joint.
  † In scientific medicine the results of all tests are expressed in metric quantities as are dosages of drugs and fluid balance charts. It is illogical, therefore, to measure size in inches.

5. If it is none of these, a degenerative, a metabolic, a parasitic, or a hormonal disorder may provide the key.

Of the multitudinous variety of lumps that are presented for diagnosis, the simplest is a *sebaceous cyst*. Manifestly the swelling is *in* the skin, but because the swelling is often comparatively small and the contents are pultaceous* it is not always possible to be certain whether it is cystic. Elementary as is the diagnosis, when a sebaceous cyst occurs in an unusual situation it is surprising how often the lump is misdiagnosed. Occasionally an obvious punctum (*Fig.* 39) settles the diagnosis without any further ado.

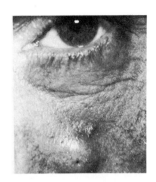

Fig. 39. The obvious punctum leaves no doubt concerning the diagnosis—sebaceous cyst, but it is by no means constantly present.

Next in simplicity of diagnosis, and even commoner, is a subcutaneous *lipoma*. A lipoma superficial to the deep fascia (the usual situation) is an elementary clinical problem, because often its lobulation can be made out, especially if the swelling can be compressed between the finger and thumb of one hand while its surface, now more prominent, is stroked firmly by the fingers of the other hand. Another sign of value is the 'slipping' sign. If the edge of the lump is pressed, the swelling slips from beneath the finger (*Fig.* 40). In the case of a subcutaneous lipoma, so regularly can this sign be elicited that it may be said

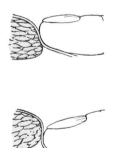

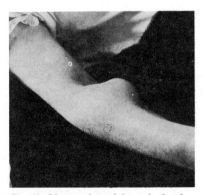

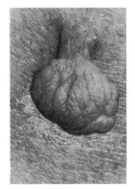

Fig. 40. The slipping sign of a subcutaneous lipoma.

Fig. 41. Lipoma situated beneath the deep fascia in front of the elbow.

Fig. 42. Pedunculated lipoma on the back.

---

* *Pultaceous.* Latin, *puls* = porridge.

to be pathognomonic* of that condition. On the other hand, a lipoma situated beneath the fascia (*Fig.* 41), or especially beneath muscle, is often exceedingly difficult to diagnose as the overlying fascia negates the slipping sign and masks the lobulation. An easily recognized variety which is not uncommon is a pedunculated lipoma (*Fig.* 42).

As a rule, a lipoma is entirely painless; from time to time subcutaneous lipomata are multiple (*Fig.* 47), and if one or more of them is painful, or at least tender, the condition is known as *adiposis dolorosa* or *Dercum's disease*. Other multiple superficial lumps comprise neurofibromatosis (*see Fig.* 58, p. 29), warts and naevi, and secondary carcinomatous nodules.

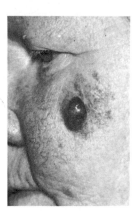

Fig. 43. Malignant melanoma on the cheek.

A malignant melanoma (*Fig.* 43) can arise in any pigmented tissue such as the anal skin or the uveal tract, but it does so most frequently in a pigmented skin mole. Unless removed very early, this tumour is of relentless malignancy (*see Fig.* 406, p. 234).

Throughout the demonstrations that follow, reference will be made to the diagnosis of lumps in various regions and particular organs, but before leaving this important subject it is necessary to demonstrate some physical signs of general application.

The Sign of Emptying. When the swelling is compressed it diminishes in size considerably or disappears; when the pressure is released, it refills slowly (*Fig.* 44). This is *the* sign of a cavernous haemangioma (*Fig.* 46), but it is also present in lymphangiomata and meningoceles, with narrow necks.

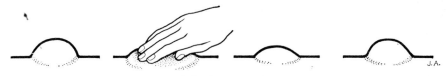

Fig. 44. The sign of emptying.

---

* *Pathognomonic.* Greek, πάθος = disease + γνώμη = signature. The signature of that disease, and none other.

FRANCIS X. DERCUM, 1865–1931, *Professor of Neurology, Jefferson Medical College, Philadelphia.*

Some Lumps for Diagnosis

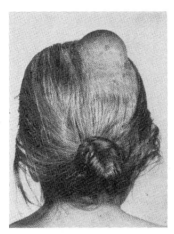

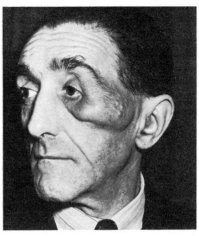

Fig. 45. The swelling appeared in a matter of weeks and is not tender or warm to the touch. It would be correct to make a diagnosis of 'probably secondary malignant disease of bone', but where is the primary? In this instance biopsy proved a bone metastasis secondary to carcinoma of the thyroid.

Fig. 46. Cavernous haemangioma extending into the orbit. The swelling gave the sign of emptying.

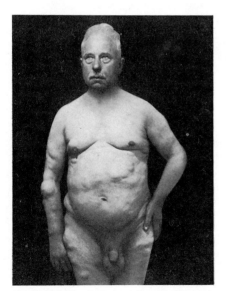

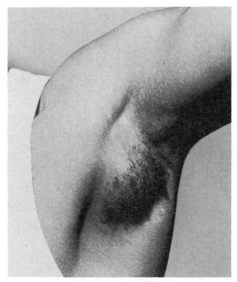

Fig. 47. Multiple subcutaneous lipomata (Dercum's disease).

Fig. 48. Axillary swelling. On palpation it shows expansile pulsation. Systolic bruit present. Aneurysm of axillary artery following trauma.

Some Lumps for Diagnosis

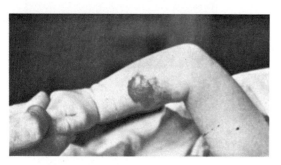

Fig. 49. Capillary angioma (strawberry naevus).

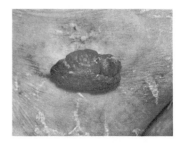

Fig. 50. Pedunculated papilloma. Slowly increasing in size, it finally outgrew its vascular supply and it has become gangrenous.

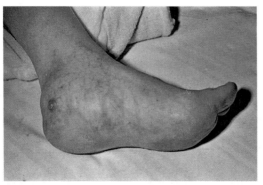

Fig. 51. Students who examined this patient concluded that the swelling was an abscess, but it is not tender, the periphery feels 'wooden' and lacks superficial oedema. It is doubtful whether the sign of local heat is present. Case of synovial sarcoma (which arises from joint synovium).

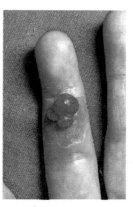

Fig. 52. Usually after a minor penetrating injury to the hand (but sometimes elsewhere) a dull red polypoid lesion resembling granulation tissue appears and persists. Diagnosis: pyogenic granuloma.

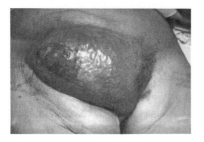

Fig. 53. The patient had noticed a lump in the groin for many years. For ten days it had been painful and for three days she had vomited incessantly. Strangulated femoral hernia with gangrene of contents (small bowel) and of overlying skin. The case presented, not in a remote area lacking in doctors, but in England fairly recently!

On a miniature scale, the sign of emptying is useful in the diagnosis of a capillary angioma (*Fig*. 49), which blanches when the skin about it is put on the stretch. In this way tiny capillary angiomata can be distinguished from de Morgan's spots. The latter are raspberry red (*see Fig*. 435, p. 250), and do not show the sign of emptying. They are of no clinical significance. At one time they were thought to suggest visceral carcinoma.

The Sign of Indentation. Certain cysts (large dermoid and sebaceous cysts) containing pultaceous material can be moulded. When the swelling is indented with the finger, in contradistinction to the sign of emptying, it stays indented. The only other lump in which indentation occurs is one formed of solid faeces.

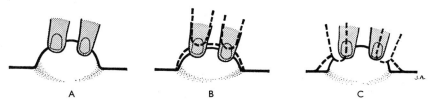

Fig. 54. A, Place the index and middle fingers on the swelling. B, Transmitted pulsation. C, Expansile impulse. The sign of an aneurysm.

Expansile Impulse. It is often a perplexing problem to decide whether the pulsation of a swelling is *transmitted* from a neighbouring artery or whether the swelling itself is pulsating (*Fig*. 48). Place the index and middle fingers over the swelling (*Fig*. 54). They will be felt to move with the swelling. If the pulsation is transmitted, the movements of the fingers during each throb of the pulse are parallel with each other. If the swelling is expansile, the fingers are felt to move apart.

Estimating the Size of an Aneurysm. The following method is helpful in deciding whether surgical treatment is necessary, notably with abdominal aortic aneurysm (Eastcott). Place the parallel index fingers ⎯⎯⎯⎯⎯⎯⎯⎯→ in the long axis of the aneurysm at its outer margins. The distance between the finger tips equals the diameter of the aneurysm.

When a stethoscope is applied over it, an aneurysm is either silent or a systolic bruit can be heard. On the other hand, an arteriovenous fistula emits a continuous murmur through systole and diastole (Rob).

It should always be remembered that a very rapidly growing vascular neoplasm, particularly a bone sarcoma, often pulsates very obviously. 'A swelling which has most of the characteristics of, but is not, an aneurysm, is a sarcoma' (Morison).

Tumour of a Muscle (*see Fig*. 6, p. 4), or any swelling situated in, or attached to, a muscle, gives one pathognomonic sign. When the muscle is relaxed the lump is movable freely across the long axis of the muscle; when contracted, this range of movement becomes abruptly limited. Sometimes the patient understands what is meant by a request to brace the muscle, or group of muscles. More often the muscle must be rendered tense by causing it to contract against resistance. Expedients for rendering individual voluntary muscles tense are discussed in Chapter 27.

CAMPBELL DE MORGAN, 1811–1876, *Surgeon, Middlesex Hospital, London.*
HARRY H. G. EASTCOTT, *Contemporary Consultant Surgeon, St. Mary's Hospital, London.*
CHARLES G. ROB, *Contemporary Professor of Surgery, E. Carolina School of Medicine, Greenville, South Carolina.*
JAMES R. MORISON, 1853–1939, *Professor of Surgery, University of Durham, Newcastle-upon-Tyne.*

Herniation of a Muscle is shown when a lump appears (due to a defect in the deep fascia) on the patient being asked to tense the muscle.

Fibrosarcoma can take varying forms in the subcutaneous tissue, fascia, or muscle. It is firm or hard in consistency, grows slowly, and typically, unless widely excised at the first operation, recurs time and again.

Desmoid Tumour is an example of the above. It occurs in the abdominal wall, often in the lower half and usually in middle-aged multiparous women and occasionally in operation scars.

Tumour of a Nerve. *See* p. 414.

Tumour of Bone (*Fig.* 45). The characteristics are discussed on p. 422.

Cutaneous Swellings giving rise to diagnostic difficulty:

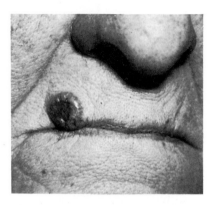

Fig. 55. Molluscum sebaceum of the lip at an early nodular stage.

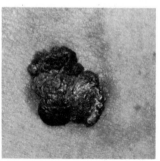

Fig. 56. Senile hyperkeratosis on the back of the hand of a patient aged 73.

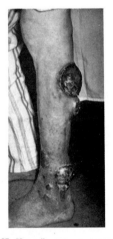

Fig. 57. Kaposi's sarcoma occurring in a Jew born in Poland.

Molluscum* Sebaceum (kerato†-acanthoma‡) is a nodule usually on the face (*Fig.* 55) varying in size from 0·5 cm up to 3 or 4 cm in diameter ('giant' variety) and firm in consistency. It must be distinguished from a wart by its being harder and less hyperkeratotic. Later, during the course of its natural regression without treatment it breaks down and ulcerates, when it is liable to be confused with an epithelioma.

---

* *Molluscum*. Latin, *molluscus* = soft.

† *Kerato*. Greek, κέρας = horn. A prefix denoting horny tissue or the cornea.

‡ *Acanthoma*. Greek, ἄκανθα = prickle+ὦμα = tumour. Excessive local development of the stratum granulosum of the skin.

Keratoma Senilis (senile hyperkeratosis) is found usually on the face or dorsum of the hands of elderly persons, especially those who have been exposed to the elements. Often solitary, the lesion is flat or elevated, greyish-brown in colour, and covered by scales (*Fig.* 56). It is an entirely benign lesion.

Pyogenic Granuloma. *See Fig.* 52, p. 26.

Kaposi's Sarcoma. Jews from Poland, Eastern Europeans and Italians are more susceptible than members of other white races but the condition is relatively common in Africa south of the Sahara Desert. Generally the tumour arises in middle life in males as multiple, symptomless, plum-coloured nodules, usually situated on the lower extremities (*Fig.* 57).

ON 'SPOT' ('SNAP') DIAGNOSIS

As a rule, lightning diagnoses are to be disparaged; often dramatic, they may prove dangerous. More reliance can be placed upon a conclusion based on data gleaned from touch as well as sight (*Fig.* 51). However, there are clinical conditions that should be apparent to the diagnostician almost immediately. Take, for instance, diffuse neurofibromatosis (*Fig.* 58). If a student palpates one nodule, ponders, and then commences examining another of these subcutaneous swellings, it usually transpires that he is not aware of this clinical entity. To the clinician familiar with one of a number of conditions an absolute diagnosis is forthcoming almost immediately. Their number increases with experience. The foundation of 'spot' diagnosis is to have encountered an exactly similar case previously.

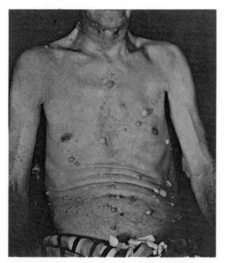

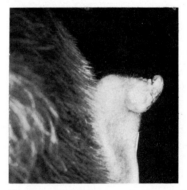

Fig. 58. When diffuse neurofibromatosis is associated with cutaneous pigmentation and the presence of multiple sessile and pedunculated tumours on the skin, the condition is known as von Recklinghausen's disease of nerve or molluscum fibrosum.

Fig. 59. A sebaceous horn growing from the ear.

Figs. 59–64 illustrate some clinical entities, which, once seen, can be diagnosed at almost lightning speed.

MORITZ KAPOSI, 1837–1902, *Professor and Director of the Dermatological Clinic, Vienna.*
FRIEDRICH D. VON RECKLINGHAUSEN, 1833–1910, *Professor of Pathology, Strasbourg.*

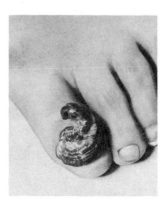

Fig. 60. Onychogryphosis* involving the big toe, the usual situation.

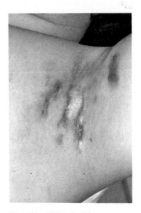

Fig. 61. Hidradenitis suppurativa, a chronic suppurative process involving the apocrine glands of the axilla (infrequently the groin).

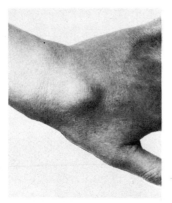

Fig. 62. Simple ganglion of the dorsum of the wrist.

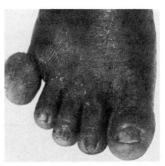

Fig. 63. Ainhum; in no other condition does spontaneous amputation of the little toe occur.

---

* *Onychogryphosis.* Greek, ὄνυξ = nail + γρύπωσις = curving.

Chapter 4

LOCAL INFLAMMATION; ULCERS AND SINUSES; SCARS

CLASSIC SIGNS OF INFLAMMATION

That *redness,* swelling, heat* and *tenderness* are the cardinal signs of inflammation was first expounded by Celsus; to these four signs can be added that described by Galen—*loss of function.*

No better demonstration of these signs can be given than in the case of a *simple boil* (furuncle). Where a boil (*Fig.* 64 A) ends and a *carbuncle* begins is nebulous, but there is no mistaking a fully developed example of the latter (*Fig.* 64 B). That the urine must be tested for sugar in cases of carbuncle and multiple boils cannot be repeated too often. Remember that ketone bodies are sometimes present in the urine of patients with a carbuncle or multiple boils, not because they are diabetic, but because of toxaemia. A virulent boil may be mistaken for *anthrax*. Even in cases where the black central scab and circumscribed surrounding vesicles make the diagnosis of anthrax (*Fig.* 65) practically certain, confirmation by bacteriological examination of the serum from a vesicle is essential. Pus and pain are absent.

A
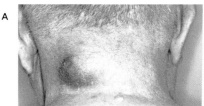
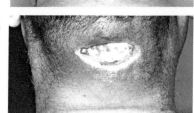
B

Fig. 64. A, A large boil at the back of the neck. B, A carbuncle at the back of the neck, a typical site.

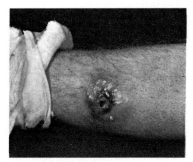

Fig. 65. Cutaneous anthrax.

ERYSIPELAS †

The most common site of origin is the face, including the lobule of the ear—sometimes infected by non-aseptic piercing for ear-rings. The lesion is rosy or crimson, with a peculiar smooth and characteristically shiny appearance.

The affected part is tender and definitely warmer than the adjacent skin. The patient's temperature rises. When the face is attacked oedema may close the eyelid (*Fig.* 66) or lids completely. Usually the regional lymph nodes are moderately

---

* In dark-skinned races this sign is replaced by shininess of the skin.

† Greek, ἐρυθρός = red + πέλλα = skin.

AURELIUS C. CELSUS, *circa* A.D. 25. *Roman encyclopaedist and medical author.*
GALEN, A.D. 130–200. *Physician successively to three Roman Emperors.*

swollen. The eruption reaches its peak on the fifth day; the brilliant erythema then changes to a livid hue, after which it turns brown and later yellow. Sometimes an exudate occurs beneath the cutis to form vesicles, later turning to pustules. Involvement of other sites tends to become forgotten, the hands and genitalia being the next commonest, then the umbilicus in young infants; finally an ulcer of the lower limb is sometimes the site of entry of the specific streptococci.

For the differential diagnosis between erysipelas and superficial cellulitis of the face, *see* p. 33.

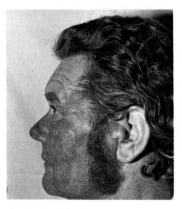

Fig. 66. Erysipelas of the face.

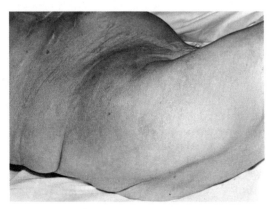

Fig. 67. Subcutaneous cellulitis spreading from infected lymph nodes in the groin.

ERYSIPELOID

Erysipeloid (fish handler's disease) occurs almost exclusively in fish and meat handlers, not forgetting seamen engaged in whaling and sealing. Three or four days after a scratch or cut, the surrounding area becomes inflamed and dark red or purple in colour. As a rule, some part of the hand is affected. The infection lies in the skin and the subcutaneous tissues, and therefore presents many of the features both of erysipelas and cellulitis, with two notable exceptions—the constitutional symptoms are relatively slight and the infection is self-limiting.

CELLULITIS

Inflammation of cellular tissue can be superficial or deep. Superficial (i.e. subcutaneous) cellulitis is more common and less difficult to diagnose.

The part affected is swollen, tense and tender. Later it becomes red, shiny and boggy. Frequently cellulitis commences in an infected wound. If a wound is not at once apparent, look for a small puncture, blister, or abrasion where organisms could have gained entrance. Examine the regional lymph nodes for enlargement. Take the patient's temperature.

In a child, where no obvious abrasion exists in the immediate vicinity, bear in mind Morison's aphorism: 'Cellulitis occurring in children is never primary in the cellular tissues, but secondary to an underlying bone infection.'

From the point of view of differential diagnosis, early superficial cellulitis may be said to have:

1. *No edge.*
2. *No fluctuation.*
3. *No pus.*
4. *No limit.*

JAMES R. MORISON, 1853–1939, *Professor of Surgery, University of Durham, Newcastle-upon-Tyne.*

In adults, when a breach of the continuity of the skin has been excluded, the most common site of origin of cellulitis is an infected bursa. The bursa thus implicated can be either an anatomical bursa (notably an olecranon or a prepatellar bursa (*Fig.* 67)), or an adventitious* bursa, the leading example of which is a bursa over a hallux valgus, known colloquially as a 'bunion' (*Fig.* 68).

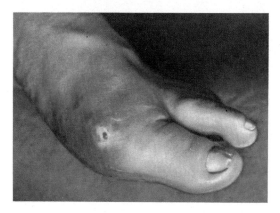

Fig. 68. Bunion—the colloquial name given to an inflamed bursa over a hallux valgus. In this case the infected bursa had ruptured through the skin.

Cellulitis of the Face is sometimes difficult to distinguish from erysipelas. The distinction is academic as the treatment is identical (antibiotics) but *Milian's Ear Sign* may prove helpful. As facial erysipelas spreads, it involves the pinna because it is a cuticular lymphangitis. On the other hand, all subcutaneous inflammations stop short of the pinna because of close adherence of the skin to the cartilage.

Cellulitis of the Orbit. (*See* p. 69.)

Ludwig's Angina † is cellulitis occurring beneath the deep cervical fascia. In many instances the floor of the mouth becomes oedematous (*Fig.* 69).

Other Examples of Deep Cellulitis are: (1) That occurring in layers of the abdominal wall after an operation for a purulent condition, especially when the drainage afforded is inadequate; and (2) Pelvic cellulitis, e.g. parametritis, that occurring in the connective tissue around the uterus.

Pyoderma Gangrenosum (Meleney's Gangrene or Ulceration). Often on the abdominal or chest wall after an operation for a septic condition, but occasionally elsewhere in which case the patient often suffers from ulcerative colitis, but sometimes without obvious cause, an area of cellulitis appears which progresses rapidly with the formation of a central purplish zone surrounded by an angry red zone. The whole area is exquisitely tender with gross oedema of the surrounding skin. Soon the purplish zone becomes gangrenous (*Fig.* 70), and unchecked the gangrene spreads widely. At first the general signs are mild unless the patient is already debilitated from the underlying disease. When the gangrenous skin sloughs an ulcer with undermined edges is left.

A Gumma, although now rare, is a great imitator, and never reaches a large size. At first firm, soon it commences to soften in the centre. Next, the overlying skin becomes infiltrated and reddish-purple. Finally, the characteristic ulcer (*see* p. 38) forms. A point in favour of the diagnosis of gumma is that it tends to occupy the middle line (*Fig.* 71).

---

* Adventitious = occurring in an unusual place.

† *Angina.* Latin, *ango* = to throttle.

GASTON MILIAN, 1871–1945, *Dermatologist, Hôpital Saint-Louis, Paris.*
WILHELM VON LUDWIG, 1790–1865, *Professor of Surgery and Midwifery, Tübingen, Germany.*
FRANK L. MELENEY, 1889–1963, *Professor of Clinical Surgery, Columbia University, New York.*

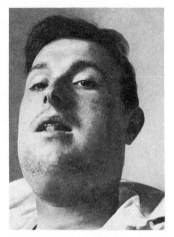

Fig. 69. Ludwig's angina. Note swelling in the submental region, and inability to close the mouth owing to oedema of the tongue and floor of the mouth. Respiratory obstruction is threatened.

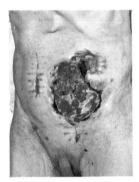

Fig. 70. Pyoderma gangrenosum of the abdominal wall after an operation for carcinoma of the colon.

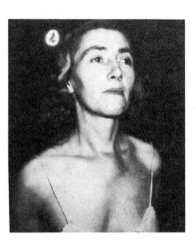

Fig. 71. Gumma over the manubrium.

CAT-SCRATCH DISEASE

This infection, due to a cat bite or scratch, is frequently misdiagnosed. It occurs about ten days after inoculation, by which time a minor breach of the skin is liable to have healed, although one should search for a primary lesion, which resembles a furuncle. The leading sign is considerable lymphadenitis *without visible intervening lymphangitis*, the axillary or inguinal lymph nodes being affected almost exclusively. The constitutional symptoms are often considerable. The diagnosis is supported by finding an enlarged spleen, but it can be confirmed only by the specific intradermal test.

ACUTE LYMPHANGITIS

Inflamed superficial lymphatic vessels can be seen coursing from the site of infection to the regional lymph nodes. Such a tell-tale red line or lines may occur in the skin of one of several regions, but is seen principally in an arm or a leg (*Fig.* 72). Sometimes the initial lesion is so minute that it cannot be found even after a careful search.

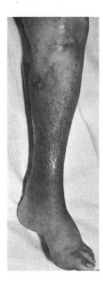

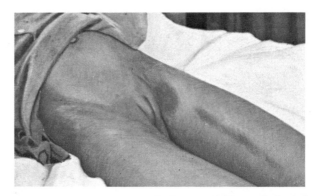

Fig. 72. Acute lymphangitis with subcutaneous cellulitis over the inguinal lymph nodes which are usually enlarged and tender.

Fig. 73. Thrombophlebitis occurring in varicose veins.

PHLEBITIS

Phlebitis and thrombosis occurring in *deep* veins have to be recognized by their effects, for there may be no physical signs of the condition itself. Phlebitis of *superficial* veins is easily recognized, and because thrombosis and phlebitis go hand in hand (thrombophlebitis) the veins feel like tender, hard cords. Varicose veins are frequently the seat of phlebitis (*Fig.* 73).

ULCERS

When examining an ulcer pay particular attention to the following:
The Shape. Is it round, oval, irregular, or serpiginous?*
The Edge. This may be sloping downwards towards the crater, undermined, punched out, or everted.
The Floor. The most typical is the slough in a gummatous ulcer, which looks like wet wash-leather (chamois leather).
The Base. Whether indurated or attached to deeper structures.
The Surrounding Tissues. Look for signs of inflammation, pigmentation, or, in the lower limbs, varicosity.

After examining an ulcer it is essential to consider its lymphatic drainage and lymph nodes. Sometimes these are obviously involved; more often a systematic and painstaking examination by palpation is required.

---

* *Serpiginous*, creeping like a serpent. Healing in one place while extending in another.

As is shown in the following diagrams, ulcers are of five main varieties:

1. A carcinomatous ulcer has everted edges which to the palpating fingers feel hard⸻⸻⸻→

2. Rodent ulcer has slightly raised edges ⸻⸻⸻→

3. The so-called 'septic ulcer', of which varicose ulcer is the commonest example, has sloping edges⸻⸻⸻→

4. The tuberculous ulcer is characterized by undermined edges⸻⸻⸻→

5. An ulcer of tertiary syphilis is punched out⸻⸻⸻→

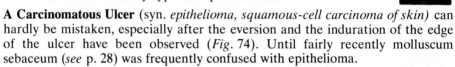

A Carcinomatous Ulcer (syn. *epithelioma, squamous-cell carcinoma of skin*) can hardly be mistaken, especially after the eversion and the induration of the edge of the ulcer have been observed (*Fig.* 74). Until fairly recently molluscum sebaceum (*see* p. 28) was frequently confused with epithelioma.

Rodent Ulcer * (syn. *basal cell carcinoma of skin*). Particularly if early, the features of malignancy are not nearly so obvious. The fact that this ulcer is commonly situated above a line joining the angle of the mouth with the lobule of the ear (*Fig.* 75) should alert the clinician. Its outline is circular, its edge, if not everted, is definitely raised, and this heaped-up edge often shows nodules possessing a peculiar pearl-like lustre (*Fig.*75). Minute venules in the edge are characteristic.

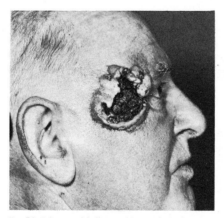

Fig. 74. A large epithelioma with a typical edge.

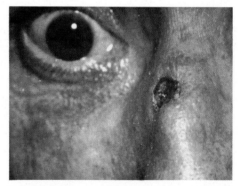

Fig. 75. A rodent ulcer usually occurs above an imaginary line joining the angle of the mouth and the lobule of the ear.

A Tuberculous Ulcer nearly always has undermined edges, this characteristic being shared only by some bed-sores. Tuberculous ulcers are usually painful.

---

* *Rodent ulcer*, so called because it gnaws the tissues (even bone) like a rat.

When *lupus vulgaris** (cutaneous tuberculosis) (*Fig.* 76) as a cause of cutaneous ulceration is suspected, take a glass slide (or a glass tongue depressor) and press it firmly over the lesion. Pressure removes the surrounding hyperaemia, and apple-jelly-like nodules (tuberculous papules) become apparent.

The Hunterian Chancre (primary syphilitic sore) (*Fig.* 77) is a painless ulcer. It is usually oval, has sloping edges, and exudes a discharge that is often bloodstained. When first inspected it is often covered by a crust, removal of which reveals the base covered with pink granulations. To the palpating fingers (protected by gloves) the ulcer is hard; even when palpated through the prepuce the hardness is apparent—it has been likened to the sensation of feeling a buried button.

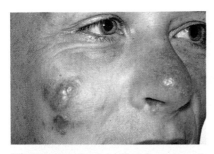

Fig. 76. Lupus vulgaris usually, but not always, is found affecting the face.

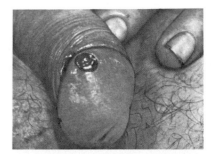

Fig. 77. Hunterian chancre.

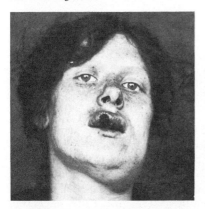

Fig. 78. Primary chancre of the upper lip with characteristic bilateral enlargement (because of crossed lymphatic drainage) of the submental and submandibular nodes. In this case the nodes are more marked on the opposite side.

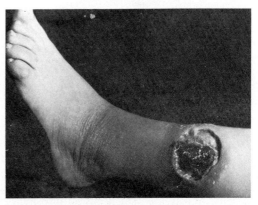

Fig. 79. Cutaneous gumma situated over the *middle two-fourths* of the leg below the knee—a characteristic situation. Compare with varicose ulcer (*Fig.* 80).

The lymph nodes of the groin can be felt slightly enlarged; 'shotty' is the term that has been given to them. By 'shotty' is implied that the nodes are hard and small. This is very different from the extravagant enlargement of the regional lymph nodes that occurs when a primary syphilitic sore is extragenital (*Fig.* 78).

---

* *Lupus vulgaris*. Latin, *lupus* = a wolf; *vulgaris* = ordinary. 'Lupus is a malignant ulcer . . . and it is very hungry like unto a wolf.' (Philip Barrow, *Method of Physicke*, 1590.)

JOHN HUNTER, 1728–1793, *Surgeon, St. George's Hospital, London. Tradition has it that he was imbued with the idea that syphilis and gonorrhoea were manifestations of the same infection and to test his hypothesis he inoculated himself by means of a scalpel and that he died of an aortic aneurysm. Dempster has revealed that a post-mortem showed atheroma of the aorta but no aneurysm or other evidence of syphilis.*
WILLIAM J. DEMPSTER, *Contemporary Consultant in Experimental Surgery, Postgraduate Medical School, London.*

A Gummatous Ulcer is unquestionably punched out and painless. The base is covered with the characteristic wet wash-leather (chamois leather) slough which may contain one or more 'islands' of normal tissue that have escaped the necrosis. Note that a similar slough occurs also in tissue undergoing post-irradiation necrosis.

A healed gumma gives a circular 'tissue-paper' scar, which is strong evidence of a previous syphilitic infection. The scar of yaws (*see* p. 529) is similar.

The characteristic punched-out appearance of gummatous ulcer (*Fig.* 79) is seen sometimes in a gravitational or a varicose ulcer (*Fig.* 80) and in trophic* ulcers, particularly perforating ulcer of the foot (*Fig.* 81) associated with tabes dorsalis and other diseases of the central nervous system or diabetic neuropathy.

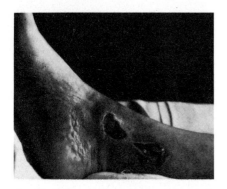

Fig. 80. Varicose ulcers are apt to appear in pigmented areas, and they tend to 'ride the vein'. They are almost confined to the *lower quarter* of the leg.

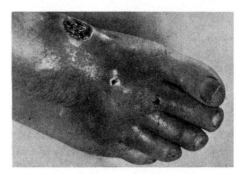

Fig. 81. Perforating ulcer of the dorsum of the foot occurring in a patient with tabes dorsalis. A smaller, deeper, ulcer is present on the sole of the foot—the typical situation.

SINUSES AND FISTULAE

A *fistula* implies a tunnel connecting two epithelial surfaces, whereas a *sinus* is a blind track opening on to the skin or a mucous surface. Several references to fistulae and sinuses in particular situations will be made later in the book.

The opening of a sinus may be situated at a distance from the underlying pathological lesion. An opening near the anus almost always is the external opening of a tunnel which has an internal opening into the anal canal or rectum (Fistula-in-ano, *see* p. 273).

A Sinus originating from a Foreign Body or in Infected Bone. Of great clinical significance is exuberant granulation tissue ('proud flesh') around the orifice (*Fig.* 82). The cause of exuberant granulations is a foreign body—any foreign body—an infected non-absorbable suture is now the commonest but bone necrosis in the depths of the sinus is an alternative cause.

The only clinical method of determining the length and direction of the track of a sinus is by probing, and this can be performed safely provided the probe has been sterilized and is used with great gentleness.

---

* *Trophic.* Greek, τροφιχός = appertaining to nutrition.

*A Sinus or Sinuses caused by Actinomycosis.** Multiple indurated sinuses especially about the lower jaw and neck, suggest *actinomycosis* (*Fig.* 83). Express a little of the discharge into a test-tube half full of water. Cork the tube and shake vigorously. If cayenne-pepper granules (*Fig.* 83, inset), so characteristic of actinomycosis, are present, they will soon sink to the bottom of the test-tube.

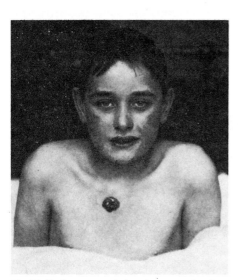

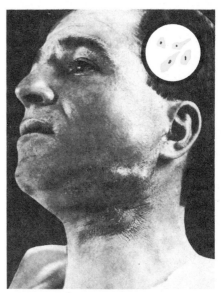

Fig. 82. Exuberant granulation tissue around a sinus. Case of osteomyelitis of the sternum.

Fig. 83. Actinomycosis of the neck. Pus expressed from one of the sinuses showed cayenne-pepper granules (the little dots within the drop of pus shown in the inset).

The Physical Characteristics of a Purulent Discharge are of very limited value in suggesting the causative organism, bacteriological examination always being required. Streptococcal pus from newly infected tissue is watery and only slightly opalescent; sometimes it is bloodstained. Staphylococcal pus is yellow and of creamy consistency. Very typical is the blue, or bluish-green, pus caused by infection by *Pseudomonas aeruginosa* (formerly called *Bacillus pyocyaneus*). The anchovy-sauce coloured pus from an amoebic abscess of the liver is very characteristic.

Odour emanating from a Discharging Sinus. Pus resulting from the activity of certain micro-organisms emits an odour; thus an infected wound, the seat of gas gangrene, emits a peculiar sickly-sweet odour, likened to decaying apples. An objectionable odour emanating from a discharging abdominal sinus or from a specimen of pus is likely to be diagnosed as '*B. coli* pus'. In fact pus resulting from the activity of *Escherichia coli* is absolutely odourless. The smell is due to the proteolytic propensities of certain anaerobic organisms derived from the lower alimentary tract, or less frequently to *Proteus vulgaris*.

---

* *Actinomycosis.* Greek, ἀκτίς = a ray + μύκης = fungus. The ray fungus.

Infection by bacteroides (which are not uncommonly the predominating organisms in cases of intra-abdominal suppuration and infections of the abdominal wall) gives rise to an odour similar to that of over-ripe Camembert cheese.

Faecal Fistula. Sometimes a 'faecal' fistula is reported when it is not fluid faeces, but foul, faecal-smelling pus that has been discharged from an abdominal wound; exceptionally such pus contains small bubbles of gas. Conversely, the passage of *large* bubbles of flatus with the discharge is unmistakable, and proof-positive that there is a communication with the bowel.

SCARS

Much can be learnt from careful study of a scar, particularly an abdominal scar. Usually a patient is aware of the nature of a previous abdominal operation, but

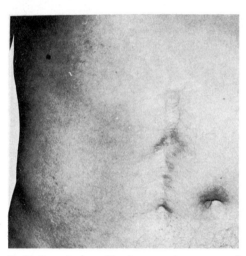

Fig. 84. Ragged scar resulting from operative treatment of a perforated duodenal ulcer in the pre-antibiotic era.

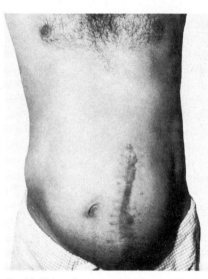

Fig. 85. This patient was stabbed in the abdomen with a knife, sustaining penetrating injuries of the small bowel. Severe sepsis followed operative treatment and an incisional hernia resulted. Note also the keloid scar.

if not, a guess as to its nature can be hazarded from the site of the scar, e.g. the customary grid-iron appendicectomy scar in the right iliac fossa.

A fine linear scar, whether on a limb or the abdomen, implies an operation wound which healed without sepsis. Such a scar is virtually invisible and cannot be reproduced photographically. Conversely, a wide ragged scar indicates a septic wound (*Fig.* 84). Such an abdominal incision if short is likely to heal soundly, whereas if long, an incisional hernia becomes a possibility or even a probability (*Fig.* 85). Moreover, if a patient with this type of scar presents with intestinal obstruction an adhesion figures high on the list of likely causes (consequent on intraperitoneal sepsis).

Another complication of sepsis following an accidental or operation wound is keloid* thickening of the scar (*Fig.* 86). Coloured races are particularly prone

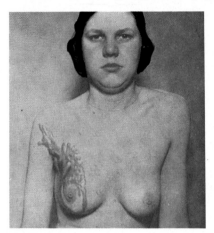

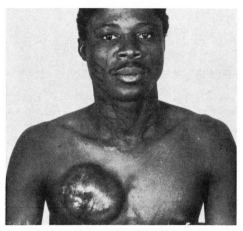

Fig. 86. Keloid developing in a scar following a burn.

Fig. 87. Dermatofibrosarcoma protuberans—a relatively benign form of fibrosarcoma.

to this (*Fig.* 85) even in the absence of sepsis. An intracutaneous lump which simulates keloid without the patient having undergone an operation previously is likely to be an example of dermatofibrosarcoma protuberans (*Fig.* 87).

---

* Keloid. Greek, χηλή = spot, εἶδοζ = form.

Chapter 5

SOME DISTINCTIVE SURGICAL STATES

SHOCK

Shock, more descriptively called 'peripheral circulatory failure', is met with frequently in surgical practice. This is not the place to discuss its aetiology. The simple concept that it is basically due to diminished blood volume (oligaemia) can be accepted here. The main signs are as follows:

The patient lies still, paying little or no attention to events around him. Rather, he stares aimlessly and apathetically straight before him. Disturbed, he will move a little, and will answer questions in a weak voice; the necessity for repeating questions often arises. Undisturbed, he soon reverts to his state of lethargy.

The pupils are dilated, and react slowly to light.

His colour is pale, and is often described as grey. Pallor is present because there is less blood than normal in and beneath the skin; grey, because what blood there is, being stagnant, contains less oxygen than usual. Sometimes in profound shock this leads to marbling of the skin of the back of the hands and the front of the legs, and to cyanosis of the lips.

Beads of sweat are often perceptible, especially on the forehead and the upper lip.

The pulse: Typically the pulse rate is accelerated and feels 'thready', i.e. less forceful than normal: this is relatively more striking than the increased rate.

The temperature is below normal.

The blood pressure is lower than usual for the particular person.

The urine is reduced in quantity and its specific gravity is raised.

Such is the typical overall picture of established shock. There are, however, exceptions—not infrequently misleading exceptions.

In shock, especially that occurring in a person previously in perfect health, even an estimation of blood pressure, which is the best measurement of the degree of shock easily available, is not always reliable. A barely palpable pulse is instinctively assumed to be a sign of low blood pressure, but in this instance it can be due to arterial vasoconstriction, in which event the central blood pressure may in fact be above normal: soon after an injury a rise in blood pressure to over 140 mm Hg is not uncommon (hypertensive pattern of shock). Also often there is no information available as to the patient's normal blood pressure before the injury. In short, an estimation of the blood pressure with a sphygmomanometer is not always to be trusted implicitly.

Thus there are occasions on which every grain of clinical evidence that can be gleaned by physical signs is of value. *A reduced rate of blood flow through the skin* can be made apparent, with practice, by the following method:

Press the thumb against the sternum and hold it there. Then remove it quickly (*Fig.* 88). Normally the time required for the blanched area to turn pink is less than a second: in cases of early shock the reaction is noticeably longer.

Coldness of the extremities: Skin temperature is best appreciated in the extremities. The best testing surface for delicate observations is the dorsal surface of the middle phalanx of the flexed finger.

In a hot climate, or if the patient, before coming under observation, has been warmed with hot-water bottles or the like (a reprehensible practice), both the last two signs may give negative results, even though the shock is profound.

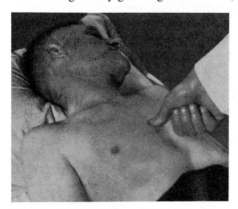 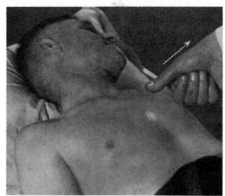

Fig. 88. In shock the skin remains blanched momentarily longer than normal.

Observing superficial veins: Inspect the dorsum of the hands and forearm. In established shock the normally visible veins will be less full than usual (collapsed) and on emptying them by upward stroking with a finger they fill more slowly than usual. To judge these criteria requires experience.

VARIETIES OF SHOCK

Collapse due to Haemorrhage. If the patient has bled externally the source is usually obvious, e.g. a compound fracture. A more difficult question is, Is the patient bleeding internally? Common examples are ruptured spleen (*see* p. 324), ectopic pregnancy (*see* p. 316), melaena due to bleeding peptic ulcer (*see* p. 297). This is one of the most momentous problems with which the diagnostician is confronted. Internal haemorrhage is sometimes difficult to recognize. As a result of haematoma formation around the bone ends and into the muscles, the blood loss in a case of multiple closed fractures may amount to several litres.

Pallor: This outstanding and constant sign is due not only to blood loss but to the concomitant vasoconstriction of cutaneous vessels. Such pallor may be so pronounced (*Fig.* 89) as to be discerned while approaching the patient. In less evident cases, especially in artificial light and/or when the clinician has not seen the patient previously, pallor is best ascertained by examining the conjunctiva of a lower lid and the fingernails—in coloured races this is the only clinical method of detecting anaemia. Unless varnished, the fingernails are the windows of the capillary network. If in doubt, press the fingernail near its free edge; about half the nail-bed blanches. Release the pressure gradually; the pristine hue spreading from the base returns almost instantaneously. Compare the colour with that of your own fingernail.

The pulse: While a progressive increase in the pulse rate (*see* p. 7) is an unrivalled confirmatory sign of internal haemorrhage, considerable haemorrhage can occur before the pulse rate *commences* to rise. This is demonstrated convincingly when a donor gives blood for transfusion: during and after the collection of blood the pulse rate and the blood pressure usually remain unchanged.

Restlessness: Due to cerebral hypoxia the patient seldom remains quite still, and tends to resent his arms and chest being covered by bedclothes.

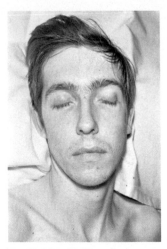

Fig. 89. Jehovah's Witness* after major surgery. Refused blood transfusion. Haemoglobin 50 per cent.

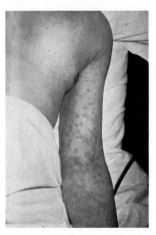

Fig. 90. Septicaemic rash following prostatectomy.

A feeling of want of fresh air, which is sometimes interpreted by the patient as choking, occurs when the loss of blood is considerable. 'Air hunger', which implies actual gasping for breath, is seldom in evidence, but occasional sighing is not uncommon.

Thirst with repeated requests for something to drink is yet another reason for the absence of tranquillity.

Burns Shock. The cause is obvious. In this instance the fluid lost is a plasma-like exudate through the burned tissues so there are no signs of anaemia, at least in the early stages.

Septic (Bacteriaemic) Shock. Occurs in advanced peritonitis (*see* p. 310) and in severe infections (septicaemia—*see below*).

SEPTICAEMIA

Improvement in the treatment of sepsis with antibiotics has led to the survival of increasing numbers of patients who would have succumbed previously. At some stage during the postoperative period, signs of shock together with intermittent pyrexia and sometimes rigors, supervene. Often the skin is warm and dry (*pink shock*). The patient looks and feels ill; indeed his condition may come to resemble that of malignant cachexia (*see* p. 48). A few instances are seen after otherwise uneventful operations without evidence of wound sepsis but most follow urinary tract operations or infections.

---

* *Jehovah's Witnesses.* A Christian religious sect which forbids the use of blood transfusion.

Although the clinical signs of septicaemia should be looked for carefully, an early blood culture is easily the most important investigation.

Enlargement of the Spleen. A minor enlargement (*see* p. 237) particularly should be sought.

A Septicaemic Rash (*Fig.* 90) or **Splinter Haemorrhages** under the nails are valuable confirmatory evidence. A good light is necessary for detection, but absence is not proof that the patient is not suffering from septicaemia.

DEHYDRATION

Clinical manifestations appear when there is fluid depletion corresponding to 6 per cent of the body weight (equal to about 4 litres in an adult weighing 70 kg). In most instances dehydration involves a loss of electrolytes (mainly, if not entirely, sodium chloride) as well as water, and many of the signs of dehydration as seen in surgical practice are due to the loss of sodium.

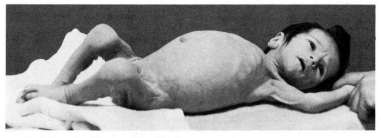

Fig. 91. Dehydration. The sign of the ridge is apparent (left upper arm).

In established cases the face is drawn and the eyes are sunken and the pressure in their anterior chambers is felt to be low. In infants the anterior fontanelle is depressed. In all dehydrated patients the tongue is coated and dry; in advanced cases it is brown in colour. With dehydration produced by loss of water only, thirst is particularly in evidence. The skin is dry and often wrinkled, making the patient look older than his years. The subcutaneous tissue feels lax. If the skin of a considerably dehydrated person is picked up between the finger and thumb and then released, instead of it springing back with normal elasticity, a ridge is formed that subsides slowly—this is the *sign of the ridge* (*Fig.* 91). The peripheral veins are small, constricted, and contain dark blood. The blood pressure is likely to be below normal. The urine is scanty, dark in colour and of a high specific gravity.

Sodium Depletion: Special Features. Excessive loss of fluid high in salt content occasioned by high intestinal obstruction with vomiting, or a duodenal or bile fistula, are almost invariably the antecedents of hyponatraemia. The features are those of dehydration described above with one exception; the patient is not thirsty.

Potassium Depletion: Special Features. Diarrhoea, whether due to a 'surgical' condition, e.g. ulcerative colitis, or otherwise, e.g. cholera, is the usual cause. Potassium loss from a newly established ileostomy is often great. Loss of mucus from a large villous adenoma of the rectum (*see* p. 276) may also lead to potassium deficiency (hypokalaemia).

The patient is listless with slow slurred speech and drowsy. There is weakness of the voluntary muscles and the abdomen is distended, so much so, that in postoperative cases paralytic ileus or intestinal obstruction may be simulated.

Electrolyte estimations performed on the blood serum are necessary to confirm a diagnosis of the above two conditions.*

BURNS

That the patient has been burnt is obvious. Diagnosis is not complete, however, without determining the extent and depth of the burn or scald. Without full diagnosis rational planned therapy is impossible. Of many methods for estimating the extent of a burn, Wallace's Rule of Nines (*Fig.* 92) is the simplest. Remember, that if areas of erythema are excluded, a burn of over 10 per cent of the body surface in children and over 15 per cent in adults will probably cause shock, and that it is important to adopt prophylactic measures before the signs described earlier in this chapter become apparent.

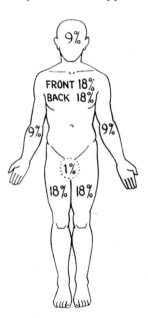

Fig. 92. The Rules of Nines; the head and upper limbs each equal 9 per cent; the front and back of the trunk and the lower limbs each equal 2×9 per cent. In children the head is relatively larger, its surface comprising up to 18 per cent in infancy.

Another useful method of calculating the extent of a burn is to compare in one's imagination the area of the front of the patient's open hand and fingers with the burnt area. If, for example, 5 hands would cover the area, the burn is approximately 5 per cent of the body surface (i.e. a hand = 1 per cent).

Depth of the Burn. At each extreme, diagnosis is easy. A first-degree burn (erythema) looks like severe sunburn. There is no mistaking the dead-white appearance of the completely destroyed skin of the third-degree burn. Compar-

---

* The diagnosis of water, sodium and potassium excess are not dealt with as they are iatrogenic. *Iatrogenic*. Greek, ἰατρός = physician+γεννάν = to produce. A morbid condition resulting from treatment.

ALEXANDER B. WALLACE, 1906–74, *Plastic Surgeon, Royal Hospital for Sick Children, Edinburgh.*

atively rarely is charring of the skin and deeper tissues seen. The difficulty lies in deciding whether part of the epithelium remains alive and is capable of regeneration, thereby obviating the need for skin grafting.

The Pin-prick Test (Jackson). Using a sterile hypodermic needle, test pain sensation (*see* p. 402) in the burnt area. If pain is present in all or part of the burn, that part is second-degree and will heal in approximately three weeks. The converse is not necessarily true; analgesia usually indicates full-thickness skin loss, but the end-organs for pain may be destroyed in deep second-degree burns with survival of some epithelial cells deep to them. Thus some second-degree burns, not requiring skin grafting, are analgesic and may be diagnosed as third-degree.

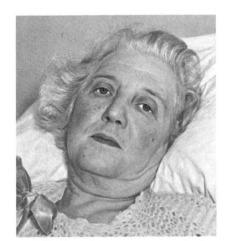

Fig. 93. Marked cyanosis.

CYANOSIS

The most usual form of cyanosis is dependent solely upon inadequate oxygenation of haemoglobin. At no time does the carbon-dioxide content of the blood play any part in this visible colour change. The degree of cyanosis is not always an accurate index to the severity of the anoxia present.

For example, when the haemoglobin content of the blood falls as low as 30 per cent (less than 5 g per dl of blood) cyanosis does not appear, even if all the haemoglobin were in a reduced state, because a minimum of 5 g per dl is required to produce visible cyanosis.

Again, peripheral vasoconstriction, by reducing the amount of blood in the surface vessels, is wont to prevent cyanosis being perceived even though a dangerous degree of anoxia is present. Thus severe oxygen want can prevail without cyanosis being apparent.

Although a mild degree of cyanosis is best perceived in the lips (*Fig.* 93), the lobules of the ears and the fingernails also should be examined in suspected cases. Even experienced clinicians vary in their ability to recognize faint blueness; for this depends, not on clinical acumen, but upon acuteness of colour perception—a very variable factor. Moreover, cyanosis is notoriously difficult to detect in coloured races. Lastly, cyanosis of a lilac hue can exist without oxygen

DOUGLAS MACG. JACKSON, *Contemporary Emeritus Surgeon, Birmingham Accident Hospital, England.*

want, and every surgical clinician will do well to be cognizant of two forms of cyanosis that are not dangerous and do not call for a freer airway, oxygen, or indeed any elaborate form of therapy.

a. Cyanosis due to cold, producing local capillary stagnation, can be most evident in the lips, nose, hands and feet without anoxia of the blood within the arterial tree.

b. Drug Cyanosis. Cyanosis of varying intensity is occasionally met with in patients undergoing sulphonamide and other therapy.

OBESITY

An excessive deposit of fat is apt to obscure intra-abdominal physical signs; it increases the difficulty of many operations, and the incidence of postoperative complications is higher in the fat than in the lean. Therefore obesity is more important to the surgeon than to the life-assurance assessor. Dr Samuel Johnson* is reported to have said: 'Sir, it is plain that if he is too fat, he has eaten more than he should have done.' In other words, in the vast majority of cases obesity is due to the ingestion of more calories than are needed for energy. The habit of overeating is usually familial as a glance at the parent of a fat child will confirm. In spite of this super-simple doctrine, it is still necessary to winnow the fatness of endocrine disorder from that of overeating.

1. Hyperinsulinism. Obesity may develop in individuals with pancreatic insulinoma (*see* p. 239). These patients learn that the symptoms of hypoglycaemia can be controlled by the ingestion of food.

2. Hyperadrenocorticism. While as a rule a deposit of fat on the trunk, and not on the limbs, has no aetiological significance, hyperadrenocorticism (*Cushing's syndrome*) should be thought of. In most cases the obesity has an abrupt onset. The face is rubicund (*see Fig. 169, p. 90) and the shape is like that of a full moon. Exceedingly characteristic are purple-red striae distentiae, mostly on the abdomen (*Fig. 94*). As the disease progresses, so the general contour becomes more and more that of a lemon on matchsticks, viz. ⟶ The wave of enthusiasm for treatment of various disorders with steroids has brought a considerable toll of additional cases.

3. Hypothyroidism should be considered if other signs (*see* p. 159) are present, but it is not a cause of extreme obesity.

4. Hypogonadism in children and adolescents usually leads to obesity (*Fig. 95*). Only rarely is the condition caused by a tumour in the hypothalamic region (craniopharyngioma), in which case the term '*Fröhlich's adiposogenitalis syndrome*' is accurate. It may follow a fractured base of skull but usually the condition is probably a variation of normal development. There are also a number of rare syndromes due to genetic defects which present with obesity and abnormal sexual development: the reader is referred to endocrinological texts for descriptions.

As a rule simple inspection and pinching up of the skin is sufficient to diagnose obesity.

LOSS OF WEIGHT: MALIGNANT CACHEXIA

That the patient has recently lost weight is suggested by his clothes, particularly the waist of the trousers, being too commodious.

Malignant cachexia is characterized by the emaciated, languid, sallow, often pallid facies, loose and wrinkled dry skin, loss of energy, appetite and weight,

---

* SAMUEL JOHNSON, 1709–1784, *celebrated lexicographer, was an LL.D. Dublin.*

HARVEY CUSHING, 1869–1939, *Professor of Surgery, Harvard University, U.S.A.*
ALFRED FRÖHLICH, 1871–1953, *Professor of Pharmacology and Toxicology, Vienna.*

and often infection of the mouth with thrush. Often the sufferer experiences little or no pain, and is apparently unaware of the grave implications of the profound loss of weight. Some seem almost optimistic, and on no account must this oblivion be dispelled by an unguarded word or a despondent facial expression or gesture. Often, too, the abdomen does not share in the obvious attenuation, but rather there is fullness due to ascites (*see* p. 242).

Why is it that advanced malignant disease is so frequently unaccompanied by pain? Cancer is a painless condition unless there is obstruction of a hollow muscular organ causing colic, or bone metastases are present, or the growth infiltrates a sensory nerve. Ignorance of this, both by the general public and by some doctors, is an important cause of delayed diagnosis.

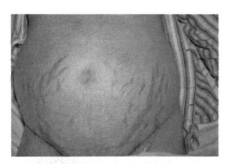

Fig. 94. Striae distentiae on the abdomen of a woman with Cushing's syndrome.

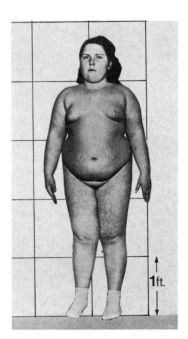

Fig. 95. Hypogonadism (note the knock-knees).

NEUROSIS

As in medicine, so in clinical surgery sometimes a suspicion arises that the patient's symptoms are functional, as opposed to organic, or, in the case of a wound (operation or otherwise) that will not heal, that the patient is deliberately tampering with it (*see* p. 528). As it is impossible to do justice here to this vast subject, all that will be attempted is to direct attention to a few practical points.

A conclusion that symptoms are due to a neurosis should not be reached until (1) the presence of relevant organic disease has been excluded by every means available; (2) positive signs of a functional disorder are present.

All too frequently, after years of observation of a patient with symptoms which must have been neurotic, fresh symptoms or signs develop which on investigation prove to be due to organic disease, very often malignant. The clinician must be on guard always to avoid missing the change in symptomatology, however tiresome the patient.

Among the most extraordinary purely functional phenomena is that known as 'glove and/or stocking anaesthesia'. The patient says the limb is numb. That he is correct there can be no doubt, for one can transfix the skin with pins (*Fig.* 96) or test for pain sensation by pinprick and the patient does not mind. However,

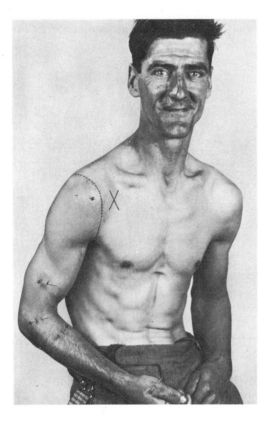

Fig. 96. The patient had a recently healed superficial scar in the palm of his right hand, for which he was claiming compensation. The skin of his right hand, arm, and forearm was anaesthetic ('glove' anaesthesia) and he actually smiled while the five pins shown were thrust through the skin distal to the line marked by the pencil. Proximal to this line (X) a touch of the point of a pin caused him to cry out.

the area of anaesthesia ends abruptly at a certain level not in keeping with any anatomical distribution of nerve supply.

Usually cases seen by the surgeon cannot be proved to be functional so easily. As aids to arrival at this difficult conclusion the following tests are helpful to some extent:

1. Test the knee jerks. They are likely to be exaggerated.

2. Touch the soft palate with a blunt object. Normally, this will cause the patient to gag unless he usually wears dentures. The patient of neurotic temperament allows the clinician to stroke his soft palate with impunity.

3. Perhaps the most difficult neurosis with which the surgeon has to contend is the hysterical joint. This usually takes the form of 'locking'. The joint is fixed

in some degree of flexion. It is sometimes possible, by suddenly diverting the patient's attention, to release the joint and extend it.

Longstanding disuse of a limb due to hysteria may present to the surgeon in two ways. First, Charcot's hysterical blue oedema—the dependent limb becomes cyanosed and swollen from lack of use. This is usually seen in the lower limb whereas in the upper limb muscle wasting consequent on disuse atrophy occurs and a radiograph shows bone decalcification similar to that seen in Sudeck's post-traumatic bone atrophy, a painful condition.

JEAN-MARTIN CHARCOT, 1825–1893, *Physician, Hôpital Salpêtrière, Paris.*
PAUL SUDECK, 1866–1938, *Professor of Surgery, Hamburg.*

Chapter 6

THE HEAD

THE SCALP

Scalp Wounds never gape unless the aponeurosis (galea* aponeurotica) has been divided. Thus it can be told at a glance whether this structure has been implicated; if it has, a compound fracture must be sought in the operating theatre.

Haematoma. A collection of blood (or pus) beneath the aponeurosis (dangerous area) tends to involve the whole area between the attachments of the occipito-frontalis muscle and fluctuation can be detected over the entire scalp, from the frontal to the occipital region. On the other hand, an effusion beneath the pericranium is limited by the suture lines, and is therefore confined to the area of one cranial bone. In the newborn such a swelling (*cephalhaematoma*) is usually found over the parietal bone. A subpericranial haematoma is often exceedingly deceptive to the palpating fingers: *it feels exactly like a depressed fracture*, because the peripheral part of the swelling is firm from coagulation of the blood, while the centre remains soft.

Haematoma connected with a Fracture of a Parietal Bone in a Child. A parent brings a child some days after a fall upon the head, having discovered a lump on the side of the head. There is a soft cystic swelling on one side of the head, not bounded by any of the suture lines of the skull. A radiograph reveals a linear fracture of the parietal bone.

Cellulitis of the Scalp. The scalp becomes swollen and boggy, and unless arrested, the infection spreads widely. One or both eyelids and, perhaps, the pinna on the affected side become swollen. The regional lymph nodes (*see* p. 53) soon become enlarged and tender.

A Localized Swelling in the Scalp can be made to move on the skull (*Figs.* 97, 98); conversely, the scalp can be made to move over a swelling springing from the skull.

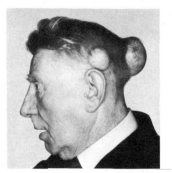

Fig. 97. Sebaceous cysts of the scalp, sometimes called 'wens'.

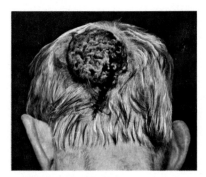

Fig. 98. Cock's 'peculiar' tumour.

---

* *Galea.* Latin = a helmet.

52

Sebaceous Cysts of the scalp (*Fig.* 97) are common. Sometimes they are single; often they are multiple so always examine the whole scalp carefully.

Cock's 'Peculiar' Tumour looks like a squamous-celled carcinoma; in the case illustrated in *Fig.* 98 it bled easily, too. It is a suppurating and ulcerating sebaceous cyst.

A Lipoma which is situated over the vertex, although apparently a localized swelling of the scalp, is wont to occur *beneath* the pericranium, and consequently its margins can be rolled on the surface of the bone (*see* the Slipping Sign, p. 23).

'Turban' Tumour is a ràre, locally malignant, relentless tumour (cylindroma) of the *skin* of the scalp that in the course of twenty years or more spreads over almost the entire scalp (*Fig.* 99) and even hangs in festoons from it. Reddish in colour, lobulated with deep crevices, and devoid of the hair of the head, its appearance is so characteristic that it can hardly be mistaken. Nevertheless it must be distinguished from a—

Plexiform Neurofibroma, which occurs *beneath* the skin. When large, it too hangs in festoons, but is, as a rule, covered by hair unless ulcerated by repeated friction and difficulty in keeping it clean. Usually it is a part of von Recklinghausen's neurofibromatosis (*see* p. 29).

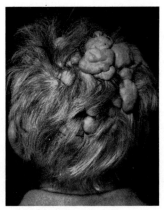

Fig. 99. Typical 'turban' tumour of the scalp present for many years.

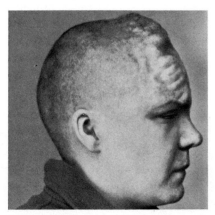

Fig. 100. Cirsoid aneurysm of the scalp. On auscultation a bruit was easily heard.

Temporal Arteritis. The patient, who is usually over 70, complains of intense headache which may have resulted in weight loss. The involved temporal artery is tender and reddened due to a segmental low-grade inflammatory arteritis. The importance of the condition is that, untreated, there is an even chance of one or both retinal arteries becoming involved with subsequent blindness. Occasionally the occipital or posterior auricular arteries are also involved.

An obscure cystic swelling implicating the scalp should be watched carefully for pulsation. The sign of emptying (*see* p. 24) (meningocele, cavernous haemangioma, and sinus pericranii*), the application of a stethoscope (bruit of a cirsoid aneurysm) (*Fig.* 100), and percussion of the swelling (pneumatocele, *see* p. 60), may have a place in the elucidation of the diagnosis.

The Lymphatics of the Scalp drain as follows:

Occipital Region. First into the nodes on the insertion of the trapezius, then into those of the posterior triangle.

---

* Sinus pericranii. A soft swelling beneath the scalp communicating with a venous sinus through a defect in the skull.

EDWARD COCK, 1805–1892, *Surgeon, Guy's Hospital, London.*

Mid-parietal Region. First into the post-auricular lymph node, and thence into the nodes of the posterior triangle.

Forehead and Anterior Parietal Region. Into the pre-auricular lymph node.

Enlarged lymph nodes situated only in the posterior triangle of the neck are most unusual apart from German measles, a common cause unlikely to be seen by the surgeon. Low-grade infection of the scalp due to *pediculosis capitis* or an infected abrasion is prone to give rise to lymphatic enlargement which simulates closely that produced by a lymphoma (*see* p. 140). The primary lesion, hidden by the hair of the head, is especially liable to be overlooked.

THE SKULL

The Anterior Fontanelle. As a rule the anterior fontanelle becomes closed by the time the infant has reached the age of eighteen months. During the first year of life an open fontanelle is a gold-mine of clinical information. Like the eyeball, it has a normal tension which can be estimated by pressing the fingers gently over the lozenge-shaped space. When the child cries, the tension is increased noticeably. In shock the normal tension is diminished. In dehydration by diarrhoea and vomiting, the fontanelle is depressed, often visibly. Considerable delay in closure is seen in several metabolic diseases, notably rickets, of which it is contributory evidence.

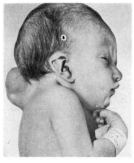

Fig. 101. Occipital meningocele.

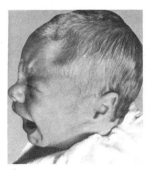

Fig. 102. Pond depressed fracture.

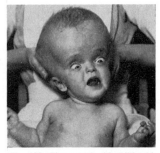

Fig. 103. Five-month-old child with untreated hydrocephalus. The somewhat bulging eyes are downcast ('setting sun' sign); the child appears always to be looking towards the floor (pressure on the orbital plates).

Meningocele is less common than its spinal counterpart (*see* p. 199) and usually it occurs in the midline. By far the most common location is through a defect in the occipital bone, although it may be found over the vault. The pouch of dura mater which comprises a meningocele may be pedunculated or sessile; it is covered either with the full thickness of the scalp or by epithelium only. The swelling to which it gives rise (*Fig.* 101) is tense, rounded, fluctuant, translucent and yields an impulse when the child cries.

Pond Depressed Fracture of the Skull is usually encountered in a neonate, and is consequent upon extreme moulding of the head during delivery or, more frequently, is a result of the application of obstetric forceps (*Fig.* 102). It can occur also during the first few months of life from a fall, or other direct injury. Such dents are comparable to greenstick fractures of long bones.

Craniosynostosis. Cranial bones are normally separated from one another at birth. A firm fibrous union usually occurs by the sixth month of life, but bony union is not completed until the sixtieth year. When one or more of the cranial sutures becomes prematurely closed, particularly before birth, deformity of the cranial vault results. Such deformities sometimes become extremely grotesque, and, as during the first year the brain increases 135 per cent in weight, the resulting constriction of the brain is the cause of a 'sugar-loaf' or 'steeple' skull with, perhaps, convulsions, mental retardation, proptosis, and visual disturbances.

The Circumference of the Head. Until a child is eighteen months of age, the circumference of the head is approximately equal to that of the thorax. This ratio is disturbed, on the one hand, by craniosynostosis and other forms of microcephaly and, on the other, by hydrocephalus. When an infant's head appears abnormally small or large, measurements of the girth of the skull at the level of the top of the pinnae and of the thorax at the nipples should be taken and compared.

Hydrocephalus (*Fig.* 103). The anterior fontanelle, normally approximately 3 cm longitudinally and 2 cm transversely at birth and progressively decreasing in size with age, is enlarged and tense. The superficial veins of the scalp are very conspicuous, which is a valuable sign in early cases of hydrocephalus or, for that matter, increased intracranial tension from any cause in infancy. The sutures may be palpably separated. Three in four cases are associated with myelomeningocele (*see* p. 199). (*See also* Arnold–Chiari Malformation, p. 200.)

The 'Setting Sun' Sign. As seen in *Fig.* 103 (which is an extreme example) the sclera is visible above the cornea at all times when the eyes are open. This sign is present in early cases even before the head circumference increases.

In an adult, especially a man past middle-age, a large cranium should incite a suspicion of:

Paget's Disease of the Skull. In addition to an examination of the trunk and the limbs (*see* p. 426) the head should be auscultated, for the thickened cranial bones are extremely vascular, and sometimes a systolic bruit is audible.

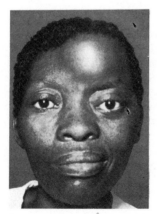

Fig. 104. Pott's puffy 'tumour', secondary to frontal sinusitis.

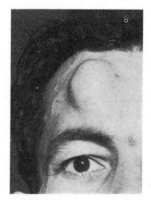

Fig. 105. A bone metastasis which felt stony hard and originated from a neuroblastoma.

SIR JAMES PAGET, 1814–1899, *Surgeon, St. Bartholomew's Hospital, London.*

Pott's Puffy 'Tumour' (*Fig.* 104) is a localized oedema over an area of osteomyelitis of the skull. In the frontal region it is due to imperfectly treated acute frontal sinusitis. About ten days after the onset considerable pyrexia with severe pain and tenderness over the sinus strongly suggests osteomyelitis. In other parts of the vault a haematoma may become infected.

Osteomyelitis of the Vault. Bone infection usually follows inadequate treatment of a compound fracture. The infection is low grade and should be suspected if a sinus or sinuses persist. A retained foreign body may be the cause of the infection or a sequestrum may form and be extruded.

Tumours of the Skull. Any of the bone tumours mentioned in Chapter 28 are occasionally seen. Exact diagnosis usually depends on biopsy.

Osteoma. A favourite site is the outer table of the frontal, parietal, or occipital bones. The swelling projects as a mound of stony-hard consistency.

Secondary Carcinoma is by far the most common tumour of the skull. It commences in the diploë, and is a blood-borne metastasis. The consistency varies from stony hard (*Fig.* 105) to very soft, depending on its vascularity. Some extremely vascular metastases show pulsation.

Meningioma, although it usually remains within the skull, occasionally forms a sessile swelling over one of the bones of the vertex. The swelling is bony hard in consistency. It is impossible by clinical means to distinguish it from primary or secondary bone tumours.

INTRACRANIAL LESIONS

To the general surgeon easily the most important pathological condition affecting the head is the injury resulting from trauma to the brain and intracranial blood vessels. Owing to the rigid skull, diagnosis must often be inferred from the signs resultant on the brain damage rather than by direct examination, although this has its place. The surgeon is thus attempting the diagnosis and localization of an acute space-occupying lesion (blood clot), whereas the neurologist is more concerned with chronic space-occupying lesions (usually neoplasms). The refinements of diagnosis of the latter do not, in ordinary circumstances, concern the general surgeon, and the medical student will be, or should be, taught the elements of neurological diagnosis on the medical wards.

In this section, therefore, only certain signs which may be found in patients suffering from trauma to the head will be considered.

It must be emphasized at the outset that, with brain injuries, the main presenting features are loss of consciousness, of lesser or greater duration and degree, and restlessness, which make localizing signs, if present, difficult to interpret. Such signs as are present, therefore, often act as an indication that active surgical treatment is necessary rather than as a pointer to the site of the lesion (blood clot). The loss of function of a cranial nerve *at an early stage* usually implies its damage, complicating a fractured base of skull.

EXAMINATION OF A CASE OF RECENT HEAD INJURY

Unless there is an obvious compound fracture of the vault, which should no more be missed than any other compound fracture, a single examination is seldom conclusive, and before it is possible to ascertain what damage has been sustained and/or to judge if progressive changes are occurring, the patient must

PERCIVALL POTT, 1714–1788, *Surgeon, St. Bartholomew's Hospital, London.*

be visited many times at frequent intervals. In this connection there is no better incentive than to remember the aphorism of Hippocrates that *No head injury is so slight that it should be neglected, or so severe that life should be despaired of.* The findings at each visit must be recorded. In all cases radiographs of the skull should be taken at the first opportunity compatible with safety, and their findings correlated with the clinical examination. Except in cases of mild concussion, which have been admitted for observation as a safety measure, the whole scalp must be shaved at the earliest opportunity. The locality of a bruise together with the site of a fracture (if seen on a radiograph) taken together constitute the most important single clue in indicating where an intracranial haematoma is situated. **1. The Patient is Unconscious.** Examine the scalp for a wound or local bruising or haematoma. Inspect the nostrils and back of the throat (compound fracture of the anterior cranial fossa) and the external auditory meatuses (compound fracture of the middle cranial fossa) for evidence of blood diluted with cerebrospinal fluid. In practice it may be extremely difficult to prove that there is such a mixture and in cases of doubt it is wise to assume that cerebrospinal fluid is present and to adopt the necessary antibiotic treatment. Compare the size of the pupils and test their reaction to light. *Make a general survey of the body for other injuries*, especially for fractures and abdominal and thoracic injuries.

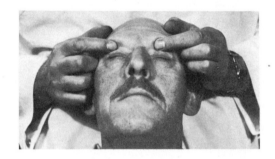

Fig. 106. Exerting pressure over the supra-orbital nerves. The left nerve is being compressed.

Coma is a state of absolute unconsciousness in which the patient does not respond to any stimulus. The reflexes are absent, including the corneal and swallowing reflexes. In *semi-coma* the patient responds only to painful stimuli and reflexes are present. To some extent the depth of unconsciousness can be judged by exerting pressure over the supraorbital nerves which, if properly applied (*Fig.* 106), is exceedingly painful, and all but deeply unconscious patients will respond to it by contracting the facial muscles of the corresponding side.

Search for paralysis. Pick up the arms and legs and allow them to fall. One side may be more flaccid than the other which suggests that there is a cerebral lesion on the opposite side. Pinch the soles of the feet; one leg may be drawn up while the other is not. This is a good test for determining if there is unilateral paralysis in an unconscious patient.

Palpate and percuss the hypogastrium for evidence of an overfull bladder.

The temperature, pulse rate and respiratory rate must be charted every half-hour; similarly, a behaviour chart must be kept at half-hourly intervals by the nurse or doctor, recording the state of consciousness and the patient's response to stimuli, questions, etc.

HIPPOCRATES, *see footnote* p. 89.

Following head injury, vomiting is common, and inhalation of vomitus is a frequent cause of death. Therefore, after the examination it is imperative *to place and have the patient kept on his side, with a clear airway* (by removing blood and mucus) during the whole of the subsequent period of observation. Due consideration should be given to the necessity for inserting an endotracheal tube. Re-examine in one hour, or sooner if called upon by the nurse in charge.

2. The Patient is Conscious or Semi-conscious. Should the patient be mentally confused, the degree of confusion at the time of examination should be recorded.

Stupor. No sensible answers can be obtained, but now and then simple commands forcibly given, such as 'hold my hand', will be obeyed.

Delirium. Although out of touch with his surroundings, relevant answers to obvious questions such as 'how old are you?', 'What is your work?' will be forthcoming. However, he is irritable when disturbed, may be aggressive, noisy, and try and get out of bed.

Confusion. Some degree of coherent conversation is possible.

If this has not been done already (when the patient was unconscious) carry out the examination detailed on p. 56. In addition, make a survey of the integrity of the cranial nerves, as described below.

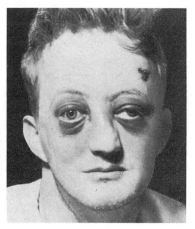

Fig. 107. Injury to the third nerve. Note the ptosis and external strabismus on the left side. The patient fell from his motor-cycle and, striking his head, sustained a fracture of the anterior cranial fossa.

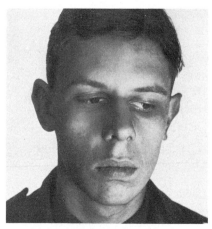

Fig. 108. Paralysis of the right fourth nerve following a head injury. When the patient looks downwards and to the left he suffers diplopia. The illustration shows the lack of rotation of the right eyeball as compared with the left.

EXAMINATION OF THE CRANIAL NERVES

When the patient is conscious the following procedures can be undertaken. In a fair proportion of head injuries cranial nerve damage (often transient) is found.

1st (Olfactory) Nerve. In lesions (abscess or tumour) involving the deep inferior part of the temporal lobe, hallucinations of smell are not infrequent; as a rule these are unpleasant. Complete anosmia is a frequent sequel to fractures involving the cribriform plate of the ethmoid. Smell must be tested on each side by occluding first one and then the other nostril. For the test highly volatile substances should be avoided; ground coffee is satisfactory.

2nd (Optic) Nerve. *Visual Fields:* Gross defects can be detected by a simple examination. The clinician and the patient face one another. While the left eye is tested, the patient covers his right eye with his right hand, and the examiner covers his own left eye with his left hand. The patient fixes his left eye on the pupil of the examiner's right eye. The test object consists of a ball of cotton wool attached to a wooden spatula. The field of vision is ascertained by moving the test object laterally, medially, and up and down.

3rd (Oculomotor) Nerve. *Movement of the Lids:* There is ptosis on the affected side (*Fig.* 107). *Eye Movements:* On asking the patient to look ahead the affected eye deviates outwards (*Fig.* 107).

The following reactions are also lost:

Reaction of the Pupil to Light. The patient is instructed to look at a distant corner of the room. The lamp should be held *out of the line of vision* 15 cm from the eye to be tested. When the light is flashed on the pupil will contract.

Reaction of the Pupil to Accommodation. The patient is requested to look alternately at the most distant object available and at the tip of the clinician's finger held 20 cm from the eye which is being examined. When the farther object is sighted the pupil dilates.

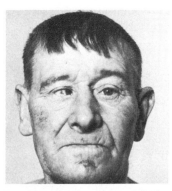

Fig. 109. Left sixth-nerve palsy following a head injury. The left eye does not follow an object laterally due to paralysis of the lateral rectus muscle.

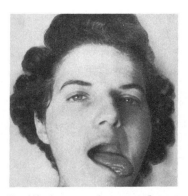

Fig. 110. Answer to the request 'Put out your tongue'. Case of paralysis of the left hypoglossal nerve.

4th (Trochlear) Nerve innervates only the superior oblique muscle. When paralysed, usually there is a slight deviation of the eyeball upwards and inwards, but the striking symptom of which the patient complains is *diplopia* (*Fig.* 108), especially when going downstairs, i.e. *on looking downwards*.

5th (Trigeminal) Nerve. *See* p. 97. A rapid test is to ask the patient to clench the teeth. The masseters can be felt to contract if the 5th nerve is intact.

6th (Abducent) Nerve. Paralysis of the lateral rectus (*Fig.* 109).

7th (Facial) Nerve. *See* p. 99. A rapid test is to ask the patient to show his teeth. Supra-orbital pressure (*see* p. 57), if it evokes a response on one side only in the unconscious patient, demonstrates facial paralysis.

8th (Acoustic) Nerve. *See* p. 84.

9th (Glossopharyngeal) Nerve. The principal sign of a lesion of this nerve is loss of taste in the posterior third of the tongue (*see also* p. 98).

10th (Vagus) Nerve. Does the palate move when the patient says 'Ah'? The vagus innervates the soft palate and in unilateral lesions the uvula moves to the opposite side.

11th (Spinal Accessory) Nerve. *See* p. 403. Paralysis of the trapezius leads to failure to shrug the shoulder.

12th (Hypoglossal) Nerve. Ask the patient to protrude the tongue (*Fig.* 110).

FRACTURED BASE OF THE SKULL

A fracture of the vault, if not obvious clinically, almost always is seen on good quality radiographs. Diagnosis of the following is more difficult, for the fracture is often not visible on an X-ray.

Fracture of the Anterior Cranial Fossa. The peculiar danger of this injury is its liability to be internally compound by implication of one or more paranasal sinuses. In this event cerebrospinal rhinorrhoea develops, with its ever-present possibility of meningitis. Moreover if the patient blows his nose or sneezes (which contingencies must be rigorously avoided) air is likely to be driven into the cranial cavity beneath the dura, and a *pneumatocele* results. Cranial percussion over the frontal bone on the more involved side is then likely to give a sonorous note, but radiographs are necessary to confirm the diagnosis.

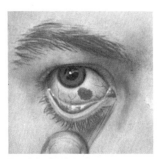

Fig. 111. Conjunctival haemorrhage from injury.

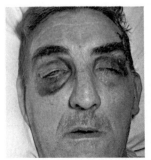

Fig. 112. Fracture of the right anterior cranial fossa. The bruising is limited by the orbital margin. A posterior limit of the subconjunctival haematoma cannot be found.

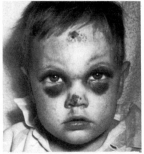

Fig. 113. Two black eyes following a fractured base of skull.

The Differential Diagnosis between Orbital Haemorrhage consequent upon a Fractured Anterior Cranial Fossa and a 'Black Eye':

1. Examine the eyelids. In a fracture the extravasated blood is limited to the orbital margin by the palpebral fascia and tends, therefore, to be circular. In 'black eye' there is no such limitation.

2. In fracture of the anterior cranial fossa the discoloration is purplish from the start, unlike the beefy redness of a recent 'black eye'.

3. Examine the conjunctiva. In 'black eye' there may be a conjunctival haemorrhage, but this is often *in* the conjunctiva (*Fig.* 111), and moves with the conjunctiva when the eyelid is moved gently by the pulp of the little finger. In fracture of the anterior cranial fossa the haemorrhage is always *subconjunctival*.

4. Ask the patient to rotate his eyes by following your finger. In 'black eye' the posterior limit of the extravasated blood can be defined. In a fractured anterior cranial fossa there is no posterior limit (*Fig.* 112), and the haemorrhage as a whole tends to be fan-shaped, the handle of the fan being towards the iris.

5. Two black eyes following one injury indicate fracture of the base of the skull (Finch) (*Fig.* 113).

Fracture of the Middle Cranial Fossa. This should be suspected when there is blood, or blood diluted with cerebrospinal fluid, escaping from the auditory meatus, which must always be examined.* The escape of blood, however, is not pathognomonic of a fracture, for it also occurs when the tympanic membrane is ruptured. However, with the latter the blood will clot, but blood admixed with cerebrospinal fluid will not do so but continues to drip. The exception to this rule is serious haemorrhage from tearing of the posterior branch of the middle meningeal artery.

Fractures of the middle cranial fossa may give rise to facial paralysis (*see* p. 99), and/or deafness, and/or nystagmus.

Battle's Sign. If there has been doubt, bruising over the mastoid process appearing a day or two after the injury, confirms a diagnosis of fracture of the middle fossa.

Fracture of the Posterior Cranial Fossa is even more menacing than fracture of the anterior or middle fossa, for one or more of the venous sinuses that groove the occipital bone are liable to be torn. Not infrequently deep coma persists from the moment of injury; soon the pupils become dilated and inactive. There is derangement of normal respiratory rhythm, culminating in Cheyne–Stokes (periodic) respiration (*Fig.* 114). In such cases, if the pulse becomes irregular it indicates a lesion of the brain-stem that will probably prove fatal.

Slowly developing clot accumulation leads to nystagmus and ataxia.

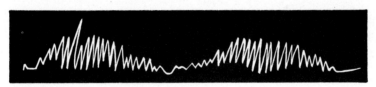

Fig. 114. A recording of Cheyne–Stokes respiration.

SIGNIFICANT SIGNS OCCURRING DURING THE PERIOD OF OBSERVATION OF A PATIENT WITH A HEAD INJURY

The clinician's aim is to decide which patients (a small minority) should be subjected to surgical intervention. In neurosurgical centres angiography, computerized tomography and other sophisticated methods of diagnosis help in reaching a decision; in other circumstances any suspicion of traumatic intracranial haemorrhage should lead the surgeon to make exploratory burr-holes because to wait until clinical diagnosis is certain is to wait until the patient is near death. Traumatic intracranial haemorrhage, which may be extradural, subdural, or intracerebral, gives rise to acute cerebral compression which also can arise from cerebral

---

* Exceptionally the ear drum remains intact with a middle fossa fracture in which case the escaping CSF may trickle down the Eustachian tube and present as cerebrospinal rhinorrhoea.

Sir Ernest Finch, 1884–1960, *Professor of Surgery, University of Sheffield.*
William H. Battle, 1855–1936, *Surgeon, St. Thomas's Hospital, London.*
John Cheyne, 1777–1836, *Physician, Meath Hospital, Dublin.*
William Stokes, 1804–1878, *Regius Professor of Physic, University of Dublin.*

oedema occurring around a major cerebral contusion or laceration.

Pulse Rate. Gradual slowing—a sign to which much attention has been directed in classic descriptions of middle meningeal haemorrhage—prevails only when the increased intracranial pressure so produced occurs very slowly. Much more commonly intracranial bleeding is accompanied by a fast pulse rate.

Temperature. Subnormal temperature due to shock from the blood loss of associated injuries is common. As the shock is treated, a moderate pyrexia of up to 38 °C with fluctuations is usual and of no particular significance. It is due to aseptic absorption of small amounts of blood.

Pyrexia of 38 °C or over, developing a few hours after the accident, indicates primary injury to the thermoregulating mechanism, and usually other signs of a midbrain lesion (e.g. decerebrate rigidity) are present.

Considerable pyrexia developing at a later period, i.e. up to three days after the accident, is due, most probably, to an intracranial haematoma, or (especially in cases of a fractured anterior cranial fossa) to meningitis, or to other infection (e.g. pneumonia).

Respiration. Rapid respiration associated with restlessness is a not infrequent accompaniment of intracranial haemorrhage. Stertorous breathing with the cheeks puffing in and out usually signifies an advanced stage of cerebral compression.

Convulsive Seizures occasionally are the first sign that something more serious than simple concussion is present. One may be fortunate enough to observe a 'fit', but rarely is the clinician so favoured: usually he has to trust to a description by the nurse. Try to find out where the fit *began*. In conjunction with the seeking of this information, it is useful to recall the localization of the various centres in the pre-Rolandic area of the cerebral cortex. In middle meningeal haemorrhage the fit is of the Jacksonian type* and unilateral. In haemorrhage from the superior longitudinal sinus the fits may be bilateral.

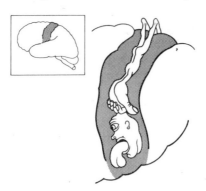

Fig. 115. Cerebral localization in the pre-Rolandic cortex (*after* Penfield). Note the relatively large area for the hand (particularly the thumb) and for the facial muscles (particularly the tongue).

Ordinary *epilepsy* (which may have caused the head injury, especially in children) may be the cause of difficulty. However, recovery is rapid and complete and usually the relatives know that the patient is an epileptic (Lewin).

Neck Rigidity. Blood in the CSF is an irritant and produces sterile meningitis. Therefore, if a patient, seen soon after the accident, is found to have slight

---

* Jacksonian epilepsy = progression of involuntary clonic movements mainly limited to one side or to one group of muscles.

Luigi Rolando, 1773–1831, *Professor of Anatomy, Turin.*
John Hughlings Jackson, 1835–1911, *Physician, The London Hospital.*
Walpole S. Lewin, *Contemporary, Neurosurgeon, Addenbrooke's Hospital, Cambridge.*
Wilder G. Penfield, 1891–1976, *Director, Montreal Neurological Institute, Montreal.*

pyrexia, a rapid pulse and rigidity of the muscles of the neck, then, probably, subarachnoid haemorrhage is the correct diagnosis. It must, however, be remembered that a fracture-dislocation of a cervical vertebra will also give rise to rigidity of the neck and a fast pulse rate, but pyrexia is absent. In any case of doubt X-rays of the cervical spine must be obtained *before* testing for neck rigidity lest irreparable damage to the spinal cord be produced by the examination. To elicit the sign, proceed as follows: with the patient lying on his back in a relaxed state, the head is flexed steadily, but gently, on the thorax until definite voluntary resistance is felt. When the sign is positive, not only is the range of flexion distinctly subnormal, but when flexion is continued beyond the point where resistance is felt, it causes pain of varying intensity.

Late neck rigidity with high pyrexia and severe headache, particularly if associated with leakage of CSF from the nose or an ear or following a compound fracture, suggests septic meningitis.

Lucid Interval. The classic sign of *Middle Meningeal* (syn. *Extradural*) *Haemorrhage* is a lucid interval. By this is meant that the patient regains consciousness and shortly afterwards lapses once more into unconsciousness. It is subject to the widest variations, from a few minutes to several days, and may be completely absent because of (1) Severe concomitant injury of the brain, or (2) Alcoholism. Remember that a drunken person is particularly liable to injury and that the stupor can be due to alcoholic poisoning, or to head injury, or to a combination of these. The most serious difficulty, however, occurs when a patient remains unconscious because of intra-cerebral injury and yet an extradural haematoma is forming at the same time. In this instance the *extradural haematoma* can be suspected by: (*a*) the presence of a haematoma of the temporalis muscle on the affected side; (*b*) the gradual onset of hemiparesis and hemiplegia; (*c*) deepening coma, perhaps accompanied by (*d*) Hutchinson's pupils (*see* p. 64).

Subdural Haemorrhage is very much more common than extradural, and is not usually associated with a lucid interval. However, like an extradural haematoma, lateralizing signs may be found to be present.

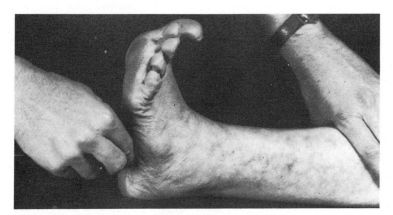

Fig. 116. Plantar reflex, extensor response—Babinski's sign (↑). The outer side of the sole from the heel forward is stroked with a blunt object. The big toe dorsiflexes and, typically, the other toes fan out.

Subarachnoid Haemorrhage has been referred to above (*see* Neck Rigidity, p. 62). A neurological examination in such a case is often indefinite for any lateralizing sign.

Intracerebral Haemorrhage can be associated with either extra- or subdural haematoma, or it may be the sole lesion. Lateralizing signs are usually absent.

Lateralizing Neurological Signs. A very characteristic feature of an extradural haematoma is the appearance of paralysis of the arm, leg and face of the contra-lateral side. If the patient is completely conscious and cooperative (unusual), weakness or actual paralysis is easily ascertained. If a large extradural clot is present, on applying the supraorbital pressure test (*see* Fig. 106) the semi-conscious individual will not respond on the affected side, but on the non-affected side purposeful movements will be made to remove the noxious stimulus. In the absence of signs of hemiplegia, the supraorbital pressure should be continued until the clinician is satisfied that movement takes place in all four limbs. When no response can be obtained, to eliminate the possibility of the supraorbital nerves being in bony grooves, and therefore incompressible, rub both cheeks vigorously, and then observe the face, particularly the corners of the mouth. Even in deep unconsciousness the corner of the mouth on the non-paralysed side tends to be drawn upwards after a 'facial massage'. When either of these tests suggests that hemiplegia is present, corroborating signs (absent abdominal reflexes, increased triceps jerks, and a positive Babinski's sign) must be sought. In comparatively early cases the arm is always more affected than the leg.

Babinski's Sign (*Fig.* 116) is most significant and (in cases of intracranial haemorrhage) the one present most frequently. It usually denotes a haematoma on the opposite side of the brain.

Difficulty in Speech. If the lesion in left-sided in a right-handed individual, the first lateralizing sign may be difficulty in speech (aphasia) if the patient is conscious; in right-handed people Broca's area usually is left-sided.

Inequality of the Pupils is of considerable localizing value. *Hutchinson's pupil*, due to compression of the third nerve against the free edge of the tentorium, is seen frequently in cases of extradural haematoma, but it occurs also in some cases of subdural haematoma. In order not to overlook this sign when it is of most value, half-hourly examinations are mandatory. As a result of increasing pressure upon the third cranial nerve, the pupil passes through the following stages:

STAGE	Pupil on opposite side to the lesion		Pupil on side on which compression commenced
1	Normal		Slightly contracted. Reacts to light
2	Normal		Moderately dilated. Reacts to light sluggishly
3	Moderately dilated. Reacts to light		Widely dilated. Does not react to light
4	Widely dilated. Insensitive		Widely dilated. Insensitive. Occasionally ptosis is present

Joseph F. F. Babinski, 1857–1932, *Head of the Neurological Clinic, Hôpital Pitié, Paris.*
Pierre P. Broca, 1824–1880, *Professor of Clinical Surgery, Paris.*
Sir Jonathan Hutchinson, 1828–1913, *Surgeon, The London Hospital.*

The first stage is seen but rarely. It is the second (*Fig.* 117) and third stages that are of signal diagnostic importance.* Widely dilated and fixed pupils on both sides indicate that death is near.

Myotonic Pupil. The patient complains of blurring of vision of one eye and is found to have a dilated pupil which reacts only sluggishly to light and on accommodation (*see* Argyll Robertson reaction p. 5). If a head injury is suspected consternation is compounded when the knee jerks are tested in *Adie's Syndrome* in which sluggish or absent tendon jerks are additional to the myotonic pupil.

When any of the above signs, and especially when a combination of them, makes a diagnosis of serious intracranial lesion probable, it is most necessary to re-examine the shaved scalp to look for a haematoma or a bruise and to review the X-rays. Should the localizing signs be on one side of the body and the haematoma or bruise is situated on the other side, that is what we should expect; but if the haematoma or bruise is situated on the same side as the paralysis, remember the possibility of a *contre-coup†* injury.

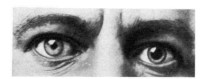

Opposite side to lesion: Normal.   Side of lesion: Dilated; reacts to light.

Fig. 117. Hutchinson's pupils: second stage.

Cerebral Irritation is almost certainly due to the presence of blood in the cerebrospinal fluid of a patient who is recovering consciousness. Usually it asserts itself about thirty or forty hours after the injury. The patient lies curled up in bed, his face turned from the light, because he hates it (*photophobia*). The eyelids are closed. The temperature is moderately raised. The patient resents being aroused. He is abusive and irritable. No further examination is necessary, or, indeed, possible.

TRAUMATIC INTRACRANIAL VASCULAR LESIONS

Blood vessels may be damaged after a blow by being stretched or by impinging on an unyielding structure (e.g. the falx cerebri). Arteries may also thrombose subsequent to hypotension due to shock caused by extracranial injuries. The syndromes described below are commoner in older patients with brittle atherosclerotic arteries and are seen 2–5 days after the injury.

Internal Carotid Artery Thrombosis. In a young patient a neck injury is the usual cause (*see* p. 387). Older patients are prone to such thrombosis with relatively minor trauma to the skull and no early loss of consciousness. In either instance the patient shows classic hemiplegia on the contralateral side with aphasia if the speech centre is on the affected side.

Carotico-cavernous Fistula. See Pulsating Proptosis, p. 79.

Venous Sinus Injury. One of the sinuses is torn by an extensive fracture easily seen on a radiograph. The site of the fracture is thus an important clue to localizing the bleeding sinus.

---

* The *consensual* light reflex is lost in the Hutchinson pupil but is present with the fixed dilated pupil of intra-ocular haemorrhage or severed optic nerve, i.e. the pupil contracts when a light is shone into the opposite eye.

† *Contre-coup.* French = counter-stroke. The transmission of a shock from the point struck to a point on the opposite side (of the head).

WILLIAM J. ADIE, 1886–1935, *Neurologist, Royal Ophthalmic Hospital, Moorfields, London.*

Superior Sagittal Sinus. The slowly developing collection of clot causes bilateral leg spasticity with ankle clonus and extensor plantor reflexes but little or no involvement of the arms.

Transverse (Lateral) Sinus. The collection of blood in the posterior fossa obstructs the circulation of CSF, causing bilateral papilloedema which is associated with diplopia due to sixth nerve palsy (*see* p. 59). The patient is otherwise well.

Cavernous Sinus Thrombosis after Injury. The thrombus is aseptic and does not show the serious systemic illness or proptosis and chemosis of the septic variety (*see* p. 70). After an anterior cranial fossa injury (the fracture often not being seen on a radiograph) the patient develops delayed bilateral third-nerve palsy including ptosis (*see* p. 59).

BIRTH INJURY OF THE BRAIN

Diagnosis rests on suspicion when one or more of the predisposing factors are present. They are severe toxaemia of pregnancy, antepartum haemorrhage, prematurity, fetal distress, difficult labour (often with forceps delivery) and precipitate labour.

Traumatic Intracranial Haemorrhage in Neonates is by far the most frequent cause of death in the newborn, the haemorrhage usually being subdural or subarachnoid. Convulsions are very common; usually they are generalized. The condition is said to be accompanied by the cephalic cry—a sharp, fretful cry, especially on picking up the child. Pyrexia or hyperpyrexia is a leading and important sign. Vomiting and failure to gain weight are frequent. The anterior fontanelle is tense and may bulge. Unilateral dilatation of the pupil is found in some cases.

Patients seen later, e.g. in childhood, often show spastic diplegia (*see* p. 440) as an end-result. In some a monoplegia or hemiplegia is found.

Chronic Subdural Haematoma in Infants, which is eminently suitable for treatment, has been overlooked because of the close simulation of the clinical picture with that of hydrocephalus (*see* p. 55). Often injury occurs during forceps delivery. The first sign is difficulty in feeding and irritability in an infant a few days old who has apparently recovered from one of the predisposing events mentioned above. Vomiting is frequent. The veins of the scalp are dilated, the anterior fontanelle bulges, and the child's head is enlarged but the eyes are not typically downcast.

CHRONIC SPACE-OCCUPYING LESIONS WITHIN THE SKULL

Intracranial space-occupying lesions comprise not only neoplasms, but chronic haematomata (together with cysts arising therefrom) and abscesses. The general surgeon, in ordinary circumstances, is concerned only with such lesions as result from trauma or the septic complications thereof. If a rigid boundary is not drawn at this point it becomes extremely difficult to avoid a long digression into methods of diagnosis not strictly of surgical interest.

Chronic Subdural Haematoma. This remote complication is of interest to the surgeon. Weeks or months after an injury a collection of blood draws fluid to it by osmosis, enlarges, and causes symptoms. Headache is usual and the patient becomes drowsy and confused. Lateralizing·signs as with an acute extradural haematoma (*see* p. 63) may be present.

Intracranial Abscess is one variety of chronic space-occupying lesion. The practitioner should have some knowledge of the possibility of an abscess complicating certain surgical conditions.

Headache and vomiting are the major symptoms of an intracranial abscess, and papilloedema is a cardinal sign and should be sought with the ophthalmoscope. A description of the technique is beyond the scope of this work. The temperature is raised unless masked by antibiotics.

The three varieties described below may follow a compound injury in which event the problem of localization is simplified. In other circumstances the following considerations apply:

Extradural Abscess is usually secondary to spread from the middle ear or from the frontal sinus. In the former the pus escapes into the extradural space through the tegmen tympani; in the latter through the posterior wall of the sinus. The signs are those of osteomyelitis localized to the bone affected. There is severe circumscribed headache, tenderness on percussion over the area involved, and in the case of the frontal region a Pott's puffy 'tumour' (*see* p. 56).

Subdural Abscess is produced by infected thrombophlebitis of the superior sagittal venous sinus spreading from an infected frontal air sinus or other septic process in the head or neck. The abscess forms usually between the occipital lobe and the tentorium, the most dependent part with the patient recumbent. The general signs of a serious infection usually are in evidence. Cortical thrombosis may cause Jacksonian epilepsy and paralyses as in extradural haemorrhage (*see* p. 63).

Intracerebral Abscess arises in one of several ways apart from trauma: (1) Otitis media with mastoiditis gives rise to an abscess of the temporal lobe or the cerebellum of the diseased side, the former being much more common. A chronic infection is more likely to result in a brain abscess than an acute infection. It is not unknown for a patient who has had a discharging ear for years to forget to mention it to his doctor. Too frequently, when he commences to vomit he is given medicine for indigestion and later, as this symptom progresses, a barium meal is ordered. Only when he collapses and loses consciousness does it become obvious that a neurological examination should have been made earlier. The patient is suffering from an *otitic brain abscess*. (2) Nasal sinusitis with or without osteomyelitis may cause an abscess of the frontal lobe. (3) Lastly, and very important, is a *metastatic abscess*, a well-recognized complication of lung abscess, bronchiectasis, or pyaemic states. It can occur anywhere in the brain, and consequently its localization is usually a problem for the neurologist.

Chapter 7

THE ORBIT

Diseases of the eye itself are beyond the scope of this work. In the surgical wards and out-patients are seen the results of trauma about the orbit and a variety of cystic and solid swellings many of which displace the eyeball forward. It is convenient to reserve the term 'proptosis' for these, and to retain the word 'exophthalmos' for the protrusion, bilateral or unilateral, associated with thyrotoxicosis.

Certain *congenital* lesions are drawn to the surgeon's attention.

Epicanthus is a concave skin fold at the medial angle of the lids (*Fig.* 118), usually bilateral and present normally in Mongolian races. When well marked, it gives an appearance mimicking squint, owing to the relatively larger amount of white sclerotic visible on the lateral, as compared with the medial, side. As the nose develops the fold becomes less pronounced.

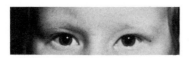

Fig. 118. Epicanthus, left.

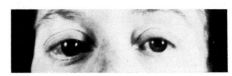

Fig. 119. Buphthalmos (right eye).

Coloboma. Notches, or colobomata, are sometimes present as congenital deformities of the lower lids. They are sometimes associated with dermoid cysts in the neighbourhood, and often form a part of the Collins–Franceschetti syndrome (*see* p. 81).

Infantile Glaucoma (Buphthalmos). * When increased intra-ocular tension develops in an infant, it causes uniform enlargement of the cornea and the sclera. General enlargement of the eye results so that it comes to resemble the eye of an ox. Although generally bilateral, when the condition is chronic and unilateral (*Fig.* 119) the patient may present on account of some other condition, the affected eye being painless, though sightless or almost so.

Depressed Fracture of the Zygomatic Bone. Because of its prominence and exposed situation, the zygomatic (malar) bone is in a vulnerable position and, as a result of a blow upon it, inward displacement (*Fig.* 120), with shattering of the related wall of the maxillary sinus, is moderately common. This injury gives rise to a triad of signs: (1) Unilateral epistaxis (from tearing of the mucous membrane of the maxillary sinus); (2) A black eye with subconjunctival ecchymosis (from forcible displacement of part of the floor of the orbit); and (3) Flattening of the contour of the cheek in its upper part, a most telling but transitory sign, for soon the depression becomes masked by the bruising and oedema of the overlying soft tissues. Thus this depressed fracture is frequently overlooked at a time when it could be elevated with comparative ease and precision. Further delay is caused by arranging for a radiograph to be taken and by waiting for a report, for it is not always easy for the inexperienced to see this fracture. A small series of additional physical signs enable a prompt diagnosis to be made without such aid.

---

* *Buphthalmos.* Greek, βοῦς:οφθαλμός = ox,eye.

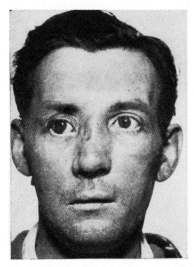

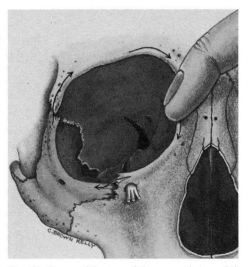

Fig. 120. Depressed fracture of the zygomatic bone. The right pupil is a centimetre below the level of the left, and the margin of the lower lid and the inner canthus are depressed correspondingly.

Fig. 121. Depressed fracture of the zygomatic bone. Palpating the orbital rim.

1. With the pulp of the index finger, palpate the entire bony rim of the orbit in a circular fashion. If a depressed fracture of the zygomatic bone is present, a definite notch, or at least an unmistakable irregularity, will be felt on the inferior border of the orbital margin at the zygomatic suture line (*Fig.* 121). This is the sign *par excellence* of this fracture.

2. Often the upper lip is anaesthetic due to implication of the infra-orbital nerve at its exit from the infra-orbital foramen.

3. Diplopia from subsidence of the floor of the orbit.

4. Blood and clot within the maxillary sinus obliterate normal translucency. (*See* p. 136.)

Orbital Blow-out Fracture. Blunt trauma to the orbit occasioned by blows by a fist or in car accidents cause compression of the orbital contents and disruption of the fragile orbital floor. Often the inferior oblique muscle is incarcerated in the fracture line, upward movement of the eyeball being lost. Those unaware of the entity are liable to diagnose an oculomotor palsy. In untreated cases, when the oedema subsides, enophthalmos (*see* p. 76) becomes apparent due to reduction in the orbital contents.

Black Eye. *See* p. 60.

Orbital Cellulitis. In view of the fact that the paper-like lamina papyracea of the ethmoid forms the major part of the medial wall of the orbit, it is not surprising that the commonest cause is ethmoiditis. Others are infection from the frontal sinus, a furuncle or other infection of the face, infection of a penetrating wound of the orbit, and, particularly in infants, infection from the gums and teeth. There is some swelling of the eyelids (*Fig.* 122). On parting the lids it will become apparent that there is proptosis and frequently chemosis* as well. Because of

---

* *Chemosis.* Greek, χήμη = cockleshell. Oedema of the ocular conjunctiva.

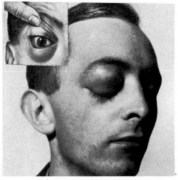

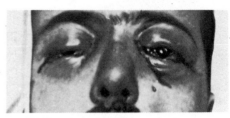

Fig. 123. Thrombosis of the left cavernous sinus; right threatened. Bloodstained lacrimation.

Fig. 122. Orbital cellulitis. The patient cannot open the eye. Inset shows the accompanying proptosis.

pressure on, or involvement of, the optic nerve, often acuity of vision is reduced. There are two outstanding dangers of uncontrolled infection of this space—thrombosis of the cavernous sinus and infection of the globe of the eye.

Thrombophlebitis of the Cavernous Sinus. Infection reaches the sinus by various routes: (1) Along the angular ophthalmic vein from infection of the face; (2) Along the lateral and petrosal venous sinuses from the middle ear; (3) Through the pterygoid venous plexus from infection of the pharyngomaxillary space (posterior variety of peritonsillar abscess; *see* p. 131); (4) From cellulitis of the orbit via the ophthalmic vein. The latent period between the appearance of the primary lesion and signs indicating involvement of the sinus is about five days. The onset is catastrophic with severe headache and rigors, followed by delirium and semi-consciousness. Oedema of the eyelids and chemosis are manifest early; to these are added proptosis, partial or complete ophthalmoplegia,* and finally dilatation and fixity of the pupil. Sometimes bloodstained tears trickle down the cheeks (*Fig.* 123). Unless checked by massive antibiotic therapy similar signs, varying from oedema of the eyelids to the fully fledged clinical picture, appear on the other side. Having regard to the free intercommunications of the cavernous sinus this tragic train of events with threat of blindness or death cannot be wondered at.

THE EYELIDS

Blepharitis is inflammation of the lid margins which are red with scales or crusts between the short and distorted lashes. It is often associated with errors of refraction or muscle balance, which must be investigated.

Trachoma† is a chronic inflammation resulting in the palpebral conjunctiva becoming studded with enlarged follicles (*Fig.* 124). As it advances the oedematous lids become partially ptosed, and epiphora is a frequent accompaniment.

Ectropion (eversion of the eyelids) can affect one or both lids. That due to senile degeneration of the orbicularis palpebrarum, or to long-standing severe facial paralysis affects only the lower lids. The eversion of the lower lid leads to epiphora (*Fig.* 125 and *see* p. 72). Scarring such as that due to burns can cause ectropion or entropion depending on its site.

---

* *Ophthalmoplegia*: Paralysis of more than one of the extrinsic muscles of the eye.
† *Trachoma*. Greek, τράχωμα = roughness.

Entropion (inversion of the lids) is a common complication of trachoma and of severe blepharitis.
Xanthelasma Palpebrarum are yellow, raised patches occurring on the skin of the upper eyelids near
the inner canthus (*Fig.* 126). These plaques occur more frequently in patients with long-standing
high blood-cholesterol levels and occasionally in a more generalized form, and are present typically
on the extensor surfaces in the region of the elbows (*xanthomatosis*).

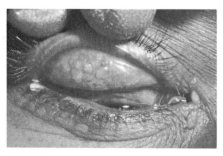

Fig. 124. Trachoma.

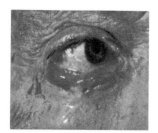

Fig. 125. Ectropion.

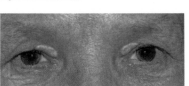

Fig. 126. Xanthelasma palpebrarum.

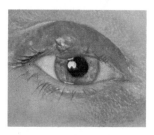

Fig. 127. Hordeolum.

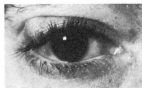

Fig. 128. Chalazion.

Hordeolum* (stye) is a suppurative inflammation of one of Zeis's glands.† In the early stage the
gland becomes swollen, hard, and painful. An abscess forms, which generally points near the base of
one of the eyelashes (*Fig.* 127). The pain is considerable until the pus is evacuated. The condition is
most common in young adults, but can occur at all times of life, especially in debilitated individuals.
Chalazion,‡ often termed incorrectly 'Meibomian cyst', is a chronic granuloma of a Meibomian
gland. Chalazia are more common in adults than in children, and are characterized by the formation
of a swelling like a bead in the substance of the lid, usually tending to expand more towards the skin
(*Fig.* 128) than towards the conjunctival surface. A small chalazion is difficult to perceive, but is
readily appreciated by passing a finger over the skin of the lid. When the ·lid is everted, the
conjunctiva related to the swelling is dark red. When the affection occurs in the upper lid, blurred
vision sometimes ensues, owing to distortion of the cornea produced by pressure of the swelling
(temporary astigmatism). From time to time secondary infection occurs. The inflammatory symptoms
are more violent than those of a hordeolum, for the gland is deeper and is embedded in dense fibrous
tissue. Pus appears as a yellow spot shining through the conjunctiva—the so-called 'hordeolum
interna'. It is exceptional for a suppurating chalazion to point cutaneously.

---

* *Hordeolum*. Latin = a barleycorn.
† Zeis's glands = the ciliary glands = the sebaceous glands of the eyelids.
‡ *Chalazion.* Greek, χάλαζιον = a hailstone.

EDUARD ZEIS, 1807–1868, *Professor of Surgery, Marburg.*
HEINRICH MEIBOM, 1638–1700, *Professor of Medicine, Helmstadt. Resigned to take up the Chair of History and
Poetic Art.*

Ptosis* *The Congenital Form* shows a very characteristic attitude of forced contraction of the frontalis, resulting in raising of the eyebrows and furrowing of the skin of the forehead (*Fig.* 129). Partial paralysis is masked by this means, but becomes manifest if the patient is asked to look upwards.

The Acquired Form is the result of paralysis of the third nerve (*see* p. 59). If bilateral, myasthenia gravis (*see* p. 91) is the usual cause.

Tumours of the Eyelid are uncommon, with the exception of rodent ulcer (*see* p. 36).

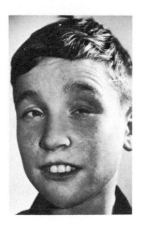

Fig. 129. Partial congenital ptosis. The furrowed brow is characteristic.

THE LACRIMAL APPARATUS

Enlargement of the lacrimal gland causes a swelling beneath the upper and outer part of the orbital rim, with bulging of the adjoining part of the upper eyelid. The fact that the swelling is below the eyebrow and that it extends into the orbit serves to distinguish it from an external angular dermoid (*see Fig.* 144).

Dacryo-adenitis. The most common cause is ascending infection, nearly always staphylococcal, in which event the pre-auricular lymph node is often enlarged. Other causes are: as a complication of mumps, or of glandular fever (search in the neck, axillae and groins for enlargement of lymph nodes, and examine the spleen for enlargement), or of herpes zoster of the lacrimal nerve.

Neoplasms of the Lacrimal Gland. Morphologically the lacrimal glands are allied to the salivary glands, because in animals that retain a patent palatine foramen some of the tears drain into the mouth, supplementing the saliva. Pathologically the lacrimal gland shares with the salivary glands the changes peculiar to Mikulicz's disease (*see* p. 105), while, like that of the salivary glands, a neoplasm of the lacrimal gland (*Fig.* 130) often proves to be a mixed tumour.

Epiphora† is due to acquired malposition of the puncta, obstruction of a lacrimal canaliculus, obstruction of the nasolacrimal duct, or dacryocystitis (*see* p. 73). Congenital obstruction of the nasolacrimal duct, consequent upon a septum or a valve in the lower end of the duct, is usually unilateral, and becomes evident about the eighth day of life. Infection of the lacrimal sac often supervenes, in which case the resulting overflow of semipurulent fluid is often mistaken for ophthalmia neonatorum. A fruitful source of epiphora is eversion of the lid from ectropion, which prevents the tears draining into the puncta. Partial epiphora (the tear that never falls, *see Fig.* 187, p. 99) commonly occurs in facial palsy, and is due to sagging of the lower lid consequent upon paralysis of the orbicularis. As a result of the sagging, the punctum does not lie at the correct angle to allow the optimum drainage of the lacrimal secretion. Finally, it is possible for the nasolacrimal duct to be compressed by a neoplasm of the maxilla, although this is unusual.

---

* *Ptosis*. Greek, πτῶσις = a fall.
† *Epiphora*. Greek, ἐπιφορά = overflow of tears.

JOHANNES VON MIKULICZ-RADECKI, 1850–1905, *Professor of Surgery, Breslau.*

Dacryocystitis. *a. Acute Dacryocystitis* is manifest by pain, oedema and redness of the skin overlying the lacrimal sac (*Fig.* 131). Epiphora is always present, and is of long standing if the acute episode follows chronic dacryocystitis. There is exquisite tenderness over the sac. Pus cannot be expressed through the punctum for two reasons: the pain on attempting to express pus is agonizing, and the more so because oedema shuts the canaliculus.

b. Chronic Dacryocystitis. When the lacrimal sac is infected, usually there is some swelling over the site of the sac. Epiphora is a leading, and occasionally the only, symptom. Light pressure over the sac causes regurgitation of fluid—mucopus or pus—through the punctum. Conjunctivitis is a usual complication. In the recently born the condition must be distinguished from ophthalmia neonatorum; this is simple, for in chronic dacryocystitis, although there is a mucopurulent discharge, there is no inflammation of the conjunctiva.

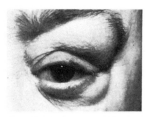

Fig. 130. Mixed tumour of the left lacrimal gland.

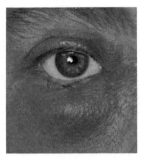

Fig. 131. Acute dacryocystitis (right).

THE ORBITAL SIGNS OF PRIMARY THYROTOXICOSIS (GRAVES' DISEASE)

It has been considered expedient to discuss the elicitation and interpretation of the orbital signs of thyrotoxicosis in this chapter rather than interrupt the continuity of the examination of the thyroid gland (Chapter 14). 'Exophthalmos' is a disorder varying from staring eyes to obviously protruding eyeballs. Both eyes are not necessarily affected (*Fig.* 132) or, in a fair proportion of patients, are unequally affected. The globes themselves are not responsible; it is the related structures that suffer in the following sequence:

Mild Exophthalmos consists merely of widening of the palpebral fissures due to retraction of the upper eyelids (*Stellwag's sign,** Fig.* 132) consequent upon tonic contraction of the striated fibres of the levatores palpebrae superioris. This creates an illusion of bulging of the eye or eyes, corrected by:

Naffziger's Method of Examination. Stand behind the seated patient and tilt her head backwards, holding it in the manner shown in *Fig.* 133, which will keep the hair out of the way. Observe the eyeballs, your plane of vision being that of the superciliary ridges. By examining the globes in this manner it is possible to confirm (*Fig.* 133, inset) or eliminate the presence of protrusion of the eyeballs. Should this test eliminate actual protrusion, that this staring look is due to lid retraction can be confirmed by von Graefe's sign.

---

* The names attached to this and the minor eye signs which follow are of academic importance only.

ROBERT J. GRAVES, 1796–1853, *Physician, Meath Hospital, Dublin.*
CARL STELLWAG VON CARION, 1823–1904, *Ophthalmologist, General Hospital, Vienna.*
HOWARD C. NAFFZIGER, 1884–1961, *Surgeon, University of California, San Francisco.*

Von Graefe's Sign. The patient should be asked to follow the finger moved up and down several times, and not too slowly. Only persistent lagging of the upper lid (*Fig.* 134) behind the corneoscleral limbus should be taken as a positive result.

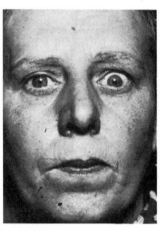

Fig. 132. Unilateral exophthalmos showing lid retraction (Stellwag's sign).

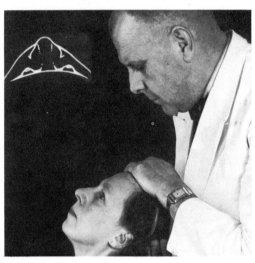

Fig. 133. Naffziger's method of looking for, or excluding, minor degrees of bulging of the globes.

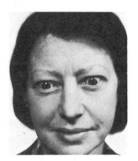

Fig. 134. Von Graefe's sign. Upper lid lag when the patient looks down.

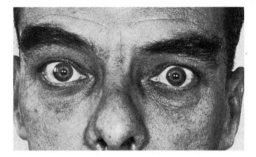

Fig. 135. Moderately severe exophthalmos of a degree fairly typical of Graves' disease. Note the inequality of the bulging.

Moderate Exophthalmos (*Fig.* 135). The bulging is due almost entirely to increased deposition of fat. On Naffziger's method of examination it is evident that eyes do, in fact, bulge. When the bulging has reached moderate proportions, *Joffroy's sign* is positive, namely an absence of wrinkling of the forehead when the head is bent down and the patient looks upwards (*Fig.* 136).

Severe Exophthalmos. Intra-orbital oedema is superadded to the increased deposition of intra-orbital fat. Clinically it embraces three components:

ALBRECHT VON GRAEFE, 1828–1870, *Professor of Ophthalmology, Berlin.*
ALEX JOFFROY, 1844–1908, *Physician to the Salpêtrière, Paris.*

a. Intra-orbital congestion disclosed by watering of the eyes, especially in the early morning, at times misdiagnosed as conjunctivitis. This is the earliest manifestation which must be sought by examining the lateral ocular conjunctiva for dilated blood vessels (*Fig.* 137).

b. Increased resistance to light pressure on the globe, indicating raised intraocular tension, is found in varying degrees.

c. Muscular paresis (ophthalmoplegia), at times revealed by double vision. The eyes should be put through their full range of movement, upwards, downwards, inwards, and outwards, and inquiry made if any of them causes diplopia. Limitation of movement, especially in an upward and outward direction, is often noticeable. Later, difficulty in convergence (*Moebius's sign, Fig.* 138) becomes evident.

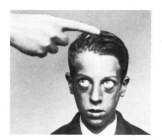

Fig. 136. Joffroy's sign.

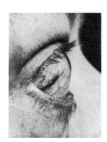

Fig. 137. Dilated conjunctival blood vessels in a case of severe exophthalmos.

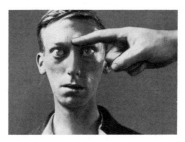

Fig. 138. Moebius's sign. Difficulty in convergence when the patient is asked to look at a near object.

A small proportion of patients with severe exophthalmos also show pretibial myxoedema (*see* p. 11), a condition never found apart from Graves' disease with exophthalmos. Exophthalmos does not necessarily decrease after successful treatment of thyrotoxicosis; on the contrary, during the first nine months following such treatment, an average of 1 mm more protuberance, as measured with an exophthalmometer, must be expected. After that time some slow recession occurs in the majority of patients. Nevertheless, the paradox obtains that in spite of slight further overfilling of the orbit there is subjective improvement in appearance due to release of spasm of the lids.

The Differential Diagnosis between Unilateral Exophthalmos and Proptosis consequent upon an Intra-orbital Mass. If the upper eyelid cannot be everted, or is everted only with difficulty, the exophthalmos is more likely to be due to thyrotoxicosis, whereas if the lid is everted easily it is more likely that the displacement of the eyeball results from the presence of an intra-orbital mass (*Gifford's sign*).

Progressive Exophthalmos supervenes comparatively infrequently and usually after otherwise successful treatment of the thyrotoxicosis with which it was associated. As its name implies, if after treatment of the thyrotoxicosis (medical, surgical, or radiotherapeutic) the exophthalmos continues to increase instead of regress, it is categorized as having entered the progressive stage and visual acuity becomes impaired by one or more of the following complications:

Chemosis. The earliest manifestation is abnormal glistening of the conjunctiva which can be thrown into folds when pressure is applied to an eyelid while the patient is asked to look to one side. Later it is only too obvious (*Fig.* 139).

Impairment of Corneal Sensitivity is a danger signal—it is a herald of corneal ulceration and all its possible inflammatory disasters.

PAUL JULIUS MOEBIUS, 1853–1907, *Neurologist, Leipzig.*
HAROLD GIFFORD, 1858–1929, *Ophthalmologist and Otologist, Nebraska University, Omaha, Nebraska.*

Exophthalmic Ophthalmoplegia. Paralysis, first of the muscles that elevate, and next of the muscles that abduct the globe, ensues. Usually the paralysis is asymmetrical.

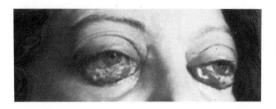

Fig. 139. Progressive exophthalmos with pronounced chemosis.

ENOPHTHALMOS

This is the opposite of exophthalmos, and it is encountered very infrequently. It is seen occasionally in cases of depressed fracture of the zygomatic bone or of the maxilla (p. 68).

PROPTOSIS: ORBITAL SPACE-OCCUPYING LESIONS

Proptosis is the first sign and, depending on the situation of the swelling, the eye may also be displaced, usually downwards, or laterally, or downwards and laterally. Many space-occupying lesions of the orbit, diagnosed clinically as a neoplasm, later prove to be one of the ill-understood granulomata.

Primary Orbital Tumours. By careful palpation of the bony margins of the orbit (*see Fig.* 121) try to differentiate a swelling arising from the bone from that in the soft tissues of the orbit or in the globe itself.

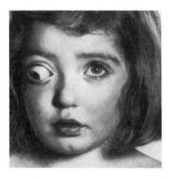

Fig. 140. Glioma of the optic nerve.

Glioma of the Optic Nerve occurs as a rule in children between 4 and 15 years of age. There is increasing proptosis (*Fig.* 140), moderate restriction of the movements of the eye and progressive visual disturbance. Unexplained scattered patches of pigmentation of the skin, especially of the trunk, are frequently present. This neoplasm can also arise in the optic chiasma, in which case the signs are identical, but, tragically, bilateral.

Innocent Neoplasms of the orbit—all of which give rise to proptosis—are a varied group, examples of which are an ivory osteoma (which usually arises from the roof of the orbit or the lacrimal bone), a dermoid cyst, and a cavernous haemangioma (*see Fig.* 46, p. 25).

The Primary Malignant Tumours of the Orbit are divided into extra-ocular and intra-ocular. Of the former, various forms of sarcoma are the most common.

The intra-ocular tumours, strictly, are outside our field, but it might be mentioned that the commonest, malignant melanoma (adults) and retinoblastoma (children) do not expand the globe until very advanced.

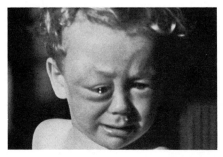

Fig. 141. Proptosis due to an orbital metastasis from a neuroblastoma of the adrenal medulla.

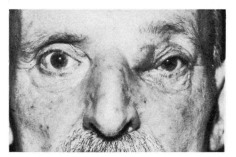

Fig. 142. Secondary deposit in the orbit from a bronchial carcinoma.

Secondary Malignant Tumours of the Orbit. Unfortunately the majority of tumours of the orbit met with in general surgical practice are metastatic. In a child a neuroblastoma of the adrenal medulla (*Fig.* 141) gives rise to an orbital metastasis relatively frequently, and in all cases of proptosis in a child, one of the first duties is to examine the abdomen. In the adult the discovery of an orbital metastasis (*Fig.* 142) should lead to an examination of the common primary sites mentioned on p. 426.

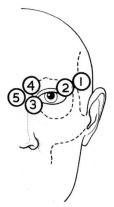

Fig. 143. The differential diagnosis of swellings situated around the rim of the orbit. 1, External angular dermoid; 2, swelling of lacrimal gland; 3, mucocele of lacrimal sac; 4, mucocele of frontal sinus; 5, internal angular dermoid.

Neoplasms of the Accessory Nasal Sinuses (*see* p. 137) tend to displace the eye as well as cause proptosis in their later stages.

Neoplasms of the Nasopharynx (*see* p. 132) rarely present with proptosis, as this implies a very advanced stage.

CYSTIC SWELLINGS AROUND THE ORBIT

A number of localized swellings situated around the upper half of the rim of the orbit (*Fig.* 143) are to a great extent distinguished from one another by differences—in some instances very slight—in anatomical position.

External Angular Dermoid. So constant is the position that it constitutes a clinical entity that can be diagnosed on sight, although it is necessary to confirm that the swelling is cystic. This sequestration dermoid, as its name implies, is situated over the external angular process of the frontal bone, which often is deeply hollowed to accommodate it. As a rule, the outer extremity of the

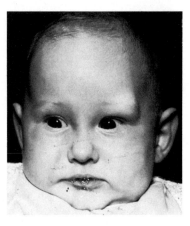

Fig. 144. External angular dermoid. The position is so constant that it allows of a 'spot' diagnosis.

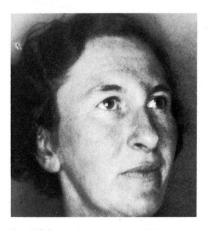

Fig. 145. Internal angular dermoid situated on the root of the nose.

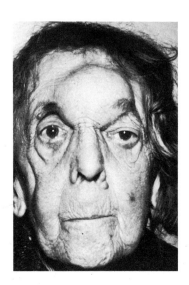

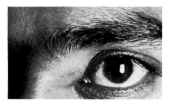

Fig. 147. Mucocele of lacrimal sac.

Fig. 146. Mucocele of the frontal sinus. The patient complained of double vision.

eyebrow extends over some part of the swelling (*Fig.* 144). The latter typical feature serves to distinguish it from a swelling of the lacrimal gland.

Internal Angular Dermoid is much less common than the foregoing. As the cyst enlarges it usually comes to lie upon the root of the nose in a more or less central position (*Fig.* 145).

Mucocele of the Frontal Sinus is a result of blockage of the frontonasal duct. The mucocele causes a swelling similar in location, but on the medial aspect of the orbit (*Fig.* 146), to that caused on the lateral aspect by the enlargement of the lacrimal gland. As it enlarges, the swelling displaces the globe.

Mucocele of the Lacrimal Sac (*Fig.* 147) is the result of similar blockage of the nasolacrimal duct.

Unilateral Pulsating Proptosis is a rare condition that always arouses much clinical interest. When an eyeball pulsates synchronously with the pulse, the following possibilities exist:

1. *Arteriovenous fistula* between the internal carotid artery and the cavernous sinus usually due to atherosclerosis but occasionally following a fractured base of skull. The pulsation ceases on occlusion of the carotid artery in the neck with digital pressure.

2. *Aneurysm of the ophthalmic artery.*

3. *Cirsoid aneurysm of the orbit.* Dilated vessels are seen coursing over the orbital margins.

4. *Rapidly growing highly vascular orbital neoplasm.*

In the first three conditions the patient notices a buzzing noise in the head and diminution of acuity of vision in the affected eye.

Chapter 8

THE EAR

The Pinna. Those who indulge in detective literature are wont to believe that by scrutinizing the cònformation of the ear hereditary tendencies, criminal and otherwise, are revealed to gifted observers. Admittedly, the shape of the pinna (*Fig.* 148) is interestingly varied, and close observation will enable the recognition of certain clinical entities to be described and illustrated.

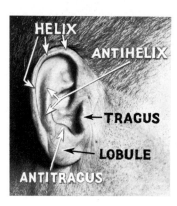

Fig. 148. The main constituent parts of the pinna.

An Accessory Auricle is a protrusion from the posterolateral aspect of the face of a core of cartilage and fibrous tissue covered by normal skin. Diminutive examples are cylindrical and erect; most are polypoid and pendulous. The usual situation is close to the tragus (*Fig.* 149). There is little doubt that the origin is by sequestration of an island of cartilage from the mandibular arch during closure of the first branchial cleft.

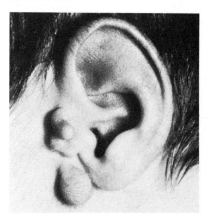

Fig. 149. Accessory auricle in a baby.

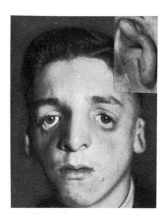

Fig. 150. Malformation of the pinnae in a patient with the Collins–Franceschetti syndrome.

80

Malformation of the Pinna. A great variety are encountered, ranging from overdevelopment to absence. Between these extremes the pinna may be misshapened in almost every conceivable way depending upon absence, under-development, overdevelopment, or aberration in fusion of one or more of the six tubercles from which it develops. Small, grossly misshapen ears are not infrequently associated with congenital atresia of the external auditory meatus, which results in deafness. Deformities of this kind are a regular feature of:

The Collins–Franceschetti Syndrome consists of congenital and familial deformities of the ears, not always bilateral, which tend not only to be placed lower than usual, but also the crumpled pinnae possess sound-catching convolutions facing in the opposite direction to normal, i.e. posteriorly (*Fig.* 150, inset). The palpebral fissures slope downwards and outwards. The lower eyelids are notched, and often without eyelashes. The upper lip is enlarged and the palate, if not cleft, is high. Micrognathia (*see* p. 89) is often present. The similarity between patients with this syndrome (*Fig.* 150) is striking, although their facial deformities vary in severity and in number. They are not mentally subnormal if the deafness is remedied early in life.

'Bat' Ears (*Fig.* 151) are, to put it mildly, self-evident.

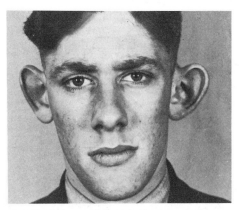

Fig. 151. 'Bat' ears. Fortunately, the deformity is reme-diable easily by a plastic operation.

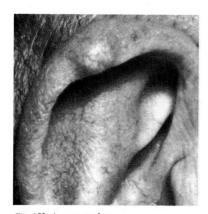

Fig. 152. A gouty tophus.

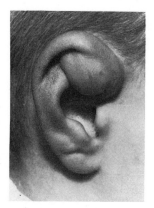

Fig. 153. Haematoma of the pinna with perichondritis.

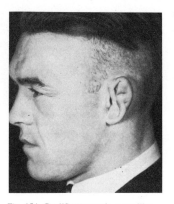

Fig. 154. Cauliflower ear in a pugilist.

EDWARD TREACHER COLLINS, 1862–1932, *Surgeon, Royal Ophthalmic Hospital, Moorfields, London.*
ADOLPHE FRANCESCHETTI, 1896–1968, *Professor of Ophthalmology, University of Geneva, Switzerland.*

Tophi are commonly present in long-standing cases of gout, and almost exclusively in males, their most typical situation being upon the helix or the antihelix (*Fig.* 152). They are also not uncommon in the olecranon bursa and in the tendon sheaths of the hands and feet. Occasionally one breaks down, ulcerates and discharges chalky monosodium biurate.

Haematoma Auris. Usually the result of injury (boxing, wrestling and rugby football account for the majority), but occasionally occurring spontaneously (in which event a disease associated with a bleeding tendency should be suspected), haematoma auris is due to an accumulation of blood between the elastic cartilage of the auricle and its perichondrium. When seen soon after the accident, it presents as a tender, discoloured, doughy swelling of typical appearance (*Fig.* 153); pain is not a feature unless suppuration supervenes, but there is a feeling of weight and discomfort. Fluctuation is seldom present as the extravasated blood has clotted.

A Cauliflower Ear (*Fig.* 154) is an unsightly deformity resulting from repeated haematoma auris with consequent necrosis of the cartilage.

Cyanosis and Frostbite. The pinna is a good site at which to look for cyanosis (*see* p. 47). Owing to its exposed position, frostbite, which is characterized by moderate swelling, redness and the formation of vesicles which are later transformed into dark scabs, is frequent. Even after the scabs have separated, the skin continues to exfoliate for a long time. Initially painless, by the time scabs form there is a feeling of heat, interrupted by shooting pain, and later by itching which causes the patient to scratch the part, thereby increasing the inflammation.

Rodent Ulcer, Epithelioma (*Fig.* 155), and *Molluscum Sebaceum* all occasionally involve the ear. These are described on pp. 28 and 36.

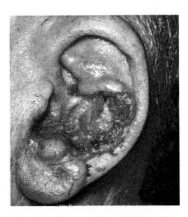

Fig. 155. Advanced carcinoma of the pinna.

Lymphatic Drainage of the Pinna and the Auditory Canal. Lymph-node enlargement due to inflammatory or neoplastic disease may affect one or more of three groups (*Fig.* 156). The preauricular node shares with the ear the drainage of the side of the face, including the eyelid (*see* p. 102), while the remaining two depots filter the whole of the scalp and posterior triangle, as well as the pinna and the auditory canal.

The External Auditory Meatus. Relatively few conditions can be diagnosed by observing the external auditory meatus, the use of a speculum being required to reveal most of the pathological states of the auditory canal and all of those involving the tympanic membrane. A consideration of the use of the auroscope is beyond the terms of reference of this work, but the student is exhorted to practise its use at every opportunity, for it is easily the most commonly used method of endoscopy in general practice.

Furuncle of the External Auditory Meatus causes intense pain, because the skin lining the canal is richly supplied with nerves and it is densely adherent to the perichondrium without the intervention of subcutaneous tissue. Not infrequently the external auditory meatus is occluded by swelling, and hearing is impaired thereby. If such be the case, the pinna should be drawn very gently upwards and backwards; this causes pain, but the meatus will be opened by the traction, and as a result hearing will be restored. When the furuncle is situated on the posterior wall of the auditory canal, post-auricular oedema is likely to result and the pinna may be displaced forwards, as in acute mastoiditis (*see* p. 85). Should the furuncle have burst recently, the pain will be lessened, and there will be a scanty, possibly bloodstained, discharge.

Otitis Externa is seen more frequently in hot damp conditions, hence its synonyms *Singapore* and *Hong Kong ear*. Itching is a feature, but pain is not marked. The skin of the external auditory canal and part of the pinna are macerated, boggy and oedematous. As with furuncle, hearing is affected if the meatus is blocked and Valsalva's experiment (p. 85) will indicate a patent Eustachian tube.

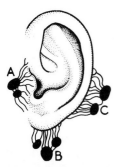

Fig. 156. The lymphatic drainage of the pinna and the external auditory meatus. A, Pre-auricular; B, Superficial cervical; C, Post-auricular.

Aural Polypus. Chronic suppuration of the middle ear sometimes is associated with an aural polypus. Usually it springs from the medial wall of the middle ear and its stalk passes through the perforation in the tympanic membrane. When long enough (a rarity) it is visible at the external auditory meatus but usually it is seen only with an auroscope.

Pre-auricular Abscess. A common cause of a pre-auricular abscess, whether it be acute or chronic (*Fig.* 157), is suppuration within, and breaking down of, a pre-auricular lymph node. Having decided that the swelling in question is an abscess, recall that the pre-auricular lymph node drains the side of the face, the pinna, and the anterior wall of the external auditory meatus. Scrutinize these regions with care, not forgetting the eyebrow and the eyelids of the corresponding side, and inquire whether the patient has had earache or an aural discharge recently. However, there is another cause of pre-auricular abscess, and particularly of a recurrent pre-auricular abscess, namely a *congenital pre-auricular sinus*—an abnormality due to imperfect fusion of the six tubercles from which the pinna is developed. Therefore, in every case where a primary focus of infection cannot be found, attention should be directed to the root of the helix where in cases of pre-auricular sinus a tiny pit can be seen (*Fig.* 158). Less often it is situated on the tragus (*Fig.* 158, inset).

Pre-auricular Ulcer is a late stage of an abscess due to a congenital pre-auricular sinus. It refuses to heal, for infection is maintained from the sinus.

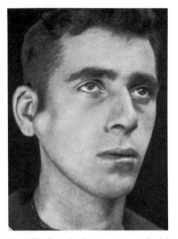

Fig. 157. Chronic abscess connected with an infected lymph node. The latter proved to be tuberculous.

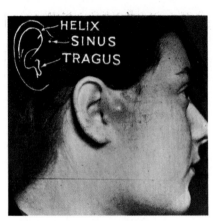

Fig. 158. Acute pre-auricular abscess due to infection of a congenital pre-auricular sinus.

THE MIDDLE EAR AND THE MASTOID ANTRUM

As noted above, examination with an auroscope is essential. It is useless to test hearing unless it is known that the auditory canal is free of wax.

Examination of Hearing (Eighth Cranial Nerve). In every case of suppurative otitis media the middle ear will contain pus and debris. Consequently there will be some degree of deafness due to impaired *conduction* of sound, i.e. *middle*-ear deafness. *A fortiori* the same is true of acute mastoiditis. In Ear, Nose and Throat clinics special apparatus should be available for measuring hearing. The practitioner proceeds as follows:

The distance at which a watch normally can be heard in the particular conditions existing in the examination room at the time must be ascertained. It is assumed the clinician's ability to hear the ticking provides a rough normal. Stand behind the patient and note the distance at which the ticking of the watch can be heard on each side. Each ear is tested separately, one being occluded while the other is being tested. If an aural discharge is present, normal hearing suggests that the discharge is due to otitis externa or to a furuncle, rather than to otitis media.

Rinne's Test. Place a vibrating tuning-fork (C512) on the mastoid process, with the limbs of the fork sloping backwards. The patient is instructed beforehand to signal when he no longer hears the sound. The still vibrating fork is then held close to the external auditory meatus. If the vibrations are still audible, then air conduction is better than bone conduction. This is the finding when hearing is normal or in perceptive deafness (*see below*), and in these circumstances Rinne's test is said to be *positive*.

If the vibrating tuning-fork applied to the mastoid process is heard *better* than when the tuning-fork, similarly vibrating, is placed close to the auditory meatus, then Rinne's test is said to be *negative*. This test is negative with *conductive deafness* when the transmission of sound through the ossicles in an

HEINRICH A. RINNE, 1819–1868, *Aural Surgeon, Göttingen.*

air-filled tympanic cavity is rendered less good by inflammatory exudate, or is definitely interrupted by erosion of one or more of the ossicles by osteomyelitis, or by ankylosis of one or more of their joints by suppurative arthritis, or by fixation of the stapes as in otosclerosis.

In *perceptive deafness* due to a lesion of the internal ear or of the auditory nerve or in the brain, air conduction is better than bone conduction but both are defective (worse than the examiner's normal hearing of the tuning-fork), or may be completely lost.

Weber's Test. Place a vibrating tuning-fork on the centre of the forehead. Normally the sound is appreciated by both ears equally, and if the patient occludes one auditory meatus with his finger the sound becomes louder on that side. Similarly, in unilateral middle-ear deafness the sound is lateralized to the affected side. If the sound is lateralized to the good ear, it suggests that the deafness in the affected ear is perceptive.

Giddiness, nystagmus and nausea are signs of involvement of the labyrinth or the vestibular nerve, special tests (beyond the scope of this work) being necessary to confirm the integrity of these structures.

Testing the Patency of the Eustachian Tubes; Valsalva's Experiment. Holding the nose so as to occlude the nostrils and blowing with the mouth shut causes air to pass up the Eustachian tubes and a crack is heard and/or a feeling of fullness is experienced in the ears.

Applying this 'experiment' as a test (applicable only when the patient is not in great pain or is not too young to understand what is required of him), ask the patient to pinch his nose, close his mouth and blow, and to let you know (by a signal with the free hand) in which ear he feels 'something give' first. If a Eustachian tube is blocked, a point in favour of otitis media as it forms part of the middle-ear cleft, the crackle on that side will be absent.

EXAMINATION OF A CASE OF SUSPECTED ACUTE MASTOIDITIS

Acute mastoiditis is a complication of otitis media. In a young child *acute* mastoiditis is the condition that must be suspected whereas in an adolescent or an adult *acute-on-chronic* mastoiditis is the usual contingency.

Acute Mastoiditis in a Young Child. The mastoid region is tender in every case of acute otitis media during the first two or three days of the attack before rupture of the tympanic membrane, but it is exceptional for acute otitis media that has been treated *adequately* to give rise to acute mastoiditis. Only when pyrexia and mastoid tenderness appear in a patient with otorrhoea of several weeks' duration, and the discharge is increasing in amount, is it justifiable to attribute these findings to acute mastoiditis (Bauer). Another important consideration is that furuncle of the auditory meatus (a condition giving rise to symptoms and signs that in some respects simulate mastoiditis) is uncommon below the age of 10 years. These facts having been assimilated, the examination should proceed as follows:

In the first place observe the patient from behind, and particularly note the angle of inclination the two pinnae make to the side of the head (*Fig.* 159). In untreated (by antibiotics) acute mastoiditis the pinna may be pushed forwards— as it may be with a suppurating posterior auricular lymph node. To exclude the

ERNST H. WEBER, 1795–1878, *Professor of Anatomy and Physiology, Leipzig.*
BARTOLOMMEO EUSTACHIO, 1524–1574, *Professor of Anatomy, Rome.*
ANTONIO M. VALSALVA, 1666–1723, *Professor of Anatomy, Bologna.*
FRANCIS BAUER, *Contemporary Otorhinolaryngologist, Walton Hospital, Liverpool.*

latter (*a*) examine the scalp for an inflammatory lesion, not omitting a search for the presence of pediculi capitis (nits), and (*b*) palpate the posterior triangle of the neck for enlarged lymph nodes (*see* p. 53).

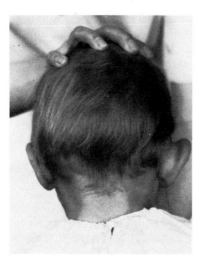

Fig. 159. Examination from the back in mastoiditis. The ear on the affected side stands out in this late untreated case.

Secondly (if the patient is old enough), test his or her hearing. In the case of a suppurating posterior auricular lymph node hearing will be unimpaired. In acute mastoiditis, unquestionable *conductive* deafness will be present on the affected side.

Thirdly: If necessary armed with a swabstick, look for a discharge. If this contains obvious mucus, the source must be the middle ear because the auditory canal does not possess mucus-secreting glands. When the canal has been cleansed a perforation of the drum must be sought with the auroscope.

Fourthly, test for local tenderness. It is valueless to seek local tenderness over the mastoid process because, as has been explained, tenderness is present in this situation both in otitis media and post-auricular adenitis. On the other hand, tenderness (after the first few days) elicited when pressure is applied over the suprameatal triangle of Macewen, which overlies the mastoid antrum, is of crucial importance, and, unless the sign is positive, a diagnosis of acute mastoiditis is not substantiated. Except in the very young, this triangular depression can be felt through the skin (*a*) by drawing the pinna forwards (*Fig.* 160), which gives access to all but the anterior limit of the triangle, and (*b*) by direct finger-pressure (*Fig.* 161), which enables the anterior limit to be felt more readily than the posterior edge of the triangle. If the first, and then the second, method is employed no stone will be left unturned to ensure that the area of tenderness is localized accurately. When acute mastoiditis develops in a fully cellular mastoid process, pus may burrow to the surface and form a subperiosteal abscess, which causes forward displacement of the pinna, described already. Rarely, the pus tracks into the digastric fossa, forming an abscess over and beneath the tip of the mastoid process (Bezold's mastoiditis), in which case fluctuation may be detected at this point.

Acute-on-Chronic Mastoiditis. Chronic mastoiditis is painless and causes a long-continued discharge via a perforated drum and conduction deafness (almost always). Its diagnosis depends on clinical evaluation by an expert and on X-ray changes which need not concern us here. Should the free drainage of pus from the mastoid antrum and the middle ear become impeded by granulation tissue blocking the perforation in the tympanic membrane, or by the enlargement of a cholesteatoma* occluding the aditus,† retention of pus under pressure ensues,

---

* Cholesteatoma. A pearly or putty-like mass of epithelium desquamated from the infected attic or antrum+cholesterol crystal. Particularly the soft variety smells abominably.

† The narrow passage leading from the mastoid antrum to the tympanic cavity.

SIR WILLIAM MACEWEN, 1848–1924, *Professor of Surgery, University of Glasgow.*
FRIEDRICH BEZOLD, 1842–1908, *Professor of Otology, Munich.*

and acute-on-chronic mastoiditis is at hand, the first and foremost symptom of which is severe pain in the ear. The first sign is *lessening* or *cessation* of the aural discharge that has been present for a very long time—in all probability for years.

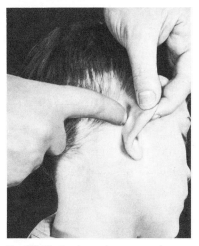

Fig. 160. Testing for tenderness over the mastoid antrum. Method *a*.

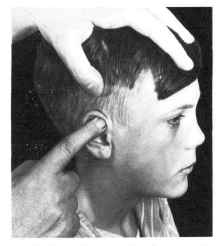

Fig. 161. Testing for a point of tenderness over the mastoid antrum. Method *b*.

The condition for which acute-on-chronic mastoiditis is most likely to be mistaken is a furuncle situated on the posterior wall of the auditory canal. A furuncle in this situation will cause very severe pain similar to that of mastoiditis, as well as narrowing of the external auditory meatus, and possibly some forward displacement of the pinna due to posterior extension of inflammatory oedema. In usual circumstances a patient with a furuncle of the auditory canal will not give a history of long-standing aural discharge; indeed, as a rule, while the pain is acute there is no discharge at all (*see* p. 83).

It is, however, possible for a furuncle of the auditory canal to occur in a patient with chronic mastoiditis, in which event, difficulties in differential diagnosis deepen. Nevertheless, with this coincidence it is improbable that the narrowing of the external auditory meatus will prove sufficient to cause the aural discharge from which the patient has suffered for years to lessen in amount or alter in consistency.

Traction on the Pinna. The crux in the differential diagnosis between these two conditions rests in gentle upward and backward retraction of the pinna. In furuncle, this sign induces such intense pain that the examiner instinctively ceases to complete the retraction: in acute-on-chronic mastoiditis little or no pain is evoked.

Complications. The usual channel for its escape being blocked, pus locked within the mastoid antrum, by a process of pressure necrosis, seeks, and not infrequently gains, an exit in one of several ways:

a. Through the tegmen (roof) = extradural abscess; subdural abscess; meningitis.

b. Through the posterior wall = thrombophlebitis of the lateral sinus.

c. Through the medial wall = labyrinthitis (severe giddiness).

Thrombophlebitis of the Sigmoid (Lateral) Sinus. The sinus lying behind and below the mastoid antrum can be implicated by the spread of thrombophlebitis from small veins of the tympanic cavity, or by juxtaposition of an extradural abscess. The classic signs in the pre-antibiotic era were a hectic temperature rising to 39 or 40 °C, followed by rigors and profuse sweating, with comparative well-being in the intervals. This no longer appertains today. As a result of antibiotic therapy there is only a moderate rise in temperature. However, sometimes tenderness along the course of the internal jugular vein can be elicited, and occasionally induration can be felt. Torticollis (*see* p. 138) is also a significant sign.

Facial Nerve Paralysis (*see* p. 99), occurring in association with otitis media either acute or chronic and whether complicated by mastoiditis or not, is a sign that treatment is inadequate and should be reviewed. It is due to the proximity of the nerve, in its bony canal, to the middle ear.

Zygomatic Mastoiditis occurs when air cells exist in the zygomatic process of the temporal bone and become infected. An inflammatory swelling in front of and above the ear may simulate parotitis, but the other signs of acute-on-chronic mastoiditis are present.

Gradenigo's Syndrome consists of signs of acute-on-chronic mastoiditis associated with homolateral paralysis of the sixth cranial nerve (*see* p. 59) and deep-seated retro-orbital pain. The abducent nerve leaves the posterior cranial fossa in a narrow sheath of dura mater and becomes compressed when air cells in the tip of the petrous apex become inflamed.

Middle Ear Carcinoma occurs as a complication of long-standing chronic mastoiditis and is rare. If a patient with an aural discharge of many years' duration continues to complain of pain when there is no evidence of acute-on-chronic mastoiditis the condition should be suspected.

Giuseppe Gradenigo, 1859–1926, *Professor of Otorhinolaryngology, Naples.*

Chapter 9

THE FACE AND JAWS

SOME CHARACTERISTIC FACIES *

The study of characteristic facies is always of profound interest and importance. Here will be described some facies of surgical interest not illustrated in other sections of the book.

The Hippocratic Facies. The eyes are sunken, but bright. The nose is pinched. There are crusts on the lips. The tongue is dry and shrivelled. The forehead is cold and clammy. It is true that the sharp nose, hollow eyes and collapsed temples are due mainly to the result of dehydration rather than of peritonitis as such, but this facial picture (*Fig.* 162), combined with a thready pulse and a grossly distended abdomen, is pathognomonic of advanced diffuse peritonitis.

Micrognathia (Pierre Robin Syndrome). The neonate has a characteristic profile (*Fig.* 163) due to a foreshortened horizontal ramus of the mandible. This renders the tongue unduly mobile and results in tongue swallowing with frequent attacks of dyspnoea and cyanosis especially if a cleft palate is also present, as is usual. Another neonatal rarity which can only be diagnosed from previous knowledge of the typical syndrome is *nasal choanal atresia*. The infant becomes cyanosed whenever it stops crying at which time it instinctively tries to breathe through its (blocked) nose. An attempt to pass a fine rubber catheter down both nostrils proves that they are blocked posteriorly at the choanae. Choking and cyanosis on feeding is also seen as the baby cannot mouth-breathe when feeding.

The Facies of Congenital Syphilis. Both congenital and acquired syphilis can produce a saddle-shaped nose, but one must not jump to conclusions. Leprosy is a common cause in the tropics. Nevertheless, a sunken bridge of the nose (*Fig.* 164) does call for more than a casual glance for other stigmata. Look for bossing of the frontal bones, interstitial keratitis (or the scars thereof), Hutchinson's teeth (*see* p. 114), or deafness. Hutchinson's triad of congenital syphilis consists of the last three.

The Facies of Cretinism in infancy is easily overlooked. The face is pale, puffy and somewhat wrinkled. The skin is dry and cold. A protruding tongue (*Fig.* 165) is especially characteristic. The anterior fontanelle remains open. In endemic cretinism the thyroid gland is palpable, if not visibly enlarged; in the sporadic variety, usually but not invariably, the atrophic thyroid is impalpable.

The Facies of Hepatic Cirrhosis (*Fig.* 166). When the disease is moderately advanced the eyes are sunken, and a variable degree of icterus is present in the watery conjunctivae. The presence of spider naevi (*see* p. 236) contributes to the suspicion that the function of the liver is impaired by cirrhosis.

'Adenoid' Facies. The concept that enlarged adenoids are the cause of a high-vaulted palate, narrow dental arch and protruding incisor teeth (*Fig.* 167) has been abandoned. The triad of defects is familial. Enlarged adenoids, however, may be coincidently present so the patient merits a full examination of the nasopharynx (*see* p. 130).

---

* A collection of facial signs suggesting a 'spot' diagnosis.

HIPPOCRATES, *by common consent the Father of Medicine, was born on the Island of Cos in the Aegean Archipelago about 460* B.C. *He lived to be over 80 years of age in an era when the average expectation of life was approximately 32 years.*
PIERRE ROBIN, 1867–1950, *Stomatologist to the Hospitals of Paris.*

CHARACTERISTIC FACIES

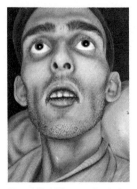

Fig. 162. Hippocratic facies. Advanced peritonitis.

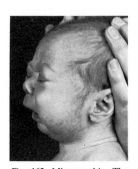

Fig. 163. Micrognathia. The profile should enable a prompt diagnosis, imperative if the infant's life is to be preserved.

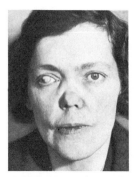

Fig. 164. Facies of congenital syphilis. Saddle-nose and scar of interstitial keratitis.

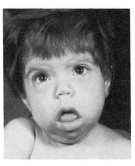

Fig. 165. Facies of a cretin. The large protruding tongue is characteristic.

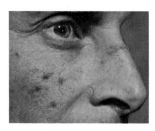

Fig. 166. Spider naevi in hepatic cirrhosis.

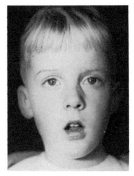

Fig. 167. So-called 'adenoid' facies.

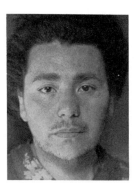

Fig. 168. Virile facies in a woman, aged 25, suffering from adrenocortical hyperplasia.

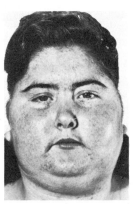

Fig. 169. Moon face of Cushing's syndrome in a female patient aged 19.

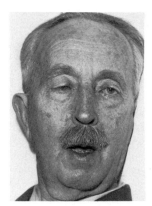

Fig. 170. Facies of myasthenia gravis. The ptosis and drooping jaw are intermittent.

The Virile Facies of a woman suffering from hyperplasia or tumour of the adrenal cortex is often so evident (*Fig.* 168) that further description is superfluous.

The Moon Face of Cushing's Syndrome (*see* p. 48). The face becomes rubicund, rounded like a full moon (*Fig.* 169) and often the lips are pursed.

Myasthenia Gravis, due to dysfunction of the thymus, and sometimes to a neoplasm thereof, is characterized by abnormally rapid exhaustion of muscles, particularly of the face. Whatever the muscular movement involved, after a rest there must be a return to power, at least in part, for the diagnosis to be made. Many patients have signs referable to the eyes (*Fig.* 170). Characteristic is intermittent ptosis, unilateral or bilateral. When this is combined with a drooping jaw, the appearance produced should bring myasthenia gravis to mind. Another earlier, more common, but less striking facies is the sneering smile consequent upon deficient action of the risorius and zygomatic muscles.

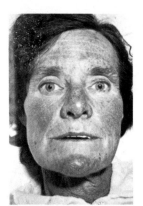

Fig. 171. Carcinoid facies.

Carcinoid Facies. An excess of serotonin secreted by the tumour gives rise to characteristic facial flushing (*Fig.* 171) only when massive liver metastases are present.

THE CHEEK

Method of examining a Localized Swelling in the Cheek

1. Observe the outside of the cheek and decide whether the swelling in question is situated in the skin.

2. Observe the buccal aspect and satisfy yourself that the swelling originates in the buccal mucosa.

3. Palpate between the finger in the mouth and thumb outside.

In the case of a swelling not in the skin and not in the mucosa, remember the sucking pad of the infant which sometimes persists. There is also an inconstant lymph node along the course of the facial artery.

Further details of examining the mucous surface of the cheek are given on p. 126, those for examining Stensen's duct on pp. 101, 103.

Accidental Vaccinia (*Fig.* 172). One of the ways in which the contagion occurs is as follows. The recently vaccinated child with a cutaneous lesion on its arm in full activity, while being carried by its

HARVEY CUSHING, 1869–1939, *Professor of Surgery, Harvard University, U.S.A.*

mother, impinges the vaccinated area against her cheek (*Fig.* 172, inset). When the scab darkens, it may be mistaken for anthrax (*see Fig.* 65, p. 31).

Idiopathic Hypertrophy of the Masseter Muscle can occur on one or both sides. Ask the patient to close his mouth and clench his teeth—the whole of the swelling hardens beneath the fingers. Request him to stop clenching—the whole of the swelling softens. Only a muscle could fulfil these responses in their entirety.

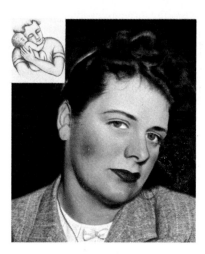

Fig. 172. Accidental vaccinia. Inset, the commonest way in which inoculation takes place.

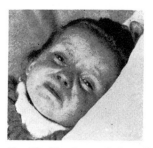

Fig. 173. The risus sardonicus of tetanus.

THE TEMPOROMANDIBULAR JOINT

Routine Examination of the Joint. The normal jaw can be opened to the extent that there is a distance of 2–5 cm between the incisor teeth, depending on age and sex. Place the fingers over the joint while the patient opens and closes his mouth; note if there is any crepitus or clicking. Crepitus signifies osteoarthrosis, and clicking suggests a loose meniscus. Auscultation over the joint may reveal significant crepitus and comparison with the opposite side may yield more valuable information than the fingers can provide. Observe whether dental malocclusion is present. Normally the upper incisor teeth lie in front of the lower when the jaw is closed. If the upper jaw is displaced backwards this relationship is lost.

Trismus. * The patient cannot open his mouth because of muscular spasm. Severe trismus may complicate any inflammatory process in the neighbourhood of the mandibular joint. Chief among these is an erupting third mandibular molar (wisdom) tooth or a dental abscess. Insert a spatula gently along the buccal aspect of the cheek, and inspect the alveolus with an electric torch.

Trismus is also seen in tetanus. The contraction of the musculature about the jaw gives the patient a painful smiling appearance—the *risus sardonicus* (*Fig.* 173)—helpful in the diagnosis of early cases.

---

* *Trismus.* Greek, τρισμός = clenching.

Displaced Articular Cartilage of the temporomandibular joint presents in one of two ways:

Clicking Jaw. On the first occasion the patient, usually a female, hears something 'snap in the ear'; subsequently, almost every time she opens her mouth she hears a click. Not unnaturally, this gets on her nerves and, on account of the phenomenon, some patients become introspective and even hypochondriacal. Occasionally the click is audible by others, for instance at the dining table.

Locking. Occasional attacks of locking occur without, or more usually with, clicking. There is sudden pain in the joint, which soon radiates to the pinna and to the skin above it, and here the pain remains located until the cartilage is reduced, or reduces itself. The patient usually is unable to close the mouth completely. The attacks are often accompanied by excessive salivation.

Dislocation of the temporomandibular joint can be either bilateral or unilateral; the former is more common, and in some cases it becomes habitual. Those cases due to dental extraction are, for the most part, unilateral.

Normally, every time the mouth is opened over a centimetre the head of the mandible leaves its socket. When the restraining ligaments are loose or broken, true dislocation occurs by the head of the mandible passing over the articular eminence.

Bilateral Dislocation. When the dislocation is bilateral the prognathous* deformity is so evident as to attract attention immediately. The mouth is open and fixed, with the lower teeth protruding. Upon examination of the mandibular joints, a distinct hollow will be seen and felt in front of the tragus.

Unilateral Dislocation. The partially open jaw is deviated to the opposite side and the small hollow noted above may be felt behind the dislocated condyle.

Ankylosis of the Mandibular Joint. Opening the mouth is restricted to a lesser or greater degree. In old-standing cases, incurred during infancy, the lower jaw atrophies (*Fig.* 174). The receding chin gives a characteristic 'shrewmouse' profile.

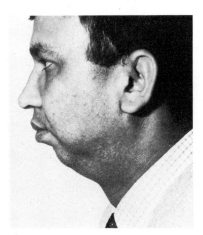

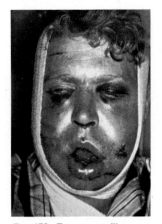

Fig. 174. The 'shrewmouse' profile.

Fig. 175. Extreme swelling soon after a severe fracture of the upper jaw. The bandage supports a fractured lower jaw.

---

* *Prognathous.* Greek, πρό in front of, + γνάθος jaw = having a projecting jaw.

Unilateral ankylosis arising later in life is not recognized so easily, and when the ankylosis is fibrous, it cannot be demonstrated by radiography. In cases of some standing, when the face at rest is viewed from in front, the facial furrows are more evident on the healthy side. The condition should not be confused with facial paralysis: Attempts to open the mouth are associated with a slight but definite deviation of the lower incisor teeth towards the ankylosed joint.

THE MAXILLA

Fractures of the Maxilla. Fracture of the zygoma is dealt with on p. 68. Other fractures of the upper facial skeleton all involve the maxilla and, if suspected, examination of the surfaces of the maxilla mentioned below will prove rewarding. Remember, however, that after an hour or two oedema will mask deformity (*Fig.* 175) except in those severe fractures in which one or both maxillae have been markedly displaced backwards in relation to the rest of the facial skeleton ('dish-face'). Always look for a break in the continuity of the upper alveolar margin and, if the patient is not edentulous, for malocclusion of the teeth.

Examination of the Maxilla. The anterolateral surface is the one most obviously available for examination, but we must go further and remember that the maxilla has five surfaces.

1. *The posterior surface* can be dismissed at once, forming as it does the anterior boundary of that deep recess, the pterygopalatine fossa, no part of the body being more completely beyond the reach of clinical methods.

2. *The superior surface* helps to form the floor of the orbit; therefore the levels of the inferior orbital margins are compared carefully. Extreme upward bulging of the floor of the orbit causes proptosis (*Fig.* 176), which in turn results in diplopia. A glance at each profile of the patient is taken in order that the relative protuberance of the eyeballs can be compared.

3. *The antero-external surface* is palpated. While this is in progress, note if there is any sign of overflow of tears (epiphora) on the affected side, and

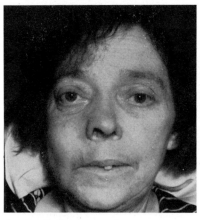

Fig. 176. Malignant upper jaw. In addition to expanding the antero-external surface of the maxilla slightly, the growth has displaced the orbital contents. Depression of the angle of the mouth on the affected side is also a typical sign (Wilson).

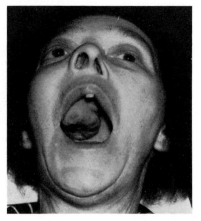

Fig. 177. Examining the upper jaw. The inferior surface of the maxilla is the hard palate. In this case of carcinoma of the maxillary sinus the corresponding side of the hard palate was involved, and the nostril was blocked.

CHARLES P. WILSON, 1900–1970, *Otorhinolaryngologist, Middlesex Hospital, London.*

question the patient about this. The nasolacrimal duct may become involved in malignant disease of the maxilla.

4. Much of the upper jaw is available for examination through the mouth.

a. Examine the teeth and compare the dental formulae; missing teeth must be accounted for—careful attention to do this may elucidate the diagnosis, e.g. in odontomata.

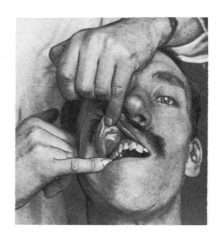

Fig. 178. Examining the buccal aspect of the upper jaw. Case of cyst of the maxilla, presumably of dental origin.

b. *The inferior surface* of the maxilla forms the major part of the hard palate. In certain cases of malignant upper jaw, the swelling can be seen (*Fig.* 177).

c. A large part of the *anterior surface* is beneath the cheek, and without the intervention of the cheek (*Fig.* 178) much more can be made out than by external palpation. Pass the index finger between the cheek and the jaw. With the thumb outside, and the finger still inside, the zygomatic process should be palpated.

5. *The medial surface* forms the lateral wall of the nostril, and by occluding the nares one at a time and asking the patient to blow through the nose, some rough idea of this surface may be obtained. If the nostril on the affected side is *not* blocked, we know at least that the medial wall of the maxilla is not bulging to any great extent. Sometimes bulging is apparent on inspection (*see Fig.* 177). Should there be unilateral nasal obstruction, a nasal speculum must be used to investigate the cause.

Finally, examine the cervical lymph nodes, and also test the integrity of the second division of the fifth cranial nerve (p. 97).

Ordinary clinical examination of the upper jaw can be supplemented by transillumination of the maxillary sinus (*see* p. 137).

Acute Osteomyelitis of the Maxilla in Infants. The baby is severely ill with high pyrexia. The first sign is the appearance of redness and swelling below the inner canthus. At this time the differential diagnosis from dacryocystitis and from orbital cellulitis is difficult. The upper and lower eyelids soon become puffy (*Fig.* 179) and there is a discharge of pus from the nostril on the affected side. Unless the infection can be arrested, it progresses subperiosteally and in a matter of about 48 hours the inflammation reaches the alveolar margin where swelling can be seen.

Burkitt's Tumour (Burkitt's Lymphoma). In many parts of tropical Africa this is easily the commonest neoplasm between 4 and 8 years of age and exceeds all others combined in this group. The

DENIS P. BURKITT, *Contemporary Surgeon, Member of External Scientific Staff, Medical Research Council, London.*

sex incidence is roughly equal and it is found in a wide belt on either side of the Equator and in New Guinea.———————————————————————————→

In 80 per cent of cases a tumour of the jaw is the first manifestation, the maxilla being involved somewhat more often than the mandible. The earliest sign is loosening of the teeth in relation to the tumour (usually the molars and premolars). Later the gums expand as the tumour growth leads to gross disfigurement (*Fig.* 180). Sometimes there are multiple swellings involving one or more maxillae and one or more mandibles.

Other manifestations, which give rise to typical physical signs are exophthalmos due to orbital tumours, ovarian tumours, retroperitoneal lymph-node masses, other bone swellings and salivary-gland tumours. As cure by chemotherapy is possible early diagnosis is important.

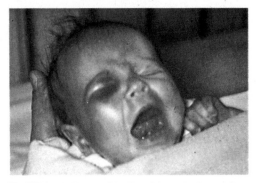

Fig. 179. Acute osteomyelitis of the right maxilla in a newborn baby.

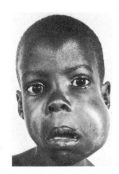

Fig. 180. An example of Burkitt's tumour.

THE MANDIBLE

Fracture of the Mandible. That the patient has fractured his jaw usually is evident. He endeavours to support the fragments with his hands. Speech is impossible, and frequently the saliva is bloodstained, because the fracture is nearly always *compound* into the mouth. Most fractures of the mandible occur in its horizontal portion. By inspection utilizing a torch within the mouth some deformity in the contour of the alveolus may be seen—frequently a tooth appears out of alignment. The gum is sometimes found to be lacerated in this situation. Should the fracture be bilateral, take immediate precautions to prevent the tongue falling back and causing asphyxia.

Fracture of the Condyle. Pain and swelling over the temporomandibular joint are the only clinical manifestations of this condition if there is little displacement of the fracture. With marked displacement the signs are those of dislocated jaw (*see* p. 93).

Examination of the Mandible for Conditions other than Suspected Fracture. The body, the angle and the inferior part of the ramus are accessible to the palpating fingers both from without and from within the mouth, where the examination is blended intimately with that of the teeth of the lower jaw. On the other hand, the upper portion of the ramus and its condyloid and coronoid processes lie deeply. With one finger inside the mouth and the fingers of the free hand applied externally (*Fig.* 181) this comparatively inaccessible portion becomes palpable.

Dental Abscess of the Mandible. See p. 117.

Median Mental Sinus allows of 'spot' diagnosis (*see* p. 29). On the point of the chin, near the mid-line, there is a painless discharging sinus (*Fig*. 182, *a*). A radiograph of the mandible reveals nothing abnormal, but a dental film of the lower incisor teeth, which on clinical examination often appear to be sound, shows an area of rarefaction around the root (*Fig*. 182, *b*); pus from a root

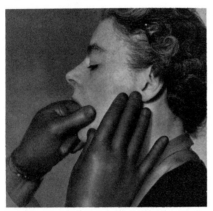

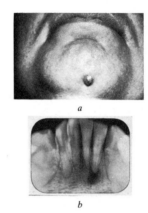

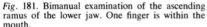

Fig. 181. Bimanual examination of the ascending ramus of the lower jaw. One finger is within the mouth.

Fig. 182. Median mental sinus (*see* text).

abscess has tracked between the two halves of the lower jaw. When the clinician is unfamiliar with this condition, almost invariably an infected sebaceous cyst is diagnosed.

Neoplasms of the Mandible. Primary neoplasms attack the mandible less frequently than the maxilla. However, carcinoma secondarily invading the mandible from the floor of the mouth is not uncommon. The principal primary neoplasm of the mandible is an *adamantinoma*, which is a slow-growing, locally malignant tumour affecting young adults more frequently in the mandible than in the maxilla. It arises from the enamel organ, and gradually and painlessly expands the bone. It feels hard at first but in advanced cases egg-shell crackling (areas of softness) can be elicited. Unaccountably it is relatively common in tropical Africa.

EXAMINATION OF THE FIFTH CRANIAL NERVE

Motor. Palpate the temporal and masseter muscles. Ask the patient to clench his teeth and note whether these muscles contract. Next direct him to open his mouth as widely as possible. If there is weakness of the pterygoid muscles of one side, the jaw will deviate to the paralysed side.

Sensory. *Trigeminal Neuralgia* begins almost invariably in either the second or third division (*Fig*. 183) of the fifth nerve. Ask the patient (usually over 60 years old) where the pain began. Sufferers can often map out accurately the distribution. 'Eating will bring it on in some persons; talking, or the least motion of the face, in others. The gentlest touch of the hand or the handkerchief will

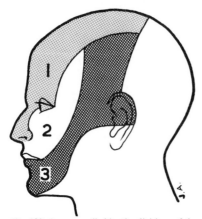
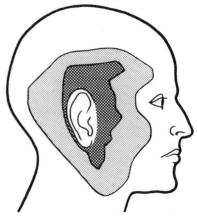

Fig. 183. Areas supplied by the divisions of the fifth cranial nerve.

Fig. 184. Frey's syndrome. Dark area, region of sweating; light area, region of hyperaemia.

bring on the pain, while strong pressure has no effect' (Fothergill). It is stabbing in nature, brief (one second) and with a dull background ache. In the earlier stages the patient believes she has toothache, and often one tooth after another, sound or carious, is removed.

During an attack the affected area is hyperaesthetic, as can be shown by stroking it with cotton-wool.

Between the attacks. Careful examination reveals one or more *trigger zones of Patrick*. Somewhere in the nerve's distribution—on the skin of the face or the mucous membrane of the cheek or gum—a hyperaesthetic area can be demonstrated, and a light touch on this initiates an attack. Curiously, the trigger is often in an area supplied by one division of the nerve, and the pain commences in another.

The Gustatory Sweating Syndrome (syn. Frey's Syndrome). This is often a sequel to an incision for suppurative parotitis. In Eastern Europe it was encountered fairly frequently (typhoid fever and typhus having been a common cause of parotitis). It is now seen occasionally after parotidectomy. The following occur while eating, especially highly spiced or sour foods and, strangely, sometimes chocolate:

1. Attacks of pain in the area supplied by the auriculotemporal nerve.
2. Unilateral facial flushing.
3. Unilateral sweating. During an attack beads of sweat stand out and trickle down the patient's cheek (*Fig.* 184).
4. Hyperaesthesia over the cutaneous distribution of the auriculotemporal nerve.

Testing Taste. Loss of taste usually results from a complete lesion of the fifth cranial nerve, following a fracture of the middle cranial fossa, an operation for trigeminal neuralgia, or an alcohol injection of the Gasserian ganglion. Another cause is a cerebral tumour in the pathway of the gustatory fibres.

Special, but simple, requirements are essential and—in order to make an unhurried examination as well as to be in possession of the necessary armamentaria—it is advisable to pre-arrange a consultation for this examination only. The patient is not allowed to speak during the examination, but is instructed to point to the appropriate card (*Fig.* 185, *right*).

The freshly washed camel-hair brush is also washed thoroughly after each of the four substances has been painted on the desired area (*Fig.* 185). Ten seconds must elapse for the patient to perceive, then he or she indicates. After each application of the four substances, first to the believed affected, and secondly to the non-affected side, the patient rinses her mouth with warm water.

JOHN FOTHERGILL, 1712–1789, *a highly successful London general practitioner*.
HUGH T. PATRICK, 1860–1939, *Neurologist, Wesley Memorial Hospital, Chicago*.
LUCJA FREY, 1889–1944, *Physician, Neurological Clinic, Warsaw. She was killed during the German occupation of Poland*.
JOHANN L. GASSER, 1723–1765, *Professor of Anatomy, Vienna*.

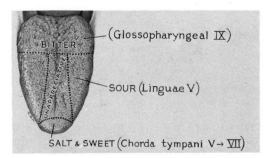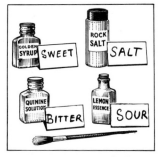

Fig. 185. Normal areas of appreciation of taste, and their nerve supplies. *Right*, the equipment for the test.

EXAMINATION OF THE SEVENTH CRANIAL NERVE

Ask the patient to shut the eyes tightly, and at the same time to show the front teeth. In case of a complete lesion of the seventh nerve the immobility of one-half of the face becomes obvious. The patient cannot shut the eye on the affected side, and in the attempt to do so the eyeballs are rolled upwards, giving rise to the well-known unsightly 'blind man' appearance (*Fig.* 186).

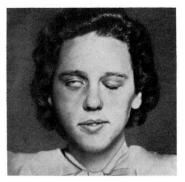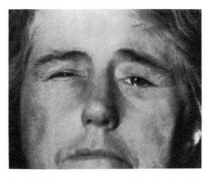

Fig. 186. Complete right-sided facial palsy following a fracture of the base of the skull. Showing the typical response to the request, 'Shut your eyes'.

Fig. 187. Showing the 'tear which does not fall' and partial paralysis of the orbicularis oculi. Case of complete removal of the parotid gland for malignant disease.

When a patient neither bears the scar of a mastoid operation nor that of an operation for removal of a parotid tumour, nor gives a history of a severe head injury, Bell's palsy is the probable diagnosis.

In cases of incomplete palsy, a more painstaking examination is required. It is advisable to divide the examination into two parts:

1. *The Examination of the Upper Face.* On the affected side the eye usually contains 'the tear which does not fall' (*Fig.* 187). Ask the patient: (*a*) To raise his eyebrows. In facial paralysis the forehead will remain smooth owing to paralysis of the occipitofrontalis. (*b*) To frown. There will be no furrowing owing to the loss of power in the corrugator supercilii. (*c*) To shut his eyes. The strength of the orbicularis oculi is tested by attempting to open the eyes against the patient's efforts to keep them shut (*Fig.* 188).

SIR CHARLES BELL, 1774–1842, *Surgeon, Middlesex Hospital, London, later Professor of Surgery, Edinburgh.*

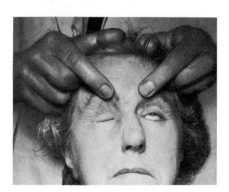

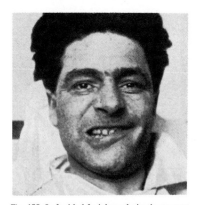

Fig. 188. Testing the strength of the orbicularis oculi. The left eye cannot be kept shut. (Same patient as Fig. 187.)

Fig. 189. Left-sided facial paralysis; the answer to the request, 'Show your teeth'.

2. *The Examination of the Lower Face*. The muscles of the lower part of the face are now tested. Ask the patient: (*a*) To puff out his cheeks. (*b*) To whistle. (*c*) To show the teeth (*Fig*. 189).

The upper facial muscles are represented on both sides of the cortex; the lower facial muscles have only a unilateral representation. Therefore it follows that in a unilateral supranuclear lesion, e.g. a 'stroke', the upper facial muscles tend to escape, i.e. the eye can be closed on that side.

Unilateral Paralysis of the Lower Lip. Paralysis of the quadratus labii inferioris results from severing the mandibular branch of the facial nerve during such operations as block dissection of the neck, excision of the submandibular salivary gland, or even during drainage of an abscess of the neck. When the patient is asked to show the teeth, the paralysis is obvious as in *Fig*. 189.

EXAMINATION OF THE NINTH CRANIAL NERVE

The sign of a lesion of the ninth nerve is loss of taste in the posterior third of the tongue (*Fig*. 185).

Trigeminal neuralgia and *glossopharyngeal neuralgia*, which is one hundred times less frequent, are alike, except for the localization of the paroxysms of agonizing pain and the areas of the trigger zones. In the latter the pain is brought on more frequently by swallowing than by any other stimulus. The trigger zones include the pharyngeal wall, the base of the tongue and especially the tonsillar region. To the patient the pain may seem to be in the ear. There is no difficulty in differentiating trigeminal neuralgia, affecting the second division of the fifth nerve, from glossopharyngeal neuralgia, but when the third division of the fifth nerve is affected, considerable care must be exercised in elucidating the exact area maximally involved.

Chapter 10

THE SALIVARY GLANDS

THE PAROTID GLAND

When a patient presents with a swelling the site of which conforms with the surface marking of the parotid gland (*Fig.* 190), proceed as follows:

Inspection. Characteristic of a general enlargement is a swelling in front of the tragus extending downwards and slightly backwards, obliterating the normal depression below and in front of the lobule of the ear (4 in *Fig.* 190).

Palpation. The following methodical technique can be recommended:

1. Lay the pulps of the fingers over the main body of the gland. Ascertain the consistency of the swelling, and whether or not it is tender.

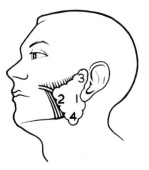

Fig. 190. The routine for palpating the parotid gland advised in the text.

2. The anterior limit of the parotid is difficult to define, but if the patient clenches his teeth the masseter muscle is thrown into relief. The gland overlies the superficial surface of this muscle to a variable extent.

3. Palpate the superior third of the gland. If there is a fullness here, make certain that it is continuous with the main body of the parotid, for the pre-auricular lymph node overlies the gland in this vicinity.

4. Lay the fingers over the inferior third. As has been stressed in the section on inspection, if the whole parotid is enlarged there is always a fullness over the postero-inferior part (4 in *Fig.* 190).

Inspection of the Orifice of the Parotid (Stensen's) Duct which lies opposite the second upper molar tooth. Retract the cheek with a spatula. If gentle pressure exerted over the gland from without causes a gush of purulent saliva, or a drop of thicker pus exudes (*Fig.* 191), the diagnosis of parotitis becomes indisputable.

Enlargement of the Deep Lobe. Very occasionally a parotid tumour involves the deep lobe only. External examination, as detailed above, suggests that the swelling is in the parotid, but it feels more deeply placed than usual. Inspection of the pharynx (*see* p. 129) reveals an apparently enlarged tonsil due to its displacement. A bimanual examination similar to that depicted in *Fig.* 199 confirms that the externally felt tumour is continuous with the swelling displacing the tonsil.

Acute Parotitis gives rise to a brawny swelling (*Fig.* 192) involving the whole

NIELS STENSEN, 1638–1686, *Migrating Danish anatomist and scientist (Copenhagen, Amsterdam, Leiden, Paris, Florence). Later he became a Bishop.*

gland. In addition, the swelling is extremely tender and the overlying skin feels warmer than that on the contralateral side. Occasionally the phenomenon displayed in *Fig.* 191 can be witnessed, but in these circumstances the pressure exerted over the gland may cause unjustifiable pain. Even when a discharge of purulent fluid down the duct cannot be seen or evoked, the ampulla of Stensen's duct may display evidence of inflammation. When it is doubtful whether there is a minor degree of redness of the ampulla, compare it with the opposite side.

Bilateral Enlargement of the parotid glands is not always due to mumps; cases of acute, subacute and chronic parotitis, consequent upon bacterial infection, occur. Painless bilateral enlargement is found in some cases of cirrhosis of the liver and some types of malnutrition.

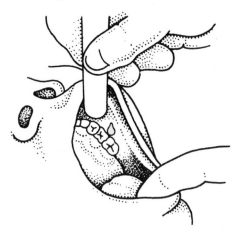

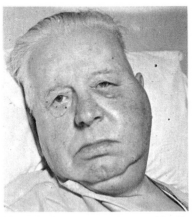

Fig. 191. Examining the orifice of Stensen's duct. Purulent saliva is seen being ejected in this case of subacute parotitis.

Fig. 192. Acute suppurative parotitis. The whole of the parotid gland is enlarged.

Chronic Parotitis. The swelling is almost, if not entirely, *painless*. Recurrent unilateral enlargement of the parotid is rarely due to a calculus; recurrent subacute and chronic parotitis are the usual causes (*Fig.* 193).

Suspected Parotid Salivary Calculus. Compared with submandibular calculus (*see* p. 105), a stone in the parotid gland or its duct is rare. If the history suggests salivary colic (attacks of pain before and during meals), followed by a swelling of the parotid, the course of the duct, which lies about one finger-breadth below the inferior border of the zygomatic bone, should be palpated for a calculus. The anterior part can be palpated satisfactorily between the finger and thumb, the finger being in the mouth (*Fig.* 194), but the major part is inaccessible by the intervention of the masseter muscle. Radiology is essential for confirmation of the diagnosis.

Differential Diagnosis of Recurrent Parotid Enlargement

1. *Idiopathic Hypertrophy of the Masseter Muscle* is described on p. 92.

2. *Pre-auricular Lymphadenitis.* The swelling is situated immediately in front of the tragus. Inflammatory oedema is wont to extend over much of the surface marking of the parotid gland, but the normal depression (*see* 4 in *Fig.* 190) is not obliterated. A primary focus of infection must be sought. Usually this is to be found in the region of the eyebrow, an eyelid (including the lacrimal gland), or the conjunctiva of the same side. More rarely, the focus is situated within the

external auditory meatus (furuncle and otitis externa, *see* p. 83). Abscess connected with a breaking-down pre-auricular lymph node is described on p. 83. Lastly, should no cause be found, remember that a lymphoma or tuberculosis may first become manifest in this situation and arrange for a biopsy.

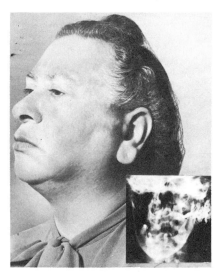

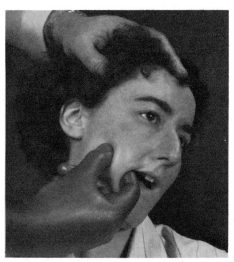

Fig. 193. Chronic parotitis. Recurring attacks of painful swelling of the parotid gland have occurred for many years. Inset: sialogram of this case, showing greatly distended ducts and alveoli (sialectasis)*.

Fig. 194. Palpating the distal third of Stensen's duct.

TUMOURS OF THE PAROTID GLAND

A Mixed Parotid Tumour (Pleomorphic Salivary Adenoma) is peculiar in remaining benign for many years and seldom (2–3 per cent) undergoing malignant change, but having a strong tendency to local recurrence if inadequately removed. It is, of course, possible for a neoplasm to arise in any part of the parotid; nevertheless most mixed parotid tumours have their beginning in a comparatively circumscribed area—a little in front of and above the angle of the jaw (*Fig.* 195).

The only other common starting-point is in the region immediately in front of the tragus. Here the differential diagnosis between an enlarged pre-auricular lymph node and a small mixed parotid tumour is impossible, unless some cause for an enlarged lymph node can be discovered. When the patient opens the mouth sometimes the forward excursion of the condyle of the mandible beneath the lump throws the swelling into prominence, and although the phenomenon has no diagnostic significance, it does enable the lump to be palpated more thoroughly.

---

* *Sialectasis.* Dilatation of the ducts and alveoli of the (parotid) salivary gland. Likened to *bronchiectasis* of the lung and probably of similar aetiology.

Occasionally a mixed tumour arising at the periphery of the gland causes difficulty in diagnosis (*Fig.* 196). Such a swelling can occur at any of the positions shown in the inset to *Fig.* 196.

Although other varieties of benign tumours arising in the parotid are impossible to distinguish clinically from the above (which form 75 per cent of all parotid tumours) an *adenolymphoma* (Warthin's tumour) is generally softer (sometimes fluctuant); tends to occur only in males not of coloured race; and is seen only after the fortieth year. These points may enable a clinical distinction, but usually histological examination of the excised swelling is necessary.

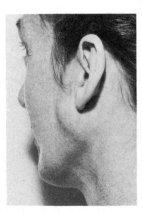

Fig. 195. A mixed parotid tumour in the most characteristic situation.

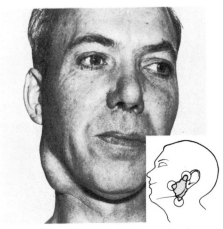

Fig. 196. This swelling in the neck proved to be a mixed salivary tumour arising from the periphery of the parotid gland. *Inset,* three situations in which peripheral parotid swellings may give rise to diagnostic difficulty.

Relatively Advanced Tumour of the Parotid Gland. As the lump is painless, it is not uncommon for the patient to procrastinate for years or even be advised by his doctor 'not to worry about it'. When the tumour has been present for some time, or is large, proceed as follows:

By testing the mobility of the tumour, endeavour to find out if it is still innocent. Remember that the clinical examination of a parotid tumour is not complete without testing the functional integrity of the seventh cranial nerve (*see* p. 99); although the nerve is related intimately to the parotid gland, its function is unimpaired unless the tumour is malignant (either *de novo* or secondarily) or, in the case of a recurrent tumour, it has been damaged at the previous attempt at removal.

Carcinoma of the Parotid Gland. As indicated, this may occur as a primary event or, rarely, complicate a long-standing mixed tumour. A painless, rapidly enlarging, recent tumour is suggestive of carcinoma, and facial palsy is proof-positive. An examination of the cervical lymph nodes is indicated; metastases occur only in advanced cases. Carcinoma is not as uncommon as is sometimes alleged; in large series some 10–20 per cent of parotid tumours are malignant.

Cyst of the Parotid. Most occur in the region overlying the angle of the mandible, and are probably derived from the first branchial cleft. The condition is far less common than adenolymphoma, which, however, is seldom so fluctuant as a true cyst. If the diagnosis is suspected needle aspiration, if

ALDRED S. WARTHIN, 1866–1931, *Professor of Pathology, University of Michigan.*

successful, will cause the swelling to disappear (cf. Cyst of Breast, p. 170). Occasionally a main branch of the parotid tree, occluded by a calculus, gives rise to a cyst.

Mikulicz's Disease is characterized by symmetrical, and usually progressive, enlargement of the lacrimal and salivary glands, with a replacement of the glandular tissue by lymphocytes. It involves the parotid, submandibular, sublingual and frequently the accessory salivary glands. Usually the disease occurs in persons between 20 and 40 years of age who at first have paroxysms of enlargement of these glands lasting from a few hours to several weeks. In a few cases regression occurs; in the majority the enlargement becomes stationary. Dryness of the mouth is a regular accompaniment of fully established Mikulicz's disease. In the beginning one gland alone, often the lacrimal, is attacked, and the diagnosis can be established only by histological examination. The disease is probably an early stage or precursor of Sjögren's syndrome in which dryness of the eyes and rheumatic joint changes are superadded to the above features.

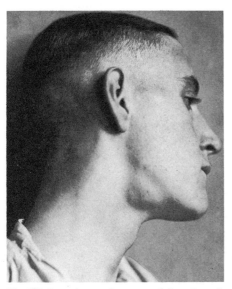

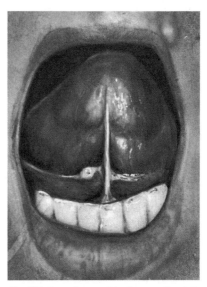

Fig. 197. Intermittent enlargement of the submandibular salivary gland. It became evident after the patient had sucked a lemon. Case of a stone in the submandibular duct.

Fig. 198. Stone impacted in the ampulla of the right submandibular duct, resulting in saliva being ejected from the left duct only.

THE SUBMANDIBULAR SALIVARY GLAND

SUBMANDIBULAR SALIVARY CALCULUS

Inspection of the Submandibular Triangle. An enlargement of the submandibular salivary gland causes a swelling beneath and in front of the angle of the jaw. When the patient volunteers the information that the swelling appears only either just before or during meals, ask him to suck a little lemon or lime juice. An interesting and diagnostic phenomenon may be witnessed (*Fig.* 197) which is proof positive that Wharton's submandibular duct is obstructed. A swelling, situated in the submandibular triangle that appears or, if present already, enlarges before one's very eyes, can be none other than a swelling of the submandibular salivary gland. On the other hand, a swelling that occupies the triangle, but remains constant in size, is not necessarily a swelling of the salivary

JOHANNES VON MIKULICZ-RADECKI, 1850–1905, *Professor of Surgery, Breslau.*
TAGE SJÖGREN, 1859–1939, *Swedish Physician.*
THOMAS WHARTON, 1614–1673, *Physician, St. Thomas's Hospital, London.*

gland and must be differentiated from other swellings of this region. Assuming that the swelling does vary in size, the next step is:

Inspection of the Floor of the Mouth. The orifices of the submandibular ducts are inspected with the aid of a torch, and the two sides compared. In about 40 per cent of cases of submandibular salivary calculus some aberration is visible on the affected side of the floor of the mouth, namely: when secondary infection has supervened the ampulla is likely to be inflamed; sometimes pus can be seen exuding from the orifice of the duct. Occasionally a stone impacted in the ampulla will be observed (*Fig.* 198).

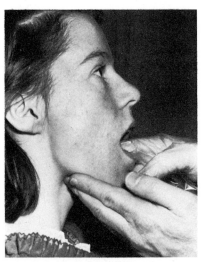

Fig. 199. Bimanual palpation of the submandibular salivary gland utilizing a disposable glove.

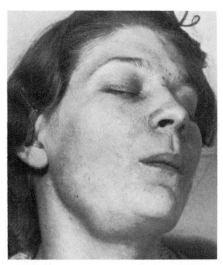

Fig. 200. Tuberculous submandibular lymphadenitis. The swelling does not vary in size and on bimanual palpation there is no contiguous swelling in the floor of the mouth.

Especially if there is no obvious abnormality present, it is essential to ascertain whether the flow of saliva from the suspected submandibular gland is impeded. This can be determined there and then in the following manner:

A dry swab is inserted under the tongue, and some lemon juice is placed on the dorsum. The patient is then asked to keep the swab in place with his finger while he moves the tongue about to taste the juice. He is then instructed to open the mouth widely, and to raise the tip of the tongue towards the roof of the mouth. The swab is removed and, quickly, the (dried) floor of the mouth inspected. Normally, saliva can be seen flowing, occasionally being ejected, from both ducts. With obstruction by a calculus there will be little or no secretion from the affected side. Finally, the fingers are placed on the skin overlying the submandibular triangle, and steady pressure is exerted on the gland. This may evoke a gush of saliva or purulent exudate when the duct is partially occluded.

Palpation of the Submandibular Salivary Gland. As there are two portions, a larger (cervical) beneath, and a smaller (buccal) above the mylohyoid muscle, there can be but one efficient method of examining the whole gland, and that is by bimanual palpation (*Fig.* 199). If it can be ascertained that there are contiguous intrabuccal and cervical swellings, this is good evidence that the swelling in question is an enlarged submandibular salivary gland.

A Method of Palpating the Submandibular Duct. Dentures, if any, are removed. The patient's head is flexed and inclined somewhat to the affected side, in order to relax the musculature. The index finger is inserted into the mouth, the pulp of the finger being placed upon the internal surface of the alveolus. The finger is passed backwards, following the alveolus until its posterior extremity is reached. The tip of the finger is insinuated between the alveolus just behind the last molar tooth and the side of the posterior third of the tongue, and rotated through a right-angle, so that the pulp is directed downwards. In conjunction with the fingers of the other hand beneath the jaw, the whole course of the duct is palpated for a calculus, from behind forwards. Sometimes this manœuvre brings on retching, but even so the information required is elicited before the patient experiences any severe discomfort.

Differential Diagnosis. *From Enlarged Submandibular Lymph Nodes.* When, on bimanual palpation (*see Fig.* 199), a cervical (as opposed to a cervical + a buccal) swelling alone is palpable, enlarged submandibular lymph nodes (*Fig.* 200) are the probable cause of the lump. Often such nodes are blended intimately with the capsule of the submandibular salivary gland.

The differentiation of the swelling from a *neoplasm* will now be discussed:

Tumours of the Submandibular Salivary Gland are uncommon compared with enlargement of the gland due to calculus and also with parotid tumours.

A Mixed Tumour presents with a slowly growing tumour of moderate size (*Fig.* 201). The lump is hard but could not be called *stony hard*. All the same, the precaution should be taken of requesting a radiograph of the region to exclude the possibility that the lump is an enlarged gland behind a calculus.

Carcinoma of the Submandibular Gland (*Fig.* 202) is rare.

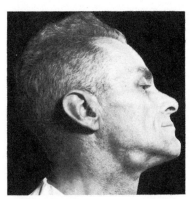

Fig. 201. This enlargement of the submandibular salivary gland, present for many months, did not vary in size. Case of mixed tumour.

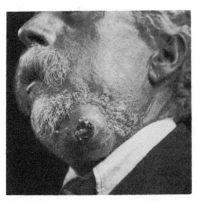

Fig. 202. Carcinoma of the submandibular salivary gland fungating through the skin.

Before concluding this subject, the possibility of a swelling in the submandibular triangle being due to a primary or secondary neoplasm of the submandibular lymph nodes must be considered. Regarding the latter, the primary growth should be situated either on the upper lip (not forgetting its buccal surface) or, far more frequently, on the anterior two-thirds of the tongue or the floor of the mouth.

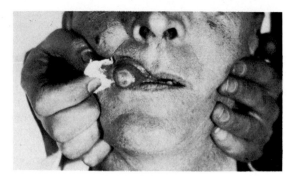

Fig. 203. Myxomatous degeneration of the left gland of Blandin and Nühn on the under-surface of the tongue.

THE MINOR SALIVARY GLANDS

The Sublingual Gland. Amidst all the affections to which the salivary glands are heir, the sublingual glands seem practically immune. An exception to the rule is Mikulicz's disease (*see* p. 105). A ranula (*see* p. 124) is a cystic degeneration of this gland.

The Inferior Lingual Gland of Blandin and Nühn. On rare occasions this gland undergoes cystic degeneration, in which event, if the normal location of the gland is known, the diagnosis is written on the face of the swelling (*Fig.* 203).

Tumours of Ectopic Salivary Glands are described on p. 127. Although known as 'ectopic', in point of fact, normally, tiny salivary glands are scattered over the palate and the nasopharynx, and neoplasms of these glands are not uncommon, while those of the named minor salivary glands (i.e. the sublingual glands; the gland of Blandin and Nühn) are of utmost rarity.

PHILIPPE BLANDIN, 1798–1849, *Surgeon, Hôtel-Dieu Hospital, Paris.*
ANTON NÜHN, 1814–1884, *Professor of Anatomy, Heidelberg.*

Chapter 11

THE MOUTH

The multiplication of instruments and apparatus designed to reveal hidden pathological conditions sometimes makes the practitioner lament that he lacks facilities for special examination. Regarding the mouth this is certainly not true. Seated in his consulting room, armed with little more than an electric torch and a spatula, he can, if he wishes, become a master of intrabuccal living pathology and diagnosis, for his opportunities are unrivalled.

THE LIPS

Clefts of the lip and palate are found in approximately one in 400 live births. Either can occur alone but often they occur together.

Cleft Lip. The hare has an upper lip cleft in the *midline.* The developmental abnormality of the lip occurring in human beings is almost invariably a *lateral* cleft, yet the inaccurate term 'hare lip' continues in general use. All degrees of cleft lip, from an interruption of the vermilion border alone to a bilateral cleft of the whole of the upper lip, are obvious.

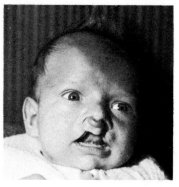

Fig. 204. Complete bilateral cleft lip and palate.

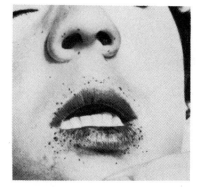

Fig. 205. The labial and circumoral pigmented spots of the Peutz–Jeghers syndrome.

Cleft Palate. In 50 per cent of cases a cleft lip is associated with a cleft palate; if the former is present the clinician should at once inspect the palate (*see* p. 127). Tripartite cleft palate and bilateral cleft lip go hand in hand, causing the premaxilla (morphologically the prognathion or snout) to jut out (*Fig.* 204), as examination of the palate will confirm.

Peutz–Jeghers Syndrome (Pigmentation of the Lips and Intestinal Polyposis). Multiple pigmented spots, varying from brown to black, on and about the vermilion surfaces of the lips (*Fig.* 205), characterize this syndrome. They are only partially obliterated by lipstick as usually applied, and are situated in an area seldom affected by freckles. Inquire regarding similar spots on the lips of relatives,

JOHN I. A. PEUTZ, 1886–1957, *Chief of Internal Medicine, St. John's Hospital, The Hague, Holland.*
HARALD JEGHERS, 1894–1968, *Professor of Medicine, Tufts University School of Medicine, Boston, Massachusetts.*

for the condition is strongly familial and is the outward sign of adenomatous polyposis of the small intestine. Such polyps bleed, intussuscept and rarely become malignant. Occult blood is present in the stool and attacks of melaena (*see* p. 20) are frequent.

Angular Stomatitis (Cheilosis*). Brownish superficial ulceration at the corners of the mouth with scabbing, which is often picked or licked off, presents but little difficulty in diagnosis. It occurs as a simple infection in children of school age ('perlèche'†). When of some standing, moist fissures appear. Always examine the related mucous surface. The fissuring of syphilis is deeper, extends on to the mucous membrane, and leaves permanent scars (*see below*). Perlèche does not extend on to the mucous surface, and heals without scarring.

Other causes of angular stomatitis are ariboflavinosis, which is prone to occur after complete or almost complete gastrectomy, sideropaenic dysphagia (*see* p. 198), or severe anaemia. Dental causes are over-closure of the mouth (*Fig.* 206) due to absence of either upper or lower teeth of dentures, and allergy to the material from which dentures are made or to lipstick.

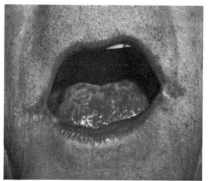

Fig. 206. Angular stomatitis due to overclosure of the mouth.

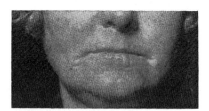

Fig. 207. Rhagades.

Rhagades.‡ White linear scars radiating from the corners of the mouth (*Fig.* 207) suggest previous syphilitic ulceration.

Returning to the lip proper:

A Primary Chancre usually is situated on the upper lip (*see Fig.* 78, p. 37).

Carbuncle of the Upper Lip. This is a dangerous situation for a carbuncle. A complication that heralds septicaemia is thrombophlebitis of the cavernous sinus. A sign of impending danger is spreading oedema from the lip to the inner canthus. When on this account the lids of one eye and then the lids of the other become closed it is probable that thrombophlebitis of the veins of the ophthalmic plexus has spread to the cavernous sinus (*see* p. 70).

With the above exceptions, it is the *lower lip* which is the site of election for pathological conditions.

---

* *Cheilosis.* Greek, χεῖλος = a lip. Cracks at the corners of the mouth.
† *Perlèche.* French, *pourlécher* = to lick.
‡ *Rhagades.* Greek, pl. of ῥαγάς = a crack.

Aphthous* Ulcer on the lip, on the tip (*Fig.* 208) or sides of the tongue, or on the mucous lining of a cheek, is common. The ulcer is a small, superficial, very painful erosion with a white floor, a yellowish border and surrounded by a narrow hyperaemic areola. Occasionally two or more are found. It usually starts in early adult life, tends to recur for some years, and is commoner in females. It is rare after the age of 50 (Sircus). Often the periodic appearance of the ulcers seems to be associated with environmental or emotional·stress. The lesion heals spontaneously in 7–14 days and is thus seen predominantly by the general practitioner.

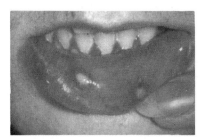

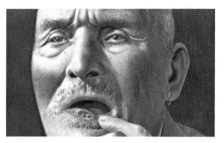

Fig. 208. Aphthous ulcers of the lower lip.

Fig. 209. Carcinoma of the lip in an elderly retired agricultural labourer.

A Median Crack in the Lower Lip is common in cold weather. In some individuals the crack becomes chronically inflamed, and bleeds readily.

Actinic Cheilitis occurs among those following an outdoor occupation in sunny climes. It gives rise to epithelial exfoliation of the lips, more especially the lower lip; small blisters recur at frequent intervals during the summer months. Actinic cheilitis recurring year after year is a precursor of carcinoma.

Carcinoma of the Lip. Ninety-five per cent of cases occur on the lower lip. The usual form is a flat ulcer appearing on the vermilion surface (*Fig.* 209) which advances slowly, remains shallow, and is surrounded by but little induration. More induration and deeper ulceration imply greater malignancy both locally and in the matter of early lymphatic metastasis.

Molluscum Sebaceum simulates a carcinoma of the lip very closely (*see* p. 28).

In order that the mucous surface of the inner aspect of the lip can be inspected, the lip must be everted fully. In addition to uncovering the full extent of an advanced neoplasm, there are two lesions that can be displayed only by this manœuvre:

A Retention Cyst of a buccal mucous gland can occur anywhere in the mucous lining of the mouth, but it does so relatively frequently on the buccal aspect of the lower lip (*Fig.* 210). The cyst is blue-domed and brilliantly translucent— signs which render the diagnosis certain.

A localized *Cavernous Haemangioma* beneath the mucous membrane of the lip simulates the above condition, but gives the sign of emptying which in this instance can be demonstrated by pressing a glass slide on to the swelling.

---

* *Aphthous.* Greek, ἄφθα, = mouth ulcer, probably connected with ἅπτειν = to set on fire. *Aphthous ulcer* is known in the USA as 'canker sore'.

WILFRED SIRCUS, *Contemporary Physician, Western General Hospital, Edinburgh.*

Examination of the Lymphatic Field of the Lips. In inflammatory and neoplastic cases examination of the lip is concluded by palpation of the cervical lymph nodes, particular attention being paid to the submental group, which are not easy to feel when only moderately enlarged.

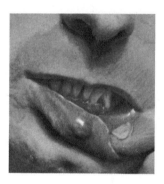

Fig. 210. Retention cyst arising in the mucous lining of the lower lip.

EXAMINATION OF THE TEETH

The task of remembering when normal eruption occurs is aided considerably by *Fig.* 211. There is a great variation in the date of eruption of teeth in normal children: some may have teeth at birth, and others none until they are a year old.

General Inspection of the Teeth. If the patient wears a denture, insist upon it being removed before proceeding with the examination. The patient is asked to show the front teeth. The anterior surface of the exposed crowns having been inspected, the lips are lifted away from the gums in order that the necks of the teeth can be scrutinized. Next the patient is requested to open the mouth, and with the aid of a spatula the more posteriorly placed teeth are examined. The use of a dental mirror is often advisable if visualization of the lingual side of a particular tooth or teeth is deemed necessary. Make a note of any carious* teeth, i.e. those with cavities due to decay. In dental practice charts similar to *Fig.* 211 are used.

Congenital Ectodermal Dysplasia is a cause of poorly calcified deciduous† teeth. In this disease the skin is very dry and the hair scanty. Poor formation of deciduous teeth is seen also in systemic affections with hypocalcaemia.

Congenital Absence of a Tooth or Teeth. When one or both lateral incisors are missing, and there is no history of a dental extraction in this region, it is more than probable that it is a case of congenital absence of the tooth or teeth concerned—an abnormality which is practically confined to lateral incisors.

Wide Spacing between the Upper Central Incisor Teeth is due sometimes to persistence of, and insertion into the palate of, the infantile fraenum of the upper lip.

Abnormally Coloured Teeth. Occasionally green teeth are seen in children who have had severe jaundice in infancy. Certain drugs, notably tetracycline (*Fig.* 212) when given in childhood cause staining of the teeth. Similar staining is seen in adults who smoke heavily and do not clean their teeth efficiently and in betel-nut chewers (*see* p. 126).

---

* *Caries.* Latin, *caries* = decay; death of tooth or bone in part.
† *Deciduous.* Latin, from *decidere* = to fall off; not permanent.

Teeth bespattered with Brown or Black Pits are due to the presence of excess of fluorides in the water the patient drank habitually during childhood and adolescence. The 0·5 parts per million used to prevent caries does not have this effect.

Transversely Ridged Teeth with curved notching due to wear are not uncommon in those who have suffered from rickets or scurvy while enamel deposition was in progress.

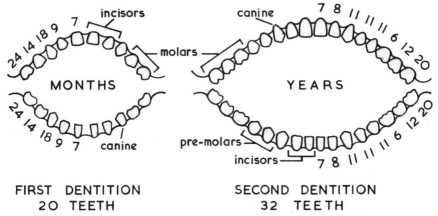

FIRST DENTITION
20 TEETH

SECOND DENTITION
32 TEETH

Fig. 211. The date of eruption of each tooth.

In a patient with symptoms referable to the stomach, examination of the teeth should never be omitted. Note particularly whether there are sufficient molars in opposition with which to carry out mastication effectively.

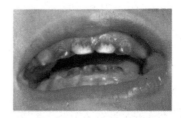

Fig. 212. Tetracycline staining of a child's teeth; recurrent urinary infections were treated with this antibiotic.

Passing now to clinical conditions of surgical importance connected with, or arising from, the teeth themselves:

Tartar consists mainly of precipitated calcium salts of the saliva. Deposits of tartar are heaviest on the lingual aspect of the necks of the lower incisors, these teeth being exposed to the salivary stream of the submandibular glands, the secretion of which is particularly rich in calcium. The relationship of tartar to pyorrhoea alveolaris is described on p. 115.

Acute Pulpitis ('toothache'). Pulp inflammation leads to a complaint that a certain tooth, usually carious, is painful. Tapping with a metal object, or rocking the tooth between finger and thumb does not cause pain as in dental abscess (*see* p. 117) but hot or cold water exacerbates the pain.

Impacted Tooth. A tooth that is prevented from erupting by the presence of other teeth is spoken of as being impacted. The third mandibular molar (wisdom) is most frequently prevented from erupting in this way, the maxillary canine and the maxillary third molar taking second and third places respectively. Absence of a canine tooth with no history of extraction nearly always implies that it lies impacted. Often such a tooth remains symptomless until perhaps late in life, when it gives rise to a painful, tender lump beneath the denture.

An Incompletely Erupted Third Mandibular Molar, which though impacted can partially erupt, is one that gives rise to severe symptoms, and is a source of danger. The tooth remains covered with a flap of gum, viz. ⸺⸺⸺⸺⸺⸺⸺⸺⸺⟶ or operculum,* which is easily overlooked if not searched for especially, permits debris to collect beneath it, with suppuration following. Incomplete eruption of a wisdom tooth is the *most common cause of trismus* (*see* p. 92).

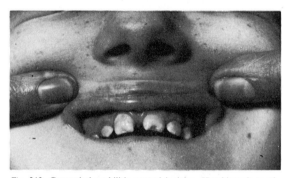

Fig. 213. Congenital syphilitic central incisors. Hutchinson's tooth, left (reader's right); screwdriver tooth, right (reader's left).

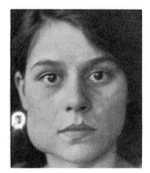

Fig. 214. A missing tooth suggested a clinical diagnosis of odontome, which later was confirmed by X-rays.

Dead (Pulpless) Tooth. A dead tooth has no living pulp. After dissolution or removal of the pulp, and closing of the pulp cavity with a filling, the dentine loses its central blood supply. For several months the tooth changes in colour slightly; it is less white than the remaining teeth. Later it becomes increasingly discoloured bluish-grey, most pronounced in the region of the gingival one-third, where the enamel is thinnest. It is insensitive to ice applied to its crown.

Hutchinson's Teeth are confirmatory evidence of congenital syphilis. The *second dentition alone* is affected. The upper central incisors are smaller than normal, broader towards the gum than at their free edge and notched (*Fig.* 213). Another characteristic tooth is the 'screwdriver' tooth (*Fig.* 213). *Moon's Turreted Molars* are dome-shaped first molars also in congenital syphilis.

Odontome. † If the case is one of a swelling in the jaw, careful attention to the dental formula (*Fig.* 211) may throw light upon the diagnosis. If a missing tooth cannot be accounted for in any other way, it is fairly good evidence that the swelling is an odontome (*Fig.* 214), a diagnosis that must be confirmed by radiography.

---

* *Operculum.* Latin, *operculum* = a lid.
† *Odontome* = a cyst or tumour arising from tooth germ.

SIR JONATHAN HUTCHINSON, 1828–1913, *Surgeon, The London Hospital.*
HENRY MOON, 1845–1892, *Dental Surgeon, Guy's Hospital, London.*

EXAMINATION OF THE GUMS

In order to examine the gums, in turn each lip must be everted fully (*Fig.* 215). Visualization of the more posterior portions of the gums requires the aid of a spatula and a torch; substitution of a dental mirror for the spatula is to be commended when a better view of the posterior part, and especially of the lingual aspect, of the gum is required. Even well-developed localized lesions often escape detection for want of running the finger along each aspect of the gum.

Healthy gums are bright pink in colour. The crenated* edge of each gum is sharply defined, firm, and closely adherent to the necks of the teeth.

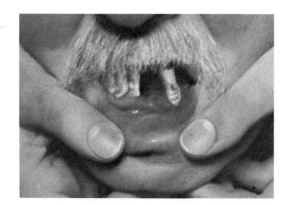

Fig. 215. 'Long in the tooth.' Tartar accumulation. Pyorrhoea present.

Receding Gums. As age advances, so the teeth appear longer, owing to recession of the gums (*Fig.* 215). Eventually, if not obscured by tartar, the rough, lustreless cementum lies exposed above the smooth, shining enamel. The process is accelerated by failing to have collected tartar removed periodically.

Pyorrhoea Alveolaris. As a consequence of recession, the periodontal membrane gives way, allowing organisms to enter and debris to collect in gingival pockets resulting from loss of adherence of the gums to the neck of the teeth. Often the teeth themselves are sound. The earliest sign of pyorrhoea alveolaris is a deep red line along the free edge of the gum, with diminution of the normal depth of crenation (*Fig.* 216). Later, if pressed, the gums bleed readily: sometimes a small bead of pus exudes. Commonly, the condition commences in relation to the incisor teeth; untreated, it spreads. Halitosis and a pink stain on the pillow (due to dribbling of slightly bloodstained saliva) are common accompaniments.

Vincent's Stomatitis (Trench Mouth) is an inflammatory condition of the gingivae and adjoining mucous membrane. In addition to an acute or subacute inflammation of the gums, there is ulceration of the gingival margins with the formation of pseudomembrane affecting particularly the interdental papillae. This is *the* characteristic sign, which, together with overpowering foetor oris, should proclaim the diagnosis.

---

* *Crenated.* Latin, *crenatus* = scalloped, viz: ⌒⌒⌒⌒

Bacteriological confirmation of the symbiotic infection by *Borrelia vincentii* and *Bacteroides fusiformis* is most desirable although many authorities hold that these are secondary invaders consequent on a virus infection.

Cancrum Oris (Noma*). Although this has virtually disappeared in Europe and North America, it is still common in Africa, Asia and South America. The commonest predisposing cause is measles, but malnutrition, gastro-enteritis, typhoid and bronchopneumonia may all act as antecedents. Three-quarters of patients fall into the age-group 2–5 years. In almost all early cases the organisms of Vincent's stomatitis (*see above*) can be isolated (Tempest).

At an early stage a painful purple-red indurated papule is found on the alveolar margin in the molar or premolar region of the mandible, maxilla, or both. Occasionally the condition is bilateral. An ulcer forms, rapidly exposing the underlying bone and extends on to the cheek or lip which is tender and swollen. There is a foul smell and in two or three days gangrene of the involved soft tissues commences leading to a well-defined slough and a hole in cheek or lip (*Fig.* 218). Soon bone and teeth sequestrate, but with modern antibiotic therapy the child usually survives to provide a problem for the plastic surgeon.

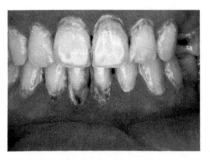

Fig. 216. Pyorrhoea alveolaris. Commencing gum retraction of the incisor teeth.

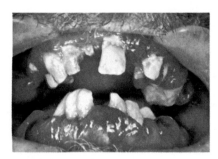

Fig. 217. The gums in scurvy.

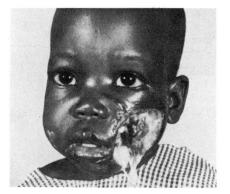

Fig. 218. Cancrum oris of the cheek at the stage of separation of the slough.

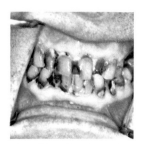

Fig. 219. Lead line in a careless painter.

Scurvy. Bleeding from the gums is a leading sign. The gums are swollen, livid† (*Fig.* 217), spongy and tender. Often the teeth become loose.

Bleeding Gums in Uraemia. The gums are not so spongy as in scurvy; in fact they look nearly normal.

---

* *Noma.* Greek, νέμειν = to devour.

† *Livid.* Latin, *lividus* = lead coloured. The original meaning has become altered, and the term has now come to signify a deep, almost purple, red.

JEAN H. VINCENT, 1862–1950, *Professor of Medicine, Val-de-Grâce Military Hospital, Paris.*
MICHAEL N. TEMPEST, *Contemporary, Consultant Plastic Surgeon, University Hospital, Cardiff.*

Generalized Hyperplastic Gingivitis at first sight simulates the gums of scurvy. However, the gums are neither so spongy nor so livid, nor are the teeth loose. Commencing in childhood, it is progressive, and, unless treated operatively, the hypertrophied gums almost bury the teeth. In some cases it is produced by drugs used in the treatment of epilepsy, e.g. epanutin.

Hyperplastic Gums of Leukaemia and Agranulocytosis. Especially in acute leukaemia occurring in a child, the gums become swollen due to extravasation of immature white cells and secondary infection. They bleed readily on being pressed but, unlike other conditions giving rise to hypertrophy of the gums, pyrexia is almost always present and the patient looks ill.

The Lead Line is seen in patients who work with lead, e.g. painters, who complain of colicky abdominal pain. The 'blue line' if inspected closely will be seen to consist of a series of grey-black dots situated about 1 mm from the free margin of the gum (*Fig.* 219) best seen with a magnifying glass. Almost identical are the bismuth and mercury lines. 'Metal' lines are now rarely encountered owing to the better protection of workers and the abolition of their use in the treatment of syphilis.

Dental Abscess. Contrary to what might be thought, X-ray evidence of an acute abscess is lacking until resorption of bone has occurred—a matter of at least ten days. Physical signs are thus extremely important in diagnosis (*see* Acute Pulpitis, p. 113). In dental abscess, pain is caused by tapping or rocking the tooth.

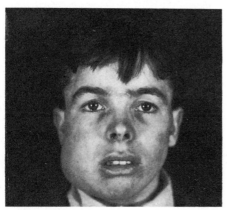

Fig. 220. Foetor, local tenderness and some degree of trismus make the diagnosis of a dental abscess (lower molar) certain.

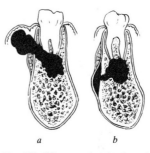

Fig. 221. When pus breaks through the lateral alveolus of the molar region, it can do so (*a*) above the buccinator muscle = a gumboil, or (*b*) below that muscle = a swollen face.

When pus generated by a carious tooth breaks through the bony alveolus and its periosteum, a process that usually takes several days, the intense throbbing pain of an undecompressed root abscess is relieved. If the muscles of mastication become involved in the extending inflammation, trismus results. In order of frequency, the various directions taken by the pus are as follows:

1. *Through the Lateral Surface of the Bone.* By passing the finger along the labial aspect of the gum a rounded, tense, tender swelling (*a gumboil*) will be felt. In chronic cases there is no tenderness, and by pressure on the swelling pus is evacuated into the mouth.

In the molar region of either jaw osseous perforation can occur either above or below the attachment of the buccinator muscle, and on this depends whether there results a gumboil (*Fig.* 221 *a*) or a swollen face (*Figs.* 220 and 221 *b*).

2. *Through the Medial Surface of the Bone.* Less commonly, the pus bursts through the medial plate of the alveolus and in the upper jaw leads to a palatal abscess. In the lower jaw a gumboil on the lingual aspect of the alveolus results.

3. *Upwards into the Maxillary Antrum.* A rare termination leading to oro-antral fistula (*see* p. 137).

Epulis * is a term applied to a swelling arising from the alveolar margin of either upper or lower jaw. There are several varieties which require microscopical examination after excision or biopsy for verification of the diagnosis.

Fibrous Epulis is a tumour of the periosteum of the alveolus, or of the periodontal membrane. It appears as a nodular mass upon the surface of the gum (*Fig.* 222), often pushing up between two teeth. The attachment of the tumour can be sessile or, more rarely, pedunculated. In colour, it is grey to slightly brighter pink than that of the normal gum; it is a non-tender swelling, elastic in consistency, and slow of growth.

Granulomatous Epulis is softer, more rapidly growing, and is of a bright red colour (*Fig.* 223). It bleeds when the teeth are brushed. Often it is found adjacent to a carious tooth or an ill-fitting denture (*Fig.* 224). Sometimes it is found, temporarily, during pregnancy.

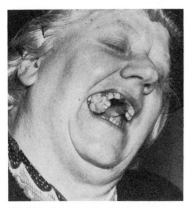

Fig. 222. Fibrous epulis.

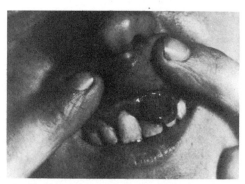

Fig. 223. Granulomatous epulis.

Giant-celled Epulis is an osteoclastoma, situated in, and expanding, the alveolus. It nearly always occurs between the ages of ten and 25 years. The swelling is painless, and is much more frequently situated in the mandible than in the maxilla.

Epitheliomatous or Carcinomatous Epulis presents the same characteristics as other buccal cancers (*see* pp. 123, 126). It is an epithelioma of the mucosa of the alveolar margin.

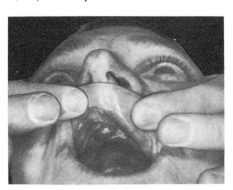

Fig. 224. Denture granuloma.

Conditions Arising from an Ill-fitting Denture. If a patient complaining of a sore gum wears a denture, examine the gums with special reference to the plate,

---

* *Epulis.* Greek, ἐπί = upon+οὖλον = gum.

which is removed for the purpose. Among the conditions directly due to an ill-fitting denture are the following:

'Prosthetic' Ulcer: An ulcer develops on the gum at a point of pressure. There is considerable erythema of the mucous membrane in the neighbourhood. Usually the condition occurs with recently fitted dentures.

Denture Granuloma (Fig. 224) = Granulomatous Epulis *above.*

EXAMINATION OF THE TONGUE

Examination of the Anterior Three-quarters. The tongue in relation to the general condition of the patient has been described on p. 8. Here abnormalities and diseases will be considered. If the history suggests a lesion, proceed as follows:

Ask the patient to put out his tongue. Abnormalities of the *dorsum* are apparent immediately.

Size of the Tongue. It is the acutely inflamed organ that commonly is larger than normal, because of oedema. Muscular hypertrophy (muscular macroglossia) is seen in cretins. Diffuse benign neoplasms are rare causes of enlargement.

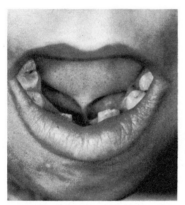

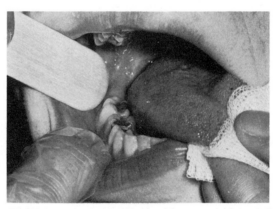

Fig. 225. Congenital short fraenum lingulae. The tip of the tongue has been rolled upwards.

Fig. 226. Displaying the lateral border of the tongue and its terminal recess. A carcinoma in this recess may be missed for want of employing this method of examination.

Restricted Mobility. Note whether the organ is protruded in the midline. If it is deviated, do not jump to a conclusion, for often the patient will deliberately rotate his tongue because he is trying to show you something on one side of it. Ask the patient to put his tongue straight out as far as he can. Decide whether there is any deviation to one side, or inability to protrude the organ to a normal extent. Lateral deviation is due either to unilateral infiltration of the lingual musculature by a carcinoma, or to a lesion of the hypoglossal nerve (*see* p. 60). In both the deviation is towards the side of the lesion. Inability to protrude the tongue fully (ankyloglossia) occurring in a patient past middle life almost invariably signifies advanced neoplastic infiltration of the lingual musculature, while in a young individual it is likely to be due to a congenitally short fraenum lingulae ('tongue-tie', *Fig.* 225), a rare condition that is revealed when the patient is asked to move the tongue upwards.

Continuing routine examination, ask the patient to rotate the tongue upwards towards the roof of his mouth revealing the *under-surface* and floor of the mouth.

The greater part of the *lateral borders* can only be seen if the cheek is retracted with a spatula and the angle of the mouth by an assistant's index finger. To grasp the forepart in a swab, and gently to pull the tongue forwards in the opposite direction, permits not only the whole of one lateral border to be seen clearly, but displays that inaccessible recess between the lateral base of the tongue and the anterior pillar of the fauces (*Fig.* 226).

Palpation of the Posterior Quarter of the Tongue and the Valleculae. A carcinoma lurking in this region can be detected easily by means of a gloved finger, and this manœuvre should be undertaken at the slightest provocation (i.e. discomfort at the back of the tongue; slight dysphagia; doubtful ankyloglossia) when no primary tumour is visible, and also to determine the extent of infiltration when only part of the neoplasm can be seen at the back of the tongue. If the patient tends to gag provide him with a surface anaesthetic tablet to be sucked.

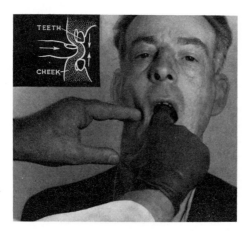

Fig. 227. Palpating the root of the tongue.

Ask the patient to open the mouth widely. Holding *all* the fingers of the left hand stiff and straight, press the fingertips firmly into the cheek (*Fig.* 227) in such a way that they intervene between the teeth (*Fig.* 227, inset). Should the patient 'bite', he will bite his cheek and not your palpating right index finger.

Lymphatic Drainage of the Tongue. No examination of the mouth is complete without systematic palpation of the cervical lymph nodes (*see* p. 139). Palpate the neck thoroughly, remembering that the anterior third of the tongue drains first into the submental nodes, the middle third into the submandibular nodes, and the posterior third into the deep cervical nodes. Cross-metastases are not uncommon, and occasionally the nodes of the jugular chain are the first to enlarge.

At this juncture, a number of clinical entities will be described, and many illustrated. True, some are rare, but unless the reader's attention is directed to them, how else can he or she recognize one or other of them should it be encountered? Especial attention is drawn to those benign conditions that simulate carcinoma.

*Leucoplakia** (Chronic Superficial Glossitis). The normal surface of the dorsum of the tongue is lost. The white colour (and its varying shades of grey) of the thickened patches of epithelium which have lost their papillae is a characteristic sign (sometimes affecting the cheek). Nowadays a history of syphilis is rare, and in one-third of all cases of carcinoma of the mouth the neoplasm is preceded by leucoplakia; on the other hand, leucoplakia is not necessarily followed by carcinoma.

Early lesions are thin, crinkled and pearly: older lesions, which are larger owing to coalescence of smaller ones, are creamy-white, thick and desquamate from time to time, leaving a beefy-red base (*Fig.* 228). When the condition is advanced we see the classic picture described most graphically by Butlin: 'the tongue looks as though it had been covered with white paint that had hardened, dried, and cracked'. Should the epithelium be shed over a considerable area a 'red glazed tongue' results. Leucoplakic plaques of long standing are so characteristic that they cannot possibly be mistaken, but frequent examinations must be made with a view to detecting the supervention of carcinoma.

In early doubtful cases of leucoplakia press a glass slide on the surface of the tongue; viewed in this manner, plaques of thickened epithelium will appear more obvious. Palpate each diseased area carefully; induration is sufficient to warrant the assumption that malignant change has occurred.

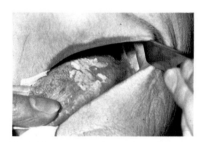

Fig. 228. Leucoplakia of the tongue.

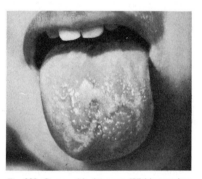

Fig. 229. Geographical tongue. Within two days the pattern changes.

Early lesions must be distinguished from one, somewhat rare, condition.

Lichen Planus offers the only difficult problem in differential diagnosis. The lingual lesions are delicate and bluish white in colour; they look like mucous membrane to which silver nitrate has been applied. It rarely occurs in the mouth alone; therefore when in doubt examine the flexor surfaces of the wrists and middle thirds of the shins for similar lesions.

Geographical Tongue (glossitis migrans) is symptomless. After an abdominal operation with peritonitis and antibiotic therapy, but occasionally idiopathically with a child, spots, rings and scallops appear (*Fig.* 229). The scallops, bright red in colour, and representing areas denuded of epithelium, are surrounded by a yellowish-white border (rings). So quickly does epithelial regeneration and fresh denudation occur that within one or two days the pattern imprinted on the dorsum changes. A cycle lasts about seven days with the idiopathic variety which may last until middle-age, but persists as long as the patient remains seriously ill with the secondary type.

'Congenital' Fissuring of the Tongue first appears towards the age of 3 or 4 years, and persists for life. As a rule there is a deepened median furrow and irregular folds occur in all directions, but *the*

---

* *Leucoplakia*. Greek, λευκός = white+πλάξ = plate.

Sɪʀ Hᴇɴʀʏ T. Bᴜᴛʟɪɴ, 1845–1912, *Surgeon, St. Bartholomew's Hospital, London.*

characteristic is that the main direction of the fissures is transverse. These fissures, which are not deep, can be made more apparent by asking the patient to put the tip of the tongue on the floor of the mouth, and then to show as much of the top of the tongue as possible, viz. ────────→
Syphilitic Fissuring of the Tongue. In contradistinction to the above, the fissures are mainly longitudinal in direction, and the intervening epithelial covering of the tongue is largely denuded.

Fissuring of Ariboflavinosis. Again the fissures are longitudinal in direction, and most are so deep as to justify the term 'crevice': the bottoms of the crevices are beefy-red. Usually the condition is associated with angular stomatitis (*see* p. 110).

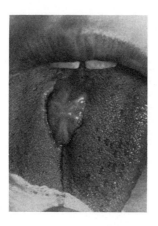

Fig. 230. Median rhomboid 'glossitis'.

Median Rhomboid 'Glossitis' is characterized by a mass, ovoid or rhomboid in shape (probably due to infection by *Candida albicans*), situated in the midline posteriorly immediately in front of the foramen caecum (*Fig.* 230). It is slightly raised, devoid of papillae and is in distinct contrast to the adjacent normal surface of the tongue and is often diagnosed in the first instance as carcinoma. On palpation, the area is slightly indurated and extends deeply into the lingual musculature.
Lingual Thyroid. See p. 160.
Haemangioma may be single or multiple, and is present from a very early age, if not from birth. However, it tends to enlarge, and gives rise to bleeding only when traumatized. The swellings (*Fig.* 231) are compressible, and when observed through a glass slide while pressure is being applied, the blue colour disappears, but returns when the pressure is removed.
Black or Hairy Tongue. Filiform papillary hypertrophy occurs at the back of the dorsum. To the elongated papillae cling tiny brown or black particles that cause the affected patch to assume an arresting furry appearance (*Fig.* 232). In about 60 per cent of cases the particles are found to contain a fungus or mould, notably the *Aspergillus niger*. It has increased in frequency with the increased incidence of buccal *Candida* infections due to elimination of the normal bacteria of the mouth in patients undergoing antibiotic treatment.

An Ulcer is Present on the Tongue. Before proceeding further, take a swab and dry the tongue thoroughly. The characters of the ulcer are then studied (*see* p. 35). Palpation of the tongue is done with a gloved finger, and whereas inspection is carried out with the tongue protruded, palpation is best performed with the tongue in, lest the contracted musculature simulates induration.

Dental Ulcer is precipitated by mechanical irritation, most commonly by a jagged tooth, but sometimes by a broken denture. In the acute stage, the ulcer, which is situated at the periphery or on the under-surface of the tongue, is elongated, often shows a slough as its base, and is surrounded by an area of erythema. Later the edges of the ulcer become heaped (*Fig.* 233), and there is distinct induration of the surrounding tissues. The relevant opposing area must be palpated for a sharp edged tooth, or, if the patient wears a denture, this must be inspected carefully. Should induration persist for longer than a week after the cause has been removed, biopsy is indicated strongly.

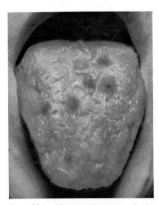

Fig. 231. Haemangiomata of the tongue. The patient complained that her saliva was bloodstained.

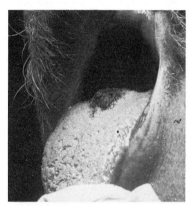

Fig. 232. Black or hairy tongue.

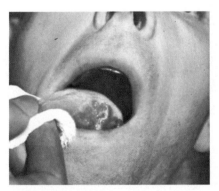

Fig. 233. Chronic dental ulcer.

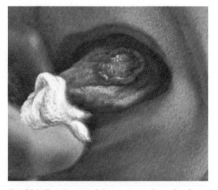

Fig. 234. Carcinoma of the tongue: ulcerating form.

Carcinoma of the Tongue. This is the most common malignant neoplasm of the mouth, and, rightly, it is in the forefront of the mind of the clinician when a patient of middle age and over complains of a lesion of the tongue. The site of election for its development is on the sides, the base and the under-surface: from the last situation it spreads to the floor of the mouth. True, the growth can commence as a wart or a nodule, but by far the most common presenting lesion is an ulcer which, by the time it is 1 cm in diameter, has rolled, everted edges (*Fig.* 234).

To dry the ulcer with a swab, and to employ a magnifying glass to observe it, sometimes unveils this characteristic when mere inspection rendered it nebulous. Be that as it may, palpation remains the main pillar that supports the diagnosis.

Are the immediate environs unmistakably indurated? If so, it is a carcinoma. That serological tests are positive for syphilis does not negate the diagnosis— lingual carcinoma can develop in the syphilitic.

Often lingual pain is referred to the ear and patients with an advanced carcinoma of the tongue sometimes present themselves with a wad of cotton-wool in one ear, complaining solely of earache. The accepted explanation is that the lingual nerve has become involved and the pain is referred to the auriculotemporal nerve.

Aphthous Ulcer of the tongue. *See* p. 111.

Primary Chancre is unusual on the tongue, but because it is unexpected in this situation, it may be misdiagnosed. It commences as a pustule, usually near the tip. This soon bursts, to form a small ulcer, and the surrounding tissue becomes indurated, but not so indurated as in the case of a penile primary chancre. As in chancre of the lip (*see Fig.* 78, p. 37), the submental and submandibular lymph nodes become enlarged, often grossly.

Gumma of the Tongue. Before it breaks down and becomes an ulcer, a lingual gumma shares with gummata elsewhere the property of providing a perplexing problem. However, that the mass thus produced is situated in the midline of the anterior two-thirds of the tongue, and is painless, helps to elucidate the diagnosis, which a serological test and, if that test be positive, a trial of antisyphilitic treatment will substantiate. On the other hand, when an ulcer forms, the characteristic 'punched-out' appearance (*Fig.* 235), the relatively small amount of surrounding induration, and above all the absence of pain, should clarify the diagnosis.

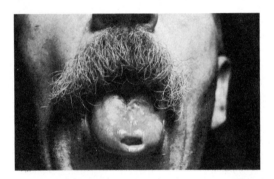

Fig. 235. Gumma of tongue.

Chronic Non-specific Ulcer of the Tongue usually is situated on the forepart of the tongue. It is an ulcer of negations. It is *not* very painful, there is *no* history of trauma, there is *no* sharp tooth to cause the lesion, there is *no* evidence of tuberculosis or syphilis, and only moderate induration is present. Without a biopsy it is likely to be diagnosed as a carcinoma.

Tuberculous Ulcer of the Tongue is now rare and usually, but not necessarily, complicates advanced untreated pulmonary or laryngeal tuberculosis. It is almost always situated on the tip or the sides of the anterior third, often multiple (*Fig.* 236), and nearly always gives rise to severe pain with impairment of mastication and articulation. The base is covered with pale granulations, and if the ulcer is large enough, the fact that its edges are slightly overhanging often can be discerned. The lingual lesions of tuberculosis are so protean* that when an unusual nodule or ulcer presents, especially if painful, tuberculosis should be suspected.

EXAMINATION OF THE FLOOR OF THE MOUTH

Ask the patient to put the tip of the tongue on the roof of the mouth and to bend the head slightly backward.

A *Ranula*† (a cyst originating in a sublingual salivary gland) can be recognized at once as an obviously translucent cystic swelling, often of a bluish tinge,

---

* *Protean.* Proteus, sea-god, fabled with the power to change into an endless variety of forms.
† So named by Hippocrates, who likened this swelling to the belly of a little frog.

situated on one side of the fraenum lingulae (*Fig.* 237), although on occasions, having filled the floor of the mouth on one side, it extends beneath the fraenum to the opposite side. Often the submandibular duct can be seen traversing the dome. Ranulae occasionally extend into the neck (plunging ranula): therefore palpate the submandibular triangle carefully from without for an extension of the swelling, and complete the examination by a bidigital palpation with the index finger of one hand in the mouth and fingers of the other hand exerting upward pressure from below the jaw.

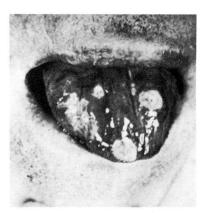

Fig. 236. Tuberculous ulcers of the tongue.

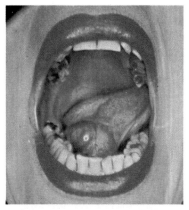

Fig. 237. A ranula is invariably translucent.

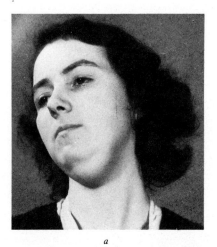

a

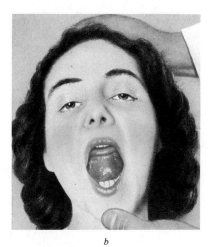

b

Fig. 238. Median sublingual dermoid cyst. a, The swelling beneath the chin; b, The swelling in the floor of the mouth.

Sublingual Dermoid Cyst can be either median (*Fig.* 238) or lateral, and either above or below the mylohyoid. When above the mylohyoid, the opaque white cyst is discernible through the normal mucous membrane; as it contains sebaceous material its opacity differs completely from the translucency of a ranula. In all cases the neck must be examined and the swelling palpated bimanually (*see Fig.* 199, p. 106). Should the cyst be median and below the mylohyoid, consider its possible relationship to the thyroglossal tract (*see* p. 162).

Carcinoma of the Floor of the Mouth. Frequently the lesion is discovered by the patient himself who, with the tip of his tongue, feels that there is something on the floor of the mouth. As the growth extends, it invades the fraenum, with the result that pain is experienced on movement of the tongue. Carcinoma of the floor of the mouth invades the lymphatics early, and spreads from the submandibular nodes to the deep cervical nodes. Untreated, it is not long before the mandible is invaded. The ulcerative form is particularly prone to become infected, often with Vincent's organisms and diagnosis is delayed in the belief that the lesion is entirely inflammatory. Once again an *indurated* ulcer in this region is almost certainly carcinomatous.

EXAMINATION OF THE MUCOSA OF THE CHEEK

The angle of the mouth is retracted, and the interior is illuminated with a torch.
Pigmented Patches. Frequently in Addison's disease, and occasionally in Peutz–Jeghers syndrome (*see* p. 109), the mucous membrane is dappled brown.
Aphthous Ulcer (*see* p. 111). A favourite site for such an ulcer is opposite the first molar tooth.
Leucoplakia. Although it attacks the cheek less often than the tongue, leucoplakia is by no means rare in the former situation.
Mucous Cyst. This is a somewhat common location (*see* p. 111).
Papilloma (*Fig.* 239) is frequently encountered on the mucous lining of the cheek.
Carcinoma of the cheek is less common than when quids of tobacco were chewed and pouched in the cheek, but it is still rife in those tropical countries where the inhabitants are addicted to betel-nut* chewing.

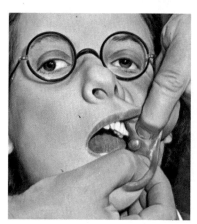

Fig. 239. Papilloma of the cheek.

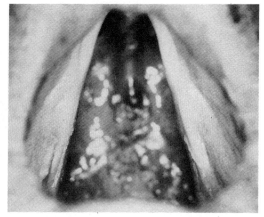

Fig. 240. Untreated cleft palate in a man aged 65 who had gone through life stoically enduring his disability.

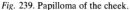

* *Betel-nut* = a few grains of the nut of the catechu palm rolled up in a leaf with quick-lime.

THOMAS ADDISON, 1793–1860, *Physician, Guy's Hospital, London.*

Further particulars of the methods to be employed in examining the cheek will be found on pp. 91 (swelling in the cheek), 101, and 103 (parotid duct).

EXAMINATION OF THE PALATE

The palatal rugae are five or six transverse ridges present on the hard palate varying in prominence in different individuals. Well developed in the newborn, no doubt to assist in sucking, as age advances they become flatter.

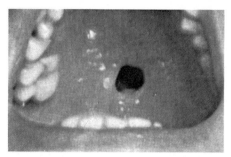

Fig. 241. A hole in the palate due to syphilis. This cause is now a rarity.

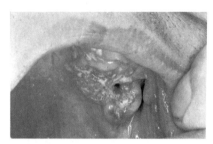

Fig. 242. Carcinoma of the palate.

Inspection of the palate is one of the very few occasions when physical examination is facilitated by an infant crying. The more the child cries the better the view obtained. If a cleft is present determine its extent, whether it involves the hard or the soft palate, or both. That the more mature patient has a hole or cleft in the palate can be suspected when he addresses you in that peculiar explosive nasal voice which accompanies a leakage of the sound waves into the nasal cavity.

Inspection of Palate. Ask the patient to tilt his head slightly backwards and to open his mouth to its fullest extent. If the light is good, the whole palate can be observed, and any abnormality detected at once (*Fig.* 240). Then ask him to say 'Ah'. Loss of movement of half the soft palate suggests a lesion of the vagus nerve (*see* p. 60) or an infiltrating neoplasm of the nasopharynx (*see* p. 132). Paralysis of the whole soft palate is found in the bulbar form of poliomyelitis. Normal movement of the whole soft palate facilitates visualization of the tonsils (*see* p. 129). The hard palate forms the inferior surface of the maxilla (*see* p. 95). *A Hole in the Middle of the Soft Palate* (*Fig.* 241) is presumptive evidence of previous syphilis (gumma). However, it is unwise to jump to a conclusion; when an operation for closure of a cleft palate has been only partially successful, a hole may be left in the middle line at the junction of the hard and the soft palate, and this is probably now a commoner cause than syphilis. Necrosis resulting from radiotherapy for a carcinoma in this region is another cause.

A Carcinoma can arise in the epithelium of the hard palate (*Fig.* 242) or the soft palate. Inability to wear an upper denture is sometimes the first symptom.

Tumour of an Ectopic Salivary Gland. The palate is the most frequent site, but these tumours may be found anywhere in the mouth or pharynx and even in the bronchi. In the beginning the tumour is symptomless and is noticed accidentally, but when ulceration occurs it becomes painful. A large proportion of these tumours are of low-grade malignancy (cylindroma) and may ultimately metastasize to the regional lymph nodes, the viscera and the skeleton. Locally, it may invade the base

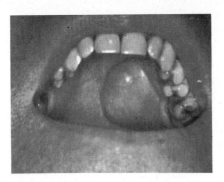

Fig. 243. Mixed tumour of an ectopic palatal salivary gland.

of the skull and implicate certain cranial nerves, causing severe pain in the distribution of the nerve or nerves involved. Mixed tumours also occur (*Fig.* 243).

Cyst of the Palate. A palatal mucous gland occasionally gives rise to a cyst similar to a cyst of other buccal mucous glands. Unless translucent, it is unsafe to assume this diagnosis.

Palatal Abscess. See pp. 117, 131.

Chapter 12

THE THROAT, NOSE AND NASAL SINUSES

Contrary to what is believed by many, much of this territory is available for clinical examination, and provided the clinician knows what to seek, and employs the correct method of seeking it, often he will be enabled to make a confident, or at least an intelligent tentative, diagnosis without the aid of specialized methods of examination.

Fig. 244. The component parts of the pharynx which, in the adult, is 13 cm in length: (A) Nasopharynx, into the lateral wall of which open the Eustachian tubes above which are the pharyngeal recesses (fossa of Rosenmüller); (B) Oropharynx; (C) Hypopharynx, which continues into the oesophagus at the level of C6 vertebra.

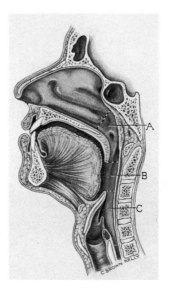

When examination by speculum, laryngeal or postnasal mirror, or X-rays is imperative, the necessity will be indicated, but details of such procedures and the resulting findings are beyond the scope of this work.
Surgical Anatomy is shown in *Figs.* 244 and 253.

THE OROPHARYNX AND THE NASOPHARYNX

Examination of the (Palatine) Tonsils. The tongue is depressed with a spatula, and, while the patient says 'Ah', the tonsils are inspected with the aid of a torch. To decide whether the tonsils (absent in the newborn) are normal in size and healthy or enlarged and/or diseased, it is necessary to display them. The best method is to depress the tongue with one spatula while the tip of a second spatula gently compresses the anterior pillar of the fauces (*Fig.* 245). This everts the tonsil from its bed. Increasing pressure will expose and open the crypts, and their content may be discharged. Pus (yellow) signifies inflammation; a whitish discharge may be normal.

BARTOLOMMEO EUSTACHIUS, 1513–1574, *Professor of Anatomy, Rome.*
JOHANN C. ROSENMÜLLER, 1771–1820, *Professor of Anatomy and Surgery, Leipzig.*

With the advent of puberty, lymphoid tissue diminishes, and the tonsils become smaller. Following recurrent attacks of tonsillitis the tonsillar lymph node (*see Fig.* 261, p. 139) is frequently palpable. Enlarged tonsils are not necessarily infected. Extensive protrusion of the tongue or its forcible depression make the tonsils appear larger. Occasionally the tonsils are so large that they almost meet in the midline but size is not important unless speech or breathing is interfered with. Unilateral enlargement may signify one of the following.

Carcinoma of the Tonsil. As a rule the patient is elderly, and severe pain radiating to the ear is frequently the chief complaint. The breath is foul and often the saliva is bloodstained: more severe haemorrhage is not unusual. Often carcinoma takes the form of an ulcer, direct palpation of which reveals characteristic induration. The tonsillar and other neighbouring lymph nodes become involved early.

Lymphosarcoma of the Tonsil. The patient is usually younger and the complaint is a lump in the throat, which, in the early stages, is quite painless. Thick speech is a common symptom. The tonsil appears large and pale and may mimic a peritonsillar abscess. Once the capsule of the tonsil has become eroded by the growth, extracapsular extension proceeds apace, and a palpable, and later visible, swelling occupies a characteristic position immediately behind and below the angle of the mandible. On this account, in spite of the fact that the cervical nodes soon become involved, a swelling in this position is likely to be an extension of the primary growth.

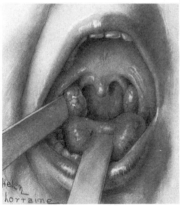

Fig. 245. By pressure against the anterior pillar of the fauces an apparently small buried tonsil may be everted from its bed. At the same time crypts are opened and their contents squeezed out.

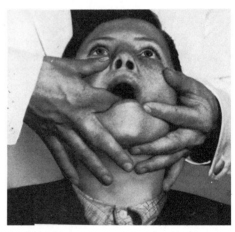

Fig. 246. Palpating the nasopharynx for adenoids.

Adenoids. The 'pharyngeal tonsil' is present at birth, persists through infancy and childhood, and undergoes atrophy before puberty. Remnants of this structure, so well marked in the very young, commonly persist into early adult life. Adenoids consist of hypertrophy of this structure. When pronounced, they form clusters of dangling 'vegetations'. Reference has been made already to the so-called 'adenoid facies' (*see* p. 89). Considerable adenoid hypertrophy causes the patient to snore loudly at night and to breathe through the mouth.

A reliable method of palpating the nasopharynx is shown in *Fig.* 246. Standing behind the seated patient (an infant is sat upon a nurse's lap) the index finger is passed into the mouth, and hooked around the posterior border of the soft palate. Swiftly, the pulp of the finger near the tip is swept over the roof and walls of the nasopharynx. The precaution to prevent the examiner's finger being bitten which has been described on p. 120, and is to be seen in *Figs.* 246 and 227, must be taken.

Alternatively, should the presence of adenoids be highly prŏbable by reason of mouth-breathing, nasal speech, nasal discharge, enlarged cervical lymph nodes, or recurrent attacks of deafness during head colds, rather than subject a young child to the psychological trauma of palpation of the nasopharynx, often it is advisable to postpone such palpation until the patient has been anaesthetized and proceed to remove the adenoids and, if need be, the tonsils, at that time. The objection to palpation of the nasopharynx of a child does not appertain with an infant.

Peritonsillar Abscess (Quinsy). The patient enters the consulting room with a handkerchief in his hand and the head held forwards and upwards. He talks as though he has a hot potato in his mouth, and makes frequent, painful swallowing movements. When asked where the pain is, he usually points to the region of the tonsillar lymph node (*see* p. 139). Some degree of trismus may make the examination difficult. Usually the abscess lies mainly in front of the corresponding faucial tonsil (*Fig.* 247). The soft palate on that side is bulging and oedematous.

A *posterior variety* of peritonsillar abscess pushes the tonsil forwards, the abscess being concealed partially thereby.

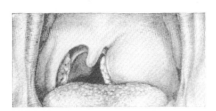

Fig. 247. Peritonsillar abscess.

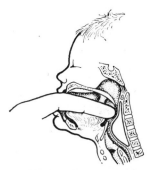

Fig. 248. Palpating an acute retropharyngeal abscess in an infant.

Acute Epiglottitis is uncommon but occasionally fatal. During early childhood there is sudden stridor, dysphagia and high pyrexia. It is usually difficult to obtain a view of the oropharynx but on doing so a bright red swelling is seen at the base of the tongue like a rising or setting sun—the inflamed and enlarged epiglottis.

Retropharyngeal Abscess is of two varieties—acute and chronic. The former, sometimes being an immediate menace to life, calls for urgent and precise diagnosis as a prelude to drainage without delay.

Acute Retropharyngeal Abscess is caused by suppuration within, and breakdown of, one or more of the lymph nodes that normally occupy the retropharyngeal space. The patient is often, but not necessarily, an infant. The apex of the abscess is opposite the glottis and interference with deglutition and respiration is caused. In order to maintain an adequate airway a child will hold its head in full extension with its mouth open—a position that is practically pathognomonic. The temperature is usually greatly raised. Note that the retropharyngeal space, which is a fascial space sandwiched between the pharynx in front and the prevertebral fascia behind, is divided completely in the midline by a strong fascial septum into a right and a left compartment; consequently the swelling of an acute retropharyngeal abscess is *always on one side of the midline*. Sometimes the abscess can be seen by depressing the tongue; it can always be felt (*Fig.* 248) as an indentable, cushion-like projection if the finger is introduced into the mouth to allow the tip of the digit to impinge upon the swelling.

Chronic Retropharyngeal Abscess. With the decline in the incidence of tuberculosis, chronic retropharyngeal abscess arising from a cervical vertebra is encountered rarely, although it is commoner in those parts of the world where the population has low resistance to tuberculosis. Such an abscess lies *behind* the prevertebral fascia and consequently occupies the midline. In this instance the symptoms of the abscess are slight compared with those of the cervical caries (*see* p. 152). Cases of chronic retropharyngeal abscess due to tuberculous retropharyngeal lymph nodes are commoner. In this instance the pus lies *in front* of the prevertebral fascia in the retropharyngeal space, and is likely to occupy the right or the left compartment as does an acute abscess, and gives rise to a unilateral swelling which, as it enlarges, causes a fullness in the neck behind the sternomastoid muscle. This outward swelling, rather than difficulty in swallowing or in breathing, first calls attention to this type of chronic abscess. The abscess can also be seen as well as felt at the back of the pharynx.

Neoplasms of the Nasopharynx. *Carcinoma*: Although it occurs relatively uncommonly the world over, in the Far East carcinoma of the nasopharynx is more common than malignant disease in any part of the body save the cervix uteri. Fifty per cent arise in the lateral wall, mostly in the fossa of Rosenmüller. The rest are divided equally between the roof and the posterior wall.

The patient presents with some of the following: (1) Slight intermittent epistaxis; (2) Nasal obstruction; (3) Pain in the ear, and not infrequently other signs of middle-ear disease due to blockage of the Eustachian tube; (4) Loss of movement of the soft palate on the affected side due to infiltration by the growth; (5) A mass in the neck (metastases in the cervical lymph nodes); (6) Cranial nerve involvement due to implication of one or more nerves at the base of the skull (*see Fig.* 276, p. 145); (7) Proptosis (*see* p. 76), due to lateral extension of the growth into the orbit, is rare.

The extremely poor prognosis is due, in part, to the lack of symptoms until late, but there is no gainsaying that often delay results from perfunctory examination by the clinician to whom the patient first reported. See again the method of digital examination of this inaccessible region on p. 130.

Juvenile Postnasal Angiofibroma is almost confined to males about the age of puberty, and when a boy presents with progressive nasal obstruction, recurrent epistaxis, a purulent nasal discharge, and on palpation of the nasopharynx, as for adenoids, a firm bosselated mass occluding the choanae* is felt, the diagnosis is certain. Mirror visualization of the postnasal space is necessary for confirmation and will reveal a reddish, firm tumour covered with normal mucous membrane.

THE HYPOPHARYNX

Carcinoma of the Hypopharynx. That hoarseness not obviously improving after more than a week calls for examination with a laryngoscope is axiomatic. Only in 20 per cent of cases is the first symptom vocal in nature.

---

* *Choanae* (posterior nares). Greek, χοάνη = a funnel.

Carcinoma of the Piriform Fossa. In a high proportion of cases a neoplasm commences in a part of the hypopharynx removed from the vocal cords, i.e. the piriform fossa, where it is notoriously silent, and often the first intimation is an enlarged lymph node behind the angle of the jaw. However, from time to time a patient presents on account of difficulty in swallowing saliva as opposed to food. The growth is beyond the reach of digital detection. Examination with the laryngeal mirror is the key to its elucidation.

Postcricoid Carcinoma. Attention is directed to the frequency with which neglected cases of sideropaenic dysphagia (*see* p. 198) result in this.

A Late Sign in Growths of the Hypopharynx. The larynx is normally mobile from side to side. When a growth has infiltrated the prevertebral fascia this mobility is reduced or absent.

THE LARYNX

Hoarseness or loss of voice is the presenting symptom of diseases of the vocal cords. Ordinary clinical examination is of no value with the exception of a search for enlarged lymph nodes. These are involved relatively late in carcinoma of the cords. Examination with the laryngeal mirror is the essential method of examination.

Laryngeal Fractures are seen increasingly with serious car accidents. Other severe injuries tend to mask the following salient features (due to fractures of the thyroid cartilage and hyoid bone and detachment of the vocal cords): (1) loss of voice, (2) local pain, (3) respiratory obstruction causing stridor (*see* p. 179), (4) subcutaneous emphysema (*see* p. 16).

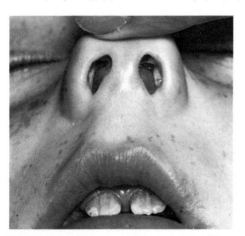

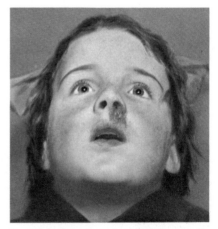

Fig. 249. Bilateral haematoma of the nasal septum following a blow on the nose.

Fig. 250. Unilateral excoriated nostril due to discharge resulting from a foreign body in the nose.

THE NOSE

A useful sign which may be present in most of the conditions described below, but particularly in *deviated nasal septum*, is elicited by asking the patient to exhale through the nose while the naris is occluded by finger pressure on the ala nasi, each side being tested in turn. Normally there is free and equal egress of air through each nasal passage.

A better view of the nasal cavities is obtained by tilting the patient's head back and elevating the tip of the nose with the thumb (*Fig.* 249).

Foreign Body in the Nose. When a child is brought by a parent with a purulent nasal discharge, and that discharge is found to be unilateral (*Fig.* 250), the first question that should spring to mind is, 'Is there a foreign body?' Simple inspection and use of the nasal speculum will usually settle this point.

Snuffles is a term reserved for a mucopurulent discharge from one or, more usually, both nostrils occurring in infants as a stringy, tenacious snot that travels in and out of the nares during inspiration and expiration, causing a characteristic noise. It is commonly associated with enlarged adenoids or deviated nasal septum, and calls for digital examination of the nasopharynx.

Nasal Choanal Atresia. *See* p. 89.

Fracture of the Nasal Bones probably occurs more often than any other fracture, except those of the wrist and the clavicle. Any blow upon the nose that causes bleeding from the nose may signify that the bone or cartilage has been broken or displaced. There are two types:

1. *Depressed Fracture* due to a blow from in front causing one, or, more usually, both nasal bones to be displaced downwards and inwards. As a haematoma often conceals the depression, both inspection and gentle palpation may fail to detect that the nasal bones have been driven inwards.

2. *Lateral Fracture.* One nasal bone is driven inwards and the other outwards, the nasal septum being involved. That the nose is crooked is sometimes obvious, at other times it requires more careful scrutiny.

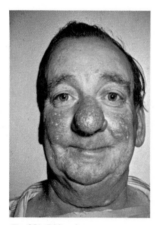

Fig. 251. Rhinophyma.

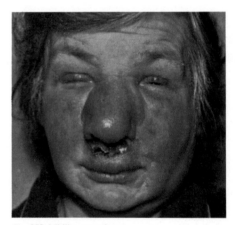

Fig. 252. Midline granuloma.

A copious fluid discharge, too thin to be pure blood, suggests a fracture of the cribriform plate of the ethmoid with leakage of cerebrospinal fluid (*see* p. 60). A sharp lookout should be kept as to whether blood issuing from the nose is diluted.

Haematoma of the Nasal Septum. Blood beneath the mucoperichondrium is due to injury except in defective blood coagulation, e.g. haemophilia. As a rule, the patient complains of headache. The mouth is held slightly open, the nostrils are splayed and the anterior end of the nose is widened.

Frequently with considerable extravasation, the skin over the tip of the nose is pale from stretching, and there is loss of sensation due to pressure on the anterior ethmoidal nerve. The haematoma is commonly bilateral (*Fig.* 249). The mucoperichondrium is very strong, and blood and pus can be locked in the septal sac for weeks, in which case the nasal cartilage, deprived of its main blood supply undergoes slow necrosis. Should the haematoma become infected, pyrexia and increased headache follow.

Rhinophyma. Dubbed by the ignorant 'bottle-nose', it is due to multiple sebaceous adenomata of the skin that cover the distal half or two-thirds (*Fig.* 251).

Midline Granuloma of the Nose. The course of this, fortunately rare, disease is divided into three stages: prodromal, active and terminal. The first stage is insidious and is characterized by a minor degree of nasal obstruction, usually unilateral, later associated with a watery nasal discharge: eventually the discharge becomes bloodstained and causes the patient to seek advice. In the second stage the obstruction increases, the discharge becomes foul and granulation tissue can be seen in the nasal passages. Spreading cellulitis of the face supervenes (*Fig.* 252): there is no pain. Sooner or later intranasal ulceration ensues, progresses and results in widespread necrosis of the nasal skeleton and the walls of the accessory nasal sinuses. Untreated, if the patient survives long enough, the whole face between the eyes and the mandible becomes destroyed.*

The Saddle-nose of Syphilis (*see* p. 89) **and Leprosy** (*see* p. 415).

New Growths of the Nasal Vestibule. Being lined by skin it is liable to the neoplasms mentioned on p. 36 and to malignant melanoma (*see* p. 24). Basal-cell carcinoma is the commonest.

THE ACCESSORY NASAL SINUSES

As shown in *Fig.* 253, the accessory nasal sinuses accessible for clinical examination are the frontal, ethmoidal and maxillary. The area of maximum tenderness for each is depicted. A unilateral purulent nasal discharge (if a foreign body (p. 134) is excluded) indicates suppuration or neoplasm of one of the sinuses.

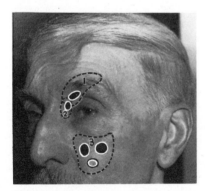

Fig. 253. Surface markings of (1) frontal, (2) ethmoidal, (3) maxillary sinuses. The black areas show where to palpate for tenderness on the cutaneous surface; white area, where to palpate from inside the mouth.

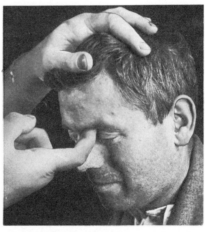

Fig. 254. Eliciting tenderness over the floor of the frontal sinus.

---

* In Brazil a similar destruction is seen due to a variety of Leishmaniasis and is known as 'espundia'.

Acute Frontal Sinusitis. Most sufferers are older children or young adults. The usual antecedent history is that in the course of a heavy cold the patient develops malaise, some elevation of temperature, and pain located over the sinus. Diving, and especially plunging feet first into water from a height, are also well-known initiating causes. Usually the localized headache commences one or two hours after rising, increases in severity towards noon, and diminishes in the middle of the afternoon; sometimes it radiates to the temporal area.

Tenderness over the affected sinus (*Fig.* 253) may be present, especially if free drainage is obstructed. To elicit tenderness the fingertip must be insinuated beneath the roof of the orbit towards the medial extremity of the sinus and pressure directed upwards (*Fig.* 254).

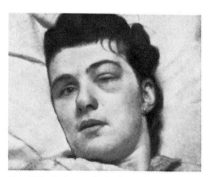

Fig. 255. Oedema of the lids of the left eye secondary to acute frontal sinusitis with ethmoiditis.

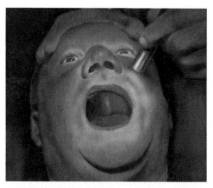

Fig. 256. In ordinary clinical practice transillumination by this method can be carried out effectively in a *darkened* room. Test first one side, then the other and compare illumination as seen through the palate.

So long as drainage can occur along the duct the symptoms remain comparatively mild; should drainage cease, often a rapid, progressive, fulminating inflammation sets in, and is heralded by an exacerbation of the general symptoms, together with oedema of the eyelids of the affected side (*Fig.* 255). Unless efficient treatment is instituted, serious complications may follow. These include orbital cellulitis (*see* p. 69), osteomyelitis of the frontal bone (*see* p. 56), extradural abscess, subdural abscess, meningitis, brain abscess and sagittal sinus thrombosis. A combination of acute frontal sinusitis and ethmoiditis is common.

Acute Suppurative Ethmoiditis *per se* is comparatively rare. Sinusitis in infants and young children is largely confined to the ethmoid, the only sinus well developed early in life. As a rule one of the acute infectious diseases, such as scarlet fever or measles, precedes its onset. The constitutional signs are slight pyrexia, sometimes accompanied by mild toxaemia. Swelling of the eyelids on the affected side occurs early and regularly. The symptoms include headache with pain radiating to the back of the eye. Unilateral nasal obstruction is present, with tenderness over the eyeball. In order to elicit tenderness over the ethmoidal cell labyrinth, pressure should be directed over the area indicated in *Fig.* 253 (2).

Chronic Frontal Sinusitis is occasionally a cause of obscure headache, the unilateral character of which is liable to be mistaken for migraine.

Acute Maxillary Sinusitis. As the maxillary antrum does not attain full development until the twelfth year, serious infections of this cavity are more likely to occur in patients past that age. Like frontal sinusitis, the most usual precursor is the common cold, but less frequent causes are infection due to extension from an apical dental abscess or as the result of perforation of the floor of the antrum during extraction of an infected tooth.

The constitutional symptoms are often severe, especially when the pus is confined by occlusion of the natural ostium. Dull throbbing pain in the cheek, and in the upper teeth when the patient stoops, is characteristic. Commonly the patient considers that he is suffering from toothache, and visits a dental surgeon. Frequently the affected side of the face is swollen and the lower eyelid is somewhat oedematous. Breathing through the nostril on the side of the lesion is impaired, and often obstructed completely. Not until the third or fourth day of the attack is a unilateral purulent discharge much in evidence. Local tenderness over the antrum is an important sign. Transillumination of the antrum is helpful (*Fig.* 256), but radiography is much more reliable.

The Differentiation of a Rapidly Growing Neoplasm from Inflammation. Several demonstrations of extreme activity of a malignant growth giving rise to local redness and increased local temperature have been described in this book. Here is a poignant example. Two patients presented, one with inflammation over the maxillary sinus (*Fig.* 257) and the other with a rapidly growing neoplasm in the same situation (*Fig.* 258). In the latter case there was neither tenderness nor softening over the swelling. The former's temperature was elevated.

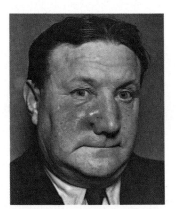

Fig. 257. Periostitis of the right maxilla with involvement of the subcutis.

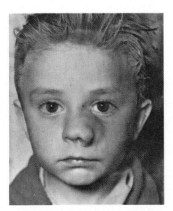

Fig. 258. Sarcoma of the left maxilla.

Chronic Maxillary Sinusitis. The essential features are a long-continued unilateral nasal discharge, local tenderness, and pain. Rhinoscopy is essential, for so often the condition is associated with nasal polypi. Transillumination and X-rays are necessary to establish the diagnosis.

Oro-antral Fistula with Prolapsing Polyp. As mentioned under 'Acute Maxillary Sinusitis' *above*, a fistula due to tooth extraction causes sinusitis which becomes chronic with polyp formation. To the patient's consternation the polyp may suddenly appear in the mouth as a soft transparent pink swelling.

Neoplasms of the Accessory Air Sinuses. The maxillary and ethmoidal sinuses are affected, rarely the frontal. At first the symptoms suggest chronic sinusitis with identical clinical findings. Later local swelling occurs (*see* Examination of the Maxilla, p. 94) and epiphora (*see* p. 72). Upward displacement of the eye (maxillary tumours) or lateral displacement (ethmoid tumours) is a late sign.

Chapter 13

THE NECK (EXCLUDING THE THYROID GLAND)

When the neck is to be examined all clothing is removed as far as the axillae, which allows the whole neck to be seen in relationship to the thorax and permits inspection and palpation of the supraclavicular fossae. When enlarged lymph nodes are found it is often necessary to examine the breasts adequately.

EXAMINATION OF THE LATERAL REGIONS OF THE NECK

The key to the lateral region of the neck is the sternomastoid muscle. Bearings are taken from this structure, first with the eye and then with the fingers.

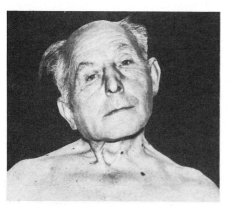

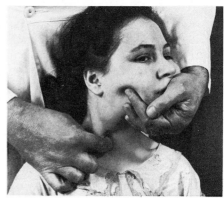

Fig. 259. Long-standing torticollis, often the sequel of a neglected sternomastoid 'tumour' of infancy.

Fig. 260. Determining the relationship of a cervical swelling to the sternomastoid.

Sternomastoid 'Tumour'. If there is a swelling obviously *in* the sternomastoid muscle, and the patient is an infant (who has usually undergone breech delivery), it is an example of the so-called sternomastoid 'tumour'.

Torticollis (Wry-neck). When one sternomastoid is tense and the head is held, even slightly, on one side, ask the patient to try to straighten the neck: if the case be one of torticollis (*Fig.* 259) he or she cannot do so, but with the attempt the sternomastoid, especially its sternal head, stands out.

Particularly in the case of a child, it is important to differentiate *ocular torticollis* due to a squint (usually involving one of the rotatory muscles of the eyeball) from a wry-neck due to shortening of one sternomastoid. The examiner clasps the head, and slowly straightens it, at the same time watching the patient's eyes. In ocular torticollis, on straightening the head a squint will become apparent.

In congenital torticollis (i.e. presenting in infancy) one-third are found to be associated with sternomastoid tumour and the rest are due to an abnormal position *in utero*, no 'tumour' being found. This variety recovers spontaneously in a few weeks (Hulbert).

In any case of torticollis of long standing, study the face critically; the features on the affected side will be seen to be, perhaps very slightly, less well developed than those of the opposite side.

Determining the Relationship of a Cervical Swelling to the Sternomastoid. Commonly, when it flanks a lateral cervical swelling the muscle becomes thin and flattened out; consequently, more often than not, by mere palpation it is impossible to determine the relationship of the swelling to the sternomastoid unless it is rendered taut. Stand behind the patient. Ask him to push his chin as hard as possible against the palm of your hand (*Fig.* 260). This makes the muscle tense. With the other hand palpate the sternomastoid from below (where it is normal) upwards, paying special attention to the anterior border.

PALPATION OF THE CERVICAL LYMPH NODES

Always conduct this examination from behind. In order that no lymph node shall be overlooked, it is well to have a routine that scrutinizes every group. *Fig.* 261 shows a useful order.

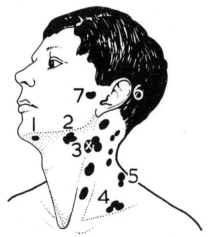

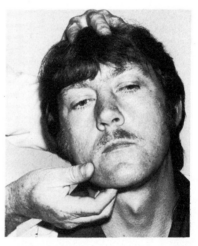

Fig. 261. Order in which various groups of cervical lymph nodes are best palpated: (1) Submental; (2) Submandibular; (3) Jugular chain; (4) Supraclavicular; (5) Posterior triangle; (6) Postauricular; (7) Pre-auricular. The node marked X is the tonsillar (jugulodigastric) lymph node.

Fig. 262. Palpating the submandibular group of cervical lymph nodes. The hand on the head enables the clinician to adjust the degree of flexion.

The submandibular nodes are rendered more easily palpable by flexion of the head (*Fig.* 262). This manœuvre is also of value in examining the supraclavicular nodes (*Fig.* 263), but in this instance a second method of examination sometimes becomes necessary (*Fig.* 264).

The lymph nodes of the posterior triangle consist of scattered nodes in the main part of this large triangle; there is also a small group of nodes situated in the apex of the triangle, and known as the suboccipital group, but attention is

KENNETH F. HULBERT, *Contemporary Emeritus Orthopaedic Surgeon, Dartford Group Hospitals, Kent.*

drawn especially to the chain of nodes lying along the posterior border of the sternomastoid.

If any of the nodes are found enlarged the possible sources of infection or of a primary growth are examined next—scalp, tongue, mouth, tonsil, ear, etc.— and particular attention is paid to the area drained by those found to be diseased (e.g. if the posterior triangle and/or posterior auricular region contain enlarged nodes, the scalp must be examined with scrupulous care). The supraclavicular nodes, particularly on the left side, may be enlarged with carcinoma of the stomach (*Troisier's sign*) or any other abdominal organ, and, increasingly, with carcinoma of the bronchus.

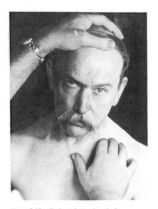

Fig. 263. Palpating the left supra-clavicular fossa from in front. If the examination is negative, in certain cases it is necessary to rise, stand behind the patient, and carry out palpation from behind.

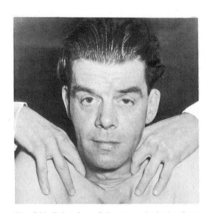

Fig. 264. Palpation of the supraclavicular fossa from behind, with the patient elevating and hunching forward his shoulders.

DIFFERENTIAL DIAGNOSIS OF A SOLID SWELLING OF THE NECK

Tuberculous Lymph Nodes. Except in populations with low immunity (e.g. the Indian subcontinent; people of African descent) this condition has become distinctly uncommon. The tonsillar node (*Fig.* 267) is often the first to become enlarged. This subject is dealt with more fully on p. 142.

A Lymphoma. Hodgkin's disease (syn. lymphadenoma) produces large, discrete, non-tender lymph nodes of firm rubbery consistency (*Fig.* 265). Palpate the axillae and the groins: the finding of a similar mass in one or both of these situations tends to support an hypothesis that will be strengthened if an abdominal examination reveals an enlargement of the spleen. Lymphosarcoma and other lymphomata cause softer but still discrete enlargements. The exact diagnosis rests on biopsy.

Carcinomatous Lymph Nodes. The leading characteristic of secondary malignant nodes (*Fig.* 266) is the stony-hard impression they impart to the palpating fingers.

On many occasions the greater cornu of the hyoid bone is mistaken for a hard fixed lymph node. In elderly subjects it tends to become ossified, when it

CHARLES E. TROISIER, 1844–1919, *Professor of Pathology, Paris.*
THOMAS HODGKIN, 1798–1866, *Curator of the Museum, Guy's Hospital, London, where he failed to obtain the post of Physician. Thenceforth abandoning medicine he became a missionary. For 36 years Hodgkin's description of the disease remained unnoticed.*

certainly does simulate a hard node: however, it lies farther forward than the lymph nodes of the jugular chain, and its true nature can be revealed by asking the patient to swallow, when the bone will move upwards.

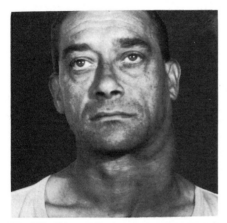

Fig. 265. This massive lymphatic enlargement is composed of rather discrete lumps which feel firm like solid rubber. A case of advanced Hodgkin's disease.

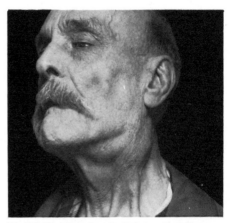

Fig. 266. These lymph nodes feel stony hard. The mass behind the sternomastoid is fixed to deeper structures. The primary growth was found on laryngoscopic examination. Case of carcinoma of the hypopharynx (see p. 132).

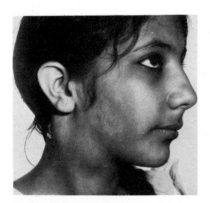

Fig. 267. Tuberculous enlargement of the tonsillar lymph node (Stage I).

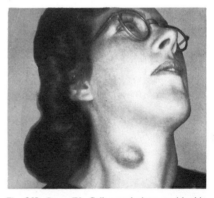

Fig. 268. Stage IV. Collar-stud abscess with skin involvement.

If the physical characteristics of the enlarged nodes leave little doubt that they are malignant, but no primary growth can be discovered easily, a search must be made of the mouth, nasopharynx, hypopharynx, and larynx, thyroid, lung fields, and external auditory canal for the primary growth. If a source is still wanting biopsy may provide a clue to the origin as silent abdominal primaries sometimes metastasize to cervical lymph nodes.

Carotid Body Tumour. *See* p. 144.

THE STAGES THROUGH WHICH A BREAKING-DOWN TUBERCULOUS CERVICAL LYMPH NODE (OR NODES) PASSES

When any infected deep cervical lymph node (or group of lymph nodes) breaks down, it passes through stages each of which possesses physical signs peculiar to itself. Tuberculosis is the usual cause for the sequence to be described, but chronic pyogenic inflammation can cause identical signs. The stages, which like Hogarth's 'Rake' pass from bad to worse, are four in number:

Stage I. The physical signs are those of a solid enlargement due to inflammation (*Fig.* 267).

Stage II. In many instances, in due course, 'the lymph node breaks down and liquefies, and the pus comes to occupy the confined space beneath the deep cervical fascia ———————————→
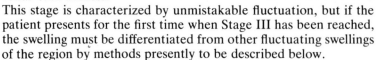
Fluctuation can be elicited but, owing to the depth of the swelling and the tenseness of the contained fluid, there may be doubt.

Stage III. After weeks or months, the dense, deep cervical fascial sheet becomes eroded, and the imprisoned pus, joyous, as it were, to escape from such a confined space, wells into the commodious compartment beneath the yielding superficial fascia, forming a collar-stud abscess. ———————————————————————→
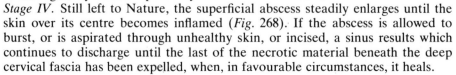
This stage is characterized by unmistakable fluctuation, but if the patient presents for the first time when Stage III has been reached, the swelling must be differentiated from other fluctuating swellings of the region by methods presently to be described below.

Stage IV. Still left to Nature, the superficial abscess steadily enlarges until the skin over its centre becomes inflamed (*Fig.* 268). If the abscess is allowed to burst, or is aspirated through unhealthy skin, or incised, a sinus results which continues to discharge until the last of the necrotic material beneath the deep cervical fascia has been expelled, when, in favourable circumstances, it heals.

Less Orthodox Cases. *a.* In a few cases the stem of the collar-stud is long: the tuberculous nodes that feed the abscess are situated some distance away, perhaps in another triangle of the neck. If the more distant areas of the neck are not palpated thoroughly for enlarged lymph nodes, such an abscess (*Fig.* 269) will perplex the clinician.

b. When, as is not rarely the case, the tuberculous process is entirely limited to a small group of nodes, and the abscess is situated directly over them, the diagnosis is far from simple, for the enlarged nodes are masked by the abscess. In such a case, provided the overlying abscess is of moderate size, try to palpate deeply behind the swelling with the finger and thumb (*Fig.* 270).

OTHER LATERAL CYSTIC SWELLINGS OF THE NECK

Cystic Hygroma is met with in infancy or early childhood (*Fig.* 271). Due to intercommunication of its many compartments, the swelling is softly cystic, and is partially compressible, but the characteristic sign that distinguishes it from all other cervical swellings is that it is brilliantly translucent. Occasionally, as a result of nasopharyngeal infection, the swelling becomes inflamed and may increase in size rapidly. Cystic hygromata, which are a variety of lymphangioma, occur also in the axilla, and rarely in the groin.

Branchial Cyst is very much more common than the foregoing, and usually it is encountered not, as one might expect, in childhood but in early adult life. Almost without exception the patient presents with a cystic swelling of the upper

---

Wᴉʟʟɪᴀᴍ Hᴏɢᴀʀᴛʜ, 1697–1764. *Celebrated engraver and painter who satirized the follies of his time in a series of engravings.*

third of the neck, deep to the upper third of the sternomastoid muscle, appearing around its anterior border (*Fig.* 272). This is the most common situation for a tuberculous cervical abscess. Occasionally the cyst becomes the seat of attacks of inflammation. When uncomplicated by inflammation, it imparts to the palpating fingers what has been described admirably as the sensation given by a half-filled rubber hot-water bottle.

If some of the fluid is aspirated pus-like material will be withdrawn from both a branchial cyst and a tuberculous abscess. With the former, when this is put in a dish and rocked to and fro, the shimmer of the lipoid content probably

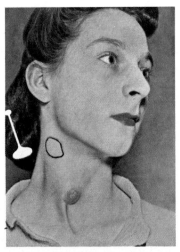

Fig. 269. Long-stemmed collar-stud abscess.

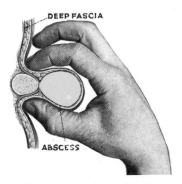

Fig. 270. By deep palpation between the finger and thumb an enlarged node can sometimes be felt beneath the cervical fascia.

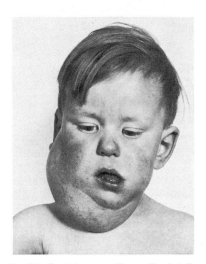

Fig. 271. Cystic hygroma. The swelling is brilliantly translucent.

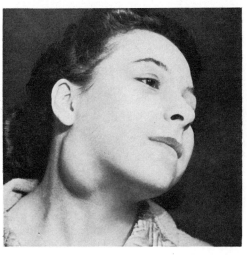

Fig. 272. A typical branchial cyst. Note its relationship to the upper third of the sternomastoid.

will be noted, and a drop placed under the microscope will show an abundance of cholesterol crystals because the lining mucous membrane contains sebaceous glands.

SOME RARER CERVICAL CLINICAL ENTITIES

Branchial Fistula. Nearly always this is congenital, and commences to discharge soon after birth. Occasionally the condition is bilateral. Commonly the orifice of the sinus is situated fairly low (*Fig.* 273). The amount of excretion varies, and it is inclined to be sticky. Branchial fistulae are prone to attacks of inflammation, especially when the small orifice becomes temporarily occluded, and the discharge becomes pent up in the commodious interior (*Fig.* 273, inset). As a rule the track is incomplete, and ends blindly in the region of the lateral pharyngeal wall. From time to time a complete fistula has an internal orifice situated just behind the tonsil. A fistula can be acquired by incision of an inflamed branchial cyst. The resulting sinus, which is usually situated in the upper third of the neck, continues to discharge, either continuously or intermittently.

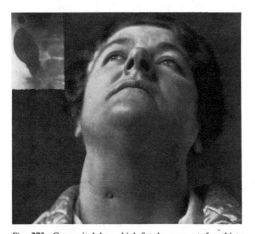

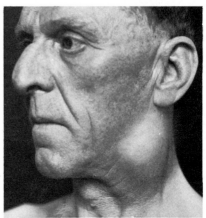

Fig. 273. Congenital branchial fistula, present for thirty years. Inset shows a radiograph after the sinus had been injected with lipiodol.

Fig. 274. This swelling has been growing slowly for several years. The lump is hard and rather smooth, and transmitted pulsation can be felt. Case of carotid body tumour.

Carotid Body Tumour is situated at the bifurcation of the carotid artery, most usually in its fork. Nearly always unilateral, it exhibits transmitted pulsation (*see* p. 27). An enlarged lymph node in this area can give rise to similar signs. Usually the swelling first becomes apparent in middle life, and increases in size very slowly. As it becomes larger, it extends upwards. It is hard, tolerably regular in contour (*Fig.* 274), and shaped rather like a potato; Hutchinson termed it 'the potato tumour'. The lump can be moved horizontally with ease, but has very little vertical mobility. A few patients complain of attacks of faintness; particularly in thin persons, pressure over the lump sometimes gives rise to slowing of the pulse rate and a feeling of faintness—carotid-body syncope. Although as a rule the neoplasm remains localized for years, eventually regional metastases occur in 20 per cent of cases, and distant metastases rarely.

SIR JONATHAN HUTCHINSON, 1828–1913, *Surgeon, The London Hospital.*

Pharyngeal Pouch. Those suffering from this condition are usually, but not necessarily, elderly, and it is commoner in men than in women. The leading complaint is regurgitation of undigested food at an unpredictable time after a meal, during swallowing of the next meal, or after turning from one side to the other at night. Sometimes the patient is awakened from sleep by a violent fit of coughing. As the pouch enlarges there are gurgling noises in the neck, especially during swallowing. Later the pouch causes a visible swelling in the neck (*Fig.* 275), usually on the left side which is softly cystic, and when pressed upon the contents of the pouch—often foul fluid—are emptied into the pharynx and mouth; sometimes this is accompanied by audible and palpable gurgling. At this stage, the symptom that transcends all others is increasing dysphagia.

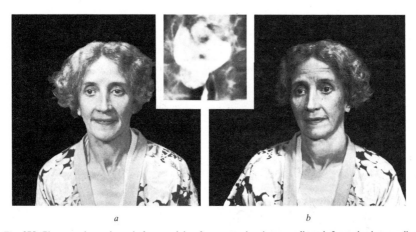

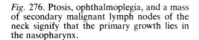

Fig. 275. Pharyngeal pouch: *a*, before, and *b*, after, water has been swallowed. Inset, barium swallow, anterior view.

Fig. 276. Ptosis, ophthalmoplegia, and a mass of secondary malignant lymph nodes of the neck signify that the primary growth lies in the nasopharynx.

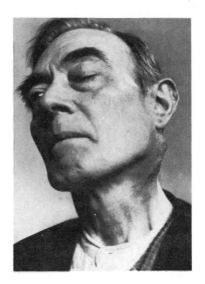

Cervical Metastases of a Carcinoma of the Nasopharynx (*see* p. 132). When a mass of metastatic cervical lymph nodes is present (*Fig.* 276), the primary growth has, almost certainly, invaded the sphenoidal fissure. Through the sphenoidal fissure pass the third, fourth, ophthalmic divisions of the fifth, and sixth nerves; these may become implicated. Armed with this knowledge a precise diagnosis of this seemingly obscure and depressing condition becomes a matter of relative simplicity.

Tumours of Nerve can arise in the vagus, the hypoglossal, the sympathetic chain, or a cord of the brachial plexus and give rise to a firm, slowly growing, painless lump which is movable vertically but not horizontally, and is inclined to displace the external carotid artery anteriorly. In the case of a tumour of part of the brachial plexus it is vital not to remove the swelling without adequate exploration, on the mistaken diagnosis of 'enlarged lymph node'. Pressure on such a swelling will often cause pain down the arm in the distribution of the affected nerve.

Laryngocele is a unilateral (occasionally bilateral), narrow-necked, air-containing diverticulum resulting from herniation of the mucous membrane through the thyrohyoid membrane where it is pierced by the superior laryngeal vessels. When distended, it forms a visible, often resonant, swelling in the neck. It should be suspected if a swelling appears when the patient blows his nose (*Fig.* 277). It occurs in professional trumpet players, glass-blowers, and persons with a chronic cough. Cervical air pouches are present in many mammals, and can be inflated voluntarily. Certain South American monkeys utilize them for howling (howling pouches).

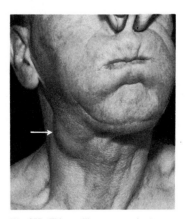

Fig. 277. This swelling appeared when the patient blew his nose (laryngocele).

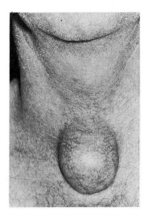

Fig. 278. A lipoma in Burns's space.

A Swelling in the Suprasternal (Burns's) Space is rare. It is rendered more prominent by asking the patient to extend the neck fully. If cystic, it is usually a dermoid, but aspiration will differentiate it from a cold abscess. Solid swellings are usually lipomas (*Fig.* 278) or enlarged lymph nodes. An aneurysm of the innominate artery exhibits expansile pulsation (*see* p. 27).

Subcutaneous Emphysema of the Neck following Rupture of the Oesophagus. *See* p. 196.

PRESSURE ON STRUCTURES AT THE ROOT OF THE NECK

Cervical Rib Syndrome (Scalene Syndrome; Superior Thoracic Aperture* Syndrome). Cervical ribs are not uncommon (0·4 per cent) and in 70 per cent the rib is bilateral. As a rule, there are no symptoms whatsoever. Conversely

---

* Paris anatomical nomenclature, which obviates the previous confusion between thoracic outlet and thoracic inlet, both of which were (and are) being used to denote this aperture.

ALLAN BURNS, 1781–1813, *Lecturer in Surgery and Anatomy, Glasgow.*

patients with symptoms and signs more frequently do not possess a cervical rib, the pressure presumably being caused by the vice-like action of the scalenus anterior and medius muscles on the structures running between them.

Normally, with the arm by the side, while the lower trunk of the brachial plexus runs straight downwards, the subclavian artery describes a smooth curve over the broad upper surface of the first rib. Should the 7th cervical vertebra possess a rib, or a fibrous band representing that structure, the curve taken by the nerve and the artery to ascend over the comparatively narrow surface of the cervical rib is much accentuated. For this reason, especially if the shoulder sags, vascular symptoms or, less frequently, nerve pressure symptoms, or both, sometimes supervene. Symptoms seldom appear before late adolescence, and in some instances they are precipitated by the patient's occupation, e.g. the postman with his bag, or by a change in occupation. Females are affected in a ratio of 2:1.

Vascular Symptoms. Pallor, coldness, or cyanosis of the hands or fingers occur. In advanced cases, partial thrombosis of the subclavian artery leads to small emboli being thrown off and peripheral gangrene, particularly of the tip of the index finger, occurs occasionally. The differential diagnosis from Raynaud's phenomenon (*see* p. 383) may prove difficult. When a cervical rib is the cause, usually these symptoms are entirely unilateral; they tend to come on towards the end of the day or at night, and are often improved by raising the limb. Also, often the radial pulse becomes perceptibly weaker when the arm is forcibly depressed by traction in a downward direction, but unfortunately, from the diagnostic standpoint, this phenomenon sometimes can be demonstrated in normal persons. More reliable is obliteration of the pulse by tensing the scalenus anterior muscle.

Adson's Deep-breathing Test depends on the fact that the scalenus anterior is an accessory muscle of respiration. Feel the radial pulse of the seated patient, who is requested to turn the head as far as possible *towards* the side of the symptoms. When asked, the patient takes a deep breath, and holds it. If inspiration causes a diminution or obliteration of the pulse, the sign is positive.

A Subclavian Murmur suggests that the artery is angulated over an obstruction.

Nerve Pressure Symptoms. It is now realized that these are rare with the cervical rib syndrome (*see* Pain in the Upper Limb, p. 466). Unlike the carpal tunnel syndrome (*see* p. 461), shooting pain is usually ulnar in distribution and such pain may be associated with aching in the shoulder or the scapular region. The pain in the elbow tunnel syndrome (*see* p. 455) has a similar distribution but the muscle weakness is strictly confined to the territory of the ulnar nerve whereas in the cervical rib syndrome the muscles affected most severely are those supplied by T.1. Thus all the small muscles of the hand suffer, but not uncommonly wasting of the thenar eminence is especially noticeable (*see* Fig. 4, p. 4) and hypothenar wasting is generally present as well. Cutaneous hyperaesthesia or sensory loss is unusual but if present is confined to the T.1. dermatome.

Examination of the Region of the Superior Thoracic Aperture. First, look and feel in the supraclavicular fossa for an abnormally elevated subclavian artery. The lump produced by the displaced artery not only pulsates, but is tender, and pressure upon it may reproduce the symptoms of which the patient complains. Next, the neck should be palpated. A well-formed, easily palpable (*Fig.* 279) (occasionally visible) cervical rib rarely gives rise to the cervical rib syndrome, but local tenderness usually is present over such a rib. In some instances the free extremity of the rib is expanded into a mushroom-like, finely bosselated, hard

ALFRED W. ADSON, 1887–1951, *Neurosurgeon, The Mayo Clinic, Rochester, Minnesota.*

bony mass. As a rule, palpation is unhelpful because a rib is either very small, or represented by a fibrous band or, more commonly, is not present.

The Costoclavicular Syndrome is encountered much less frequently than the cervical rib syndrome. Vascular symptoms predominate. As individuals grow older the muscles normally responsible for holding the clavicle away from the first rib, viz. the sternomastoid, trapezius and levator scapulae, relax. From time to time, and especially when the patient has a congenitally narrow interval between the first rib and the clavicle, the subclavian artery becomes compressed in this vice. This syndrome can be segregated from other syndromes affecting the superior thoracic aperture, as follows: The patient is instructed to stand at military attention. The volume of the pulse is noted. He is then instructed to abduct the arm to a right-angle, and finally to raise it above the head. If the costoclavicular syndrome is the cause of the symptoms, the pulse will weaken perceptibly in the last position.

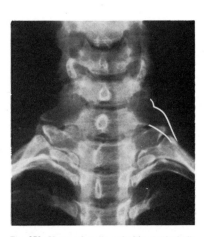

Fig. 279. X-ray of easily palpable cervical rib (left side)—same patient as in *Fig.* 4, p. 4.

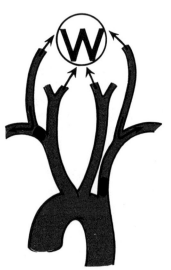

Fig. 280. The cause of the subclavian steal syndrome; the sites of blockage in the subclavian arteries are shown in black. W = circle of Willis.

ARTERIAL OBSTRUCTION IN THE NECK

Atherosclerosis (*see* p. 378) is the usual cause. Due to blockage in one or more of the internal carotid and vertebral arteries there is a deficient anastomotic circulation in the circle of Willis. Depending on the site of major obstruction one of three syndromes may develop:

    1. Obstruction at the origin of an internal carotid artery (which comprises about two-thirds of cases of this type) leads to a classic hemiplegic stroke if complete, or a transient hemiplegia if incomplete ('little stroke'). In the latter instance surgical treatment is possible and it is important to realize that the finding of a systolic murmur on auscultation over the affected artery indicates the need for a more intensive investigation by arteriography.

    2. In approximately a third of patients the obstruction is at the origin of a vertebral artery from the subclavian, or in the subclavian artery itself. Giddiness initiated by neck movement is a leading symptom and again a systolic murmur in the lower neck is a most important sign. Subclavian arterial obstruction may be characterized by a history of intermittent claudication (*see* p. 378) affecting the arm.

    3. A variety of (2) is the *Subclavian Steal Syndrome*; when the obstruction is in the subclavian artery *use of the arm* on the affected side may lead to a reversal of blood flow in the ipsilateral vertebral artery (*Fig.* 280) with resultant brain-stem ischaemia. Giddiness and a murmur are noted

---

THOMAS WILLIS, 1621–1675, *Physician, Oxford. First noticed the sweet taste of diabetic urine and described myasthenia gravis.*

as in (2) above but in addition the sign described by Javid is positive—compression of the common carotid artery in the neck on the affected side (the left in 3 of 4 cases) leads to a decrease in the retrograde vertebral flow (the circle of Willis anastomosis being reduced) and this in turn leads to a diminution of the radial pulse. In this syndrome, too, the blood pressure in the affected arm (as measured by a sphygmomanometer) is lower than on the normal side.

THE CERVICAL SPINE

It will be stressed in Chapter 31 how necessary it is to examine the cervical vertebral column in painful conditions of the upper extremity; conversely no examination of the cervical spine is complete without examining both upper limbs.

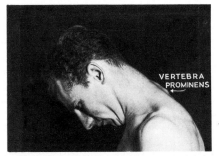

Fig. 281. Flexion. In the normal patient the chin can be placed on the chest.

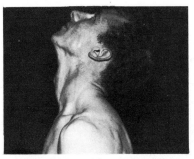

Fig. 282. Extension. The normal patient can look directly at the ceiling.

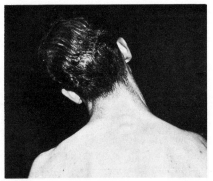

Fig. 283. Lateral bend. The ear can reach half-way to the shoulder.

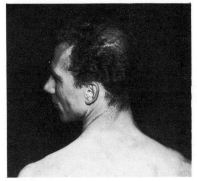

Fig. 284. Rotation. The chin almost reaches the plane of the shoulder.

TESTING MOVEMENTS OF THE CERVICAL VERTEBRAL COLUMN

The patient is seated. After duly noting if he holds his neck stiffly or in a crooked position (torticollis, *see* p. 138), ask him to point to the site of the pain, if such is the complaint. The pointing finger passes to the side or to the back of the neck, and at this juncture it is advisable for the clinician to view the neck from the side

HUSHANG JAVID, *Contemporary Professor of Surgery, Rush Medical College, Abraham Lincoln University, Chicago.*

and from the back, at the same time requesting the female patient to lift her back hair with her fingers or a comb. Unless there is some acutely painful contraindication, notably a suspected fracture, the next step is:

Testing Movements of the Cervical Vertebral Column (*Figs.* 281–284). The neutral position (*see* p. 437) is the position of ease as when one stands or sits. Nodding forwards and backwards takes place at the atlanto-occipital articulation. Flexion occurs mostly in the lower segments of the cervical spine. Lateral bend is the prerogative of the mid-segment, while rotation is the function of the atlanto-axial articulation. As age advances the movements of the neck, especially extension, become more restricted. Flexion suffers least in this way.

Palpation and Percussion are carried out in the same way as described in the section on the dorsolumbar vertebral column (*see* p. 204).

Cervical Spondylosis.* It is probable that the primary lesion is a degeneration and loss of height of one or more intervertebral discs. This causes undue mobility at the level of the affected disc which evokes osteophytic reaction and the deposition of transverse ridges of new bone at the intervertebral level causing a radiological appearance of 'osteoarthritis'. Pressure by an osteophyte on a nerve root is responsible for the symptoms. Spondylosis is essentially a radiological diagnosis, and 65 per cent of persons over the age of 50 years show such radiographic changes which are in fact, little more than a sign of advancing age, and a more reliable one than that of greying of the hair. When cervical spondylosis is the cause of painful symptoms referred to the upper extremity, a number of the following peculiarities are likely to be present. In a quarter of the patients there is a history of a remote head or neck injury. The intervertebral spaces affected most often are C.5–6 and/or C.6–7. The pain is *not* usually experienced mainly or exclusively in the periphery of the upper limb; there is also pain (though not necessarily at the same time) in the posterior part of the scalp and in the shoulder. Wasting of the muscles of the hand is rare. Weakness or absence of the biceps tendon jerk indicates a lesion of the 6th cervical nerve root, and of the triceps tendon jerk a lesion of the 7th cervical nerve root, the latter being commoner.

A Confirmatory Sign that Cervical Spondylosis (or Prolapsed Disc) is the Cause of Pain is to hold the neck in hyperextension and then to ask the patient to cough; if this induces the pain, it supports the diagnosis.

    The distribution of the pain tends to be inconstant and this, together with the age of the patient, helps in narrowing down the probable cause of the symptoms, for the diagnosis is necessarily one largely of exclusion. Other causes of pain in the upper limb (*see* p. 466) should always be eliminated early in the diagnostic endeavour.

Prolapsed Cervical Intervertebral Disc. The patient is younger than the usual sufferer from spondylosis. The symptoms come on in attacks, with intervals of complete freedom.

    While, in a few instances, there is a remote history of a relevant injury, as a rule the initial attack rises in a less dramatic manner; for instance, while stretching on wakening from sleep. Typically there is a temporary phase of a

---

* *Spondylosis.* Greek, σπόνδυλος = a vertebra + ωσις = a suffix denoting a morbid process.

stiff neck, with the head tilted away from the side of the symptoms, and exacerbations of sharp, shooting pain, which after a few days spread gradually to the lateral aspect of the shoulder, to the lateral aspect of the upper limb, and along the radial border of the forearm to the wrist. ⟶
Only occasionally does the pain radiate to the digits, but should it do so it is the thumb, index and middle fingers that are affected. The pain is made worse by coughing, sneezing, or jolting of any kind.

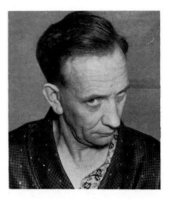

Rigidity of the Muscles of the Neck of the affected side is often present.

Muscle Tenderness affecting the trapezius and the muscles at the back of the neck is common.

Tendon Jerks. Sometimes the triceps jerk (C7) is lost, or the biceps tendon jerk (C6) is weakened.

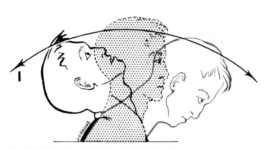

Fig. 285. Whiplash force and recoil, common type. Forcible hyperextension is followed by flexion recoil.

Fig. 286. Whiplash injury of the neck. Characteristic posture when postponed symptoms develop.

Spinal Cord Involvement by Cervical Spondylosis and Disc Protrusions. (*See* p. 218.)
Whiplash Injury of the Neck. A parked or slowly moving motor-car is rammed from behind. As the occupant's body is thrown forward, the head is thrown backward, and on recoil is pitched in the opposite direction (*Fig.* 285), these propulsions being the more violent because restraining muscles are off their guard. When the collision is head on, the lashing forces are reversed. Whiplash injury to the neck also can occur by striking the head against a low beam while walking or running, or by receiving a punch on the chin.

The ligamentum nuchae is torn. Rarely, the tip of the 7th cervical spinous process is fractured. Except, perhaps, for mild shock, nothing amiss is noted at the time, but the next day some pain in the neck occurs. About 10 days later symptoms due to cervical nerve-root irritation commence. The patient develops a 'crick in the neck'. Unilateral occipital headache commonly follows. Sometimes there is blurring of vision.

Because of the characteristic posture, the diagnosis can be strongly suspected as the patient enters the consulting-room. The head is held rigidly; it is tilted away from the painful side, the chin is turned towards the painful side, and usually the head is held in slight flexion (*Fig.* 286).

Palpation demonstrates tenderness over the lower cervical spinous processes, and especially over the interspinous spaces. Soft crepitus (effusion) sometimes can be felt over the lower part of the ligamentum nuchae.

The biceps jerk frequently is absent on one or both sides.

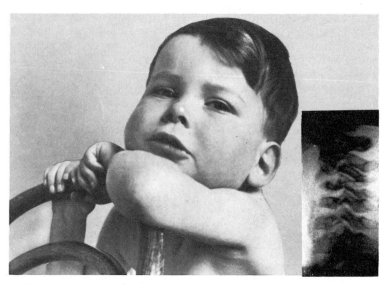

Fig. 287. Rust's sign. Inset radiograph shows caries of the 3rd and 4th cervical vertebrae.

Fractures of the Neck. (*See* p. 217.)

Pott's Disease of the Cervical Spine is now comparatively rare except in communities with a low resistance to tuberculosis and living in poor economic conditions. The patient holds the head stiffly, either thrust forward or, more rarely, held in a wry-neck position. To spare turning the head (atlanto-axial articulation) the patient's eyes rotate to follow one's movement, as for example when recording the history. If asked to look at an object on the wall to the right or to the left, it is the *body* that is rotated. *Rust's sign* is often present: with every change of position, and often when the patient is seated, he supports his head with the hands (*Fig.* 287). The general signs, and some of the local signs, are similar to those of Pott's disease of the thoracolumbar region (*see* p. 212).

Abscess Formation. An abscess connected with the body of a cervical vertebra is wont to give rise to a chronic retropharyngeal abscess (*see* p. 132).

PERCIVALL POTT, 1714–1788, *Surgeon, St. Bartholomew's Hospital, London.*
JAN N. RUST, 1775–1840, *Surgeon, St. Lazarus Hospital, Cracow, Poland.*

Chapter 14

THE THYROID GLAND

Inspection. In thin young women, the isthmus of the *normal* thyroid gland sometimes is apparent, particularly on swallowing. Otherwise the normal gland is not visible. Inspection should never be hurried, for it is a highly important method of obtaining information regarding swellings of the gland. Sometimes it is obvious that the whole gland is enlarged (*see Fig.* 299, p. 160).

In obese and bull-necked individuals, inspection of the thyroid is rendered easier by the patient throwing her head backwards, and pressing her occiput against her clasped hands (Pizzillo) (*Fig.* 288).

Because of the attachment of the thyroid gland to the larynx, a swelling will always *rise with deglutition*, unless the gland is fixed by neoplastic infiltration or inflammation. When there is a swelling that *may* be within the thyroid capsule, ask the patient to swallow. A thyroid swelling moves upwards, after which it descends again.

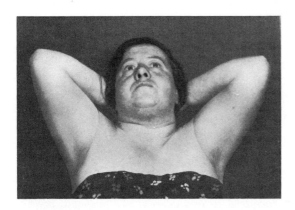

Fig. 288. Pizzillo's method of making the thyroid gland more prominent in cases where a short neck or a thick layer of subcutaneous fat renders inspection unsatisfactory.

Palpation. Routine palpation should be conducted from behind. To relax the musculature, instruct the patient to lower the chin. Using both hands, place the thumbs upon the nape of the neck. In this way, a considerable portion of the fingers comes to overlie the right and left lobes of the gland (*Fig.* 289). Commence systematic palpation of the whole of the gland by determining the limits of the lower edges of the lobes, if necessary requesting the patient to swallow.

Can the normal thyroid be felt on palpation? In a reasonably slender person it can be felt as a smooth firm structure that moves upwards as he or she swallows.

Having determined definitely the shape and position of the lower limits of an enlarged thyroid, palpate the anterior surfaces of the lobes. These are examined

GIUSEPPE PIZZILLO, *Professor of Medicine, University of Palermo.*

one at a time, and, in order to relax the overlying sternomastoid muscle, the head is inclined slightly to the side being examined.

In some instances information can be gained by asking the patient to extend the neck, instead of flexing it. In this position the gland becomes more prominent and more accessible, despite the increased tautness of the sternomastoid muscles.

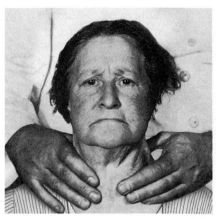
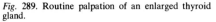

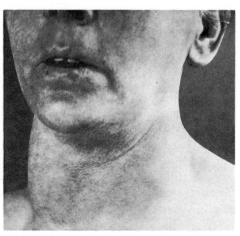

Fig. 289. Routine palpation of an enlarged thyroid gland.

Fig. 290. Secondary thyrotoxicosis. An adenoma has been present in the right lobe of the thyroid gland for 25 years. The patient is dyspnoeic and breathes through the open mouth. On the slightest exertion, she gasps.

When the whole thyroid gland is enlarged, determine whether its surface is smooth (as is found in primary thyrotoxicosis and in colloid goitre) or bosselated (characteristic of multinodular goitre). Ordinarily, unless the goitre* is very large, it can be displaced laterally with the finger, thus making it apparent that the muscles slide freely over the swelling. Fixation suggests malignancy which has broken through the thyroid capsule, or thyroiditis, or scarring due to a previous operation.

Especially *when a swelling is localized* to one portion of the gland, further examination is best conducted from in front, with the clinician seated. With the fingers define the limits of the swelling and decide in which lobe and at which pole it is situated, or whether it is in the isthmus. Record your findings (*see Fig.* 2, p. 3).

Having demonstrated that a swelling is the enlarged thyroid or is situated therein, the clinician must decide the following questions:

Firstly, and most important, is the swelling obstructing the trachea? This is uncommon, but vital because of the danger of asphyxia.

Secondly, are there signs of thyrotoxicosis, either of the primary type (*below*) or of the less usual secondary type (p. 156)? In practice this is easily the most frequent complication.

---

* *Goitre.* Latin, *guttur* = the throat.

Thirdly, is the goitre malignant (p. 156)? If so, tracheal obstruction may be present in addition.

Fourthly, does the swelling extend behind the sternum (retrosternal goitre) (p. 157)? This is also uncommon, but tracheal obstruction may be caused.

Finally, is there evidence of myxoedema (p. 159)?

TRACHEAL OBSTRUCTION

As the patient breathes a harsh noise is produced by the passage of air through the partially obstructed air-passage (stridor). If the obstruction is slight the noise can only be detected if listened for carefully in a quiet room. Later, dyspnoea, cyanosis and restlessness make the diagnosis obvious.

Kocher's Test. Slight compression on the lateral lobes produces stridor. If this test is positive it signifies that the patient has an obstructed trachea.

Narrowing of the trachea is found in carcinoma of the thyroid, retrosternal goitres, the 'scabbard' trachea of long-standing multinodular goitre and in Riedel's thyroiditis. *See also* Dysphagia Lusoria, p. 198.

Riedel's Thyroiditis is characterized by tracheal obstruction in the presence of a small goitre that is always stony hard and often irregular in contour. It should be thought of if the patient, usually male, is below the age at which such signs would point to scirrhous carcinoma, but the diagnosis must be confirmed by biopsy.

HYPERTHYROIDISM

Primary Thyrotoxicosis (Graves' Disease; Exophthalmic Goitre). Signs of hyperthyroidism are often obvious enough to be recognized at a glance but they can be so masked as to escape attention. Most patients are relatively young females, and almost invariably the thyroid gland is enlarged symmetrically. Rarely there is no enlargement either in the neck or retrosternally (*latent hyperthyroidism*).

Exophthalmos. In more than half the patients with primary thyrotoxicosis eye signs are present. These are discussed fully on pp. 73–76.

Weight Loss may be obvious and in any case should be asked about.

The Skin is moist. As a prelude to examining the pulse at the wrist, take the opportunity to feel the hands. In Graves' disease the hands, particularly the palms, are inclined to be hot and moist. These patients find hot weather intolerable, but exhibit increased tolerance to cold.

The Pulse should next be counted. In hyperthyroidism the rate is increased; probably it will be exaggerated by the nervousness occasioned by the examination. In addition attention should be paid to the regularity of the pulse or otherwise. When it is both rapid and irregular, auricular fibrillation should be suspected and an electrocardiogram obtained. Early cases are frequently mistaken for an anxiety state. A helpful method of differentiating is to arrange for the pulse rate to be taken while the patient is asleep. In thyrotoxicosis the *sleeping pulse rate* is still fast; in anxiety state it is within normal limits.

Tremor. A fine tremor of the hands is almost invariably present. Ask the patient to place her hands straight out in front and spread the fingers or ask her to put out her tongue, and to keep it out for half a minute.

A Thyroid Thrill is almost pathognomonic of Graves' disease, but it is present only in comparatively

THEODOR KOCHER, 1841–1917, *Professor of Clinical Surgery, University of Berne.*
BERNHARD M. C. RIEDEL, 1846–1916, *Professor of Surgery, Jena, Germany.*
ROBERT J. GRAVES, 1796–1853, *Physician, Meath Hospital, Dublin.*

advanced cases with greatly increased vascularity of the gland. The hand must be laid quite lightly over the lateral lobe, otherwise it is the transmitted pulsation of the carotid arteries that will be felt. Auscultation will often reveal a systolic murmur.

Secondary Thyrotoxicosis develops in long-standing cases of multinodular goitre or adenoma of the thyroid. Examination reveals less tremor and a less clammy skin than with primary thyrotoxicosis. Of cardinal importance is that *eye signs, including exophthalmos, are almost invariably absent.* Auricular fibrillation is common; at times it is the presenting evidence of thyrotoxicosis. Usually the heart is enlarged, and occasionally by the time the patient presents there are signs of cardiac decompensation such as oedema of the ankles, dyspnoea (*Fig.* 290) and orthopnoea.* The patient nearly always has had a non-toxic lesion for many years, and consequently is older than the average sufferer from primary thyrotoxicosis.

THE MALIGNANT THYROID

This is not necessarily a disease of the elderly: in a young patient (including children) in whom extravagant lymph-node enlargement is often found, a papillary carcinoma is the usual cause: in middle age a follicular growth is likely and in the old an anaplastic tumour. It should be suspected in the following circumstances:

1. A rapidly enlarging solitary swelling in the thyroid. Sudden increase in size associated with *pain* indicates a haemorrhage within the capsule and does not necessarily denote malignancy.

2. Hardness of part or whole of the swelling which can be likened to that of an unripe apple.

3. A change in a long-standing goitre which commences to enlarge much more rapidly than previously.

4. Loss of mobility of the gland which fails to move upwards on swallowing as usual, and there is also loss of lateral mobility.

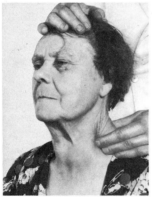

Fig. 291. Seeking the pulsation of the carotid artery. Berry's sign. The pulsation could not be detected in this case of carcinoma of the thyroid.

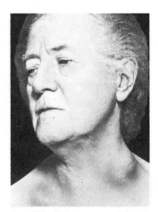

Fig. 292. Enlargement of lymph nodes in a patient with carcinoma of the thyroid.

---

* *Orthopnoea.* Greek, ὀρθός straight+πνοιά = breath. Inability to breathe except in an upright position.

5. *Berry's Sign.* When the gland enlarges it displaces the carotid tree backwards and outwards. Consequently, in many cases of large goitre the pulsation of the carotid artery can be felt behind the posterior edge of the swelling. The displaced artery is much less in evidence when the thyroid is the seat of malignant disease, for it tends to become surrounded by the tumour (*Fig.* 291).

6. Tracheal obstruction (*see* p. 155).

7. When a patient with a goitre is found to be suffering also from Horner's syndrome (*see* p. 404) or hoarseness (recurrent laryngeal nerve palsy) it suggests that the goitre is malignant and has spread locally.

8. Lymph-node enlargement (*Fig.* 292). Occasionally a comparatively young patient presents with enlarged lymph nodes in the neck, usually unilateral, and the primary growth in the thyroid is so small that it is impalpable. Biopsy is then the only method of arriving at the correct diagnosis.

RETROSTERNAL GOITRE

A retrosternal goitre is found particularly in short-necked individuals. Any thyroid enlargement can come to lie partially retrosternally. In most instances the enlargement is an adenoma. Rarely does the whole of an enlarged thyroid lie in the superior mediastinum. In this instance there is no thyroid gland to be felt in the neck but when the intrathoracic pressure rises while coughing the goitre may be seen; this is termed a *plunging goitre.*

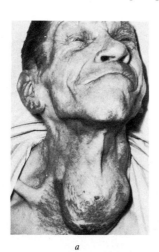 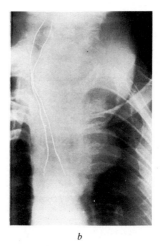

a	*b*

Fig. 293. Retrosternal goitre. Although the enlarged thyroid is very obvious on inspection, a large part of it is retrosternal and causes the patient to extend the head in order to provide a clear airway. The X-ray shows the extreme tracheal narrowing in this case.

Sometimes a goitre situated wholly within the thorax eventually becomes toxic, and because the swelling is not visible, the symptoms to which it gives rise are attributed to heart disease or neurosis. Again, the dyspnoea which a retrosternal goitre occasions may be mistaken for asthma. Mindful of this,

SIR JAMES BERRY, 1860–1946, *Surgeon, Royal Free Hospital, London.*

meticulous clinical examination sometimes renders X-ray demonstration of the presence of a retrosternal swelling of confirmatory value only (*Fig.* 293).

Dilated veins over the upper part of the thoracic wall due to pressure upon the internal jugular veins occasionally provide a clue to the diagnosis; rarely oedema of the face ensues from the same cause. Occasionally, tilting the head strongly to one side produces a sensation of dyspnoea (*Fig.* 294).

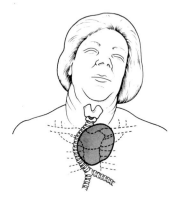

Fig. 294. Cause of dyspnoea when the head is tilted to one side.

Inquire if the patient is troubled with *nocturnal* dyspnoea. Information may be forthcoming that an attempt to sleep on one side produces such difficulty in breathing that the patient always sleeps on the other side.

Deviation of the trachea when there is no obvious thyroid enlargement (*see Fig.* 363, p. 194) is a sign of great moment as confirmatory evidence of a goitre below the superior thoracic aperture.

Slight difficulty in swallowing is sometimes present, but it is never a major complaint.

Of all the methods of diagnosis, palpation performed carefully during deglutition is the most reliable, and usually in this way a retrosternal goitre can be differentiated from a mediastinal neoplasm.

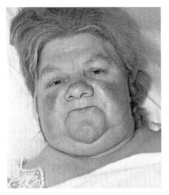

Fig. 295. Myxoedema. The malar flush is a burgundy colour. The hair of the head is dry and scanty. Note the oriental slant of the eyes.

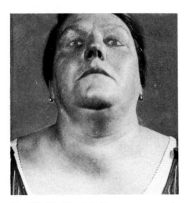

Fig. 296. Hashimoto's disease.

HYPOTHYROIDISM

Cold hands, mental slowness, puffiness of the eyelids, and perhaps ill-marked outer halves of the eyebrows should awaken in the mind of the clinician the possibility of myxoedema. The patient feels the cold weather intensely. If the hands are warm to the examiner's touch, a diagnosis of myxoedema is as likely to be wrong as is the diagnosis of hyperthyroidism when the patient's hands are cold. In established cases the face has a bloated look, with the eyes narrowed by puffiness (*Fig.* 295), giving a somewhat oriental appearance. The complexion is waxy-yellow, with a burgundy flush of the cheeks (*Fig.* 295). Only in advanced cases is there a substantial loss of hair. The voice is like that of the recording of a worn disc on a gramophone that needs speeding up. The pulse is slow. The temperature is often subnormal. Examine the supraclavicular fossae for pads of fat and the region overlying the 7th cervical vertebra for a fatty 'hump', but their absence does not disturb the diagnosis. On palpation, the skeletal muscles seem hard, and the pseudomucin-laden subcutaneous tissues everywhere are firm and podgy (pseudo-oedema). Owing to pseudo-oedema it is often most difficult to be certain whether the thyroid gland is palpable in the neck. This is in contrast to the examination of an infant suffering from sporadic cretinism (*see* p. 89), where one can feel the rings of the trachea so plainly that it is possible to be confident of an absence of the gland.

See also Pretibial Myxoedema, p. 11.

Myxoedema Coma. Hypothermia is a terminal complication of long-standing untreated cases. Nearly always it supervenes during mid-winter, and is sometimes preceded by epileptiform convulsions. Characteristic of hypothermia (whether due to myxoedema or otherwise) is that the unconscious patient's skin is reminiscent of touching the skin of a toad—deadly cold. The rectal temperature falls as low as 24 °C.

Hashimoto's Disease (Struma* Lymphomatosa) is not uncommon. Usually the first symptom is a lump in the neck. On inspection the whole gland is enlarged; nevertheless, one lobe is often larger than the other (*Fig.* 296). On palpation the thyroid is found to be of rubbery consistency with bosselations so much less pronounced than those of a multinodular goitre that they may be described as mere undulations. It is characteristic of Hashimoto's disease that the contour of the gland can be defined clearly, but often the hardness suggests carcinoma. Symptoms of mild hypothyroidism are usually present. It is seen predominantly in females who have just passed the menopause. Special blood tests show antibodies to the thyroid gland.

THYROID ENLARGEMENT IN THE EUTHYROID † PATIENT

Notwithstanding the above considerations, remember that the majority of patients with thyroid disease do not, at any rate in the first instance, exhibit complications. It is convenient to deal with these conditions in chronological sequence.

Goitre in Infancy is seen in areas of endemic goitre (*see below*), or is due to a teratoma of the thyroid, or to therapy for thyrotoxicosis administered to the mother during her pregnancy. The excessive secretion of thyrotropic hormone is carried to the fetus via the placental blood and the response is that the thyroid gland hypertrophies (*Fig.* 297). Conversely, untreated thyrotoxicosis in pregnancy leads to classic Graves' disease in the newborn infant.

---

* The River Struma rises in Bulgaria and flows into the Aegean Sea. Along its banks is an endemic goitre area. *Struma* is an alternative term for goitre.

† Euthyroid. Greek, εὖ well+thyroid = normally functioning thyroid, neither hyper- nor hypo-thyroid.

HAKARU HASHIMOTO, 1881–1934, *Director of the Hashimoto Hospital, Miyo, Japan.*

Lingual Thyroid. Reverting to ascertaining whether a thyroid gland is present in front of the trachea, remember that when the thyroid occupies an aberrant position, it is often the only thyroid and can be situated anywhere in the thyroglossal tract from the foramen caecum of the tongue to where the isthmus of the normal thyroid should be situated. Therefore, when confronted with a central swelling at the back of the tongue (*Fig.* 298) or a swelling believed to be a thyroglossal cyst ascertain by palpation whether a thyroid gland is present in the normal situation.

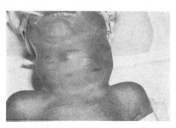

Fig. 297. Congenital goitre. The thyrotoxic mother was given prolonged therapy during her pregnancy.

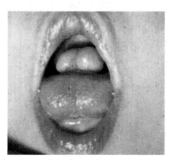

Fig. 298. Lingual thyroid.

Physiological Hyperplasia of Puberty* is almost confined to females. The thyroid gland is enlarged evenly, and feels comparatively soft. With the passage of a few years the enlargement subsides gradually, and has all but disappeared by the twenty-first year. However, all goitres of puberty that do not subside completely must be considered potential colloid goitres.

Mensuration of the Thyroid at three-monthly intervals is sometimes of value, particularly in cases of goitre of puberty. Measurements are taken with a linen tape-measure around the neck at the level of maximum swelling. In assessing any increase in size due allowance should be made for natural growth of the patient at this age.

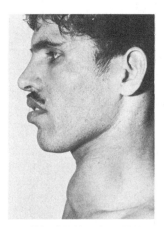

Fig. 299. Colloid goitre. Uniform enlargement of the whole thyroid is present.

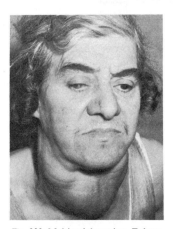

Fig. 300. Multinodular goitre. Enlargement of both lateral lobes and of the isthmus can be seen.

Colloid Goitre. Usually the patient presents between the ages of 20 and 30 years,

---

* Some physiological hyperplasia occurs also during pregnancy and at the menopause.

i.e. after physiological hyperplasia should have subsided. The whole of the thyroid gland is affected, and as a rule the deformity is most obvious (*Fig.* 299). On palpation, the swelling is found to be elastic and tolerably smooth.

Multinodular Goitre is occasionally sporadic but usually endemic in regions where the drinking water is deficient in iodine. In such localities many of the children (girls more than boys) have a visible and palpable smooth, soft, symmetrical enlargement of the thyroid gland, but after puberty many of these enlargements subside. In a proportion, varying from district to district, the goitre continues to enlarge, and becomes multinodular (*Fig.* 300). The whole gland is studded with rounded swellings, varying in size. At times these nodules can be palpated in a thyroid that seems otherwise normal; more often the whole gland feels replaced by rounded bosselations, sometimes alike in consistency, at others varying from hard to fluctuant. When a nodule, or a conglomeration of contiguous nodules, is very hard—much harder than the remainder—there are two possibilities: (*a*) carcinomatous change has taken place: (*b*) calcification has occurred. Neither is infrequent in long-standing cases. Radiography is required to settle this differential diagnosis.

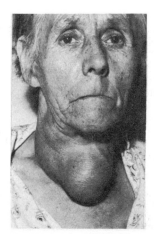

Fig. 301. Large adenoma of the right lobe of the thyroid gland.

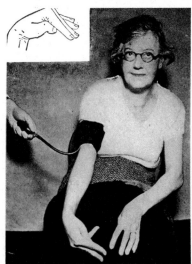

Fig. 302. Tetany; the 'obstetrician's hand'.

Adenoma. This, the commonest affection of the thyroid gland in non-goitrous areas, tends to produce an asymmetrical enlargement of the gland (*Fig.* 301). If the swelling is visible it will be seen to move upwards when the patient swallows. Define the lump and make out its relationship to the rest of the thyroid gland. Next, ascertain its relationship to the trachea which is displaced in extravagant cases.

Subacute (de Quervain's) Thyroiditis. The patient, who may have had an antecedent upper respiratory infection, complains of pain in the region of the thyroid gland which often radiates to the ears and is associated with pain on swallowing. It usually is found in a female aged 40–60 who exhibits a low-grade pyrexia. Examination reveals a tender finely nodular moderate enlargement of the gland with overlying redness of the skin. Untreated, spontaneous recovery takes place over a period of two to three months.

FRITZ DE QUERVAIN, 1868–1940, *Professor of Surgery, Berne, Switzerland.*

THE PARATHYROIDS

An enlarged parathyroid gland is hardly ever palpable upon clinical examination. It can be found only by exploration when the whole thyroid gland has been displayed at operation. However, in suspected cases of hyperparathyroidism, particularly in examples of recurrent renal calculus and in osteitis fibrosa cystica (*see* p. 427), an attempt should be made by systematic palpation to discover a possibly enlarged parathyroid before setting in motion appropriate special investigations. Nevertheless, a palpable swelling, in the presence of hyperparathyroidism, is more likely to be a coincident thyroid adenoma than a parathyroid adenoma.

Parathyroid Tetany, an uncommon complication of thyroidectomy, occurs most frequently from 1–5 days after operation, but occasionally mild forms of this condition are not recognized for several weeks. It is due to hypoparathyroidism consequent upon the removal of two or more parathyroid glands. The first symptoms are tingling and numbness of the lips, nose and the extremities, sometimes accompanied by circumoral pallor.

The Chvostek–Weiss Sign. With a percussion hammer, gently tap the 7th nerve as it emerges in front of the external auditory meatus. In tetany, tapping the hyperexcitable nerve provokes a brisk muscular twitch on the same side of the face.

Trousseau's Sign. A sphygmomanometer cuff is placed around the arm and the pressure raised to 200 mm Hg. If tetany is present, in five minutes typical contractions of the hand are seen—the fingers are extended except at the metacarpophalangeal joints, and the thumb is strongly adducted, the combined effect of which is to produce the so-called 'obstetrician's hand' (*Fig.* 302).

In severe cases painful cramps of the hands, feet and indeed all the muscles of the body occur. Strong adduction of the thumbs is almost always present, and this, coupled with extension of the feet, constitutes the 'carpopedal spasm'. Occasionally spasm of the muscles of respiration culminates in severe dyspnoea, and the patient is not only in great pain, but is in mortal dread of suffocation. Blurring of vision due to spasm of the intra-ocular muscles is common. Even if the symptoms are mild, prolonged unrectified hypocalcaemia gives rise to cataracts.

THE THYROGLOSSAL TRACT

Thyroglossal Cyst can appear at any time of life, and in contradistinction to a branchial cyst (*see* p. 142) it is often encountered in early childhood.

Differential Diagnosis. As a rule, the diagnosis is tolerably simple. Certain difficulties are met with from time to time; the chief of these results from a peculiar liability of these cysts to infection.

Bearing in mind that it is seldom large enough to exhibit definite fluctuation (or that its contents are too tense for this sign) and that it is seldom translucent, *the* sign of a thyroglossal cyst depends on its anatomical connection via the thyroglossal duct with the base of the tongue. A thyroglossal cyst thus *moves upwards when the tongue is protruded*. Request the patient to open his mouth. Grasp the swelling between the finger and thumb (*Fig.* 303*a, b*). Then instruct him to put out his tongue: to put it in and put it out again. As the tongue is fully

FRANTIŠEK CHVOSTEK, 1835–1884, *Physician, Josefsakademie, Vienna.*
NATHAN WEISS, 1851–1883, *Physician, General Hospital, Vienna.*
ARMAND TROUSSEAU, 1801–1867, *Physician, Hôtel-Dieu, Paris.*

protruded a certain amount of movement of all swellings in this region is to be expected, but in the case of a thyroglossal cyst the upward tug is unmistakable. With an adenoma of the thyroid isthmus this sign is negative but the swelling will be found to move upwards on swallowing.

A diagnosis of thyroglossal cyst is not complete without determining the presence of a thyroid gland in its normal position (*see* Lingual Thyroid, p. 160).

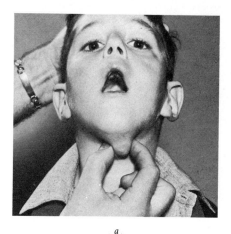
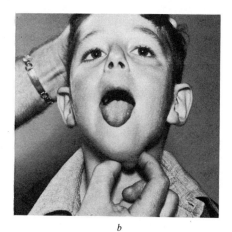

a   b

Fig. 303. If a swelling is a thyroglossal cyst, the upward tug when the patient fully protrudes his tongue is characteristic. Note that the mouth must be open at the commencement of the test when the swelling is grasped.

Special Clinical Features of Thyroglossal Cysts at Various Levels

1. Suprahyoid. A thyroglossal cyst situated immediately above the hyoid bone (*Fig.* 304) must be distinguished from a median sublingual dermoid cyst (*see* p. 125).

2. Subhyoid (*Fig.* 305) is the commonest site for a thyroglossal cyst.

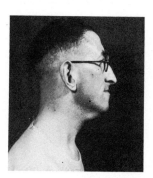
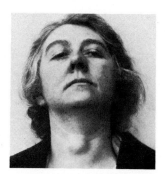

Fig. 304. Suprahyoid thyroglossal cyst.   *Fig.* 305. Subhyoid thyroglossal cyst.

3. At the Level of the Thyroid Cartilage. It is often stated that the swelling cannot be a thyroglossal cyst unless it is strictly in the midline. The exception to this rule is a cyst in relation to the ala of the thyroid cartilage. The thyroid cartilage, shaped like the prow of a ship, in the course of its development sweeps the thyroglossal tract to one side, usually to the left. This deviation makes the differential diagnosis from an enlargèd lymph node more difficult, but the manœuvre shown in *Fig.* 303, segregates these two conditions.

4. At the Level of the Cricoid Cartilage. Thyroglossal cysts at this level are less common than any of the foregoing, and they tend to assume the midline once more. It is here that the differential diagnosis between a thyroglossal cyst and an adenoma of the isthmus of the thyroid, which has been referred to already, must be made.

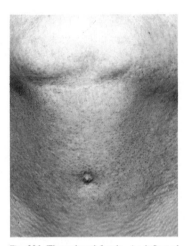

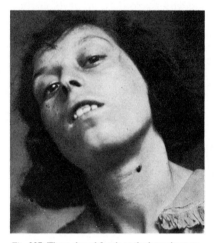

Fig. 306. Thyroglossal fistula. An inflamed cyst was incised in early childhood and the discharge continued. Attacks of inflammation recurred at frequent intervals.

Fig. 307. Thyroglossal fistula at the lateral extremity of a scar following incomplete removal of a thyroglossal cyst.

A Thyroglossal Fistula can result from bursting (or incision) of an inflamed thyroglossal cyst. More often, it is an aftermath of local removal of a cyst as opposed to extirpation of the whole of the thyroglossal tract. Usually it is situated strictly in the midline (*Fig.* 306), but in cases following incomplete removal of the thyroglossal tract the fistula may present itself at one or other extremity of a transverse scar (*Fig.* 307).

Chapter 15

THE BREAST AND AXILLARY LYMPH NODES

The breasts are examined while the patient, undressed as far as the waist, sits upright. This position is undoubtedly best for examination of the axilla (*see* p. 174) but the supine position is sometimes better for examination of the breast itself. If you are in doubt after examining the patient sitting upright, ask her to lie flat and re-examine the breasts, palpation of which against the underlying chest wall may enable a confident diagnosis.

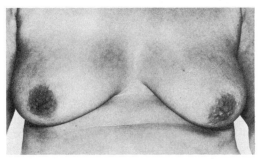

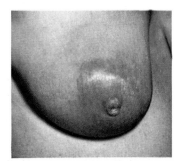

Fig. 308. Retraction of the nipples, present since the breasts developed. The patient had no complaints regarding the breasts.

Fig. 309. Mastitis carcinomatosa.

ROUTINE EXAMINATION OF THE BREASTS

Inspection. If the skin over the breast is reddened, inquire if the patient has lactated recently. Observe the level of the nipples (*see Fig.* 3, p. 4): remember that sometimes the left breast normally hangs slightly lower than the right.

The Nipples. If retraction is observed (*Fig.* 308), ask the patient how long this has been present; it is of cardinal importance only if it is recent (*see Fig.* 3, p. 4), when it indicates that neoplastic or inflammatory fibrosis is proceeding in the breast. A lump in a breast subject to *long-standing* nipple retraction may be a carcinoma, but often it is a chronic abscess caused by a blocked duct.

Close inspection of the nipple may reveal a crack, which is sometimes of considerable diagnostic importance in cases where a deep-seated breast abscess is in question. In this connection one should not hastily conclude that, because the breast looks inflamed, a more serious condition can be ruled out. In cases of mastitis carcinomatosa (*Fig.* 309) the proliferation of carcinoma is so rapid that heat and redness are present. A dry eczema of the nipple which often itches strongly suggests Paget's disease (*Fig.* 310).

The areola should be inspected and the degree of pigmentation, if any, noted. Remember that the specialized glands of Montgomery are subject to the same affections, notably retention cyst (*Fig.* 311) and abscess, as other sebaceous glands.

Sir James Paget, 1814–1899, *Surgeon, St. Bartholomew's Hospital, London.*
William Montgomery, 1797–1859, *Professor of Midwifery, Dublin.*

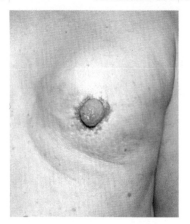

Fig. 310. Paget's disease of the nipple.

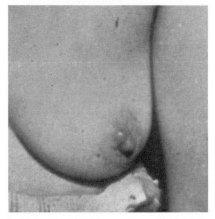

Fig. 311. An inflamed retention cyst of Montgomery's follicle. If this is incised, a chronic sinus will result.

The remainder of the skin of the breast now receives attention.

Visible veins coursing over both breasts are of no diagnostic significance, but if such veins are discerned on one side only, usually it indicates that there is an active lesion in that breast. Also look for alteration in the quality of the skin (*peau d'orange*) (*Fig.* 312). The earliest manifestation of this phenomenon (which is due to skin oedema consequent on blockage of the lymphatics by cancer cells) is seen best with the aid of a magnifying glass (*Fig.* 313). *Peau d'orange* is rendered more obvious by squeezing the skin gently (*Fig.* 314). By the time a breast cancer has ulcerated through the skin (*Fig.* 315) the diagnosis is obvious even to the most inexperienced medical student. The *ulcer* has the characteristics of an epithelioma (*see* p. 36). Another visible manifestation in a late case is the presence of *nodules* in the skin wide of the tumour.

When the arms are raised fully above the head, visible signs of carcinoma (e.g. tethering of the skin) frequently become more apparent.

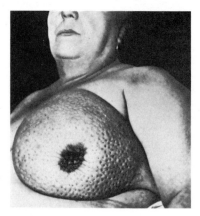

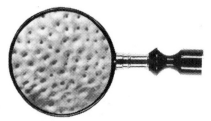

Fig. 313. *Peau d'orange* is conspicuous when viewed through a magnifying glass.

Fig. 312. Very advanced *peau d'orange*.

Palpation. If the patient has noticed a lump, ask her to find it herself, before you attempt to do so. Commence by examining the opposite breast. Next, palpate the four quadrants of the breast systematically between the pulps of the finger and thumb.* A useful routine is shown in *Fig.* 316. The normal breast gives a firm lobulated impression with nodularity a feature, particularly before the periods. In fat patients (and after the menopause when fat is laid down in the breasts) expect to feel both lobulation and nodularity less easily.

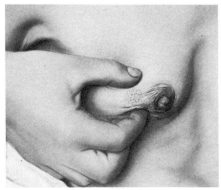

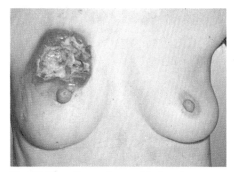

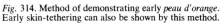

Fig. 314. Method of demonstrating early *peau d'orange*. Early skin-tethering can also be shown by this method.

Fig. 315. Ulcerating carcinoma of the breast.

Next, palpate directly behind the nipple, during which manœuvre it should be noted whether any secretion can be expressed from the nipple (*see* p. 171).

Proceed in exactly the same manner on the affected side mentally comparing the texture of both breasts. If a lump is present note:

Its position—in which quadrant of the breast. The breast occupies the interval from the 2nd to the 6th ribs. Swellings situated above or below these levels (unless in a pendulous breast) are unlikely to arise from breast tissue.

Consistency and shape—hard or soft, regular or irregular, and so on.

Fixity to the skin is tested by gently pinching up the overlying skin: this should be done systematically over the whole surface of the lump if large. If small the method depicted in *Fig.* 314 is better. The principal exception to the infallibility of this sign of malignancy is when the lump is situated immediately behind the nipple. A swelling in this situation, whatever its nature, is usually superficially adherent, because, if it is not an integral part of the duct mechanism, some or all of the twenty or so ducts that are about to open upon the surface of the nipple, of necessity, traverse the substance of the swelling. *Consequently, the most benign of lumps may be attached to the nipple.*

Fixity to deep structures (the pectoralis fascia). Testing for attachment of a given lump to the structures underlying the breast is necessary in deciding whether the lump is malignant (although benign inflammatory masses are occasionally fixed) and in staging a carcinoma (*see* p. 176). Ask the patient to place her hand lightly

---

* Many textbooks still teach that the breast should be palpated with the flat of the hand. This is much less sensitive and derives from a mistranslation of the French text of Velpeau.

ALFRED A. L. M. VELPEAU, 1795–1867, *Professor of Clinical Surgery, Paris.*

upon her hip with the thumb behind; feel the pectoralis major; it is quite loose and soft. Pick up the lump between the fingers and try its mobility, first in a horizontal, then in a vertical direction. Now ask the patient to press her hand firmly into the side, which contracts the pectoralis major (*Fig.* 317). Try the mobility of the lump once more in two planes. Note that the mobility of the normal breast upon the pectoral muscle is limited to a certain extent by the full contraction of the muscle, and it requires a certain amount of experience to appreciate minor degrees of pathological fixity.

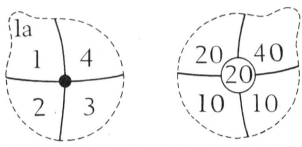

Fig. 316. (*Left*) The order of palpation of the quadrants of the breast. It should be noted that the upper and outer quadrant includes the axillary tail (1*a*). A lump in this region may be difficult to differentiate from an enlarged axillary lymph node and vice-versa. (*Right*) The relative frequency of carcinoma in the various quadrants (approximate) and centrally.

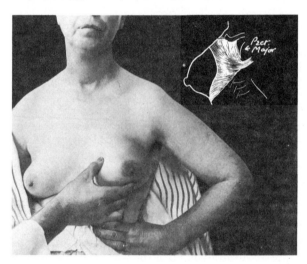

Fig. 317. Testing a lump in the breast for fixity to deeper structures. The patient presses her hand firmly into her side. This puts the pectoralis major into full contraction.

Swellings towards the periphery of the lower outer quadrant lie on the serratus anterior. Ask the patient to place the hand of the affected side upon your shoulder, and to press. This contracts the serratus anterior (*see also Fig.* 663, p. 405).

Examination of the Lymphatic Field of the Breast. *See* p. 174.

At the conclusion of every examination of a tumour of the breast where the signs leave little doubt as to malignancy the liver should be examined for the presence of metastases (*see* p. 235).

ACCESSORY METHODS OF EXAMINING THE BREAST IN SPECIAL CIRCUMSTANCES

Examination in the Pendulous Position. Especially when the breasts are large and pendulous and a lump in one of them is placed deeply it is well worth requesting the patient to stand and, leaning forward, to support herself with her outstretched arms resting on the arm of a chair or a couch or on a table, according to her height. In this way the breasts can be inspected (*Fig.* 318), and palpated in the hanging position in which the greatest enemy to effective palpation of the breast tissue—namely, mammary obesity—is to some degree circumvented.

Radiology. Although radiological investigations and their indications are beyond our briefing some mention must be made of the value of this method in suspected breast cancer. In the presence of an undoubted lump its removal for histological examination is essential if the physical signs of cancer are not conclusively present. Only when there is doubt whether a lump is actually present (notably in a fat breast) should it be recalled that breast carcinomata almost always can be demonstrated on X-rays taken with the appropriate technique (mammography).

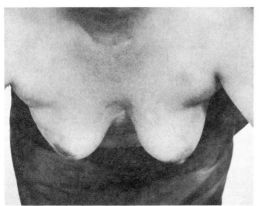

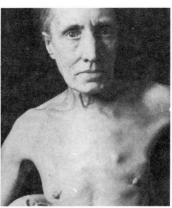

Fig. 318. The dependent position for examination of the breasts. In this case the right breast is tethered by a scirrhous carcinoma.

Fig. 319. This hard, rounded lump was neither attached to the skin nor to the pectoral muscle. There were no palpable lymph nodes in the axilla. The patient's age made the clinician wary. Operation showed a typical carcinoma.

Record of the Clinical Examination of the Breast. The record of the examination may be entered conveniently in the graphical manner (*see Fig.* 2, p. 3). The breast is divided into four quadrants, and a triangle represents the axilla. The clinical findings registered in this way form an accurate record that is more valuable than much description.

So ends the description of the routine examination of the breasts, with special reference to mammary carcinoma, the earliest sign of which is a comparatively small, hard lump in the breast, *unattached* to the skin and mobile within the breast tissue in which it is embedded (*Fig.* 319).

THE CHARACTERISTICS OF NON-CANCEROUS LUMPS

Fibro-adenosis* Is common in women between 20 and 40 years of age, and especially in spinsters, nulliparae and those who have not suckled a baby. Often the whole breast, indeed both breasts, are inclined to be 'lumpy' and they may

---

* Formerly known as 'chronic interstitial mastitis', a misnomer as there is no inflammation present.

be slightly tender. At other times the lumpiness is confined to a sector of the breast. In still other cases there is an ill-defined lump which can be felt on palpation between the fingers and thumb in an otherwise tolerably normal breast. Such a lump is wont to be painful and somewhat tender during menstruation, whereas cancer, in the early stages, is painless.

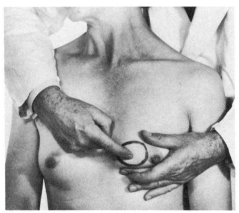
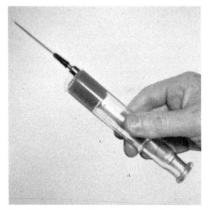

Fig. 320. Testing a lump in the breast from behind for fluctuation.

Fig. 321. Typical yellow-green fluid obtained on aspirating a cyst associated with fibro-adenosis.

The differential diagnosis between fibro-adenosis and early carcinoma of the breast is sometimes exceedingly difficult, particularly in a large breast in which the ill-defined lump may be deeply situated. This is not surprising seeing that both these common conditions can coexist, especially in pre-menopausal patients. Therefore if, after a thorough examination (including mammography, see p. 169), no conclusion can be reached, it is safer to assume that a carcinoma is present, and leave the diagnosis to be settled at an early operation.

Cyst of the Breast. If a history of menstrual pain suggests fibro-adenosis (the usual precursor of a cyst) endeavour to elicit fluctuation. This is best undertaken by standing behind the patient and placing the arms over the patient's shoulders. With one hand the lump is fixed; with the index finger of the other hand (the displacing finger) fluctuation is sought (*Fig.* 320). In addition to a cyst, an abscess (tenderness over a chronic abscess is sometimes absent) and a lipoma of the breast, all give a positive sign of fluctuation, while in the case of a very tense cyst this sign may be absent.

The Aspiration Test. If the history and physical signs suggest that the swelling is a cyst in association with fibro-adenosis an attempt should be made to aspirate it. If typical yellow-green fluid (*Fig.* 321) is found, it is excellent treatment to empty the cyst completely, after which the breast is carefully re-examined to make certain that the swelling has disappeared totally. An added precaution is to have the fluid scrutinized microscopically for cancer cells. Abbe noted in 1903 'There is probably no experience of the surgeon that yields him greater pleasure than to see the profound gratitude of patients who have come to him expecting no less than mammary amputation and to be told when the mammary cyst is aspirated that they are well.'

ROBERT ABBE, 1851–1928, *Surgeon, New York.*

Fibro-adenoma. Usually the patient is a woman under 30 years of age and the small lump is firm in consistency. A fibro-adenoma is rounded or ovoid; many of the larger examples are gently undulating in contour. This absolutely benign neoplasm slips beneath the fingers so readily that unless it is held between finger and thumb securely, it is liable to be lost within the breast ('breast mouse'). ─────────────────────────────→

Even a tumour that is smooth, and when moved neither causes the slightest dimpling of the skin nor any apparent drag on the breast tissue, can prove to be a carcinoma. The patient illustrated in *Fig.* 319 is a case in point, but her age was against the diagnosis of fibro-adenoma.

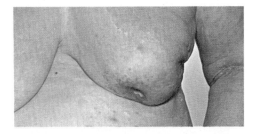

Fig. 322. Sarcoma of the breast.

The firmness of a fibro-adenoma is due to the fibrous tissue it contains. As a rule the proportion is high, and the tumour is known more corectly as a *hard fibro-adenoma*: in a few cases the amount of fibrous tissue is relatively small, and the tumour is then known as a *soft fibro-adenoma*. Soft fibro-adenomata are frequently bilateral, and they tend to occur in women over 30 years of age.

Fat Necrosis. Many women with breast cancer state that they noticed the lump after injury to the breast. There is no doubt that trauma has drawn attention to the painless lump. Fat necrosis is indistinguishable clinically from an early carcinoma without lymph-node enlargement. In recent cases bruising of the overlying skin is a point in favour of the diagnosis of fat necrosis but can also be found with a traumatized carcinoma. Procrastination is therefore unwise, and early biopsy must be advised.

Galactocele. If the patient is, or recently has been, lactating, and a cystic swelling without obvious signs of acute inflammation is present, the *aspiration test* (*see above*) should be attempted. Milk will be drawn off and the swelling will disappear if it is a galactocele.

Sarcoma (Serocystic Disease of Brodie). This comparatively rare condition accounts for ½ per cent of breast tumours. The striking clinical feature is a tendency to grow rapidly, and to attain great size and yet remain localized within the breast. The surface of the tumour is unevenly bosselated (*Fig.* 322) with areas of softening and even fluctuation in the larger convexities. The overlying skin is thin and tense, and large veins can be seen coursing beneath it. Exceptionally, the skin becomes eroded from friction, and the tumour protrudes as a fungating mass, but as a rule it is neither adherent to the skin nor to deeper structures. The axillary lymph nodes are not enlarged, except secondarily to infection. In about 15 per cent of cases the tumour gives rise to distant metastases.

A DISCHARGE FROM THE NIPPLE

When there is a history of *bleeding from the nipple*, it is not exceptional for the patient's vest to show tell-tale evidence (*Fig.* 323). Therefore look at that part of the under-garment or brassière that has been in contact with the nipples prior to the examination. Apart from the serosanguineous discharge from the denuded skin in cases of advanced Paget's disease of the nipple and a scanty seropurulent discharge oozing from a cracked nipple, the discharge comes from a lactiferous duct. Such a discharge can be bright red blood, dark altered blood, yellow serous

Sir Benjamin Brodie, 1783–1862, *Surgeon, St. George's Hospital, London.*

fluid, green-coloured fluid, opalescent fluid and occasionally crystal-clear fluid. Opalescence can be due to milk or pus. It is therefore extremely important to be furnished with a glass slide so that if the opportunity presents to collect a drop, or several drops, of the fluid expressed, the specimen can be examined for the presence of red blood cells, cancer cells, and pus cells.

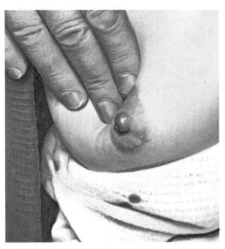

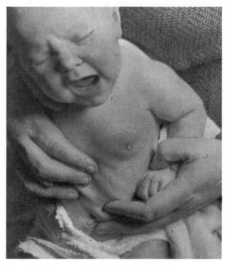

Fig. 323. Duct papilloma of the breast with retention cyst. Pressure over the cyst causes a blood-stained discharge to appear at the nipple. (The bloodstain on the patient's vest was present before the examination was commenced.)

Fig. 324. Acute mastitis in a male infant.

A Discharge of Bright Red Blood is due most frequently to a benign duct papilloma, but it can result from a duct carcinoma, and rarely from carcinoma occurring in a lactating breast. Diagnosis depends therefore not upon the presence of a discharge, but what can be learned from palpation of the breast and on microscopical examination of the discharge.

A Discharge of Dark Altered Blood is frequently the result of a duct papilloma causing obstruction to a duct, and the blood becoming pent up for a varying period.

A Discharge of Slightly Bloodstained Fluid in the presence of a sizeable cystic swelling in one quadrant of the breast strongly suggests an intracystic papilliferous carcinoma (Disease of Réclus), a rarity.

A Discharge of Clear Yellow Serous Fluid with a lumpy breast is often due to fibro-adenosis with retention cysts but can also occur in women who are on the contraceptive pill.

A Thick Green Discharge is not at all uncommon. It is due to *duct ectasia*, i.e. generalized dilatation of the major lactiferous ducts beneath the nipple due to a chronic inflammatory process which may lead to nipple retraction (*see* p. 165), sometimes bilateral.

A Milky Discharge can continue after weaning. Its presence is an indication for more efficient suppression of lactation.

In every case of discharge from the nipple the whole breast is palpated in the

PAUL RÉCLUS, 1847–1914, *Parisian Surgeon.*

usual manner. If no lump or other striking abnormality is detected, or when pressure over a segment of the areola (*Fig.* 323) does not readily produce a bead of discharge, the breast is held firmly against the chest wall by an assistant in such a way as to stretch the areola transversely, while the clinician presses the edge of the areola with his finger in a 'round the clock' manner. As a rule the bead exudes from one duct only.

ACUTE INFLAMMATIONS OF THE BREAST

Mastitis of Infants. The diagnosis of acute mastitis of infants is obvious by inspection alone (*Fig.* 324). On the third or fourth day of life, if an infant's breast is pressed lightly a drop of colourless fluid can be expressed. A few days later there is often a slight milky secretion which finally disappears during the third week. This is popularly known as 'witch's milk'. The explanation is that the hormone stimulating the mother's breasts reacts also upon the mammary tissue of the fetus. The condition is as common in the male as in the female. This physiological activity may lead to true mastitis by retrograde infection. Even so, usually it resolves; occasionally suppuration ensues.

Mastitis of Puberty. One breast is tender, slightly swollen, and inflamed. Curiously, the condition is usually seen in boys and is hardly every bilateral.

Mastitis of Mumps occurs in both sexes. Usually it is unilateral.

Bacterial Mastitis of Adult Women of child-bearing age is by far the most common variety. It usually occurs when lactation has been inefficiently suppressed. Only occasionally is it bilateral. A few cases are seen in non-lactating women.

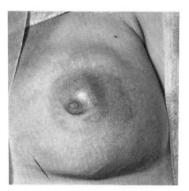

Fig. 325. Acute mammary abscess.

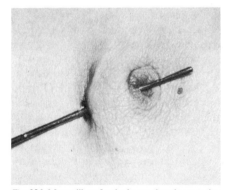

Fig. 326. Mammillary fistula due to chronic retraction of the nipple. A probe has been inserted into the fistula, the patient being anaesthetized prior to an operation.

It frequently goes on to suppuration (*Fig.* 325). The affected breast, or more usually mainly one quadrant, presents the classic signs of acute inflammation. Examine the nipple carefully for a crack or abrasion, a finding that is comparatively rare. Most breast abscesses are due to staphylococci entering the lactiferous ducts: such infection is favoured by a retracted or poorly developed nipple. Palpate the inflamed breast with extreme gentleness, the object being to ascertain which portion is most indurated, for there will lie the maximum purulent accumulation. In late cases fluctuation may be obvious. When the breast is not as tender as might be expected, but the induration is greater and the history is somewhat prolonged, it is expedient to try to eliminate the possibility of mastitis carcinomatosa, that galloping cancer of young, or pregnant, or lactating women.

Subareolar Mastitis results from an infected gland of Montgomery (*see Fig.* 311), or a furuncle of the areola.

CHRONIC ABSCESS OF THE BREAST

Chronic Intramammary Abscess is often a very difficult condition to diagnose. When encapsulated within a thick wall of fibrous tissue it cannot be distinguished clinically from a carcinoma, skin tethering or *peau d'orange* being present.

In countries where tuberculosis is rife, tuberculosis of the breast is not rare. When a patient presents with a purulent sinus connected with a breast abscess and enlarged axillary lymph nodes consider the possibility. With no enlarged lymph nodes think of actinomycosis (*see* p. 39).

Chronic Subareolar Abscess usually is associated with retraction of the nipple, and unless the retraction is remedied the condition recurs time and again, in spite of incision of the abscesses.

Mammillary* Fistula (Atkins) presents as a recurrent abscess that points and discharges on to the areola, and continues to discharge for weeks at a time. It is due to a fistula from a lactiferous duct involved by duct ectasia (*see* p. 172) or in relation to a chronically retracted nipple (*Fig.* 326).

EXAMINATION OF THE AXILLARY LYMPH NODES

The patient should be seated as for examination of the breast. The right axilla is palpated with the left hand, and vice versa. In all patients with suspected breast disease *both* axillae must be examined. Let us assume that the left axilla is to be palpated first. The various groups of lymph nodes are illustrated in *Fig.* 327. A, B, and C are palpated from in front, while D, E, and the supraclavicular lymph nodes (not shown in *Fig.* 327) are palpated from behind the patient.

Central Group (*Fig.* 327 A). Raise the patient's arm from her side, and pass the extended fingers of the right hand high up into the apex of the axilla, directing the palm towards the lateral thoracic wall (*Fig.* 328). The patient's arm is now brought to her side, and the forearm rests on the examiner's forearm, the arm hanging loosely in this position (*Fig.* 329). The non-examining hand is now free to be placed upon the patient's right shoulder, and serves to steady and control subsequent manœuvres. To make certain that the highest limit has been reached, once again the fingers in the axilla are pressed upwards. The hand should then be cupped, and the finger-pulps pass downwards with a firm, sliding movement, until they are well below the level of the axillary outlet.

When one or more of the central axillary lymph nodes are enlarged, they will be felt momentarily imprisoned between the thorax and the examining fingers (*Fig.* 330): the number, size, consistency and mobility or fixity are noted.

Lateral Axillary Group (*Fig.* 327 B). These lie on the axillary vein, and the most lateral nodes of this group lie distal to the pectoralis minor, where they are comparatively accessible. Raise the arm again, this time slowly, and while raising the arm (and lowering it, if necessary, until the optimum position has been

---

* *Mammilla*. Latin = a nipple.

SIR HEDLEY ATKINS, *Contemporary Emeritus Professor of Surgery, Guy's Hospital, London.*

reached) palpate around and beneath the insertion of the pectoralis major for an enlarged node lying on the third part of the axillary blood vessels.

Interpectoral Group (*Fig.* 327 C) is next examined. The patient's arm is elevated, and the fingers are insinuated beneath the pectoralis major. This time the pulps of the fingers are directed forwards. On lowering the arm as shown in *Fig.* 329 the pectoralis minor muscle frequently can be detected, and between the two muscles are situated the interpectoral nodes.

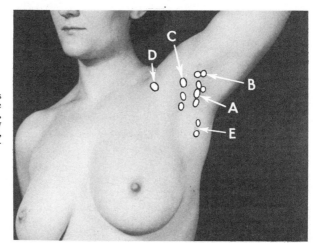

Fig. 327. The axillary lymph nodes from a clinical standpoint and the order in which they are palpated. A, Central group; B, Lateral axillary group; C, Interpectoral group; D, Infraclavicular group; E, Subscapular group.

Infraclavicular Group (*Fig.* 327 D). Enlargement of lymph nodes lying on the clavipectoral fascia should be suspected when there is obliteration of the infraclavicular hollow or where there is unilateral prominence of veins in this region. The area is palpated and compared with that of the opposite side.

Subscapular Group (*Fig.* 327 E). These, lying on the posterior axillary fold, are best examined from the back (*Fig.* 331). Standing behind the patient, the examiner palpates the antero-internal surface of the latissimus dorsi, and if these lymph nodes are enlarged they will be found at the bottom of the fold. The apex of the axilla should also be palpated from this aspect, which gives good access to the more posterior of the central group.

Examination of the Supraclavicular Fossae. *See* p. 139.

Conclusions. The findings should be recorded graphically. Indurated enlargement of a lymph node or nodes in any of the groups detailed above signifies that metastasis has occurred, and if the enlarged node is tethered, the eventual prognosis is poor. One must be mindful that lack of palpable evidence of lymph-node involvement is no guarantee that metastasis has not occurred. Indeed, in approximately 50 per cent of cases of carcinoma of the breast with impalpable lymph nodes histological scrutiny of the specimen obtained by regional block dissection shows a carcinomatous deposit in one or more of the nodes removed. It must also be mentioned that the chain of lymph nodes along the internal mammary vessels is not clinically accessible.

Note that shotty enlargement of the axillary lymph nodes often occurs in fibro-adenosis.

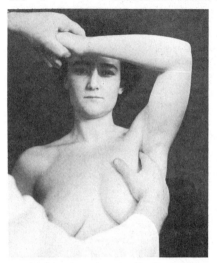

Fig. 328. Examining the axilla (I). The arm is raised, and the fingers are inserted as high as possible.

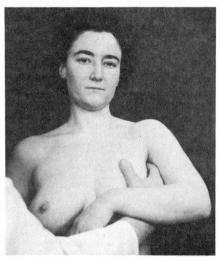

Fig. 329. Examining the axilla (II). Note that the patient's arm rests comfortably over the examiner's forearm so that the pectoral muscles are relaxed.

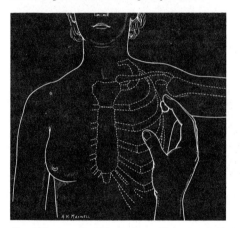

Fig. 330. A node high in the axilla momentarily imprisoned between the thorax and the examining fingers.

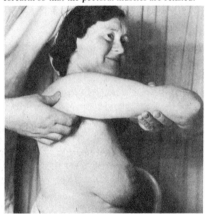

Fig. 331. Examining from the back, the subscapular lymph nodes lying in the posterior fold of the axilla.

Sometimes it is difficult to be sure whether a given lump is situated in the axillary tail of the breast, or whether it is due to metastases in the lowermost of the pectoral group of nodes (*Fig.* 332).

When the axillary lymph nodes are the seat of bacterial invasion (often due to an infected lesion of the hand or arm) they are wont to break down and form an axillary abscess (*Fig.* 333).

CLINICAL STAGING OF BREAST CANCER

It is insufficient to diagnose carcinoma of the breast. To advise appropriate treatment suitable for a given patient, the surgeon should estimate how early or advanced is the growth. From this more refined diagnosis the average prognosis can be deduced.

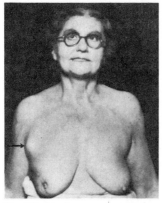

Fig. 332. Massive secondary involvement of the lowermost pectoral group of lymph nodes. There is a primary neoplasm visible in the breast proper, causing retraction of the right nipple.

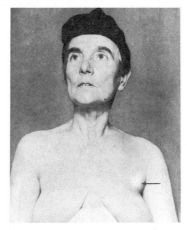

Fig. 333. A tender swelling under the left pectoralis major is present. Temperature raised. Subpectoral abscess.

Two forms of clinical staging are in use, the first simpler, but the second more desirable by virtue of the greater detail possible.

The International Classification. Four stages are recognized:

I. A lump is present, perhaps with slight tethering to the skin. Paget's disease without lymph-node enlargement falls into this category.

II. In addition, there are mobile enlarged lymph nodes in the ipsilateral axilla, or the nipple is recently retracted, or the lump is tethered to the skin.

III. The tumour is extensively adherent to skin (including *peau d'orange*), or to underlying muscle, or is ulcerating, or ipsilateral nodes are fixed.

IV. There are distant metastases (including skin nodules), contralateral or supraclavicular nodes, or a lump in the opposite breast, or liver, bone, or lung metastases.

The **TNM** *Classification* has been sponsored by the International Union Against Cancer. **T** refers to the characteristics of the tumour, **N** of the lymph nodes, and **M** denotes the presence or absence of metastases.

T_1. Size 2 cm or less with no fixation or nipple retraction. Paget's disease with a lump showing these characteristics is included.

T_2. Tumour more than 2 cm diameter but less than 5 cm, or less than 2 cm, but with tethering of overlying skin or retraction of nipple.

T_3. Tumour more than 5 cm diameter but less than 10 cm, or less than 5 cm with infiltration or ulceration of skin, or *peau d'orange* over tumour, or fixation to muscle.

T_4. Any size tumour with infiltration or ulceration of skin wide of tumour, or *peau d'orange* wide of tumour, or chest-wall fixation, or tumour larger than 10 cm.

N_0. No palpable axillary lymph nodes.

N_1. Axillary lymph nodes, palpable but mobile.

N_2. Axillary lymph nodes, fixed to each other, or to other structures.

N_3. Supraclavicular lymph nodes movable or fixed, or oedema of arm.

M_0. No evidence of distant metastases.

M_1. Distant metastases including skin wide of breast, opposite breast or nodes, or other metastases.

Note that the growth is given the highest number in each series which can be applied. Thus the lesion depicted in *Fig.* 319 would be staged T_1, N_0, M_0, while that in *Fig.* 332 would be T_2, N_2, M_0. It is a good exercise for the student to work through the illustrations of breast cancer in this chapter and stage them as far as the data allow.

THE MALE BREAST

The examination of the male breast is carried out in the same manner as in the female.

Mastitis. Reference has been made already to mastitis of infants and mastitis of puberty affecting males. In adults traumatic mastitis occurs among soldiers carrying heavy equipment strapped across their shoulders.

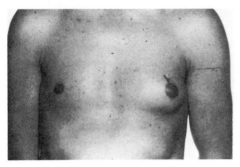

Fig. 334. Gynaecomazia in an adolescent.

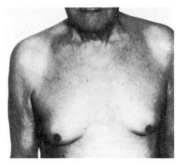

Fig. 335. Oestrogen gynaecomazia following treatment of carcinoma of the prostate.

Fig. 336. Carcinoma of the breast in a man who did not report it until the skin became ulcerated and painful. In male patients this delay in seeking advice is the rule, rather than the exception.

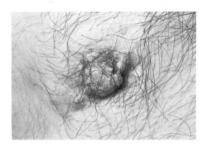

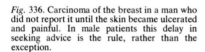

Gynaecomazia

a. *Idiopathic.* Hypertrophy of the male breast may be unilateral or bilateral. The breast (or breasts) enlarges at puberty, and sometimes presents the characteristics of a moderately developed female organ (*Fig.* 334). Usually the enlargement regresses in 6–12 months.

b. *Hormonal.* Enlargement of the breasts has often accompanied oestrogen therapy,* particularly for carcinoma of the prostate (*Fig.* 335). It can also occur as a result of a teratoma or a chorionepithelioma of the testis, in anorchism, and after castration. In *leprosy* it is likely that testicular atrophy is the cause of the gynaecomazia commonly seen. The contents of the scrotum must therefore always be examined.

c. *Associated with Portal Cirrhosis.* Gynaecomazia sometimes occurs in patients with liver damage which results in incomplete destruction of circulating oestrogens thereby stimulating the breast to hypertrophy. The liver should always be examined.

Fibro-adenosis is not rare in men. It can occur on one or both sides. In unilateral cases fibro-adenosis can be distinguished from carcinoma by the occurrence of a small disc-shaped, movable, firm, tender swelling beneath the areola. Usually the tenderness diminishes after two months and the hypertrophy is all but gone in six months.

Fibro-adenoma is not exceedingly rare, and presents the same clinical features as in the female (*see* p. 171) except that the lump is not elusive in the small male breast.

Carcinoma, which accounts for about 1 per cent of all cases of carcinoma of the breast, has an evil reputation: many cases are far advanced when the patient first presents. Primarily this is due to the fact that so often the patient does not seek advice for months or years (*Fig.* 336). Secondly, the breast is so small that the enlarging growth reaches the extramammary tissue much sooner than in the female. On the other hand, the signs of malignancy (hardness of the lump, skin tethering, *peau d'orange*, and fixity of muscle, *see* pp. 166–8) are more easily detected.

---

* Unprotected workers engaged in the manufacture of oestrogens are liable to develop gynaecomazia.

Chapter 16

THE THORAX (INCLUDING OESOPHAGUS)

The thorax is considered fully in medical works so no purpose would be served by embarking upon a detailed consideration of physical signs connected with lung and heart disease. Attention will therefore be focused on particular points significant to the surgeon.

First consider a condition of such great urgency that the patient's life is hanging in the balance, and the chances of recovery rest largely upon the clinician's diagnostic acumen and prompt action.

Laryngeal or Tracheal Obstruction. Stridor,* dyspnoea, cyanosis and restlessness (fighting for breath) are cardinal signs of obstruction of the major air-passage. The larynx moves forcibly up and down with respiration and, especially in an adult, the accessory muscles of respiration can be seen to contract violently with each attempted inspiration (*see Fig.* 347, p. 185). Simultaneously the distended jugular veins become empty and indrawn, only to billow forth again when inspiratory gives place to expiratory effort. On baring the thorax another characteristic sign is seen:

The Sign of Recession. The lower end of the sternum, together with the adjacent costal framework, the supraclavicular fossae and epigastrium, is sucked in during inspiration. This is especially noticeable in young children, e.g. in diphtheria, now a rarity. In older children and adults, owing to the greater rigidity of the chest wall, gross recession is rarely in evidence, but retraction of the intercostal spaces usually is evident in comparatively thin subjects. Considerable and consistent recession is a sure sign of respiratory obstruction, except where the patient is recovering from an anaesthetic and is still under the effects of a muscle relaxant.

THORACIC DEFORMITIES

Much information can be obtained from general inspection of the thorax, and an astute surgeon will not fail to notice the thoracic build and respiratory expansion of the patient in every relevant case. Chronic bronchitis is a pointer to the likelihood of complications after anaesthesia, particularly atelectasis (*see* p. 193). **Pectus Excavatum** (funnel chest) and **Pectus Carinatum** (pigeon chest) are both due not to rickets, but to a congenital elongation of the costal cartilages so that the sternum is pushed forwards or backwards (Abrams). In the former the lower sternum forms a fixed irreversible deformity (*Fig.* 337) which, if severe, causes the patient to suffer from dyspnoea on exertion and renders him liable to respiratory infection. By pressure upon the heart, funnel chest sometimes causes a systolic murmur and degrees of exertion intolerance, which have been mistaken

---

* *Stridor* is a harsh noise produced as respiratory air passes through a partially obstructed main air-passage.

Leon D. Abrams, *Contemporary Cardio-Thoracic Surgeon, Queen Elizabeth Hospital, Birmingham.*

for heart disease. Rarely more serious effects are observed, culminating in heart failure. In the latter there is a keel-like protuberance of the body of the sternum (*Fig.* 338).

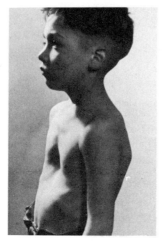

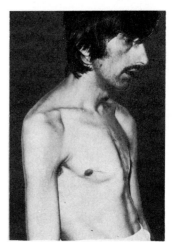

Fig. 337. Pectus excavatum (funnel chest).

Fig. 338. Pectus carinatum (pigeon chest).

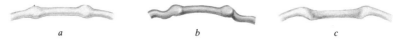

a   b   c

Fig. 339. Deformities of the sternocostal junction. *a*, Rickety rosary; *b*, Harrison's sulcus; *c*, Scorbutic rosary.

Deformities of the Sternocostal Junction. The rachitic chest, resulting from impaired mineralization of bone consequent upon vitamin-D deficiency, is first seen in infants between 6 and 18 months of life as a **rickety rosary**, produced by bead-like enlargement of the ribs at their junction with their cartilages (*Fig.* 339 *a*).

Later the softened ribs encourage the development of a **Harrison's sulcus**. This groove occurs at the costochondral junction (*Fig.* 339 *b*), the lower ribs appearing caved in.

The Scorbutic Rosary due to vitamin-C lack differs from that produced by rickets in that the sternum is displaced backwards (*Fig.* 339 *c*).

Slipping Rib. The pain is referred to the exact position of the incompletely tethered rib, usually the tenth, the cartilage of which can be moved upwards so as to override the ninth (*see Fig.* 341 (*inset*)), and this movement causes pain. Usually the patient is a young woman.

CLUBBING OF THE FINGERS

This (*Fig.* 340) is a sign of chronic anoxia from any cause; it is important to the surgeon in assessing the patient's fitness for anaesthesia. It is common in patients with bronchial carcinoma and may be associated with bronchiectasis and, as Hippocrates described, with a chronic discharging empyema sinus. It is also seen with advanced (notably congenital) heart disease, cirrhosis of the liver and

EDWIN HARRISON. 1779–1847, *Physician, St. Marylebone Infirmary, London.*
HIPPOCRATES, *see footnote p. 89.*

chronic colitis. The over-curving of the nails is the result of bulbous enlargement of the nail-beds with, in later cases, lateral expansion of the terminal phalanx resulting in a drumstick appearance. In established cases the fingernails are curved longitudinally like a parrot's beak. *Hypertrophic pulmonary osteo-arthropathy* consists of clubbing, together with symmetrical swelling of joints (particularly ankles, wrists, or knees) which feel hot on palpation. The commonest cause (80 per cent) is bronchial carcinoma, in 6 per cent of which it occurs.

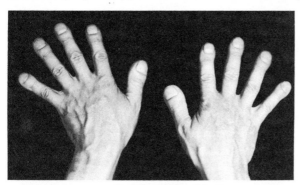

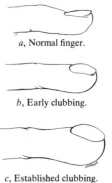

a, Normal finger.

b, Early clubbing.

c, Established clubbing.

Fig. 340. Clubbing of the fingers.

COUNTING RIBS

Often it is necessary to know which rib is injured or diseased. Running the finger downwards from the suprasternal notch, a transverse ridge can be felt, and often seen—the angle of Louis (sternal angle). The finger, moved to the side along this ridge, will pass directly on to the second rib. Ribs are counted from this point (*Fig.* 341). Posteriorly, ribs may be counted upwards, starting with the twelfth, which can usually be felt, but in obese individuals only with difficulty. When the arm rests by the side, the lower angle of the scapula lies upon the seventh rib. The spine of the scapula lies over the third rib or third intercostal space, but the scapular surface markings are not absolutely reliable guides.

THORACIC INJURIES

Injuries of the thorax occur frequently and severe injuries are seen increasingly with motor-car accidents.

Fractured Rib. Ask the patient, who is stripped to the waist, to take a deep breath. If a rib or ribs are fractured, pain is likely to be experienced in the region of the fracture before the zenith of inspiration, and he at once clasps a hand to the injured part to support it. Careful palpation along each rib in this region will often reveal local tenderness and evidence of a breach of bony continuity, especially in a thin subject. Such evidence is occasionally more reliable than a radiograph. In fat or muscular individuals, particularly when the fracture is situated somewhere in the middle ribs (quite a common situation), the compression test is valuable.

The Compression Test. The base of one hand is placed over the sternum, and the base of the other over the spine; the thorax is then gently compressed

ANTOINE LOUIS, 1723–1792, *Surgeon, Hôpital Charité, Paris. A notorious achievement was to perfect the guillotine, which was first used in 1792 in the execution of a highwayman. Some attribute the description of the angle of Louis to* PIERRE LOUIS, *1787–1872, Physician, Hôpital la Pitié, Paris.*

anteroposteriorly (*Fig*. 342). When a rib has been fractured this manœuvre causes pain at the site of the lesion.

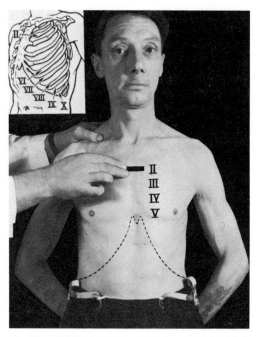

Fig. 341. Method of counting ribs. The angle of Louis is found; this is opposite the second costal cartilage. Bearings are taken from this point.

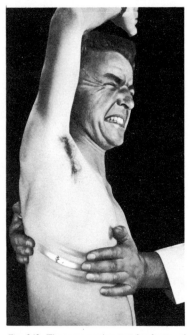

Fig. 342. The compression test for fractured rib. Commence with 'fairy-like' pressure.

In every case of fractured rib the clinician must keep a sharp look-out for signs of concomitant injury of a lung (*see below*), and on the left side for signs of a rupture of the spleen (*see* p. 324), which are also sometimes delayed.

Fracture of the Sternum. The posture is characteristic: the body is bent forwards with the shoulders rotated inwards, and the head held forwards and downwards. Thanks to the comparative accessibility of the sternum to the palpating fingers, the deformity associated with a fracture of this structure is usually detected without difficulty. The spinal column must be examined for a concomitant injury (*see* p. 216).

Injury of a Lung. There are two early signs, the presence of either of which leaves no doubt that the underlying lung has been implicated in the injury. The first is *haemoptysis*: if even a small quantity of frothy bright-red blood is expectorated it is proof that contusion or laceration of lung tissue with escape of blood into the alveoli or bronchioles has occurred. In every case of thoracic injury an early question should always be, 'Have you coughed up any blood?'

The second is the presence of *subcutaneous emphysema*. The physical characteristics have been described on p. 16. Following a thoracic injury it can make its appearance in two ways: (*a*) As a result of traumatic rupture of pulmonary tissue air passes beneath the visceral pleura to the hilum of the lung, and thence, via the mediastinum, it appears in the neck. Extreme instances of this variety are to be seen when a wound or rupture of the trachea or large bronchus allows a communication to exist with the areolar tissue of the mediastinum. Quickly the whole of the subcutaneous plane of the neck and face becomes distended with air. (*b*) Following laceration of the adjacent lung by a fractured rib or by a stab wound (*Fig.*343) emphysema appears over the site of injury and spreads for a varying distance around the site of fracture. This variety of subcutaneous escape of air may or may not be associated with a pneumothorax.

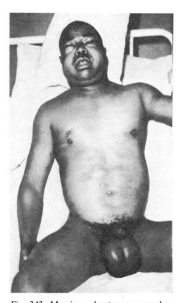

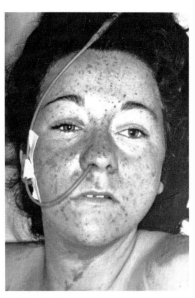

Fig. 343. Massive subcutaneous emphy-sema involving the scrotum, the neck, and the face, resulting from a stab wound of the thorax above the right nipple.

Fig. 344. Traumatic asphyxia, following a traffic accident.

Minor degrees of subcutaneous emphysema are common following thoracic operations.

Contusion of the lung may lead to the signs of pneumonia a few days after an injury. This diagnosis is beyond our province.

Haemothorax and Haemopneumothorax are common complications of compression injuries of the thorax with fracture of a rib or ribs. Sometimes the onset is insidious, and consequently the possibility of blood or air (frequently in combination) accumulating in the pleural cavity should be suspected for three or four days, even after a fracture of a single rib. Reliable signs for their detection are dullness on percussion in the case of haemothorax, hyper-resonance above this in the case of haemopneumothorax, and absence of breath sounds. Signs of shock (*see* p. 42) are present if blood loss has been sufficient. The diagnosis must be confirmed by the typical radiological appearances.

Traumatic Asphyxia occasionally complicates compression injuries of the thorax. Petechial haemorrhages, due to extravasation of blood from compressed venules, are seen in the skin, confined mainly to the face and neck (*Fig.* 344), although they may be seen to a lesser extent on the thorax. The conjunctivae are bright red from conjunctival haemorrhages. In rare severe instances the face is purple.

Stove-in Chest. Several ribs are fractured with a resulting local indentation of the chest wall. If this lesion is uncomplicated by flail chest (*see below*), its efforts on respiration are not severe. Blood loss may be marked.

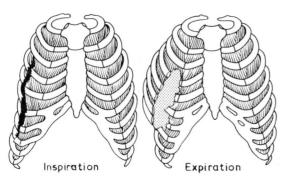

Inspiration   Expiration

Fig. 345. Paradoxical respiration. The comminuted fractured ribs are displaced inwards during inspiration and outwards on expiration or cough.

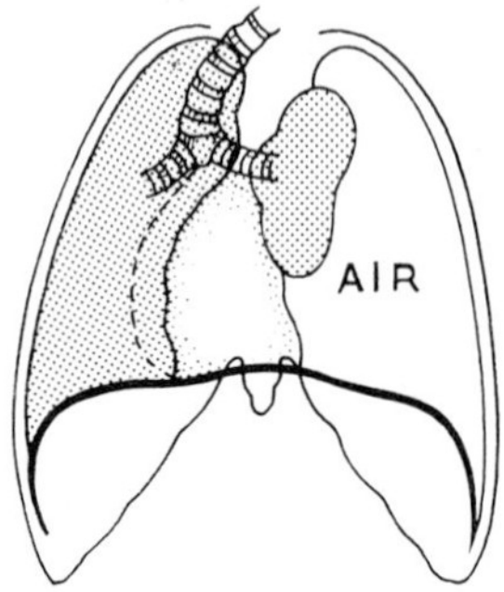

Fig. 346. Tension (valvular) pneumothorax showing displacement of the mediastinum and trachea.

Flail Chest. A crushing injury resulting in comminuted fractures of three or more ribs, each with a fracture posteriorly *and* at, or near, the costochondral junction, causes a flail chest. An even more dangerous variant is when a number of ribs or costal cartilages are fractured on either side near the sternum, rendering the sternum flail. In either case the flail segment is sucked in during inspiration and driven out during expiration; the breathing is therefore paradoxical, the injured side of the thorax moving in while the uninjured side moves out (*Fig.* 345). This results in air being shunted from the injured to the uninjured side and back again, rather than being exhaled, with progressive accumulation of carbon dioxide which, together with loss of effective cough and resulting accumulation of tracheobronchial secretions, produces unmistakable dyspnoea and cyanosis. The increasing anoxia and carbon-dioxide retention result in increased dyspnoea and more pronounced paradoxical movement with rapid deterioration of the patient's condition—a vicious cycle that can be broken only by urgent appropriate treatment.

Tension (Valvular) Pneumothorax. Blood as well as air is extravasated into the pleural cavity, but the air decidedly predominates. The cause is laceration of the lung communicating with a branch of the bronchial tree. This permits air to enter the pleural cavity from the lung during inspiration, but it does not permit its escape during expiration—hence the term 'valvular'. Increasing dyspnoea and cyanosis are leading features. Absence of breath sounds, hyper-resonance, cardiac displacement, pallor and poor pulse are classic signs. As the air accumulates in the pleural cavity, so the mediastinum and trachea tend to become more and more displaced (*Fig.* 346).

Bronchial Tear. After a severe accident the patient develops a tension pneumothorax which is treated by tube drainage. A continuing massive leakage of air indicates that a main bronchus has been torn and that urgent thoracotomy is essential. Many patients present with massive subcutaneous emphysema (*see* p. 182) extending even into the scrotum.

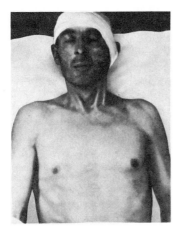

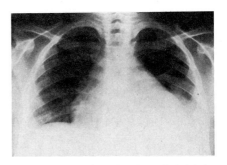

Fig. 348. An X-ray showing the typical globular enlargement of the heart in cardiac tamponade.

Fig. 347. Blast injury. Appearance of the chest in full inspiration, showing fullness of the lower thorax and overaction of the accessory muscles, notably the sterno-mastoid.

Blast Injuries due to high explosives are borne, to a great extent, by the lungs. In patients who survive, the symptoms and signs are few: consequently, the condition may be overlooked, especially when other lesions are in evidence. Always suspect the presence of lung injury in every patient involved in an explosion. An expanded appearance of the lower chest is a fairly regular accompaniment (*Fig.* 347).

Open Wounds of the Thorax. A 'sucking' wound of the thorax indicates that the pleura has been opened. Bloody froth issuing from the wound, coupled with respiratory distress, suggests a tension pneumothorax.

Cardiac Tamponade. In a penetrating wound of the pericardium the heart will almost certainly be wounded, in which case bleeding will occur into the pericardium. As the amount of blood in the pericardium increases so, *pari passu*, is the heart compressed, and the circulation fails correspondingly. The pulse rate becomes faster and the pulse pressure progressively weaker. Pulsus paradoxus is present, i.e. the pulse feels weaker when the patient inspires. The veins of the face and neck become engorged, and the dimensions of the area of cardiac dullness increase (*Fig.* 348). The heart sounds are faint and muffled on auscultation. This condition occasionally occurs with a closed injury.

Contusion of the Heart. After a blunt injury to the front of the chest, the patient complains of precordial pain and weakness; a low blood pressure is noted without the other signs of tamponade mentioned above. An electrocardiogram will show changes similar to those of coronary thrombosis and a physician should be asked to interpret this and manage the case.

Traumatic Rupture of the Aorta. This serious injury is becoming commoner in this age of traffic accidents. A proportion of patients reach hospital alive in severe shock and, if conscious, complaining of intense chest pain which may be attributed to concomitant fractured ribs. Radiography is essential for diagnosis but Powley has described an important physical sign which may be observed during the time necessary to arrange arteriography; as the mediastinal haematoma spreads to the root of the neck, the neck measurement may increase by as much as 10 cm in 2–3 hours. The normal size of the neck is obtained from the patient's shirt collar. The blood pressure measured in the upper extremities may be raised, that in the lower extremities is reduced.

PHILIP H. POWLEY, *Contemporary Surgeon, Princess Margaret Hospital, Swindon, Wilts.*

SOLID SWELLINGS OF THE THORACIC CAGE

Non-specific Costochondritis (Tietze's Disease) is common. The patient, in civil life nearly always a woman, complains of a varyingly painful swelling of the chest wall. More often than not she considers that the lump is in the breast, and this is the real cause of the concern, which may be shared by her medical attendant. The most common cartilage to be affected is the second. On careful palpation it becomes quite evident that the swelling in question is caused by an expansion of the cartilage as it joins the rib. This disease also occurs in military recruits in whom it appears to result from carrying heavy equipment strapped to the chest.

Tuberculous Costochondritis. Only a very small proportion of cases prove to be tuberculous. Unless the patient has other evidence of tuberculosis, shows a positive dermal test, or has a swelling that is larger and more defined than a diffuse expansion of the costochondral junction, it is impossible to diagnose the tuberculous variety in its early stages, for there are no characteristic radiological changes. Later, the presence of fluctuation (cold abscess) makes diagnosis easier.

A Neoplasm of that Portion of a Rib lying Beneath the Breast also causes apparent enlargement of the breast. *Fig.* 349 shows a case in point. If the hand be placed over the breast the whole breast will be found to be movable on the swelling behind it; this is the method by which is settled the important question, 'Is the swelling in, or behind, the breast?'

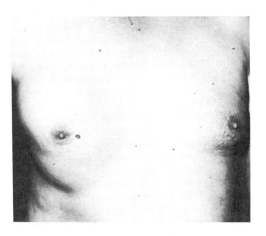

Fig. 349. A tumour of the rib causing apparent enlargement of the right breast in a young adult male. After surgical excision it proved to be a chondrosarcoma on histological examination.

Neoplasm of the Rib. If it is remembered that swellings involving the skin and soft tissues (e.g. sebaceous cyst, p. 23, lipoma, p. 23) can occur in the chest wall, it becomes comparatively easy to recognize that a bony hard swelling lies in the long axis of a rib and is expanding the rib. Confronted with a hard swelling of a rib which is unlikely to be caused by excessive callus around a fracture, one should ask oneself the basic question, 'Is this neoplastic swelling primary or secondary?' In practice the great majority are secondary.

Secondary Carcinoma of a Rib is associated particularly with primary carcinoma of the breast or of the bronchus (*Fig.* 350), but it can originate from any primary, particularly those mentioned on p. 425. Pain and local tenderness are marked and may be present long before a swelling is manifest. Spontaneous fracture of a rib, the seat of a secondary carcinoma, occurs rather frequently.

ALEXANDER TIETZE, 1864–1927, *Chief Surgeon, Allerheiligen Hospital, Breslau.*

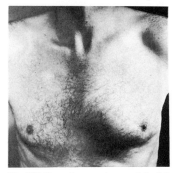

Fig. 350. Secondary carcinoma of the left 5th rib in a patient with carcinoma of the bronchus.

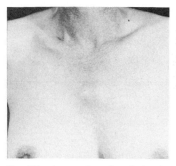

Fig. 351. A secondary deposit in the sternum. The patient had complained of painless haematuria for some months. Case of carcinoma of the kidney.

Primary Rib Tumours are not rare. The conditions considered on pp. 424–6 can occur. Chondrosarcoma (*Fig.* 349) is the commonest. If a primary source cannot be found a biopsy should be carried out.

Neoplasms of the Sternum are considerably less frequent than those of the ribs. Secondary tumours are much more likely (*Fig.* 351). Primary tumours are distinctly rare.

Lymphoma of an Internal Mammary Lymph Node. As it enlarges it causes a solid swelling in one of the upper intercostal spaces near the sternum (*Fig.* 352); the costal cartilage is sometimes involved in the swelling. This may be the presenting lesion of these conditions.

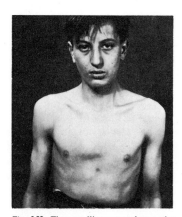

Fig. 352. Firm swelling centred over the fourth right intercostal space. This was the presenting sign in this patient with Hodgkin's disease. Note that he looks ill.

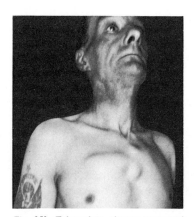

Fig. 353. Tuberculous abscess connected with the third right costal cartilage.

CYSTIC SWELLINGS OF THE THORACIC WALL

A patient with a cystic swelling connected with the deeper layers of the thoracic wall is presented. After confirming that the swelling fluctuates, apply the following tests: ask the patient to cough, and by inspection and palpation note if there is any impulse.

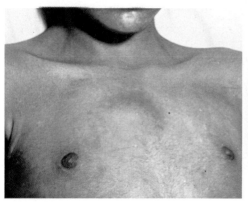

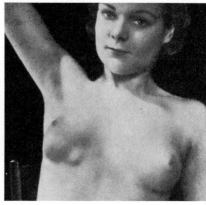

Fig. 354. Tuberculous abscess originating in an internal mammary lymph node in an Indian. The abscess is about to burst through the skin (*see* p. 142).

Fig. 355. A retromammary tuberculoma connected with a tuberculous internal mammary lymph node. Mistaken by several observers for a breast lump.

Cold Abscess arising in the Thoracic Wall. *When the swelling is situated anteriorly* and there is no evidence of gross underlying pleural effusion (*see* Empyema Necessitans, p. 189) there are two possibilities: (*a*) that the abscess has originated in a tuberculous rib or costal cartilage, in which case it is likely that a portion of the diseased rib will be found to be expanded. In *Fig.* 353 the enlarged third rib can be seen, as also (overlying the sternum) the swelling caused by the abscess. Should, however, the related ribs and costal cartilages look and feel normal, it is probable that: (*b*) the site of origin of the abscess is a tuberculous internal mammary lymph node (*Fig.* 354). Sometimes the related costochondral junctions can only be palpated adequately after the abscess has been aspirated. The internal mammary chain of lymph nodes does not extend below the sixth intercostal space; a cold abscess below this level is almost certainly not of lymph-node origin.

A cold abscess of the lateral thoracic wall is uncommon.

When the swelling is situated posteriorly there are three possible sites of origin: (1) a tuberculous rib; (2) a tuberculous dorsal vertebra; (3) a perinephric abscess, often secondary to a tuberculous pyonephrosis. The latter two conditions are confirmed or eliminated by examining the spine in the case of (2), and in the case of (3) by excretory pyelography.

Occasionally a cold abscess of the thoracic wall is partly reducible into an extrapleural pocket of the abscess cavity.

Retromammary Abscess. The *acute type* results from suppuration in deep lobules of the breast, and pus burrowing posteriorly comes to lie between the breast in front and the pectoral fascia behind, viz.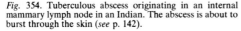

In the *chronic variety* the pus occupies the same plane, but it arises in a tuberculous costochondral junction or in a tuberculous lymph node of the internal mammary chain (*Fig.* 355). Retromammary pus tends to gravitate to the lower and outer quadrant of the breast which it displaces forward, thereby creating an illusion of enlargement.

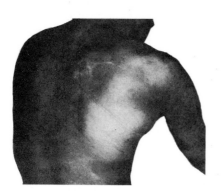

Fig. 356. Empyema necessitans in an African.

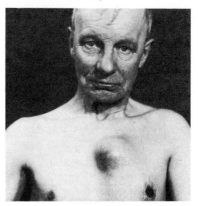

Fig. 357. Aortic aneurysm eroding the thoracic wall. The patient had little complaint. His Wassermann reaction was strongly positive.

Empyema Necessitans. Although now rare in Western Europe and North America, this (*Fig.* 356) is still encountered in some parts of the world. Almost always the swelling appears on the anterior or lateral aspects of the thorax, somewhere between the third and sixth intercostal spaces. Fluctuation is obtained readily. If the flat of the hand is laid over the swelling and the patient is asked to cough, usually a fluid thrill can be felt. With the flat of the hand still in position, exert moderate pressure on the swelling. Contrary to what might be thought, it is exceptional for the empyema to be completely reducible into the thoracic cavity, probably because today most cases occurring in urban communities are the result of seepage along the needle track of a previous aspiration. When it occurs on the left side, sometimes the purulent collection transmits the cardiac pulsation and has been mistaken for an aneurysm.

Aortic Aneurysm. A syphilitic aneurysm may give rise to a swelling near the sternum (*Fig.* 357), but it is unlikely that such a pulsating swelling will cause diagnostic perplexity.

A Hernia of the Lung is a great rarity: it gives rise to a completely reducible tympanitic cystic swelling, usually at the apex of the lung, i.e. at the root of the neck above the clavicle.

DISCHARGING SINUSES OF THE THORACIC WALL

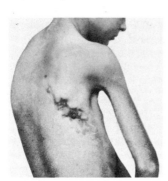

Fig. 358. Chronic empyema sinus of seven years' duration. The opening is at a comparatively high level. The patient had clubbing of the fingers.

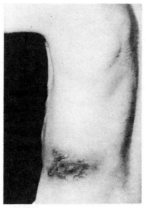

Fig. 359. Actinomycotic sinus arising from the lung.

Chronic Empyema Sinus. An empyema has been drained, but the sinus continues to discharge indefinitely (*Fig.* 358). Among the causes are ineffectual drainage, underlying lung disease, a retained drainage-tube, osteomyelitis of ribs, tuberculosis and actinomycosis. The elucidation of the problem is impossible without the aid of radiography and other diagnostic adjuvants. Nevertheless, at the clinical examination note the level of the sinus, palpate the bony thorax around it for undue callus formation, and examine the pus.

Actinomycotic Sinus. The surrounding skin is apt to present a dusky appearance (*Fig.* 359) because of involvement, not of the skin, but of the underlying subcutaneous tissues. Perhaps the most notable feature of this lesion is the curious linear puckering that appears in the area about the sinus or sinuses. The correct diagnosis can only be made as described on p. 39. In more than half the cases the pulmonary infection is secondary to actinomycosis elsewhere.

Sinus resulting from a Tuberculous Rib or a Tuberculous Internal Mammary Lymph Node. The preceding abscess has been considered on p. 188.

RETROCLAVICULAR SWELLINGS

Reference is made here to swellings situated in the supraclavicular fossa plunging beneath the clavicle to fill the infraclavicular fossa rather than to enlarged lymph nodes in this situation. These often present difficulties in diagnosis. A tumour of one of the cords of the brachial plexus is liable to be mistaken for a deep-seated lipoma or an enlarged lymph node. Indiscriminate excision is disastrous for the function of the arm. A stony-hard mass in this deep recess beneath the clavicle may prove to be not a mass of malignant lymph nodes but a bone tumour arising from the first rib. An X-ray is necessary for accurate diagnosis.

CARCINOMA OF THE BRONCHUS

This disease has increased in frequency so alarmingly that it is incumbent upon the clinician to be highly alert concerning its possibility, particularly in those with a long history of heavy smoking. Tobacco staining or clubbing of the fingers (*see* p. 180) are data which should arouse suspicion.

Early diagnosis in a curable stage is a matter for the chest physician who usually invokes the aid of a surgeon skilled in the use of the bronchoscope. Unfortunately, the neoplasm is often highly malignant and metastasizes early, the patient presenting with a metastasis. It used to be said that syphilis was the great imitator (of other diseases), but with the decline in untreated venereal disease carcinoma of the bronchus has taken over this unenviable role.

The following are the more frequent manifestations seen by the surgeon:

Bone metastases, in the ribs (*see* p. 186), long bones (*see* p. 426), or back (*see* p. 214). Pain is the leading feature in the great majority of patients, with a swelling appearing as a late sign.

Pathological fractures are not infrequent, particularly in the long bones and vertebrae (*see* p. 434).

Loss of appetite and weight should, in the first instance, suggest cancer of the stomach. In many cases, carcinoma of a bronchus is found to be the culprit.

Enlarged lymph nodes in the neck (*see* p. 140) or axillae (*see* p. 174) of male patients are frequent. Typically they are stony-hard in consistency. It is not unknown for enlargement of other nodes (e.g. groin, *see* p. 251) to be the first sign.

Recurrent laryngeal nerve paralysis (hoarseness) in the absence of thyroid cancer (*see* p. 156) often proves to be due to carcinomatous deposits originating in a bronchus.

Malignant enlargement of the liver (*see* p. 235) or *ascites* (*see* p. 242) are occasional presentations.

Secondary nodules of growth in the skin, single, or few in number, or multiple, are sometimes the first sign. They are of hard consistency, vary in size from a couple of centimetres in diameter down to minute swellings which can only be discerned by running the pulp of the index finger over them, and have appeared in a matter of days or weeks (cf. multiple lipomata, *see Fig.* 47, p. 25).

Superior vena caval obstruction (*see below*).

Pancoast's Syndrome results from a growth commencing in the apex of the lung, and, as it is silent for a long period, it is the harbinger of death. It comprises three or more of the following manifestations: distension of the veins of the neck (pressure on the superior vena cava); swelling of the face from the same cause; Horner's syndrome (*see* p. 404) from pressure on the sympathetic chain; shooting pains down the arm. Later a lower brachial plexus lesion develops (*see* p. 405).

PRESSURE ON THE SUPERIOR VENA CAVA

Visible engorgement of the veins of the neck is usually an indication of metastases in the posterior mediastinum pressing upon the superior vena cava, but it can be due to other causes such as a primary neoplasm, or a cyst pressing upon this great venous channel, or cicatricial contracture following a stab wound (*Fig.* 360).

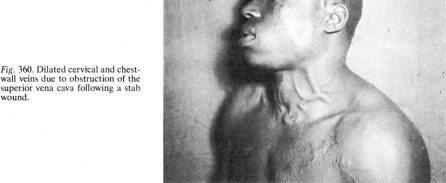

Fig. 360. Dilated cervical and chest-wall veins due to obstruction of the superior vena cava following a stab wound.

EXAMINATION OF A PATIENT WITH SUSPECTED ACUTE PULMONARY INFECTION

When called to a patient whose history suggests postoperative atelectasis, pulmonary infection, or a subdiaphragmatic abscess, as well as when confronted

HENRY K. PANCOAST, 1875–1939, *Professor of Roentgenology, University of Pennsylvania, Philadelphia.*

with one whose sudden upper abdominal pain might be pleuritic in origin, adopt the following routine:

1. Look for evidence of cyanosis (*see* p. 47).

2. While counting the patient's pulse rate and taking the temperature (if this has not been recorded within the past half-hour) focus your attention on the respiratory movements. Are the respirations laboured? Do they appear painful? Then proceed to count the respirations. For those whose memory for figures is not a strong point the following table is of value:

1st year	...	...	...	35–45 per minute
1–2 years	...	...	...	20–45
3–4 years	...	...	...	20–40
4–5 years	...	...	...	20–30
Adults	...	...	...	16–20

3. Bare the chest, and observe the respiratory excursions, noting particularly if both sides of the lower chest expand equally. Then ask the patient to breathe deeply and continue the observation, directing the eyes first to the movements of the clavicles (apices), then to the movements of the upper abdomen (bases), and lastly to the more obvious lateral movement of the costal margins. Does one side expand less well than the other? To assess this point, move to the foot of the bed for a few moments.

4. Place the hands over the costal margins, as shown in *Fig.* 361. The fact that one side expands less well than the other becomes evident even in a case where doubt existed, or when no inequality was observed on inspection.

5. Further examination by percussion, auscultation and X-ray is beyond our briefing.

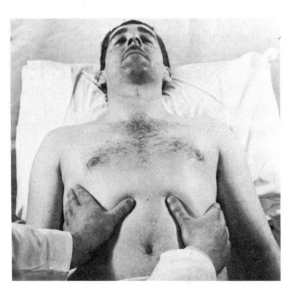

Fig. 361. Ascertaining respiratory excursions. Commence during expiration with the thumbs opposed: normally inspiratory widening of the subcostal angle occurs equally on both sides.

CLINICAL DIAGNOSIS OF POSTOPERATIVE CHEST COMPLICATIONS

Although facilities for early X-ray of patients are now fairly universally available, the practising surgeon will find it an advantage to be able to make a tentative diagnosis early, and thereby institute immediate treatment particularly in pulmonary embolism in which a premonitory small embolus, unless treated, often heralds a fatal large embolus.

In order of probable times of onset after the operation the following are the conditions commonly encountered:

1. Venous Air Embolism is not the almost unheard-of rarity it is alleged to be by some. It is considered first as it can occur at any time after the commencement of an operation or diagnostic procedure. In fatal cases in which the diagnosis is unsuspected, death is often attributed to pulmonary embolism or coronary thrombosis. Even at necropsy, air embolism is often missed because of slovenly technique. Air can be sucked into the venous system during operation or in procedures such as open heart operations, arteriography, or blood transfusion, but the most common cause is permitting the bottle of an intravenous infusion set to run dry.

The onset is usually abrupt, with deep inspirations, coughing expirations, cyanosis, then a few gasping breaths succeeded by unconsciousness and cessation of respiration. The pulse becomes imperceptible and the blood pressure falls to an unrecordable level. A stethoscope applied to the precordium reveals *the 'mill-wheel' murmur*—a churning and splashing that masks the true heart-sounds. If the pulps of the fingers are placed over the jugular vein, bubbles of air sometimes can be felt moving beneath.

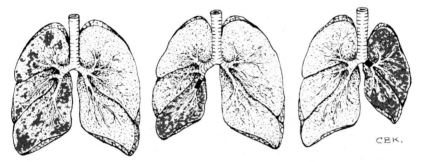

Fig. 362. The three types of atelectasis. Note the site of the plug of mucus (black) in the second and third varieties.

2. Inhaled Vomitus—Aspiration Pneumonia. In spite of the universal adoption of methods of prevention from time to time prophylactic measures evade effective application, and the unconscious or semiconscious patient vomits, and inhales the vomitus. Probably the highest incidence of this regrettable occurrence is in connection with head injuries, but the recovery period following general anaesthesia—particularly short anaesthetics in poorly prepared patients—accounts for many cases. On the other hand, owing to the great attention that is paid to gastric aspiration in cases of intestinal obstruction, once the patient has left the operating table this complication is infrequent. Occasionally vomitus is inhaled by a fully conscious person, more especially by young children in the early stages of a severe systemic infection, one cause of 'cot death'.

Called to a dyspnoeic patient recovering from a general anaesthetic, the smell of vomitus and, perhaps, the presence of some of it on the pillow may direct one's thoughts to this little-discussed subject. In the absence of a more obvious cause for the dyspnoea and cyanosis (e.g. a cervical haematoma following thyroidectomy) the first thing to do is to prise open the mouth, draw forward the tongue, and insert a finger far back into the laryngopharynx. This presence of mind has resulted in the hooking out of a piece of food, or even a denture. If the insertion of an airway does not improve matters immediately, assume that vomitus is filling the trachea and bronchi, and unless it is removed mechanically by all means available, in a very short period of time the patient will succumb.

3. Collapse of the Lung (Atelectasis). This is by far the most frequent postoperative pulmonary complication. There are three varieties (*Fig.* 362); each is essentially the result of blockage of some part of the bronchial tree with a plug, or plugs, of inspissated mucus. If permitted to persist, infection of the uninflated portion of the lungs soon follows. In about 80 per cent of cases atelectasis is right-sided and nearly always occurs during the first 24–48 hours after operation.

Lobular (Segmental) Atelectasis is usually basal. In the early stages there are little or no constitutional disturbances. Pyrexia and cough do not appear until infection supervenes. The most valuable early sign is the presence of sonorous rhonchi over the base, or more usually throughout the lung field on the affected side. If early and effective treatment is not instituted the condition is liable to be followed by bronchopneumonia and, indeed, most instances of 'postoperative pneumonia' are of this variety.

Lobar Collapse. There is a moderate elevation of temperature, followed by a sudden rise to 39 °C or more. The other leading feature is dyspnoea. Pain in the chest is comparatively rare. On examining the bared chest, respiratory movement is likely to be less active on the side (*see Fig.* 361).

Massive Collapse is comparatively rare. In addition to a plug of mucus, it can arise as a result of inhaling a foreign body. Unlike the foregoing, it is more frequent on the left side, due to the conformation of the left bronchus. Cyanosis of the nail-beds will almost certainly be present. In typical cases there is very restricted movement or immobility of the thorax on the involved side. The following signs should be sought early:

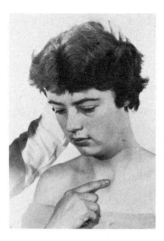

Fig. 363. Palpating the suprasternal notch for tracheal deviation.

a. The trachea is displaced to the side of the lesion. If the index finger is placed in the suprasternal notch (*Fig.* 363) and the head is flexed, deviation of the trachea can be detected readily.

b. The heart is displaced towards the side of the lesion (apex beat).

c. The sternomastoid sign may be present on the side of the lesion: the sternal head of this muscle is more tense than its fellow as it is an accessory muscle of respiration.

4. Pulmonary Embolism. The patient is commonly old, obese, or otherwise unfit, although the condition can occur, tragically, in the young and fit patient and, rarely, in children. In surgical wards usually he or she underwent an operation seven to ten days previously, and up to the time of the catastrophe was progressing favourably. Female patients on the 'contraceptive pill' are particularly liable. On the medical side cardiac disease is the most significant factor associated with the combination of phlebothrombosis decubiti and pulmonary embolism. As a rule pulmonary embolism is unheralded by signs of peripheral venous thrombosis (*see* p. 389).

According to its size, lodgement of an embolus in the pulmonary arterial tree brings about a varying train of events:

a. Arrest at the Bifurcation of the Pulmonary Arterial Trunk. Suddenly the patient cries out. There is a feeling of impending death from suffocation and usually a great desire to defaecate. Profound shock causes the patient to become pale and to sweat profusely. The blood pressure falls; the pulse becomes feeble and irregular, or imperceptible. If, as is usual, the right heart fails, pallor gives place to cyanosis and death occurs in a few minutes. In fatal cases in categories (*a*) and (*b*), if a post-mortem is carried out, in two-thirds evidence is found of previous lesser emboli which, perhaps, should have been detected by the ancillary investigations mentioned below.

b. Arrest in the Right or Left Pulmonary Artery is characterized by a similar onset, but the patient rallies, and if he survives for an hour or more the blood pressure remains low. Sweating, pallor, tachycardia, increased respiratory rate* and moderate pyrexia are leading signs. With treatment, some of this category of patient can be saved, so it is important to know that the diagnosis is one of exclusion; the electrocardiogram does *not* show changes of coronary thrombosis; the chest X-ray is *normal*. In doubtful cases, if facilities are available the diagnosis can be confirmed by scanning the lungs after the intravenous administration of human albumin labelled with radioactive iodine *or* by pulmonary angiography.

c. Arrest in a Large Branch of the Pulmonary Arteries. The onset is quite dissimilar to either of the above. The patient experiences a sudden pain in the chest, because a segment of the lung has become infarcted. The severe generalized thoracic pain to a large extent passes off, but more localized pain on taking a deep breath, or on coughing, takes its place. The respiratory rate and temperature are raised. At every visit (and the patient should be visited frequently) the sputum pot should be inspected; in about 40 per cent of cases the patient coughs up blood or clot, the latter being particularly characteristic.

d. A Shower of Small Pulmonary Emboli gives rise to symptoms and signs identical with bronchopneumonia. This type of case usually shows the signs of phlebothrombosis decubiti.

In categories (*c*) and (*d*) a third of patients will undergo a fatal episode of pulmonary embolism if untreated.

THE OESOPHAGUS

So far as direct physical examination is concerned, no organ is more inaccessible than the oesophagus. Nevertheless, by the application of indirect physical signs, much can be ascertained—in some instances a reasoned diagnosis can be made by their aid alone. This must be confirmed by radiology and oesophagoscopy.

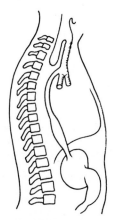

Fig. 364. Congenital atresia of the oesophagus—usual configuration.

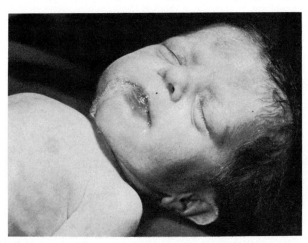

Fig. 365. Frothy saliva pours almost continuously from the nose and mouth. This is pathognomonic of congenital atresia of the oesophagus.

CONGENITAL ATRESIA OF THE OESOPHAGUS

It is computed that this occurs once in every 800 births. In 90 per cent of cases the configuration of the deformity is that shown in *Fig.* 364. It will be seen that the upper pouch ends blindly, while the lower pouch communicates with the trachea. Recognition within 48 hours of birth and subsequent surgical rectification

---

* The patient, dyspnoeic due to pulmonary embolism, prefers to lie flat (Gibson).

RONALD GIBSON, *Contemporary Physician, Brompton Hospital, London.*

is the only hope of the infant's survival. The diagnosis is not difficult. The newborn babe regurgitates all its first and every feed. If this happens and *food* spills into the lungs, pneumonia follows. Therefore every neonate should have sterile water for the first feed, so that if atresia is present the infant will not have to undergo the necessary operation with the added complication of pneumonia. In addition to immediate regurgitation of the first feed, the infant appears to salivate profusely. Actually there is no increase in production, but as none can be swallowed, saliva pours from the mouth and the nose almost continuously, and because it is mixed with air bubbles it assumes a frothy character (*Fig.* 365). This copious outpouring of frothy saliva is *the* sign of oesophageal atresia: to no other condition does this phenomenon appertain. When the fistula is fully patent, in addition to the above signs the infant's abdomen becomes distended because an excessive amount of air is swallowed, and if regurgitation of stomach contents occurs the foam may become bile-stained. The diagnosis can be confirmed simply: a soft rubber catheter is introduced into the oesophagus through the nose, and if an obstruction is encountered 10 cm from the nostril the diagnosis is practically certain. In this event, all attempts at feeding must be stopped forthwith.

The Syndrome of Cyanosis on Feeding a Newborn Infant

1. A large diaphragmatic hernia permitting abdominal contents in the left pleural cavity may cause bile-stained vomitus (sometimes with blood) accompanying respiratory embarrassment on feeding, but no frothing. Bowel sounds are heard on auscultation of the left half of the chest, and with a large hernia breath sounds are absent. The abdomen may appear flatter than usual (scaphoid) as much of its contents ————————————→ are in the chest. An X-ray is necessary to confirm the diagnosis. Urgent surgical treatment is, on occasion, necessary.

2. Oesophageal Atresia (*see above*).
3. Dysphagia Lusoria (*see* p. 198).
4. Micrognathia (*see* p. 89).
5. Choanal Atresia (*see* p. 89).

SPONTANEOUS RUPTURE OF THE OESOPHAGUS

If the diagnosis can be made early and the patient subjected to immediate operation, death, otherwise inevitable, can sometimes be avoided. Eighty-five per cent of the patients are males, and a high proportion have a history of alcoholism. Following a heavy meal there is vomiting, and during one of these expulsive acts the oesophagus ruptures in its lower third. Agonizing pain is experienced usually in the left (occasionally the right) side of the lower thorax, radiating to the back. Note particularly that, unlike many conditions from which rupture of the oesophagus must be differentiated, vomiting *precedes* the pain. As a rule vomiting ceases with the onset of the rupture, but should it continue, the vomitus is likely to be streaked with bright red blood. There is insatiable thirst, and the pain is so intense that morphine fails to relieve it. In many instances subcutaneous emphysema appears in the suprasternal notch and spreads around the neck; when sought, crepitus often can be detected here within an hour of the rupture.

In really early cases examination of the thorax reveals no physical signs, for the gas and fluid are confined to the mediastinum. When, after a matter of a few hours, the extravasated gas and fluid burst through the parietal pleura a hydropneumothorax results, and the general course is swiftly downhill, with dyspnoea, cyanosis, and rapidly increasing circulatory failure.

REFLUX OESOPHAGITIS

Reflux oesophagitis, the most common affection of the oesophagus, can occur apart from a hiatus hernia, but in about 80 per cent of cases it is associated with this (*see* p. 264). The typical sufferer is short, with a tendency of obesity, and as a rule gives a long history of episodic attacks and reports only when the symptoms have become severe and more or less continuous.

Pain is a leading symptom. Pain in the back, between the shoulders, in the presence of a known hiatus hernia denotes oesophagitis; such pain seldom bears a definite relationship to meals, although it is sometimes provoked by taking hot fluids, hot food, or alcohol. The pain is wont to wake the patient during the night; often it is relieved by sitting upright, and sometimes by taking alkalis.

Heartburn with regurgitation of small quantities of acid material is very common, especially when lying flat or stooping.

Absence of Tenderness. The complete absence of tenderness in the epigastrium or in either hypochondrium is helpful in differentiating the condition from an upper abdominal lesion.

Dysphagia is rather a frequent symptom of oesophagitis. The patient says that the food becomes arrested for some moments at the level of the lowest part of the breast bone. This occurs long before any cicatricial stenosis has developed, and at this time it is due, in all probability, to oedema of the mucous membrane. Later, as stenosis due to fibrosis ensues, it becomes progressively worse.

INCREASING DYSPHAGIA AS A SOLE SYMPTOM

Undoubtedly the diagnosis can be ascertained only by radiological examination and by oesophagoscopy. Nevertheless there are certain points to which attention must be directed at the preliminary clinical examination.

Ask the patient where he thinks the food is arrested. If he is intelligent, he can often indicate the point at which he thinks 'the stoppage' is occurring, this often being the site of the lesion. Examine the mouth. Palpate the neck, particularly for enlarged lymph nodes, paying especial attention to the supra-clavicular fossae (*see* p. 139). Examine the abdomen (enlarged liver), and look for signs of wasting as evinced by laxity of the subcutaneous tissues.

Carcinoma of the Oesophagus. This is the commonest cause of increasing dysphagia, being particularly common in the Far East and tropical Africa. Men over 45 years of age are the most frequent victims, but a third are women. In advanced cases regurgitation (oesophageal pseudo-vomiting) is fairly common. The regurgitated material is alkaline, mixed with saliva, and possibly streaked with blood.

Prominent among the non-malignant causes of increasing dysphagia are the following:

Achalasia of the Oesophagus (Mega-oesophagus)* occurs principally in women over 40 years of age, but it is not limited to that sex or to that time of life. More often than not the patient only seeks relief after the symptoms have been present for many years. The long history is helpful in differentiating the condition from carcinoma, as also is the unique feature that dysphagia is equally in evidence

---

* The widely employed term 'cardiospasm' is inaccurate, for the spasm lies just above the cardia. The condition is common in South and Central America where it occurs as a complication of Chagas's disease (South American trypanosomiasis) of which, it has been estimated by the World Health Organization, there are 7 million cases in this part of the world. Some 10 per cent develop complications affecting the heart, oesophagus or colon.

CARLOS CHAGAS, 1879–1934, *Brazilian Physician.*

when swallowing fluids or solids. As a result of probably years of undernourishment, the patient is sometimes reduced to a state of chronic ill health, rendering normal activities impossible.

Sideropaenic Dysphagia.* The patient is nearly always a middle-aged woman. Typically she complains of choking, or fear of choking, and delayed swallowing of food localized at the level of the cricoid cartilage. Close examination provides clues to the diagnosis, but not all the following are necessarily present:

Moderate Pallor.

Lips and Corners of the Mouth are cracked, giving the mouth a pursed appearance. This angular stomatitis or cheilosis (*see* p. 110) is often accompanied by increased salivation.

Tongue is usually devoid of papillae, smooth, and pale, but rarely inflamed.

Finger-nails are brittle, and tend to be spoon-shaped (koilonychia†).———→

Spleen is only occasionally enlarged, as in other iron-deficiency anaemias.

Koilonychia, an inflamed tongue, and cheilosis are not unusual in sideropaenia‡ *per se*, and thus the syndrome can only be set apart by the presence of the characteristic dysphagia. Instrumental examination of the laryngopharynx and the oesophagus is necessary as the condition is premalignant and postcricoid carcinoma may have supervened.

Globus Hystericus is quite common. Again, the patient is almost invariably female and complains that food seems to stick at the level of the cricoid cartilage. However, she is not anaemic and clinical examination of the neck together with instrumental examination of the laryngopharynx and a barium swallow reveal no abnormality. The stigmata of neurosis (*see* p. 49) may be present.

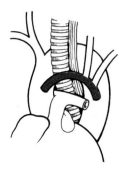

Fig. 366. The usual anatomical configuration of a vascular ring. The accessory aorta is shown in red. The left common carotid and subclavian arteries usually take their origin from it.

Pharyngeal Pouch (*see* p. 145) is also sometimes a cause of dysphagia.

Dysphagia Lusoria§ (Vascular Ring). The oesophagus and trachea are surrounded by an arterial ring (*Fig.* 366) due to failure in the normal disappearance of parts of the primitive aortic arches. Usually the ring does not obstruct the tubes passing through it at birth, but as these grow relatively more rapidly than the arteries, dysphagia and stridor may appear in a matter of months or years. A baby thus affected will lie with its neck extended, as in this position the pressure on the trachea is reduced. Flexion of the neck brings on the stridor.

---

* This syndrome was first described in 1919 by Paterson and Kelly. It is also known (correctly but clumsily) as the Paterson–Kelly–Plummer–Vinson syndrome and (incorrectly but commonly) as the Plummer–Vinson syndrome.

† *Koilonychia.* Greek, κοῖλος = hollow+ὄνυξ = a nail.

‡ *Sideropaenia.* Greek, σίδηρος = iron+πένης = poor.

§ *Lusoria.* Latin, *lusus* = a jest. Originally described as a jest of nature.

DONALD R. PATERSON, 1863–1939, *Ear, Nose and Throat Surgeon, Royal Infirmary, Cardiff.*
ADAM B. KELLY, 1865–1941, *Ear, Nose, and Throat Surgeon, Victoria Infirmary, Glasgow.*
HENRY S. PLUMMER, 1874–1937, *Physician, Mayo Clinic, Rochester, U.S.A.*
PORTER P. VINSON, 1890–1959, *Physician, Medical College, Virginia, U.S.A.*

Chapter 17

THE BACK

SPINA BIFIDA

Failure of the fusion of the cartilaginous bars forming the vertebral arch results in a defect of the spinolaminar component of the vertebral column. Usually it affects one vertebra only, most commonly in the lumbosacral region; less often, a meningocele occurs in the cervico-occipital region (*see* p. 54).

Spinal Dysraphism* presents in four forms:

Myelocele is the outcome of failure of the neural as well as the vertebral arch to close. This produces an oval, raw, uncovered defect communicating with the central canal of the spinal cord. This variety is fairly common, but the infant is stillborn, or dies shortly after birth.

Syringomyelocele is comparatively rare. Through the bony defect bulges a cystic swelling formed, not of the membranes of the cord only, but by gross dilatation of the central canal (hydromyelia). Such a state of affairs is associated with gross paralyses below the lesion. Little wonder, then, that clinical interest is mainly centred around the other varieties, which are:

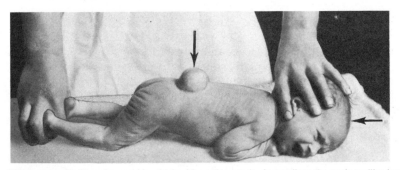

Fig. 367. A transmitted impulse could be obtained from the anterior fontanelle to the cystic swelling in this case of meningocele.

Meningocele. There is a protrusion of meninges through a defect in the spinolaminar segment. The sac contains cerebrospinal fluid only. In very early life the most reliable sign that the swelling is a meningocele is that it is entirely covered by healthy skin (*Fig.* 367). This variety is relatively favourable but unfortunately comprises only 10 per cent of cases.

Myelomeningocele. In England and Wales 2500 babies are born alive with this defect each year, a formidable problem as surgical treatment is now feasible in favourable cases. The normally developed spinal cord or cauda equina lies within the sac, sometimes adherent to the serous lining of the protruding swelling. The sac is not entirely covered by skin, but is surmounted by unepithelized meninges (*Fig.* 368). Not unexpectedly, in a matter of days or weeks, if untreated, the sac ruptures, the underlying spinal cord looking like granulation tissue.

---

* *Dysraphism.* Greek, δυσ = bad+ῥαφή = seam. Defective fusion.

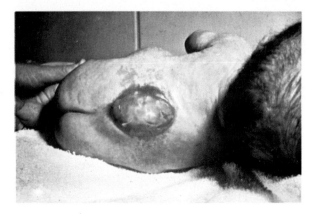

Fig. 368. Myelomeningocele in a neonate. Note that hydrocephalus is also present.

Further Clinical Examination. When the swelling is intact, transmitted impulse can be sought from the swelling to the anterior fontanelle (*Fig.* 367): if present it signifies that a wide-mouthed channel communicates between the cerebrospinal canal and the swelling. This does not constitute fluctuation (*see* p. 12). The swelling is brilliantly translucent and, in cases of myelomeningocele, occasionally the cord or nerves can be seen as dark shadows within the sac. If it was not obvious on the first sight of the patient, one should now measure the head to exclude hydrocephalus (*see* p. 55). Hydrocephalus, which develops in some three-quarters of otherwise successfully treated cases, is never a result of the operation (as was thought formerly) but is a manifestation of the Arnold–Chiari malformation (displacement of the hindbrain (rhombencephalon) and herniation into the spinal canal of the cerebellar tonsils, which obstruct the free circulation of cerebrospinal fluid).

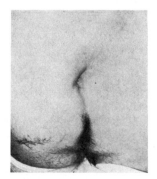

Fig. 369. Post-anal dimple.

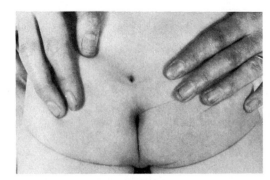

Fig. 370. Congenital sacrococcygeal sinus.

Lastly, one should seek signs of paralysis of the lower extremities, kypho-scoliosis (*see* p. 203), other congenital defects and note whether the anus is patulous, all of which are indications that surgical treatment is probably not worth while, the infant being doomed to a life of mental deficiency, paralysis and urinary incontinence.

JULIUS ARNOLD, 1835–1915, *Professor of Pathological Anatomy, Heidelberg.*
HANS CHIARI, 1851–1916, *Professor of Pathological Anatomy, Strasburg.*

Spina Bifida Occulta is due to failure of the vertebral arches to unite, but there is no protrusion of the coverings of the spinal cord. Most instances are detected radiologically in investigating patients with low back pain but a local patch of hair, a naevolipoma, or a dimple sometimes marks the site of the defect—in no other situation does Nature call attention to a deep-seated abnormality in such a brazen way. The dimple (post-anal dimple (*Fig.* 369)) is caused by a fibrous band—*the membrana reuniens*—which unites the deep layers of the skin to the spinal theca. The membrana reuniens neither stretches nor does it grow, but remains stationary in length while the body increases in stature. The skin is pulled upon at one end and the theca and the spinal nerve roots at the other, possibly producing such conditions as foot-drop and weakness of urinary and anal sphincters *appearing for the first time in childhood or adolescence.* When dimpling occurs very early in fetal life it progresses apace, and at birth a pit of varying depth results. This is known as:

Congenital Sacrococcygeal Sinus (*Fig.* 370). Should the sinus expand intraspinally, to form a dermoid cyst, the symptoms and signs are often primarily those of a cauda equina tumour. A sacrococcygeal sinus, which is rare, is sometimes mistaken for a pilonidal sinus (*see* p. 274), which is common but is never found at birth.

EXAMINATION OF THE BACK

This is best carried out first with the patient standing and then lying down.

A. EXAMINATION STANDING

Inspection. Proper inspection requires exposure of the entire posterior aspect of the patient from head to foot, and removal of the shoes to avoid the effect of high or unequal heels. The arms hang loosely by the side.

Landmarks are noted—the vertebra prominens, the spinous processes, the angles of the scapulae, the posterior iliac spines and crests. In many women the dimples of Venus are visible (*Fig.* 371): they overlie the sacro-iliac joints.

The lateral contour of the back is inspected. Normally there is a lumbar lordosis (*Fig.* 372 *a*), more marked in the female. In many conditions characterized by spasm of the sacrospinalis muscle this is lost (*Fig.* 372 *b*) notably

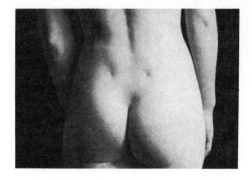

Fig. 371. The dimples of Venus mark the sites of the sacro-iliac joints.

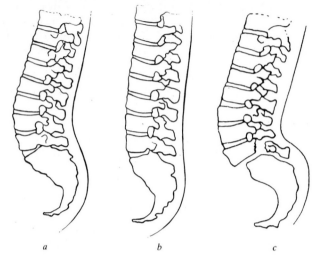

Fig. 372. Illustrating the lateral contour of the back. *a*, Normal; *b*, In conditions associated with sacrospinalis spasm; *c*, Spondylolisthesis.

prolapsed lumbar intervertebral disc and early Pott's disease. Increased lordosis (*Fig.* 372 *c*) denotes spondylolisthesis (*see* p. 216).

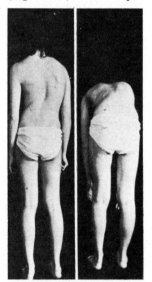

Observe the symmetry of the body—whether one half is more prominent than the other. This can be done by comparing the two sides of the trunk with reference to an imaginary line prolonged upwards from the gluteal cleft. In this way scoliosis is detected. Now direct the patient to lean forwards and cross the arms over the chest so that the hands rest on opposite shoulders. A postural deformity disappears in this position whereas a fixed deformity appears greater (*Fig.* 373).

Sometimes the spinous processes of the vertebrae are not very prominent, and it may be difficult to detect scoliosis; ask the patient to fold his arms and lean forwards, and then run the finger firmly down the vertebrae without hurting him. A red line on the skin results, and the curve of the spine becomes evident.

Scoliosis.* Note whether the curve is single (*see* Fig. 381), S-shaped (*Fig.* 373), or more complex. Record the findings diagrammatically. Endeavour to determine which type of scoliosis is present.

Fig. 373. Advanced idiopathic kyphoscoliosis in a girl aged 14.

POSTURAL. Usually the curve is single—it disappears when the patient bends forward.

Postural Scoliosis in Infancy. A small proportion (5–10 per cent) of cases progress to the more serious idiopathic kyphoscoliosis mentioned *below*. The

* *Scoliosis.* Greek, σκολίωσύ = lateral curvature of the vertebral column.

PERCIVALL POTT, 1714–1788, *Surgeon, St. Bartholomew's Hospital, London.*

clinician should be on the look-out, especially if the mother states that 'the baby always screws round one way'. If the baby is suffering from congenital postural scoliosis it will not spontaneously bend away from the side of the concavity when lying on its abdomen. Skin wrinkles on the trunk on this side are also typical. ────────────────→

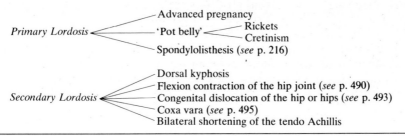

In this variety the female-to-male ratio is 2:3 and the curve is convex to the *left* in the thoracic region.

COMPENSATORY scoliosis is due to a cause that is usually obvious: (*a*) torticollis; (*b*) pneumonectomy or thoracoplasty; (*c*) short leg; or (*d*) deformed hip. That due to a short leg usually disappears when the patient sits, but comparative measurements of the length of the lower limbs are required.

STRUCTURAL (FIXED) scoliosis is always accompanied by rotation of vertebrae, i.e. there is an element of kyphosis (*see below*) as well. The main causes are congenital (e.g. hemivertebra), asymmetrical paralysis of the intercostal muscles (especially that following poliomyelitis), and the most common variety, idiopathic (*Fig.* 373). The latter affects adolescents with a female-to-male ratio of 7:1 and in 90 per cent the curve is convex to the *right* in the thoracic region.

Kyphosis.* When kyphosis is present, pay particular attention to its type, whether it is a gentle curve or an angular deformity, having in mind the following aetiological table:

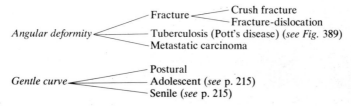

Angular deformity
- Fracture
  - Crush fracture
  - Fracture-dislocation
- Tuberculosis (Pott's disease) (*see Fig.* 389)
- Metastatic carcinoma

Gentle curve
- Postural
- Adolescent (*see* p. 215)
- Senile (*see* p. 215)

Lordosis.† The normal lumbar curve is exaggerated. That the depth of the normal lumbar furrow (*see Fig.* 371) produced by that curve is increased is best seen in an oblique light while viewing the patient's back in the usual way. On the other hand, gross lordosis is perceived at once when the patient is viewed from the side. While a protuberant belly produces lordosis, lordosis can cause a protuberant abdomen, and the clinician must decide which is primary. Lordosis, which is less common than kyphosis, can be primary or secondary.

Primary Lordosis
- Advanced pregnancy
- 'Pot belly'
  - Rickets
  - Cretinism
- Spondylolisthesis (*see* p. 216)

Secondary Lordosis
- Dorsal kyphosis
- Flexion contraction of the hip joint (*see* p. 490)
- Congenital dislocation of the hip or hips (*see* p. 493)
- Coxa vara (*see* p. 495)
- Bilateral shortening of the tendo Achillis

---

* *Kyphosis*. Greek, κύφωσις = a knuckle; a hunchback.
† *Lordosis*. Greek, λόρδωσις = curvature of the vertebral column in a forward direction.

Continuing with the examination:

The Pointing Test. The patient should point to the place where pain is experienced. If this cannot be reached, the pointing finger must be helped. An exquisitely tender area may i idicate a torn muscle fibre or bundle. This area is marked on the skin. At the conclusion of the examination, sometimes it is of value to repeat the test. The visible skin mark can be used as a check of the patient's sincerity.

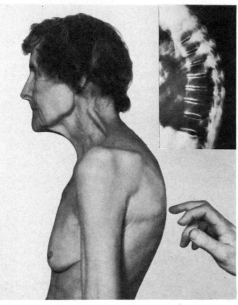

Fig. 374. Percussing the spinous processes of the vertebrae. A patient with senile osteoporosis complaining of backache.

Palpation is of particular value in determining spasm of muscles that flank the spine. A spastic muscle feels firmer than normal. It is short, and therefore it causes concavity of the spine towards the side of muscular contraction (*see Fig.* 381). Tenderness may be due to local pathology or to irritation of the spinal nerves that supply the part. Next examine the spinous processes and the interspinous notches with the index finger. It is often valuable to commence this part of the examination by running the finger down the whole length of the spinous processes, commencing at the vertebra prominens.

Vertebral Percussion. The spinous processes are struck with the percussing finger (*Fig.* 374) or a knee hammer. Commence at the vertebra prominens, and percuss each spinous process down to the second sacral. Tenderness over a particular vertebra indicates disease. The method is of particular value in the dorsal region.

Testing Spinal Movements. *Flexion* is the principal movement to be tested.

Most of the movement of true flexion of the spine occurs in the lumbar region; comparatively little in the thoracic, while in the cervical region normal flexion merely consists of the obliteration of the anatomical forward convexity. Flexion of the spine *per se* is largely apparent and much of this movement occurs at the atlanto-occipital and hip joints.

Ask the patient to bend forwards and endeavour to touch his toes, keeping the knees straight. The degree of flexion is measured by the distance between the fingertips and the ground (*Fig.* 375) or as shown in *Fig.* 376. With a young

TESTING THE MOVEMENTS OF THE THORACOLUMBAR VERTEBRAL COLUMN

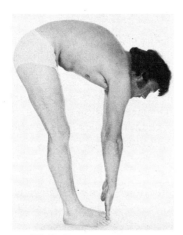

Fig. 375. Flexion.

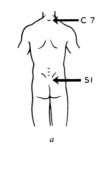

a

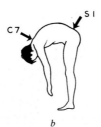

b

Fig. 376. With the patient in the neutral position, measure the distance between the spinous processes of C7 and S1 vertebrae (*a*) with a tape measure. Now ask him to bend forward as far as possible (*b*). In the normal adult male the tape should record an increase of 10 cm between the two processes.

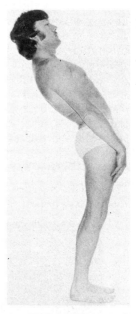

Fig. 377. Extension. An angle of 30° with the vertical is possible in the normal patient.

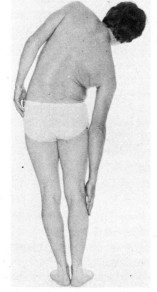

Fig. 378. Lateral bend. An angle of 35° is normal.

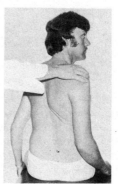

Fig. 379. Rotation. A 45° angle with the coronal plane is normally attainable.

child, the test can be carried out without tears by dropping a coin or toy upon the floor and watching him pick it up. A normal child will pick up the coin by flexing the spine. Should the child reach for the coin very cautiously by bending the knees it is obvious that spinal rigidity is present.

Extension. Ask the patient to lean backwards as far as possible (*Fig.* 377), and observe whether this movement causes pain.

Lateral Bend. The patient slides each hand in turn down the thigh (*Fig.* 378). Limitation of this movement only suggests osteoarthrosis or early ankylosing spondylitis.

Rotation. To obtain reliable results, the patient must be seated on a low backless stool or on a couch (*Fig.* 379). If on a stool, he should plant his feet on the floor; if on a couch, he must be seated so that the popliteal spaces rest on the edge of the couch. Thus the buttocks are anchored. The examiner then grasps the shoulders and rotates the patient's trunk to the right and to the left.

B. EXAMINATION WITH THE PATIENT LYING DOWN

Prone. The presence of muscular rigidity and the detection of areas of localized tenderness are best ascertained in this position.

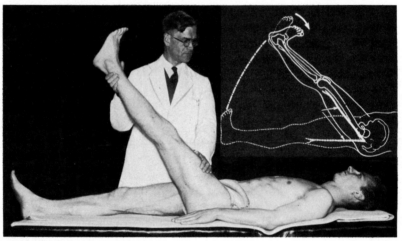

Fig. 380. The straight-leg-raising test. Note the position of the clinician's hands. Normally the leg can be raised to 90° (slightly less as age advances).

Supine

In Cases of Scoliosis. Measurements of the length of the lower limbs (*see* pp. 486 and 491), and exclusion of deformities of the hip joint are carried out.

In Cases of Suspected Tuberculous Spondylitis. Palpate the abdomen, particularly the iliac fossae, where a psoas abscess may be felt as a swelling.

In Cases of Sciatica. The ankle jerks (S1) should be tested; often the jerk on the affected side is diminished or absent. The knee jerk (L4) is affected infrequently. Look particularly for a dropped big toe as lesions of L5 nerve root cause paresis of the dorsiflexors of the foot, and particularly of the great toe. In lesions of S1 there is no such paresis.

*The Straight-leg-raising Test.** First ascertain that there is no compensatory lordosis by insinuating a hand beneath the lumbar spine (*see* p. 490). With one hand grasping the ankle and the other placed on the front of the thigh, to keep the knee straight, the leg is raised until the patient experiences pain, as evidenced by watching his face (*Fig.* 380) or until the normal excursion is accomplished. During the procedure watch the lumbar curve, a change of which invalidates the test. If the test produces pain below the normal full excursion, the angle at which the pain was experienced is recorded. The test is repeated, and as this angle is approached, additional care is exercised, and at the very first twinge of pain the hand resting on the thigh is moved to the fore-part of the foot, and the forefoot is dorsiflexed (*Fig.* 380, inset). Dorsiflexion of the foot affords additional traction to the sciatic nerve and aggravation of the pain therefrom suggests irritation of one or more of the nerve-roots that go to form the sciatic nerve.

The results of applying the straight-leg-raising test in some of the conditions considered in this chapter are as follows:

1. In rigid kyphosis of adolescents (*see* p. 215) the raising is limited to 60° by tight hamstring muscles.

2. If pain is evoked under 40° it suggests that it is due to *impingement* of a protruding intervertebral disc on a nerve root. When pain occurs only after the limb has reached a considerably higher level, it indicates that it is caused by *tension* on a nerve root that is abnormally sensitive from a cause not necessarily an intervertebral disc lesion.

Rectal or Vaginal Examination. Their importance cannot be over-emphasized in the search for a neoplasm or other possible cause of pain in the back.

LOW BACK PAIN

Sufferers from this extremely common condition throng general practitioners' surgeries and flood orthopaedic clinics. In the following section the causes are discussed and the elicitation of relevant physical signs described.

The Prolapsed Intervertebral Disc Syndrome. This may be due to extrusion of the disc in younger patients or to pressure on nerve roots by osteophytes (spondylosis, i.e. osteoarthrosis) in older persons. The first symptoms commonly appear in three ways: (*a*) Low back pain; (*b*) Sciatica; (*c*) Lastly (*a*) and (*b*) may occur in combination, appearing either simultaneously, or one following the other (usually (*a*) before (*b*)). Various combinations of acute and gradual onset also occur.

Pain at first is located in the buttock. Soon it spreads to the back of the thigh and then increases in severity and radiates down the leg, sometimes to the great toe or to other toes. Pain with a distribution as wide as this must be due to involvement of one or more roots of the sciatic nerve (L4–S3).

Characteristic Stance. In the throes of an acute attack the standing patient leans forward, so that the normal lumbar cavity is obliterated. The hip and knee joints on the affected side are flexed and only the ball of the foot touches the floor.

---

* Laza K. Lazarevic, a Yugoslav physician, first described this sign in 1880. It is usually ascribed to E. C. Laségue, a French physician, who in fact learnt it from one of his pupils, J. J. Forst, who described it independently in 1881.

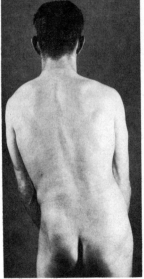

Fig. 381. Prolapsed intervertebral disc (L3–4), showing sciatic scoliosis. The patient walked with his left hip joint flexed.

Often lumbar scoliosis from muscular contraction is present (*Fig.* 381), the convexity usually, but not always, being directed to the side of the prolapsed disc (*sciatic scoliosis*).

While many of the following signs are present at all stages of an attack, it must be emphasized that the diagnosis does not hinge on any particular sign.

Muscle Spasm. Spasm of the sacrospinalis is present uniformly. It is more in evidence on the side of the lesion.

Pain is distributed along the 4th and 5th lumbar or the 1st sacral dermatome, according to whether the L3–4, L4–5, or L5–S1 disc protrudes.

Spinal Movements. Both flexion and extension of the spine are grossly diminished. Even in the acute phase, lateral flexion and rotation are comparatively free.

Local Tenderness. It is usual to find deep tenderness 5 cm lateral to the midline, the tenderness being more pronounced on the side of the protrusion, should that be unilateral (Armstrong).

Vertebral Percussion. Tenderness is sometimes localized to the spinous process or processes in juxtaposition to the lesion.

Straight-leg-raising Test. See p. 207.

Coughing and Sneezing. Usually lower extremity pain is increased when intraspinal pressure is raised by these expulsive acts.

Femoral Nerve Stretch Test. If pain is felt in front of the thigh (unusual) indicating that the protruding disc is L2–3, ask the patient to lie on the abdomen again, and flex the knee ——→ of the affected side. Should this manœuvre reproduce the pain complained of, it is confirmatory evidence that a nerve-root component of the femoral nerve is being stretched over the disc.

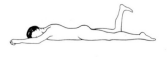

Remission of Symptoms. Complete remission of symptoms between attacks is characteristic of lumbar disc lesions. If a history of continuous low back pain or of sciatica is obtained, another cause should be suspected strongly and sought by all means available.

JAMES R. ARMSTRONG, *Contemporary Emeritus Orthopaedic Surgeon, St. Thomas's Hospital, London.*

THE SACRO-ILIAC JOINTS

From the standpoint of clinical examination this joint is extremely inaccessible, for it is completely protected by bone, except at one small area where the articular (so-called 'auricular', because it is ear-shaped) cartilage becomes subligamentous. This area, which is situated one finger's breadth medial to and one finger's breadth below the posterior superior iliac spine affords the principal opportunity of ascertaining whether the joint is tender.

The Pointing Test. Ask the patient to point to the site of maximum pain. Typically the finger points to the surface marking of the sacro-iliac joint, which sometimes is identified so conveniently by a dimple (*see Fig.* 371).

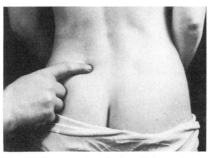

Fig. 382. Palpating the left sacro-iliac joint. When no dimple overlies the joint, locate the posterior superior iliac spine and take bearings from this point.

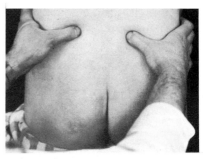

Fig. 383. Deep comparative palpation of the sacro-iliac joints. Exercising considerable pressure, first one thumb and then the other passes over the joint. The left thumb is performing the movement at the time of the photograph.

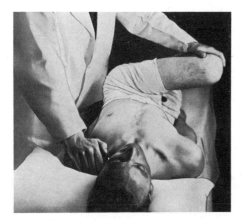

Fig. 384. The 'pump-handle' test.

Forward Bending. Ask the patient to bend forward and endeavour to touch the toes (*see Fig.* 375). Usually, but not necessarily, this movement is performed hesitatingly and incompletely. If it is *pain* that prevents flexion of the back, again ask the patient to put his finger on the place that hurts him most. Now request the patient to sit and bend forward (*see Fig.* 386). In sacro-iliac lesions this movement is now comparatively free, because the pelvis is supported.

Rotation of the vertebral column (*see Fig.* 379) is extremely important. In sacro-iliac affections it always brings on, or intensifies, pain at the affected joint.

Palpation. Tenderness over the sacro-iliac joint and nowhere else strongly suggests a lesion of this joint. Especially when the overlying dimple is present, the joint (*Fig.* 382) is located easily. In other circumstances it is best to follow the iliac crest in a backward direction until the posterior superior iliac spine is reached, and then take bearings from this eminence as described already. A good practical method is, with the patient sitting erect, to place the thumb just medial to the posterior iliac spine and, while exerting pressure, ask the patient to bend forward slowly. By his so doing the thumb passes over the joint cleft (*Fig.* 383) and when it reaches the portion unprotected by bone, if the sacro-iliac joint is involved the patient will flinch and exclaim, 'That is the place'.

The Straight-leg-raising Test. Except in cases of sacro-iliac tuberculosis where abscess formation has involved the nerve trunks, the straight-leg-raising test can be performed to its full extent with, perhaps, the production of slight pain in the region of the affected joint at the zenith of the arc of elevation.

The 'Pump-handle' Test. With the patient supine and commencing on the pain-free side, grasp the limb just below the knee, and in order to steady the trunk, with the free hand grasp the shoulder on the same side. Fully flex the hip and the knee joints, then, by firm pressure, direct the flexed knee steadily towards the opposite shoulder (*Fig.* 384). This completed without undue discomfort to the patient, proceed to perform the test on the suspected side. The test is positive if pain is experienced in the sacro-iliac joint.

The main affections of the sacro-iliac joint are, in order of frequency, sacro-iliac strain, sacro-iliac arthritis, and sacro-iliac tuberculosis.

Sacro-iliac Strain. The great majority of patients with pain localized to a sacro-iliac joint are said to be suffering from 'sacro-iliac strain', but it must be admitted that the causative pathology is unknown. The above tests for sacro-iliac pain are positive but straight leg raising is normal as are the X-rays and the blood-sedimentation rate.

Sacro-iliac Arthritis is uncommon. It may be a complication of Reiter's disease (*see* p. 439), in which it is present clinically in 20 per cent of cases. It is unusual for the sacro-iliac joints to be spared in ankylosing spondylitis (*see* p. 214) and some patients with ulcerative colitis exhibit clinical sacro-iliac arthritis. In a number of instances no cause can be found. Needless to say, other major joints should be examined for evidence of similar involvement.

The leading symptom is painful stiffness of the lower part of the back, most in evidence first thing in the morning, and usually of a band-like distribution across the sacrum and buttocks. Sometimes there is a limp or, if the condition is bilateral, a slightly stiff, waddling type of gait.

Tuberculosis of the Sacro-iliac Joint is rare, but its occurrence is one of the important reasons why all patients with persistent low back pain should have an X-ray examination. Contrary to all other forms of joint tuberculosis this is a disease of young adults. In only about half is the pain localized, mainly in the region of the sacro-iliac joint. Low central backache, pain in the groin (which is likely to be attributed to arthritis of the hip joint), and sciatica are frequent. During the stage of intra-articular abscess formation the pain is severe, and starting pains (*see* 'night cries', p. 213) are typical. When the pus has eroded the ligamentous covering of the joint, it manifests itself as a fluctuating swelling, and, intra-articular tension being relieved, the pain ceases. About 65 per cent of the abscesses appear over the sacro-iliac joint; the remainder track forward into either the groin or the iliac fossa.

Exceptionally, such an abscess appears in the femoral triangle.

THE LUMBOSACRAL JOINT

Lumbosacral Strain. The patient is often between 25 and 50 years of age, and usually female. The pain, which is situated near the top of the sacrum, is of a nagging character, and often radiates to the front and lateral aspect of the thigh. It increases by bending forward, as in many household tasks, and is especially in evidence at the end of the day. Routine examination is mostly negative, but positive information is forthcoming if attention is focused on the lumbosacral articulation in the following ways:

There is a slightly increased concavity of the lumbar curve and some spasm of spinal muscles during active movements of the spine. Forward bending is limited *both when standing and sitting*.

Request the patient to lie flat on her back on the examining couch while the clinician becomes otherwise occupied for a few minutes. Note the posture assumed. Often the patient finds lying flat on the back intolerable, and after a short while flexes both knees and hips.

The Straight-leg-raising Test can be performed with freedom on either side, but with some pain located in the lumbosacral region at the zenith of the elevation.

The patient should now be examined prone, with four pillows beneath the pelvis. This opens up the gaps between the lower lumbar spinous process and facilitates palpation (*Fig.* 385) of the supraspinous ligaments. The greatest tenderness is elicited either just below or just above the spinous process of the 5th lumbar vertebra. Sometimes a depression denoting damage to, or laxity of, the supraspinous and interspinous ligaments (*sprung back*) contrasts sharply with the normal resistance of intact ligaments between the lumbar vertebrae higher in the series.

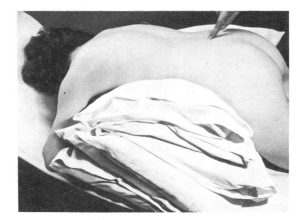

Fig. 385. Lumbosacral strain. With four or five pillows beneath the abdomen, the lower intervertebral spaces are rendered more accessible while the palpating finger is directed particularly to the space below and the space above the 5th lumbar vertebra in the middle line.

LOW BACK PAIN WITHOUT PHYSICAL SIGNS

It must be admitted that, in practice, of patients with the complaint of low back pain, at least half fall into the category of 'no physical signs'. If, after a reasonable trial of simple methods of treatment, a radiograph is ordered, it is always normal or shows a condition which does not account for the pain (e.g. spina bifida occulta, *see* p. 201). An additional confirmatory scientific test is that the blood sedimentation rate is normal.

Fibrositis, Myofascial or **Back Strain, Lumbago,** and **Muscular Rheumatism** are terms which can be applied (with tongue in cheek) in these circumstances, provided that the methods of physical examination so far considered (including rectal and vaginal examination) have been carried out conscientiously with negative results and that X-rays are normal. Physiotherapy often relieves the pain, although it would be pretentious to claim that the treatment has cured the condition, as the cause is not known. In this connection it may be added that various manipulative methods of treatment are not to be scorned; although the reasoning behind the treatment is illogical, it does produce good results on occasion.

If pain persists, consider the following:

Malingerer's Low Back Pain. The patient usually has a good reason (compensation) for persistence of pain. Helpful in the diagnosis is that the expression 'agony' is often used, yet the patient shows no sign of severe suffering. A frequent additional complaint is headache. An inquiry into the general health is liable to evoke an account of many and varied symptoms elsewhere. Depression and anxiety states are common—the province of the psychiatrist. Two tests are of value in confirming functional backache.

1. *Aird's Test.* The standing patient is asked to touch his toes with the knees straight. If flexion of the spine is greatly reduced, ask the patient to sit down on

an examining couch and touch his toes. If his pain has a non-organic basis he will be able to do so with ease; it requires no genius to realize that the spinal flexion is identical with that necessary to touch the toes when standing (*Fig.* 386).

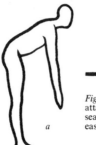
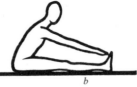

Fig. 386. *a*, Degree of forward flexion commonly attainable by a malingering patient; *b*, On being seated the same patient can touch his toes with ease! (*After Aird.*)

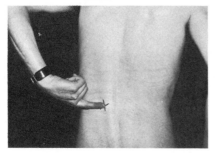

Fig. 387. Without hesitation the patient points to the same spot as he did at the first examination. Undoubtedly a case of genuine pain.

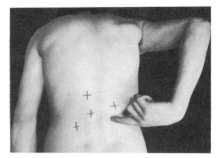

Fig. 388. Migratory localization of maximum site of pain; probably malingering or possessed of a high degree of 'compensitis'.

2. *Magnuson's Test.* Ask the patient to point to the site of the pain and mark the area. Then look at the patient's throat, examine him rectally, and perform any relevant examination of parts well away from the site of the alleged pain. By this expedient the patient's attention is diverted (from his back) for several minutes. The examination of the back is then resumed. If the man experiences real local pain, assuredly its position will remain steadfast (*Fig.* 387). If he is malingering, he may not remember the exact place where he located the pain (*Fig.* 388), or which area or areas he said were tender.

SPECIFIC CAUSES OF SPINAL DEFORMITY

Pott's Disease (Tuberculous Spondylitis). The most common (about 40 per cent) variety of bone and joint tuberculosis is in the spine. The symptoms and signs vary according to the level of the lesion, which commences in the cancellous bone of a body of a vertebra adjacent to an intervertebral disc; the commonest region to be affected is the lower thoracic and upper lumbar. Certain symptoms and signs occur in all regions:

Pain is nearly always localized to the site of the lesion; occasionally it is referred, e.g. along an intercostal nerve or nerves. Its absence should not mislead the clinician, for the disease can progress with so few symptoms that the patient follows his calling until the onset of paralysis, or the formation of a large abscess.

PAUL B. MAGNUSON, 1884–1968, *Professor of Surgery, North-western University, Chicago.*
PERCIVALL POTT, 1714–1788, *Surgeon, St. Bartholomew's Hospital, London, described painful deformity of the spine with paraplegia, which he considered to be due to tuberculosis.*

Night Cries occur in children caused by pain resulting from relaxation during sleep of the involuntary muscular spasm that splints the intervertebral joint.

Evening Pyrexia is likely to develop as the disease progresses, and with it lassitude, anaemia, and poor appetite—all of which are signs of toxaemia.

Muscular Rigidity. Protective muscular spasm, especially of the sacrospinalis, develops early. In the adult flexion is greatly reduced; in a child the coin-dropping test (*see* p. 206) is regularly positive.

A sign peculiar to the thoracolumbar region is: 'if a deepened midline spinal sulcus is seen about the tenth thoracic vertebra you have noticed the first sign of Pott's disease in its earliest stages at the most frequent site. This deepened sulcus is due to increased muscular tonicity of the sacrospinalis muscles; it is Nature's plaster cast' (Jardine).

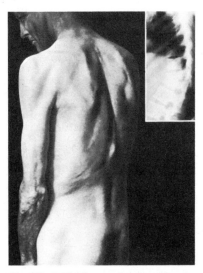

Fig. 389. Pott's disease. Angular deformity. Inset, collapse of a vertebral body.

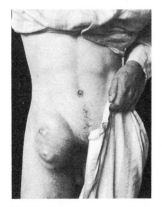

Fig. 390. Psoas abscess from Pott's disease of a lumbar vertebra. The patient had so few symptoms that he did not report before the abscess had reached these dimensions.

Angular Deformity. It is not long before the anterior portion of the vertebral body most affected softens and collapses, producing the characteristic angular deformity. To see the prominence (of the spinous process) so caused to the best advantage, the patient should be viewed from an oblique angle (*Fig.* 389).

Vertebral Percussion reveals tenderness over the process or processes concerned in the angulation.

Referred Pain. Pain from spinal lesions sometimes is referred to other sensory fibres proceeding to the same nerve root. Thus Pott's disease has been mistaken for pleurisy, appendicitis and sciatica. This emphasizes the necessity for routine examination of the back when pain is situated in the abdomen or thorax.

Abscess Formation. An abscess connected with an upper thoracic vertebra is wont to point in the mediastinum, and may rupture into the pleural cavity. Alternatively, it follows the course of an intercostal nerve and points in the lateral aspect of the chest (*see* p. 188). In the lower thoracic and upper lumbar regions the pus enters the psoas sheath and tracks downwards causing a mass in

FRANCIS E. JARDINE, 1886–1956, *Surgeon, Royal Infirmary, Edinburgh.*

the iliac fossa. Later, it points beneath the inguinal ligament, and if its contents are not aspirated the abscess spreads subcutaneously (*Fig.* 390).

Paraplegia is caused by compression of the spinal cord by granulation tissue, oedema, or extreme kyphosis. Muscular weakness in the lower extremities is followed by exaggerated reflexes, ankle clonus and finally paralysis. Formerly common, paralysis now supervenes in only a small and decreasing proportion of cases, due to more efficient treatment.

Non-tuberculous Spondylitis. The frequency with which the vertebrae are attacked by tuberculosis tends to obscure non-tuberculous osteitis of the spine which, like Pott's disease, is the local manifestation of a general disease. Like osteomyelitis of a long bone, the onset of non-tuberculous spondylitis is either acute or subacute but, unlike that condition, the infecting organism is far from stereotyped.

Obviously the nature of the infecting organism cannot be diagnosed by clinical methods, but often it can be strongly suspected. For instance, in communities where typhoid is common, typhoid spondylitis occurring many months after the illness is by no means a rarity in adults. On the other hand, in rural communities where goats are kept, spondylitis due to brucellosis occurs from time to time. Therefore, in a child, always examine the spleen and the lymph nodes for enlargement. In areas where hydatid disease is endemic it can cause spondylitis. Apart from actinomycosis, other less well-known fungus infections, notably coccidioidomycosis,* attack the vertebral column. The latter is endemic in California, Central America, and in parts of Canada. Intradermal tests and biopsy alone can differentiate this infection from tuberculous spondylitis.

Post-traumatic Kyphosis (Kümmell's Disease) is a prerogative of the adult spine. Following an injury to the vertebral column and apparent recovery, weeks or months later painful kyphosis of the thoracic region develops due to osteoporosis culminating in a collapse of a body of a vertebra. It is thus the result of an unrecognized fracture of a body of a vertebra.

Angular Kyphosis due to a Metastatic Tumour in a Vertebra.

The body of a vertebra is a favourite site for a carcinomatous deposit, the lumbar vertebrae being rather more commonly involved than the others. The primary growth can be situated in any of the organs listed on p. 425, but with vertebral metastases the breast, bronchus and the prostate are the most frequent sites of origin. Often the clinician knows that the patient has had a carcinoma treated.

Most secondary deposits in bone are osteolytic, and in the spine such bone destruction commonly results in vertebral collapse and spinal cord compression. A few secondary deposits—particularly some of those of prostatic origin—are osteosclerotic, producing new bone by osteoblastic activity. In this instance pathological fractures do not occur, but the spinal cord or nerves become compressed.

Usually there is a short, sometimes an abrupt, history of pain in the back, and often in the case of an osteolytic metastasis suddenly the vertebra collapses, possibly as a result of slight trauma. On examining the back an angular deformity may be apparent. In untreated cases after a period varying from a few days to weeks, the pain becomes worse and neurological signs commence in the legs.

After secondary carcinoma, lymphoma (including multiple myelomatosis, *see* p. 424) is the most common neoplastic condition to involve the spine.

Ankylosing Spondylitis ('Poker' Back) occurs predominantly in males of military age. When the disease has developed fully the patient's stance is characteristic. The back forms a continuous curve from the base of the skull to the sacrum. The lower abdomen is protuberant (*Fig.* 391). Often the knees are bent to maintain balance. Chest expansion is permanently and grossly reduced. When the condition is developing the chief complaint is low backache and/or buttock-ache typically on rising

---

* Coccidioidomycosis mainly affects cattle, sheep, dogs, cats and some rodents in the form of purulent mesenteric lymphadenitis.

HERMANN KÜMMELL, 1852–1937, *Professor of Surgery, Hamburg.*

in the morning. Tenderness over bony prominences usually is present. The common sites for such tenderness are the ischial tuberosities, the greater trochanters, the anterior superior iliac spines and the heels. In early cases there is tenderness over the manubriosternal joint. Iritis is a relatively common complication. The coexistence of non-specific urethritis or Reiter's disease (*see* p. 439) always should be investigated by an appropriate prostato-urethral examination. Very frequently ankylosing spondylitis is associated with sacro-iliac arthritis (*see* p. 210). In severe cases spinal fractures are relatively frequent.

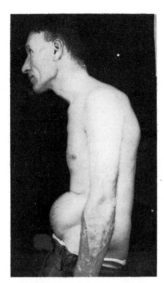

Fig. 391. Ankylosing spondylitis.

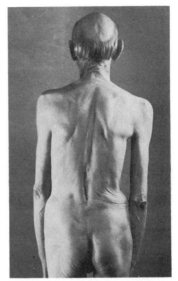

Fig. 392. Spondylolisthesis. Demonstrating the transverse loin creases.

Adolescent Kyphosis (Scheuermann's Disease). Unlike postural kyphosis, the curvature cannot be straightened by muscular effort. The parents complain that the child (13–16 years of age) is becoming increasingly round-shouldered. Inspection reveals a rounded thoracic kyphosis and in pronounced examples a compensatory lumbar lordosis, which in middle life becomes the seat of low back pain. Straight leg raising (*see* p. 207) is usually limited by tight hamstring muscles.

Calvé's Disease is rare. In a child a single vertebra collapses, probably due to eosinophilic granuloma (*see* p. 425) with resultant kyphosis.

Kyphosis in the Elderly. *Senile Kyphosis* is a common deformity characterized by a gradually increasing stoop with a forward thrust of the neck. There is no pain, unless associated with other spinal disease.

Senile Osteoporosis. Usually the patient is thin, and a woman (*see Fig.* 374), sometimes with peculiar dietary habits.

Paget's Disease of Bone. Almost without exception, there are signs elsewhere (*see* p. 426).

Finally, kyphoscoliosis may be part of *von Recklinghausen's neurofibromatosis.* The deformity commences in early middle life, and in middle-aged and elderly patients, look for the characteristic nodules (*see Fig.* 58, p. 29).

HOLGER W. SCHEUERMANN, 1877–1960, *Radiologist, Sundby Hospital, Copenhagen.*
JACQUES CALVÉ, 1875–1954, *Director, La Fondation Franco-Américaine, Berck-sur-Mer, France.*

Spondylolisthesis.* The affected vertebra (usually the 5th, but sometimes the 4th, lumbar vertebra) slips forwards because of a stress fracture of the pars interarticularis. It is found in about 5 per cent of radiographs, the patient having no symptoms referable to the condition. Symptoms occur when the relevant spinal nerves are carried forward with, and become constricted by, the edge of the slipped vertebra.

The awkward gait occasioned by *considerable* spondylolisthesis is reminiscent of that of bilateral congenital dislocation of the hips—an erroneous conclusion that can be disproved easily (*see* Trendelenburg's Sign, p. 495). The signs are increased lumbar lordosis (*see Fig.* 372 *c*) associated with a transverse loin crease or creases (*Fig.* 392) of the skin and subcutaneous tissues in the immediate vicinity of the subluxation, which often become apparent when the patient is viewed from the lateral aspect, the sacrum appearing to extend to the waist. On running the finger down the lumbar spinous processes, as the lowest process in the series is reached, suddenly the finger sinks into a deep recess, and as it emerges therefrom it encounters a sharp ridge, viz. ⎯⎯⎯⎯⎯⎯⎯⎯⎯⎯⎯⎯⎯⎯⎯⎯⎯⎯⎯→ which is the superior border of the sacrum. Where symptoms arise, the first complaint is of low back pain and stiffness after exercise. Restriction of flexion, as demonstrated by bending, is present. Pain referred to the 4th or 5th lumbar dermatome is not infrequent.

FRACTURED SPINE

In 84 per cent of cases of fracture of the spine occurring in civil life, the spinal cord is undamaged (Nicoll), and consequently these fractures should not necessarily be enshrouded with the atmosphere of calamity that sometimes prevails. With *stable* fractures there is no danger of the undamaged cord being damaged whereas with *unstable* fractures this danger exists. Preliminary clinical examination is thus best conducted by rolling the patient gently on to one side without twisting the vertebral column so that three or four persons are required to turn the patient, one being delegated to control the head. In addition radiological examination is essential in suspected cases.

1. Fracture of a Spinous Process (10 per cent) nearly always occurs near the cervicothoracic junction where the processes are long and thin. Usually, because the spinous process gives attachment to the sacrospinalis, violent muscular contraction produces an avulsion fracture. There is sudden considerable pain extending from the neck to the shoulder, aggravated by flexion or rotation of the neck. Pressure over the fracture produces exquisite tenderness. Lateral mobility of the process can sometimes be elicited.

2. Fracture of a Transverse Process (30 per cent) is confined to the lumbar region. While it can result from a blow on the loin (the urine should be examined for the presence of blood), usually it is produced by violent muscular action. The processes give attachment to their powerful muscles—the psoas, quadratus lumborum and the deeper part of the sacrospinalis which, when they contract

---

* *Spondylolisthesis.* Greek, σπόνδυλος = a vertebra+ὀλισθάνειν = to slip. In this instance, slipping forwards.

Ernest A. Nicoll, *Contemporary Regional Advisor on Postgraduate Education, Sheffield Regional Hospital Board.*

strongly, as in suddenly flexing or twisting, can snap one or more of the processes. The back is very painful and acutely tender to one side of the middle line. Pressure over the spinous processes is not painful. Any attempt at movement results in muscular spasm. If a patient with this injury (or **1** above) is told that he has a 'fractured spine' neurosis resulting in continuous backache on exertion is a frequent aftermath.

3. Fracture of a Lamina (5 per cent) is difficult to detect, and is often associated with a fracture of a transverse process or processes. The lesion occurs in the lowest part of the lumbar spine.

4. Compression (Crush) Fracture of a Body of a Vertebra (30 per cent) is commonly confined to the thoracic and lumbar regions. It is produced by hyperflexion such as would be occasioned by a heavy fall of coal on to a miner's shoulders while his back is bent.

Stable Compression Fracture (interspinous ligament intact). Occasionally slight kyphosis ⎯⎯⎯⎯⎯⎯⎯⎯⎯⎯⎯⎯⎯⎯⎯⎯⟶ is visible. Pressure on the spinous process evokes unmistakable tenderness.

Unstable Compression Fracture (interspinous ligament torn). At the moment of impact the articular facets slide on one another, separate, and then, on recoil, do not necessarily slide back into correct position, and so become locked. The spinal column is unstable and the contents of the spinal canal are exposed to future injury unless the locked facets are unlocked and the spine fixed. It is highly important to recognize this condition, which can be diagnosed entirely by clinical examination. Irrespective as to whether or not kyphosis is visible or palpable, on running the finger down the spinous process *a gap can be felt between two adjacent spinous processes.*

5. Burst Fracture (10 per cent) is due to a weight falling on the head (cervical spine) or to a fall from a height (lumbar spine) so that a compression force is applied vertically and the involved vertebra bursts ⎯⎯⎯⎯⎯⎯⎯⎯⎯⎯⎯⎯⎯⎯⟶ Almost all these fractures are stable although painful.

6. Fracture-dislocation (10 per cent). Air travel, motor-cycling, coal-mining, and horse-riding account for many of these injuries that result from violent hyperflexion of the spine. The interspinous and other ligaments are ruptured allowing the posterior intervertebral joints to dislocate. The angular deformity can always be felt as an unmistakable gap between the spinous processes ⎯⎯⎯⎯⎯⎯⎯⎯⎯⟶ of the implicated vertebrae. Fifty per cent of fracture-dislocations of the vertebral column are associated with damage to the spinal cord (usually in the neck), or the cauda equina, causing varying degrees of paraplegia or tetraplegia.

SPECIAL FEATURES OF INJURIES OF CERVICAL VERTEBRAE

Flexion Fracture. Typically this is the result of diving into shallow water and striking the head on the bottom. Usually the 5th vertebra is fractured. If the injury is neither fatal nor complicated by tetraplegia, the patient can walk without supporting his head with his hands. Movements of the neck are almost completely restricted by pain. There is acute tenderness over the spinous process of the affected vertebra, which may be somewhat more prominent than normal.

Hyperextension Partial Dislocation. Relatively minor falls or blows on the forehead may result in sufficient hyperextension of the neck to rupture the anterior longitudinal ligament. ⟶
The patient, often over 40 years of age, sometimes has a tell-tale bruise on the forehead. Partial paraplegia may accompany this seemingly minor injury.
Paraplegia associated with Cervical Spondylosis or Prolapsed Disc. The above mechanism may be the cause, the spinal canal being narrowed by an osteophyte or the disc protrusion. Thus partial paraplegia occurs without rupture of the anterior longitudinal ligament.

Occasionally a laterally protruded disc causes the *Brown-Séquard Syndrome*. With pressure on one side of the spinal cord there is dissociation of loss of power and loss of sensation: thus the leg that exhibits most muscular weakness reveals little or no loss of pin-prick sensibility, whereas the relatively strong leg shows diminished response to painful stimuli. The phenomenon is, of course, explained by the decussation of the sensory fibres in the spinal cord and is also caused by spinal tumours.
Fracture of the Atlas. If not fatal immediately, the patient supports his head in his cupped hands, and is unable to nod. He complains of severe occipital headache.
Fracture of the Odontoid Process is another result of a diving accident. Usually, immediate death occurs from damage to the brain-stem. When the contents of the neural canal escape damage, not only can the patient walk, but he holds his unsupported head erect. However, he is quite unable to rotate the head and on opening the mouth a prominence is visible in the pharynx. Unless the condition is diagnosed and the head and neck are completely immobilized, the patient is in dire danger of sudden death. Routine radiographs are often unhelpful, the clearest views being obtained with the mouth widely open.
Subluxation of the Atlanto-axial Joint due to softening of the transverse ligament of the atlas in septic processes, notably retropharyngeal abscess and tonsillitis, occurs in children, but is a rarity. Again, the patient supports the head with the hands and will not perform nodding actions. The dangers are as above.

In summary therefore, leave no diagnostic stone unturned if a child or adult complains of pain in, and/or exhibits limitation of movement of, the neck after an injury, however trivial.

THE SPINAL CORD

In an adult the cord ends at the lower border of the 1st lumbar vertebra, to give place to the cauda equina; above this level, therefore, a lesion is of the spinal cord, and below this of the cauda equina. In the case of the spinal cord, one of the first thoughts of the clinician is 'At what level is the lesion?' The student is referred to works on neurology for help in answering this question. Tumours are also out of our field. Remember, however, that a child, complaining of backache in whom none of the signs or X-ray changes of Pott's disease (*see* p. 212) can be found, may be suffering from a spinal tumour, and obtain a neurological opinion.

INJURIES OF THE SPINAL CORD

The complication of a fractured vertebra that transcends all else in importance is injury to the spinal cord. In civil life most injuries are due to indirect violence, and the most common site of the lesion is about C6, due to force applied from above. The second most frequent site (due to force applied from below) is in the region of L1. The thoracic region is seldom involved.

In a conscious patient who is known to have sustained an injury to the vertebral column, the immediate recognition of a concomitant injury to the spinal cord is seldom a problem. Provided the aid of the simple tests given below

CHARLES E. BROWN-SÉQUARD, 1818–1894, *successively Professor of Medicine at Harvard and Paris.*

is involved, no particular difficulty cloaks the recognition of a spinal injury in a comatose patient. *The* difficulty is in the case of multiple injuries, now common as the result of high-velocity automobile accidents. A bleeding head or a fracture of an extremity attracts so much of the clinician's attention that injury to an internal organ or to the spine is overlooked.

At this juncture let it be assumed that a patient with suspected injury to the spine is about to be admitted. The clinician on duty should proceed as follows:

If possible, examine the back as described on p. 216 to save unnecessary movement. Look and feel for an angular deformity and/or a gap between the spinous processes as described on p. 217, remembering that such findings are rare and occur only in gross fractures; incidentally, signs of local bruising should also be noted.

A. In a Conscious Patient continue thus:

Motor Power. Ask the patient to move his legs. If he can draw up both legs, one can be certain that there is no serious damage of the spinal cord. If only one leg is drawn up, do not jump to the conclusion that there is a unilateral lesion. Examine the immobile thigh and leg for local injury, remembering particularly fractured neck of the femur.

When the patient cannot move either of his legs:

Test the movements of the arms. If the arms are paralysed, their position may be the key to the level of the lesion.

Level of C5. * Arms completely immobile by the sides.

Level of C6 and C7. The unopposed action of the muscles supplied by the 5th and 6th cervical segments (deltoid, biceps, brachioradialis) leads to a characteristic posture of the upper limbs ⟶ with the arms abducted and the elbow flexed to a lesser or greater degree depending on the exact level of the injury.

Level of C8 and T1. The upper limb functions more or less fully with the exception of those muscles innervated by T1 so that a claw hand similar to that of Klumpke's paralysis results (*see* p. 405).

Level of T2. Often there is contraction of the pupils, owing to irritation of the ocular motor fibres which leave the spinal cord at the segment above.

The abdomen should be inspected. Distension due to temporary bowel paresis is frequent with cervical cord injuries. When respiration is purely *abdominal* (diaphragmatic) it implies that the intercostal muscles are paralysed. The lesion is situated, therefore, above T2.

Before completing the abdominal part of the examination percuss the bladder: retention of urine is usual when the spinal cord is damaged. A lesion above T6 results in paralysis of the muscles of the abdominal wall. Between T6 and T12 the lower the lesion, the more the muscles of the abdominal wall will be spared. In relevant cases consider the possibility of a fractured pelvis (*see* p. 330). *Sensation* should be tested with a pin. A band of hyperaesthesia at the level of

---

* *Above C5.* Transection is fatal because all the respiratory muscles, including the diaphragm (supplied by the phrenic nerve), are paralysed. This occurred in judicial hanging.

the lesion, with anaesthesia below, is indicative of a grave injury to the spinal cord.

Reflexes. At this stage the reflexes below the level of the lesion are in abeyance, as is described in the section on spinal shock (*see below*).

B. In an Unconscious Patient the absence of deep reflexes and failure to obtain reflex movement to painful stimuli such as pinching in the lower part of the body, yet being able to obtain responses over the arm and shoulder, indicates a concomitant lesion of the spinal cord. If no response is obtained at any level, the examination must be repeated at intervals. In these circumstances no conclusion can be drawn until consciousness or semi-consciousness is regained, or responses are obtained over the upper extremities, whichever should happen first.

Injury to the spinal cord manifests itself in three forms, namely, cord concussion, cord transection and root transection. The first can terminate in complete recovery, or give place to the second or to the third, or a combination of the second and third.

Cord Concussion (a state of *spinal shock*) gives rise to a sensory loss, *flaccid* paralysis and visceral paralysis (abdominal distension due to paralytic ileus, retention of urine) below the level of the lesion. When raised, the affected limb falls like a log. Reflexes are in abeyance. In addition to testing the usual reflexes, the anal reflex provides a valuable sign.

The Anal Reflex. In normal circumstances, when a finger is inserted into the anal canal the finger is gripped tightly by the external sphincter. When this reflex is lost the anus remains open ('yawns') for several seconds. For obvious reasons this must be tested in the dorsal position (*see* p. 267).

Eight hours after its onset cord concussion commences to regress. The condition is completely reversible, and when present alone (a rarity, it must be stressed) complete recovery can be expected within 7–10 days.

Cord Transection. As a result of the trauma, the cord can be wholly or partly transected. At first the signs are those of cord concussion. As this passes off, the part of the spinal cord below the lesion, bereft of the controlling influences of the brain, acts as an independent unit in that it mediates reflex activity. In a matter of hours the anal reflex returns. The *penile reflex* becomes active (erection occurs on slight cutaneous stimulation of the organ). In 1–4 weeks the stage of spinal shock passes off. The flaccid paralysis becomes spastic (extensor plantar reflex*), tendon reflexes return and become much exaggerated, clonus is present, retention of urine is usual, lost sensation never returns. *The presence of anal and penile reflexes in the absence of sensation below the injured segment is diagnostic of cord transection*, and enables a decision to be reached that the lesion is anatomical and irreparable long before spinal automatism ensues.

The Reflexes of Spinal Automatism. Pinch the skin of the dorsum of the foot vigorously. In normal individuals the withdrawal from the noxious stimulus is a quick one—all the joints of the lower extremity flex. When the spinal cord has been transected, and the stage of spinal shock is waning, the first sign of returning function in that part of the cord isolated from the brain by transection is contraction of the hamstrings with flexion of the big toe. A few days later, when the stage of spinal shock has passed off completely—

The Flexor Withdrawal Reflex of the Lower Extremities is obtained. In the paraplegic the reaction is *slower* than normal, and while the hip, knee, and ankle joints flex, the big toe moves *upwards*. If the

---

* Babinski's Sign–*see* p. 64.

lesion is above T12 and the patient is lean, it will be seen that the muscles of the abdominal wall participate in the flexor reflex by contracting slowly.

An Incomplete Lesion. Riddoch originally postulated that an incomplete lesion is suggested when the stimulus (pinching the dorsum of the foot) brings on less pronounced flexion than when the lesion is complete, and the semiflexion thus produced is followed after a time by extension. Guttman has shown that this paraplegia-in-extension sequence depends on the presence of sepsis (pressure sores, urinary infection) and the posture in which the lower limbs have been maintained after the accident. An incomplete lesion (approximately 40 per cent of cases) must be diagnosed by the findings on neurological examination, e.g. the Brown-Séquard Syndrome (*see* p. 218).

Root Transection differs from cord transection in that the paralysis remains flaccid.

Haematomyelia implies a focal extravasation of blood within the spinal cord, the result of trauma without a fracture. Usually the cervical region is affected and the lesion is incomplete. Apart from transection following a fracture, there is no condition in which a lesion of the spinal cord develops so rapidly as haematomyelia.

Traction Birth Injury of the Spine occurs particularly during delivery of the aftercoming shoulders and head in breech delivery. The paraplegic infant lies in a characteristic position with the legs limp and everted in a frog-like posture. There is no involuntary motor response or cry of pain in response to stimulus. The bladder soon becomes palpable.

INFLAMMATION OF THE SPINAL MENINGES

An epidural (extradural) abscess may be associated with a furuncle or be a sequel of acute pyogenic osteomyelitis of a vertebra. Pain starts in the back with exquisite localized tenderness. Vertebral percussion (*see* p. 204) is positive. After a day or two the pain radiates forward on one or both sides owing to pressure on nerve roots (cf. herpes zoster, *see* p. 319) and mimics intra-abdominal or intrathoracic disease. By this time the patient has a high pyrexia, is manifestly severely ill, and may exhibit rigors. Antibiotics may mask the other signs of acute osteomyelitis (*see* p. 417) but spinal tenderness and rigidity remain undoubtedly present. At an early stage the first signs of paraplegia are present (extensor plantar reflexes, weakness of the legs, urinary retention).

CAUDA EQUINA LESIONS

A space-occupying lesion within the neural canal below the level of the 1st lumbar vertebra compresses the cauda equina. Such lesions comprise tumours, Pott's disease, fracture-dislocation of the lumbar spine, and protrusion of L4–5 or L5–S1 intervertebral disc.

Sensory Signs. One of the most salient features of a lesion of the cauda equina is an area of saddle-shaped hyperaesthesia, and later of anaesthesia, which, as its name implies, represents an area over both buttocks, the anus and the perineum. This can be tested with a pin, starting near the anus and working laterally until normal sensation is appreciated.

Motor Signs are a *flaccid* paralysis of the muscles of the leg below the knees.

Reflexes. The ankle jerks are absent, but the knee jerks are often accentuated owing to the weakness of the opposing hamstrings.

GEORGE RIDDOCH,1888–1947, *Neurologist, London Hospital. Pioneer of the modern treatment of traumatic paraplegia.*
SIR LUDWIG GUTTMAN, *Contemporary Director Emeritus and Founder, National Spinal Injuries Centre, Stoke Mandeville Hospital, Bucks.*

Bladder Symptoms. Since the sacral reflex arc is concerned in emptying of the bladder, its interruption by compression of the cauda equina usually causes *retention of urine with overflow.* Even after a severe lesion of the cauda, reflex micturition is sometimes established later, the reflex being mediated through the vesical plexus.

Anal Sphincter Relaxation. See p. 220.

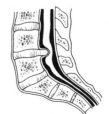

Cauda Equina Lesion due to Massive Prolapsed Intervertebral Disc is rare. The extruded disc material impinges upon, and compresses, the cauda equina causing *bilateral* sciatica, viz. ————————————————————→

The straight-leg-raising test is often positive at a low angle (but this may not be found if the extruded disc is lying free and not pressing on the emergent nerve roots), the ankle jerks are absent, there is weakness of the legs, but, above all, added to these signs there is hyperaesthesia of the saddle-shaped area referred to above. In many instances there is an abrupt onset of paralysis within a few days, in which event the condition is a surgical emergency.

Chapter 18

NON-ACUTE ABDOMINAL CONDITIONS

Since the first edition of this work the gradual and recently accelerating development of ancillary methods of investigation (particularly radiology) have enabled the clinician to diagnose non-acute abdominal disease at earlier stages. A careful history followed by efficient physical examination by the methods to be described will lead to an accurate tentative diagnosis in the majority of patients, but ancillary investigations will be required in almost all.

GENERAL PRINCIPLES IN THE EXAMINATION OF THE ABDOMEN

The patient should lie flat on the back. In passing, it is almost unbelievable how often a presumably intelligent person, when requested to lie on his back, will promptly roll on to his abdomen. As a rule, one pillow is sufficient, but always ascertain that the patient's head and neck are quite comfortable. Round-shouldered persons and those short of breath when lying flat or with ankylosing spondylitis require more than one pillow. Have the abdomen bared completely and the blanket sufficiently low (*Fig.* 393) to display the inguinal and femoral rings. When a patient, particularly a young man, realizes that he is about to be examined, sometimes he arches his back and blows out his chest—no doubt to demonstrate his manly proportions. Tell the patient to relax and breathe through the mouth, and by trying to insinuate your hand between the couch and the patient, make certain that his back is resting comfortably upon the couch.

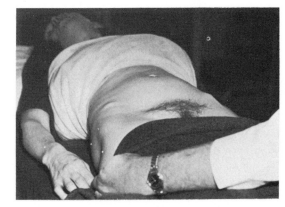

Fig. 393. Before commencing the examination of the abdomen, ensure that the whole abdomen, including the inguinal and femoral rings, is exposed.

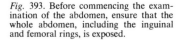

THE VALUE OF INSPECTION

Inspection. A great deal of information can be gathered from inspection (*Fig.* 394). In the demonstrations that follow, an endeavour will be made to bring out particular points that are revealed thereby. A common error is to

223

skimp this important part of abdominal examination. Look carefully for a visible swelling and for erythema due to hot-water bottle applications, the latter being evidence of fairly severe pain and of its location.

Palpation. Continue in a calm, methodical frame of mind, and instead of placing the hand upon the abdomen unceremoniously, pay very careful attention to several preliminary details.

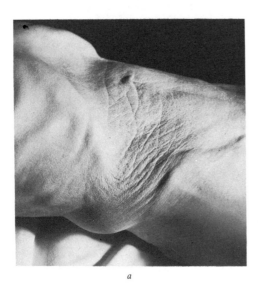
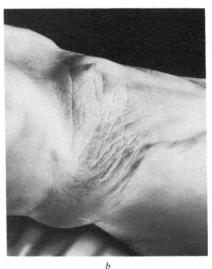

a   *b*

Fig. 394. By patiently watching the abdomen for about a minute (*a*) this swelling appeared, accompanied by visible peristalsis passing from left to right. (*b*) Case of pyloric stenosis due to carcinoma.

1. Routine palpation of the abdomen should be carried out with the flat of the hand. It is the flexor surfaces of the fingers, used collectively, that form the active palpating agent; the tips of the fingers take no part in the manœuvre. In order that the hand may impinge upon the abdomen at the correct angle, it is essential for the forearm to be maintained in a strictly horizontal plane. As beds and couches vary in height, the examiner, if need be, must sit on a suitable chair or even kneel upon the floor, no matter how undignified this may appear (Emerson).

2. The great enemy of efficient palpation is muscular rigidity. The hands must be warm, at least as warm as the patient's skin, otherwise he will certainly contract his abdominal muscles. To wash your hands in hot water before the examination is an excellent expedient. Especially in cold weather, it is a good practice to commence palpating with a blanket or the patient's under-garment intervening between the abdomen and the hand. The patient's confidence is thus obtained, and, realizing that he is not going to be hurt, he tends to relax the abdominal muscles.

3. Ask the patient to breathe quietly and rather deeply through the mouth and keep the arms loosely by the sides. Request him to 'drop the jaw'—this ensures that the mouth is open and it seems to help in obtaining general muscular

CHARLES P. EMERSON, *Contemporary Professor of Medicine, Boston University School of Medicine, Boston.*

relaxation. Tell the patient that he is not going to be hurt. Some relax better when they are engaged in conversation. Experience, and to some extent native wit, will reveal what manner of individual the clinician is palpating.

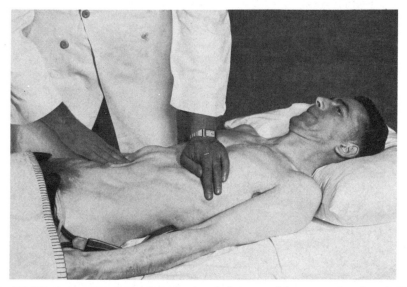

Fig. 395. With the base of the left hand pressing upon the lower part of the sternum, thoracic respiration is impeded and the abdominal muscles relax.

Overcoming Rigidity in Refractory Cases. In spite of ingenuity and subterfuge, the abdominal wall sometimes continues to remain unrelaxed. In such cases Nicholson's expedient is of considerable value. The base of the palm of the left hand is placed upon the lower part of the sternum and increasing pressure is exerted. Eventually the examiner is leaning quite heavily upon the chest, with the result that the patient breathes abdominally, while his thorax is comparatively still. When he draws in his breath his abdominal muscles necessarily relinquish their tonicity, whereupon the right hand seizes its awaited opportunity (*Fig.* 395).

To continue with examination of an average case:

Technique of Routine Palpation. If pain is experienced in any particular part of the abdomen, begin by palpating the region diagonally opposite. For example, if the pain is located in the right iliac fossa, commence palpating the left hypochondrium and work round, palpating each quadrant in turn, ending with the region of which the patient complains. During this manœuvre there should be cooperation between the hand and the mind. When the hand is over a particular region the mind should visualize the anatomical structures beneath, and while each quadrant is being palpated the examiner's eyes should be turned towards the patient's face, for if he winces when one area is palpated, and not another, obviously it is a sign of considerable diagnostic moment.

Deep Palpation. During the routine palpation of the abdomen just described no attempt is made to palpate deeply; this is reserved as a confirmatory measure in particular instances. The first essential is to overcome the resistance of the

NEVILLE J. NICHOLSON, 1901–1967, *Surgeon, County Infirmary, Louth, Lincolnshire.*

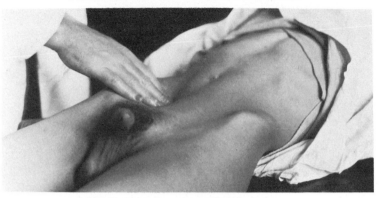

Fig. 396. Deep palpation in the right iliac fossa.

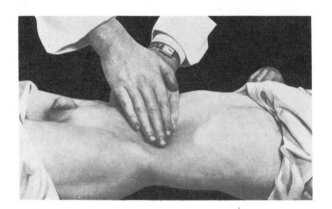

Fig. 397. Using both hands, one superimposed upon the other, pressure is distributed evenly and the method is effective, particularly in deep palpation.

abdominal wall. Even a tense abdominal wall tends to relax during expiration or the pause between expiration and inspiration. Continuing palpation, advantage is taken of each period of relaxation for the forepart of the hand to sink progressively deeper and deeper into the abdomen. The position of the hand and fingers during deep palpation depends upon which viscus the clinician is attempting to palpate and at what distance that viscus is situated from the surface—usually the angle of inclination must vary with the thickness of the subcutaneous tissue. Deep palpation is not conducted with the flat of the hand, but rather with the flexor surfaces of the fingers with the hand tilted at a slight angle, viz. ————————————————→

By gentle, even pressure, which becomes progressively deeper and deeper (*Fig.* 396), valuable information, unobtainable by any other method, is sometimes forthcoming. When an indefinite lump is present the technique shown in *Fig.* 397 sometimes proves useful.

Percussion is of value in certain conditions, as indicated on p. 227.

Auscultation (*see* pp. 301, 312) is of occasional value (*see also* Mesenteric Ischaemia, p. 229).

EXAMINATION OF AN INTRA-ABDOMINAL SWELLING

Inspection. If there is a visible lump, note particularly if it moves on respiration. In the endeavour to elucidate the nature of a lump in the abdomen, the first step is to exclude a swelling in the abdominal wall (*see* p. 245).

Palpation. Note the consistency and shape of the lump; whether it is regular or irregular; mobile or fixed to the posterior abdominal wall and whether it moves on respiration. An examination in the knee-elbow position should be resorted to in obscure cases, and occasionally this is very helpful, particularly in deciding whether pulsations are transmitted from the abdominal aorta to an overlying swelling, or whether the swelling itself is pulsatile. If the swelling arises from the pelvis, a bimanual rectal or vaginal examination (*see* pp. 280, 284) is essential. This is an excellent opportunity to set forth a simple, yet fundamental and unwavering rule: *Never express an opinion upon a tumour arising out of the pelvis until the bladder has been emptied by a catheter.*

There is one physical sign that occasionally proves helpful in obscure intra-abdominal swellings, and that is the *sign of a mesenteric cyst.* The lump moves in a plane from the right hypochondrium to the left iliac fossa, but not in the plane at right angles (AB) to this. ⟶

Percussion. This will demonstrate whether the lump contains gas, i.e. is part of the gastrointestinal tract or an abscess connected therewith.

In the demonstrations that follow, the physical signs of swellings connected with particular organs will be considered. So far as tumours are concerned, the abdomen is indeed a temple of surprise, and it is by our diagnostic humiliations when the abdomen is opened that we learn.

EXAMINATION OF A SUSPECTED GASTRIC OR DUODENAL CASE

While the history and a barium meal radiological examination are all-important in the diagnosis of a non-acute lesion of the stomach or duodenum, physical examination is indispensable, and sometimes yields invaluable information.

Examine the Teeth particularly for evidence of pyorrhoea. Record the number of teeth present, particularly the molars. Are the latter sufficient to effect adequate mastication? If the patient has a dental plate, ask him whether he can chew his food properly with it. In a surprising number of cases the patient replies that he removes his teeth when he eats!

Pyloric Stenosis. If, from the history, this is suspected, particular attention should be directed to watching for visible peristalsis passing from left to right in the epigastrium (*see* Figs. 394*b* and 398).

The Sign of Splashing (Succussion Splash). Splashing is of value only when the stomach, under normal conditions, would be empty—that is, *three hours after a meal.* The hand is laid over the stomach, and short, sudden, dipping movements are made. A gurgle suggests incomplete emptying of the stomach due to pyloric obstruction.

A Visible Lump. In the course of observing the epigastrium, occasionally a lump, almost invariably due to a carcinoma of the stomach, can be seen in the epigastric notch descending at each inspiration and disappearing during expiration.

Palpation. In very thin individuals the normal pylorus sometimes can be felt but a barium meal X-ray is essential to confirm that the lump is not that of an early carcinoma which is usually painless on palpation and feels like a cotton-reel lying transversely. Note that the absence of a lump by no means excludes carcinoma of the stomach. A neoplasm of the stomach often possesses transmitted pulsation from the abdominal aorta, and usually it moves with respiration. The mobility of the lump is important when assessing the resectability of the neoplasm.

Trousseau's Sign of Wandering Thrombophlebitis (*see* p. 394).

Carcinoma of the Stomach: Seeking Secondary Deposits

Troisier's Sign (*see* p. 140).

Examine the Liver. The edge of the liver should be examined with great care for the presence of metastases. If the liver edge is irregular and/or the abdomen seems full, it is necessary to ascertain if there is ascites (*see* p. 242).

Examine the Umbilicus for a hard nodule (*see* p. 250).

Rectal Examination. When carcinoma of the stomach is strongly suspected this is a *sine qua non* to exclude the presence of a transcoelomic implantation of metastases into the rectovesical pouch (rectal shelf of Blumer, *see* p. 277).

Vaginal Examination. Bear in mind that Krukenberg's ovarian tumours are another manifestation of transcoelomic implantation of cancer cells.

Suspected Pyloric Stenosis of Infants. The earliest sign of dehydration—lack of normal skin turgescence (*see* p. 45)—should be sought. Depression of the anterior fontanelle is in evidence only in advanced cases. This completed, proceed with the examination of the abdomen.

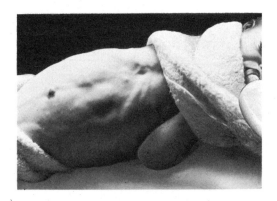

Fig. 398. Visible peristalsis. A wave could be seen passing from left to right. Case of hypertrophic pyloric stenosis in an infant.

Inspection. To observe an infant's abdomen for visible peristalsis, a good plan is to place it upon a table and arrange for it to be fed. More often than not it is necessary to watch for some time for waves of peristalsis (*Fig.* 398) which commence at the left costal margin, roll across the upper abdomen, to disappear beneath the medial border of the right rectus muscle. The most likely time for this phenomenon to appear is at the end of the feed, or some minutes afterwards.

Should the patient vomit (projectile vomiting is characteristic) the infant must be fed again while *the* sign of hypertrophic pyloric stenosis (the presence of a lump) is sought.

FRIEDRICH KRUKENBERG, 1871–1946, *Ophthalmologist, Halle. Wrote a classic thesis on malignant tumours of the ovary at the age of* 24 *years.*

Palpation. For this purpose it is best to employ the *left* hand to feel a hypertrophied pylorus and to have the baby sucking at the *left* breast (*Fig.* 399) or, if the baby is bottle-fed, resting on the mother's *left* arm. The stage is now set for palpating for a lump in the right hypochondrium. Employing this technique, the fingers rest upon the diminutive abdomen in such a way that with minimum adjustment the pulps of the index and middle fingers come to overlie the pylorus (*Fig.* 399). Palpation must be firm and deep, and it is better to maintain steady pressure than to make repeated digs. Usually it is necessary to exhibit patience and then, rather suddenly, the pylorus, which has been likened to an olive, is felt to harden beneath the fingers. If the lump is felt write in the patient's notes 'I have felt a lump'. If in doubt repeated examination is necessary. Only occasionally is an X-ray required to establish the diagnosis (*Fig.* 399, *inset*). With the administration of parenteral fluids there is no urgency with such cases. Where the symptoms point to pyloric obstruction, but no lump is felt, think of hiatus hernia—a possibility that at once becomes a probability if there is blood in the vomit.

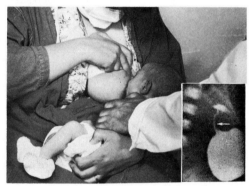

Fig. 399. Palpating the pylorus of an infant for hypertrophy. The examiner is seated. *Inset:* radiograph in a doubtful case after feeding the infant with a dilute barium solution.

Suspected Duodenal or Gastric Ulcer or Hiatus Hernia. In a fair majority of patients with upper abdominal pain peptic ulcer, hiatus hernia, or gallstones are the cause and in these clinical examination is usually unrewarding. *Fig.* 400 shows the salient features for the location of pain and, in some instances, tenderness. Exceptions are frequent and X-ray investigation is mandatory.

Mesenteric Ischaemia. The history suggests a peptic ulcer but investigations are negative. If the patient is middle-aged or elderly remember that the origin of the superior mesenteric artery is prone to atherosclerosis and that the pain after meals may be due to a relative lack of oxygen in the small bowel when engaged in peristaltic activity ('abdominal angina'). The essential clinical clue is the presence of a systolic murmur on auscultation of the upper abdomen. Complete mesenteric vascular occlusion (*see* p. 308) often occurs at a later stage.

EXAMINATION OF THE GALLBLADDER

Acute Cholecystitis. *See* p. 298.

Examination of a Case of Chronic Cholecystitis. The subjects of this disease are often fat, middle-aged, multiparous women, and this is so well known that it must be added that gallstones are not uncommon even in thin men.

The Detection of Jaundice (*see* p. 231). Needless to say it is not necessary for the patient to be jaundiced in order to diagnose gallstones. Deep, unmistakable jaundice associated with this condition means that a gallstone is, or has been, obstructing the *common* bile duct. On the other hand, slight transient jaundice can be accounted for by infection—for instance by cholangitis, which may be associated with inflammation of the gallbladder.

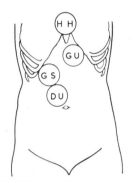

Fig. 400. Typical sites of pain with duodenal ulcer (DU) which comes on ½–2 hours after food, gastric ulcer (GU) which occurs shortly after eating, gallstones (GS), worse after fatty foods, and hiatus hernia (HH), worse on lying flat.

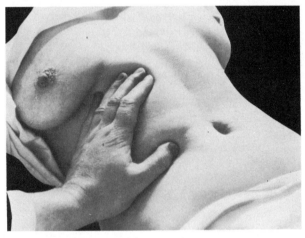

Fig. 401. Murphy's sign (Moynihan's method).

Observe the abdomen. Not infrequently a brownish stain is seen in the epigastrium and right hypochondrium due to the application of heat, usually in the form of hot-water bottles, to relieve the pain. Ask the patient to show you where she experiences the pain. She will point to the right hypochondrium. Now ask where the pain goes to, and she will often run her finger round to the right scapula.

Murphy's Sign (Moynihan's Method). Place the left hand on the costal margin in such a manner that the thumb lies over the fundus of the gallbladder (*Fig.* 401) and exerts moderate pressure. Ask the patient to take a deep breath. The sign is positive if the patient 'catches her breath' when the descending diaphragm causes the inflamed gallbladder to impinge against the pressure of the thumb (temporary inhibition of respiration when inspiration is nearing its zenith).

Apparent Enlargement of the Gallbladder. A swelling is felt in the region of the organ. Consider the following:

1. Acute cholecystitis, *see* p. 298.
2. Mucocele. The swelling is painless and there is no jaundice.
3. The patient is jaundiced. *See* Carcinoma of the Head of the Pancreas, p. 232.
4. The swelling seems very hard. Consider carcinoma of the gallbladder, or a liver metastasis or a primary liver tumour.

Differential Diagnosis between an Enlarged Gallbladder and a Hydronephrosis. This question can be decided clinically (although radiological confirmation is desirable) by the method demonstrated in *Fig.* 26, p. 14; place the hands as shown and with the displacing hand exert *gentle* upward movements with the pulps of the fingers acting in harmony. If the swelling in question is a hydronephrosis, the watching hand will appreciate the upward lift imparted to the swelling. On the other hand, a large gallbladder will be unaffected by those movements.

JOHN B. MURPHY, 1857–1916, *Surgeon, Mercy Hospital, Chicago.*
BERKELEY G. A., LORD MOYNIHAN OF LEEDS, 1865–1936, *Professor of Surgery, Leeds.*

EXAMINATION OF A JAUNDICED ADOLESCENT OR ADULT

Jaundice is very liable to be overlooked in artificial light. Lesser degrees often can be discerned by a yellow tinge of the sclerae of the eyes before pigmentation is seen in the skin. Sometimes very slight yellow discoloration can be detected by examination of the posterior portion of the hard palate in daylight. When sufficiently deep to be observed in the skin, the abdomen will display it to advantage.

Itching often accompanies jaundice. The presence of scratch marks on the chest or abdomen sometimes gives a clue to the diagnosis when the patient is examined in artificial light or if the jaundice has faded. The itching, due to an accumulation of bile salts in the blood, sometimes precedes jaundice.

Virus Hepatitis is the commonest cause of jaundice in the USA and Great Britain. Young patients are attacked more often than the middle-aged or elderly. As a rule, the condition commences abruptly with nausea, sometimes vomiting, general malaise and mild pyrexia. Then, in about three days, the patient becomes jaundiced. The liver becomes palpable and tender. Occasionally the jaundice occurs in a more severe form, rendering the condition more difficult to differentiate from that due to one of the extrahepatic causes of biliary obstruction.

Virus hepatitis can follow blood transfusion or plasma infusion. *Syringe Jaundice* is another variety. The incubation period is remarkably long—60–135 days. If it can be proved that the syringe and the hollow needle used were not freshly boiled or autoclaved, legally the doctor in charge may be held responsible for having caused the virus infection. At the present time drug addicts are frequent sufferers.

When jaundice thought to be due to virus hepatitis does not clear within a reasonable period (say, a fortnight), the diagnosis should be reviewed.

Jaundice consequent upon Gallstones. When a patient gives a history of a recent attack of pain (within 48 hours) consistent with biliary colic, and especially if previous attacks have occurred, jaundice due to gallstones must be given first consideration.

Such jaundice can arise in two ways. In about half there is a stone or stones in the common bile duct, and one of them is causing obstruction to the flow of bile into the duodenum. In the rest, it is due to concomitant infection of the intrahepatic bile ducts (cholangitis).

The icteric tinge ranges from pale lemon to bright orange, and it may *vary in intensity from day to day*. In cases due to impaction of a stone in the common bile duct the jaundice, while varying in intensity, in the aggregate is likely to become darker, and occasionally it assumes a greenish hue. In such cases the urine becomes correspondingly dark, while the stools become very light coloured, if not almost white (*see Fig.* 35, p. 20). At the commencement of an attack, tenderness in the right hypochondrium is likely to be present. As a rule, the gallbladder is impalpable. Pyrexia occurs in one-third of cases. Usually the pyrexia is mild, although there may be one or two 'spikes' of elevated temperature in prolonged cases. All jaundiced patients tend to lose weight.

Oriental Cholangiohepatitis. In China, Japan and Hong Kong cholangitis is commonly due to long-standing stones in the bile ducts associated with infestation by the Chinese liver fluke (*Clonorchis sinensis*) which infests freshwater fish eaten raw. By the time the patient seeks relief, often the urine is the colour of a strong infusion of tea, secondary infection of the obstructed ducts has occurred, and the patients are frequently acutely ill and toxic. The gallbladder is often palpable, because the stones are present only in the ducts (*see* Courvoisier's Sign, p. 233).

Congenital Choledochus Cyst is a rare condition affecting females four times more commonly than males. The symptoms and signs seldom appear before the age of 6 months, and in 50 per cent of cases are delayed until early adult life. There are attacks of jaundice, usually accompanied by upper abdominal pain and, if infection of the stagnant bile occurs, by pyrexia. In 90 per cent of cases a palpable cyst is present, the physical signs of which are identical with those of a pancreatic cyst (*see* p. 238).

Hereditary Spherocytosis* (Acholuric† Familial Jaundice). While occasionally the jaundice appears soon after birth or in very early life, more often its appearance is delayed until childhood, or even adult life. Once the disease has manifested itself, the patient suffers from periodic crises of red blood-cell destruction. Such crises are characterized by pyrexia, abdominal pain, nausea, vomiting and extreme pallor. This is followed by jaundice, which varies in intensity, and at its height is a daffodil hue. There is often a family history. On examining the abdomen the spleen will be found to be enlarged, and in thin subjects it can be palpated with ease. A number of these patients have small pigment stones in the gallbladder which may account for severe pain. Chronic ulcers of the legs are common in adult sufferers.

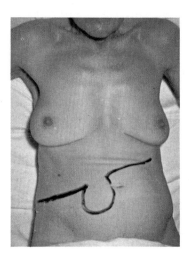

Fig. 402. Profound jaundice in a woman aged 70. There had been no abdominal pain, only slight epigastric discomfort. The outline of the enlarged gallbladder has been marked out with a skin pencil. Case of carcinoma of head of pancreas.

Jaundice due to Carcinoma of the Head of the Pancreas. One characteristic feature should be noted especially—the jaundice is steadily progressive. The icteric tinge becomes deeper and deeper until the skin and conjunctivae assume almost a mahogany hue (*Fig.* 402). The stools become putty-coloured, and remain so. In more than two-thirds of cases there is relentless, dull pain in the epigastrium, which precedes the jaundice and continues week in, week out. In less than one-third the growth commences in, or very near, the ampulla of Vater, in which event the onset of jaundice is painless, or almost so. Occasionally with this variety, necrosis of portions of the growth occurs, pent-up bile escapes into the duodenum, and variations in the depth of jaundice, together with pyrexia, mimic the waxing and waning that characterize the jaundice of calculus obstruction of the common bile duct.

---

* *Spherocytosis.* The red cells, instead of being biconcave, are biconvex. They are very fragile, and burst easily.

† *Acholuric* = without bile in the urine. In this condition the circulating bilirubin is insoluble in water, and is not filtered by the glomeruli.

ABRAHAM VATER, 1684–1751, *Professor of Anatomy and Botany, Wittenberg, Germany.*

Courvoisier's Sign. If in a jaundiced patient the gallbladder is enlarged, it is *not* a case of stone impacted in the common bile duct, for previous cholecystitis, which existed when the stone was in the gallbladder, must have rendered the gallbladder fibrotic and incapable of dilatation. There are many exceptions to this sign (apart from the fact that in a fat patient the enlarged gallbladder may be impalpable), the most notable of which are: double impaction, when there is one stone in the cystic and another in the common bile duct, and Oriental cholangiohepatitis (*see* p. 231).

JAUNDICE IN INFANCY

Icterus Neonatorum. Between the second and the fifth days of life about 1 in 6 of all newly born infants develop jaundice which reaches its zenith in three or four days, and then fades gradually. The liver is not enlarged, neither are the stools clay-coloured nor the urine deeply bile-stained. This so-called 'physiological' jaundice is deepest and most prolonged in premature infants.

Erythroblastosis Fetalis (Icterus *Gravis* Neonatorum). The baby is *born* jaundiced, the condition being brought about by a Rh-positive fetus in the uterus of a Rh-negative mother. At the present time the diagnosis can be made during pregnancy by testing the mother's serum for antibodies, and so arrangements can be made for exchange transfusion of the affected infant *in utero* or soon after delivery. Unless remedied early, the jaundiced infant may die suddenly of kernicterus.*

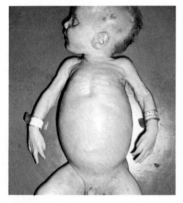

Fig. 403. Congenital atresia of the common bile duct.

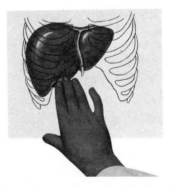

Fig. 404. Occasionally the free edge of the normal adult liver can be felt to override the fingers during inspiration.

Congenital Atresia of the Bile Ducts. Sometimes a slight icteric tinge is present at birth. More usually the jaundice does not appear for two or three days. Occasionally it is delayed for one or more weeks. Unless the atresia can be remedied, the jaundice becomes deeper and deeper (*Fig.* 403), the urine more and more bile-stained, and even the tears and saliva are yellow. From birth the stools are almost white, but after two weeks they may become faintly yellow. This does not necessarily signify that the atresia is incomplete, because in profound jaundice a small amount of bile pigments is excreted by the intestines. Gradually the liver becomes larger and larger, and on palpation feels

---

* *Kernicterus* = fixation of bile pigments in the basal ganglia of the brain.

LUDWIG COURVOISIER, 1843–1918, *Professor of Surgery, Basle, Switzerland.*

unduly hard. Nutrition is well maintained, especially if the baby is given feeds containing but little fat. Unrelieved, death results, but the child may survive for a surprising length of time (up to six years—Sherlock).

Omphalitis. Infection of the umbilicus is liable to give rise to spreading infection along the incompletely obliterated umbilical vein, and occasionally hepatitis, resulting in jaundice, supervenes. Severe infection elsewhere is also liable to produce jaundice.

EXAMINATION OF THE LIVER

During infancy until about the end of the third year the normal liver extends one to two finger-breadths below the costal margin. During inspiration, at this period of life, the extreme edge of the normal spleen is also palpable.

In healthy thin adults occasionally the edge of the liver can be felt a finger-breadth below the costal margin (*Fig.* 404). As a rule, however, and especially when the patient is well covered, the normal liver is impalpable. Consider now the enlarged liver. Inspection is not of great value, although, on occasions, the edge of a large liver can be seen to move downwards on inspiration. Reliance, therefore, must be placed on palpation. With a thin patient who relaxes easily there is no difficulty in detecting an enlarged liver. If in doubt or when a well-developed right rectus muscle hinders palpation, proceed in the following roundabout manner.

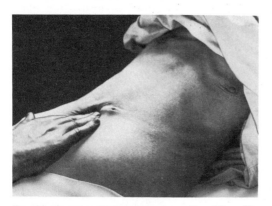

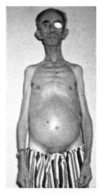

Fig. 405. Examining the free edge of an enlarged liver. The fingers·have just overridden the liver edge, which can be seen. In this case of secondary carcinoma the free edge felt irregular and was stony hard.

Fig. 406. Gross enlargement of the liver and a glass eye (which has been worn for, maybe, many years) is practically pathognomonic of secondary melanoma, the primary growth having been in the uveal tract.

Palpating an Enlarged Liver. Lay the hand on the right iliac fossa with the fingers pointing towards the left axilla. Every time the patient expires, slide the hand a little nearer the right costal margin (Osler). Progressing in this way, a time is reached when the edge of an enlarged liver strikes the hand as the patient inspires. In this event, keeping the hands stationary, ask the patient to take a deep breath, and while inspiration is in progress the fingertips will be felt to ride over the free edge of the liver (*Fig.* 405). At the moment of impact of the fingers with the liver edge the character of the organ is noted. Once the liver edge has been felt distinctly, working from right to left, the lower border of the liver is defined as far as possible and outlined with a skin pencil.

DAME SHEILA SHERLOCK, *Contemporary Professor of Medicine, Royal Free Hospital School of Medicine, London.*
SIR WILLIAM OSLER, 1849–1919, *Professor of Medicine successively at McGill University, Montreal; University of Pennsylvania, Philadelphia; Johns Hopkins University, Baltimore; and Regius Professor of Medicine, Oxford.*

Attention is directed now to the upper surface of the organ. Commencing in the right mid-axillary line at about the fourth interspace, percuss and obtain a clear resonant note. Then work downwards until the resonance is supplanted by dullness. Here mark the upper border of the liver. The anterior and posterior thoracic walls are examined similarly. Note that hydatid cyst or amoebic abscess often cause hepatic enlargement in an upward, rather than in a downward, direction.

Secondary Carcinoma of the Liver (*Figs.* 406, 407). Jaundice with stony-hard irregular enlargement of the liver edge nearly always signifies secondary carcinoma in the liver. Ascites (*see* p. 242) of a lesser or greater degree is often apparent.

Primary Carcinoma of the Liver is extremely common in some parts of the world, notably in many parts of Africa and in Malaya and Hawaii. The findings are as noted in the paragraph above, although occasionally one can appreciate that there is a single large swelling in the liver with surrounding secondaries. The presence of a systolic murmur on auscultation over an apparently solitary swelling suggests that it is a primary carcinoma.

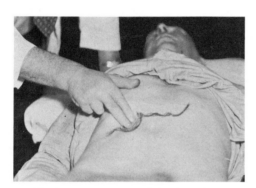

Fig. 407. Secondary carcinoma of the liver with a large bosselation in the region of the gallbladder. Typically each metastasis is umbilicated.

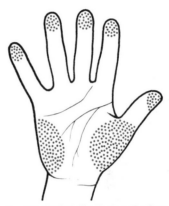

Fig. 408. Typical distribution of palmar erythema, namely over the eminences and the pulps of the fingers.

Hepatic Cirrhosis (Laennec's cirrhosis*). Usually the patient is middle-aged and frequently (particularly in the USA), but not necessarily, alcoholic. The liver is firmly and evenly enlarged. Nodularity of the organ may be apparent in a thin patient. Only exceptionally, in the atrophic type, is there no enlargement. Palpable enlargement of the spleen (*see* p. 236) is strong evidence that haematemesis is due to portal hypertension consequent on cirrhosis and not to a peptic ulcer. Lack of body hair is often a noticeable feature in a patient with established portal hypertension. Haematemesis due to this cause is found in the following categories (Hunt):

MILD CIRRHOSIS is quiet and of long duration. In some cases there are repeated attacks of slight jaundice with epigastric pain and vomiting. The stigmata mentioned below are absent.

---

* *Cirrhosis.* Laennec introduced the term from the Greek κιρρός = tawny, as the nodules are orange-yellow in colour.

RENÉ T. H. LAENNEC, 1781–1826, *Professor of Medicine, Collège de France, Paris. Invented the stethoscope in* 1819.
ALAN H. HUNT, 1908–1970, *Surgeon, St. Bartholomew's Hospital, London.*

MODERATE CIRRHOSIS. The spleen usually increases in size *pari passu* with the rising portal hypertension. If they have not been noticed on the face (a common situation) while taking the patient's history, look for:

Spider naevi (*see Fig.* 166, p. 90) not only on the face, but on the neck, shoulders and upper arms (territory of the superior vena cava). Spider naevi consist of branching arterioles which, with a magnifying glass, can be seen to pulsate. Also examine the hands for:

Palmar erythema, which is less commonly encountered than the foregoing, and, when present, is very characteristic. The hands sometimes show Dupuytren's Contracture (*see* p. 478), feel warmer than usual, and the palms are bright red, especially in the areas depicted in *Fig.* 408. By contrast, the fingernails are deathly white. The fingers may show clubbing (*see* p. 180).

SEVERE CIRRHOSIS. The patient is jaundiced and ill. Look for dilated superficial veins issuing from the umbilicus. These are numerous, and radiate in many directions, forming a *caput medusae* (*see* p. 18). In the male, examine the testes. Due to inability of the failing liver to neutralize circulating oestrogens, the testes atrophy. For the same reason, occasionally, gynaecomazia (*see* p. 178) supervenes. Ascites (*see* p. 242) will be found.

Liver Insufficiency—Hepatic Coma. When the liver cells are so damaged as to render them incapable of synthesizing ammonia into relatively harmless urea and uric acid, this develops. The high absorption of protein nitrogen, such as is occasioned by a large amount of blood in the intestinal tract following haemorrhage from oesophageal varices, often precipitates insufficiency, which may also arise simply from replacement of liver cells by fibrosis. Foetor hepaticus, a sweetish, musty odour, is noticeable. Soon there is ataxia and a flapping tremor of the outstretched hands, so coarse that it can be likened to the beating of the wings of a hovering hawk waiting to pounce. Rigidity of the limbs is usual and ankle clonus can be elicited as the encephalopathy advances. This stage of excitability lasts a varying time, and unless, by treatment, the absorption of excessive amounts of protein nitrogen can be reduced and noxious by-products neutralized, stupor, followed by coma, supervenes. Frequently repeated convulsions herald early death. Ten per cent of patients who have undergone otherwise successful portacaval anastomosis for portal hypertension suffer from episodic stupor and confusion at some stage of their postoperative course. The ingestion of a large meal of meat is liable to precipitate such an attack.

EXAMINATION OF THE SPLEEN

This is not the place for a discussion on the causes of the enlarged spleen. Methods of detecting splenomegaly will be detailed. If an enlargement is found, the stigmata of hepatic cirrhosis (*see* p. 235) should be sought, also lymphadenopathy in the neck, axillae, groins, and epitrochlear regions indicating a lymphoma.

An Enlarged Spleen as an Intra-abdominal Swelling. An enlarged spleen moves freely with respiration, and has a sharp anterior edge which is always directed downwards and inwards. Often this edge is notched, ⟶ but not necessarily so. A splenic tumour is dull to percussion, and this dullness is continuous with the normal splenic dullness, which may also be increased upwards.

The usual difficulty in differential diagnosis is between an enlarged spleen and an enlarged left kidney. In the case of the spleen there is always a small space between the posterior edge of the organ and the sacrospinalis muscle.

Palpation for Minor Enlargement. The left hand is placed over the lateral aspect of the costal margin, and, whilst exerting a certain amount of even compression, at the same time it draws the skin and subcutaneous tissues downwards and forwards over the ribs towards the expectant fingers of the right hand. This leaves a loose fold of skin under the costal margin. The right hand lies on the abdominal wall just below the margin of the ribs, with the fingertips pointing towards the spleen (*Fig.* 409). Keep the hands still, and do not expect to feel anything abnormal until near the end of inspiration. Just before the zenith of inspiration, draw the hands slightly together and dip a mere trifle with the right fingertips. If the spleen is palpable the fingertips will be felt to ride momentarily

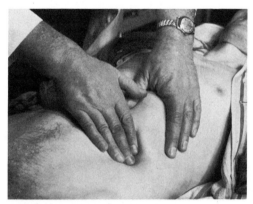

Fig. 409. Bimanual palpation of the spleen.

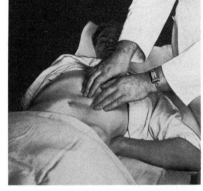

Fig. 410. Palpating the spleen from above.

over its edge. The spleen must be one and half times larger than normal before it can be detected by clinical methods* (Blackburn).

The most potent cause of failure to detect an enlarged spleen is that the organ is sought more superomedially than it should be. In other words, the spleen lies more laterally than we are inclined to think when visualizing its position.

Method of Palpating the Spleen from Above can be employed when the foregoing routine method is unsuccessful. A pillow is placed beneath the knees. The patient's left fist under the lower ribs pushes the spleen forward (Middleton). The clinician stands on the left side of the patient's head and places the fingers of both hands over the left costal margin (*Fig.* 410). The patient is instructed to take a deep breath, and if the edge of the spleen is not felt during expiration, the hands are moved farther downwards and laterally, and the process is repeated.

Kenawy's Sign is found relatively frequently with the splenomegaly associated with bilharzial fibrosis of the liver (Egyptian splenomegaly) but may be present in any type of portal hypertension. Auscultation, the stethoscope being applied beneath the xiphoid process, reveals a venous hum louder on inspiration. The phenomenon is probably due to engorgement of the splenic vein, and the hum is louder during inspiration because the spleen is then compressed.

---

* Traditionally it was taught that the spleen must enlarge 2–3 times before it becomes palpable. Blackburn has refuted this with radiological studies of experimentally induced malaria in volunteers. Moreover McIntyre has shown that in college freshmen the normal spleen was palpable in 3 per cent and remained palpable for 3 years in a third of these.

CHARLES R. B. BLACKBURN, *Contemporary Professor of Medicine, University of Sydney.*
WILLIAM S. MIDDLETON, *Contemporary Medical Director, Veterans Administration, Washington, D.C.*
O. ROSS MCINTYRE, *Contemporary, Department of Medicine, Dartmouth Medical School, Hanover, New Hampshire.*
MOHAMMED R. KENAWY, *Contemporary Professor of Medicine, University of Cairo, Egypt.*

THE PANCREAS

The oesophagus, thymus and the adrenals excepted, no organ of the body is so completely inaccessible to physical examination as the pancreas; therefore, nearly all of its diseases must be suspected by an indirect approach.

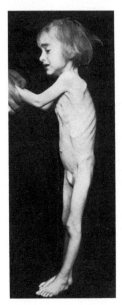

Fig. 411. Fibrocystic disease of the pancreas in a child aged 2 years.

Fibrocystic Disease of the Pancreas is but one manifestation of a congenital disease that renders the mucus of all mucus-secreting glands very viscid (*mucoviscidosis*). Viscid mucus obstructs the pancreatic ducts, giving rise to steatorrhoea (*see* p. 21) with bulky, most obnoxious stools. Viscid mucus also obstructs the bronchioles, and results in respiratory difficulty, bronchiectasis and possibly pectus excavatum (*see* p. 179). The sweat glands excrete sweat containing much more sodium chloride than normal. Thus, in hot weather, as a consequence of excessive electrolyte loss, dehydration is likely to supervene. Sufferers, if they survive infancy, not infrequently develop portal hypertension.

If an infant or child, in spite of a voracious appetite, wastes (*Fig.* 411), has a chronic cough and passes bulky and most offensive-smelling stools, think of fibrocystic disease of the pancreas. Confirmation of the diagnosis rests in chemical examination of the sweat for excessive sodium chloride content.

Chronic Relapsing Pancreatitis is a relentless, progressive disease characterized by:

Attacks of Pain almost identical with that of biliary colic, but instead of lasting minutes, the attacks last three to four days. So intolerable does the pain become that 50 per cent of the patients so afflicted become alcoholics or drug addicts; conversely, chronic pancreatitis favours those who imbibe too freely.

Mallet-Guy's Sign. With the patient lying on the right side in the knee–chest position palpation of the left subcostal region may evoke tenderness not otherwise found (*Fig.* 412). The explanation is that the overlying organs fall to the right in this position, exposing the body and tail of the pancreas to direct palpation.

Jaundice supervenes in only 15 per cent of cases but diabetes is present in 30 per cent. Steatorrhoea (*see* p. 21) should be looked for, but it is late in appearing. Loss of weight is sometimes alarming.

Pancreatic Ascites. In a small minority of cases pancreatic fluid escapes from the duct system to cause clinical ascites (*see* p. 242). The essential clue is that the ascitic fluid contains a high level of amylase (*see* p. 299).

Pancreatic Cyst is not uncommon in chronic pancreatitis. Here is a condition of the pancreas with objective signs. The cyst usually gives rise to a swelling above the umbilicus, best seen when viewed laterally (*Fig.* 413). The cyst is round, smooth, usually tense and almost always immovable. A pseudo-pancreatic cyst is a collection of fluid in the lesser sac, that not infrequently follows an attack of acute pancreatitis.

Carcinoma of the Pancreas. In an early case of carcinoma commencing in any part of the pancreas, those who rely mainly on radiographic and laboratory investigations to provide the diagnosis will go unrewarded. The symptoms, the physical signs (meagre as they may be), and, above all, awareness of the possibility of this affliction are the only stanchions upon which the diagnosis rests. The principal value of scientific methods is to rule out other possibilities.

PIERRE MALLET-GUY, *Contemporary Professor of Clinical Surgery, Faculté de Médicine, Lyons.*

Carcinoma of the Head of the Pancreas has been considered already under the heading of Jaundice, p. 232.

Carcinoma of the Body or Tail of the Pancreas is exceedingly difficult to diagnose early because of the absence of jaundice. Severe or almost intolerable epigastric pain is the principal symptom.

An Epigastric Mass (not the liver) is palpable in one out of three patients with carcinoma of the body of the pancreas.

Anaemia is not so much in evidence as in cases of carcinoma of the stomach.

Thrombophlebitis Migrans of the lower extremities (Trousseau's sign of wandering thrombophlebitis, *see* p. 394) is often the first striking sign of carcinoma of any part of the pancreas.

Diabetes is occasionally the first sign. The condition should be suspected when an elderly person develops diabetes and, in spite of adequate treatment, continues to lose weight (Lawrence). The pancreas is a common site for malignant disease in diabetics.

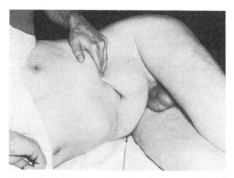
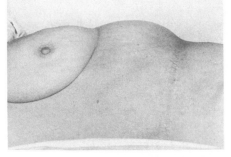

Fig. 412. Mallet-Guy's sign—tenderness over the tail and body of the pancreas in the right knee–chest position.

Fig. 413. The swelling of a pancreatic cyst viewed from the side.

Functioning Islet-cell Tumour of the Pancreas (Insulinoma). This rare tumour is never large enough to be palpated. It secretes excess insulin causing attacks of hypoglycaemia which occur at irregular intervals, becoming more frequent and more severe. Each fully fledged attack can exhibit four phases—in the beginning the attacks do not necessarily progress beyond the first or second phase.

Phase 1. Often the symptoms simulate a duodenal ulcer, awakening the patient in the early hours of the morning with vague abdominal discomfort and a feeling of being unwell.

Phase 2. In the early morning or before luncheon there is a sudden feeling of great hunger, followed quickly by trembling, sweating, dizziness, and blurring of vision.

Phase 3. Sluggish mind, inarticulate speech, incoordinated movements, diplopia and symptoms of hallucinations.

Phase 4. Fits indistinguishable from epilepsy, passing into semiconsciousness or coma, with dilated pupils and muscular spasticity, sometimes amounting to decerebrate rigidity. Sometimes the fits are unilateral, and mislead the clinician into believing that they are due to an organic intracranial lesion such as a subdural haematoma.

Diagnosis rests on the finding of a very low blood-sugar level *during an attack*.

SUSPECTED RECURRENT OR CHRONIC APPENDICITIS AND THE DIFFERENTIAL DIAGNOSIS THEREOF

The methods of examination to be employed differ very little from those dealt with fully in the early pages of this chapter. Deep tenderness at or near McBurney's point (*see Fig.* 507, p. 290) is the only positive physical sign.

The diagnosis is largely one of exclusion. Constipation, particularly in young females, is a common cause of lower abdominal pain. All patients should thus be

ROBERT D. LAWRENCE, 1892–1968, *Physician, King's College Hospital, London.*

questioned regarding their bowel habit. Rectal examination may reveal a loaded bowel, even in persons who state that they have a daily bowel action.

Secondly, a history of scalding on micturition, or of pain reminiscent of ureteric colic (*see* p. 340), should suggest to the clinician that radiographic investigation of the urinary tract is essential.

The third relatively common cause of chronic pain in the right iliac fossa is a tubo-ovarian abscess (*see* p. 318). Less common causes are as follows:

Amoebic Typhlitis.* When confronted with a patient who has resided in the tropics and has signs of recurrent inflammation in the right iliac fossa, consider the possibility of chronic amoebic colitis. In amoebic typhlitis there are *two* characteristic localized zones of tenderness, one over McBurney's point and one over an exactly comparable point in the left iliac fossa. The latter has been named aptly by Manson-Bahr 'the amoebic point'.

Tuberculous Mesenteric Lymphadenitis. The patient is usually, but not necessarily, a child. The pain is usually central, not severe, and almost constant. The abdomen is somewhat protuberant and there is tenderness on deep pressure in the right iliac fossa. Occasionally, on deep palpation, enlarged mesenteric lymph nodes are discernible as firm, discrete, tender, bean-like objects most frequently to the right of, and near, the umbilicus. If these signs are in evidence the clinician's duty is to order radiographs of the chest and to perform a skin-test for tuberculosis.

Crohn's Disease (Regional Ileitis) *see* p. 310.

EXAMINATION OF A COLONIC CASE

A history of diarrhoea or alternating constipation and diarrhoea strongly suggests that the large intestine is diseased. Blood and/or mucus (slime) in the stools is a most suggestive point. Needless to say, digital examination of the rectum (*see* p. 267) is essential.

Examination of a Case of Chronic Constipation; Suspected Chronic Intestinal Obstruction. Time spent in inspecting the abdomen is seldom wasted; in this instance it frequently brings a rich reward. In most cases of carcinoma of the colon with early (chronic) obstruction, there is a slight fullness in the right iliac fossa only apparent when looked for especially.

Arrange the patient on the examination couch carefully, so that one anterior superior iliac spine is not higher than the other, and an imaginary line through them is precisely at right-angles to the long axis of the examining couch ensuring that the patient is lying quite 'square' and is comfortable and relaxed.

Observe the abdomen intently. Compare the left with the right iliac fossa. A fullness of the right fossa due to a distended caecum is better seen than felt. The caecum is distended in most cases of obstruction to the large intestine (*see* p. 302). When there is even the slightest fullness in the right iliac fossa percuss the area. If a resonant note is obtained, the suspicion of a distended caecum is strengthened. Commence palpation in the right iliac fossa. If on deep palpation gurgling is heard, the suspicion is increased.

Palpate each of the remaining quadrants of the abdomen systematically.

When a lump in the line of the transverse colon inclining to the left of the middle line presents, the question arises: ⟶
'Is this a growth of the stomach, or is it a carcinoma of the colon?' If gurgling can be elicited on the left side of the lump assuredly the pyloric end of the stomach is obstructed (*see* the Sign of Splashing, p. 227).

---

* *Typhlitis* = inflammation of the caecum.

Sɪʀ Pʜɪʟɪᴘ Mᴀɴsᴏɴ-Bᴀʜʀ, 1881–1966, *Physician to the Hospital for Tropical Diseases, London.*

When a lump is detected in the line of the large intestine, frequently it is necessary to eliminate the possibility of a faecal mass. This can be indented by digital pressure if large enough but this is unusual. If in doubt, re-examine the patient after a bowel washout. If the mass has disappeared it must have been faecal.

Especially in thin patients, the normal pelvic colon can often be rolled beneath the fingers—a state that gives a characteristic sensation to the examining fingers.

Chronic Colonic Diverticulitis. The patient is often over the age of 60 years. The history is one of exacerbations and remissions; the exacerbations last a few days to more than a week, and the remissions for months or even years. Pain situated in the left iliac fossa is the typical complaint; it becomes worse on defaecation or on being jolted, as when riding in a vehicle. Periodic loose stools with the passage of some mucus are rather common during the attack.

Frequently the patient is obese. Palpation of the abdomen reveals tenderness in the left iliac fossa. Sometimes a thickened, tender, pelvic colon can be palpated in the left iliac fossa or on bimanual examination. When the patient is obese, deep tenderness in the left iliac fossa is the only physical sign that can be elicited.

Haemorrhage per Rectum. At least 20 per cent of patients with colonic diverticulitis pass blood per rectum and severe rectal bleeding is more common with diverticulitis than with a colonic or rectal neoplasm.

Suspected Ulcerative Colitis. The onset is in the third, fourth and second decade, in that order. Occasionally, it is encountered in childhood. The first symptom is watery diarrhoea occurring in a person of previously normal bowel habit. Mucus (sometimes bloodstained) is present in the stools (*see Fig. 38*, p. 20). The disease progresses by relapses and remissions. In untreated cases of some standing the patient becomes wasted, and severely anaemic from loss of blood. Often during the attacks there are 10–20 stools a day, accompanied by tenesmus. The frequency of the motions and the degree of invalidism go hand in hand, and are usually proportional to the extent of the involvement of the colon. When the whole colon is involved often the patient cannot work, and in an extreme case is so weak as to be partially or wholly bedridden. The only sign on abdominal examination is deep tenderness over the portion of the colon that is involved and this is by no means invariably present. Digital examination of the rectum is comparatively uninformative; the rectum is empty, may be ballooned, and if it is implicated, it is tender and may impart a sensation of heat to the examining finger. Sigmoidoscopy and radiography are indispensable in confirming the diagnosis.

Signs which indicate that a Patient with Ulcerative Colitis requires Urgent Surgical Treatment. The patient is ill with tachycardia, high intermittent pyrexia and severe diarrhoea. Lack of improvement in the general condition after 48–72 hours of intensive medical treatment suggests that the time has come for surgical intervention. An abdominal X-ray at any stage showing dilatation of the transverse colon (toxic megacolon) indicates that perforation is imminent. Later the abdomen becomes clinically distended and tenderness or rigidity attest that the colon has perforated. Severe blood loss is an unusual indication for surgery.

Congenital Megacolon (Hirschsprung's Disease) is the commonest cause of intestinal obstruction in the newborn and is more frequent in the male (4:1). In 90 per cent the signs appear within three days of birth; only in

1 per cent are they delayed until past the first birthday. The infant fails to pass meconium during the first two or three days, and then only after the insertion of a little finger or a tube into the rectum. Subsequent motions are sometimes characteristic (*see* p. 21). As a rule, by the third day abdominal distension is unmistakable, and loud borborygmi and visible peristalsis are much in evidence. In some cases, as the abdominal distension progresses, the distended flanks proclaim that the obstruction is of the large intestine (*Fig.* 414). In others the distension is indistinguishable from that occurring in partial obstruction of the lower ileum.

Rectal Examination. The anus is normal but the rectum is empty and contracted; depending on the length of the aganglionic segment, the finger may enter dilated bowel above the neurogenic obstruction. The findings are illustrated in *Fig.* 499, p. 282. Usually after the withdrawal of the finger, flatus and, in neonates, a gush of meconium are passed which may lead the clinician to conclude that all is well.

Acquired Megacolon. The symptoms arise, not soon after birth, but when the child is older. In a few cases, on inspection of the anus an anal fissure (*see* p. 273) is found to be present. In every instance, on rectal examination the finger encounters a scyballous mass, which is contrary to what is found in Hirschsprung's disease.

Megacolon in Chagas' Disease. Although acquired, in this tropical disease, the dilated bowel is due to the same cause as Hirschsprung's disease (absence of parasympathetic ganglion cells). The findings on rectal examination are thus the same as in the congenital variety but the condition is found at any age. *See* footnote on p. 197.

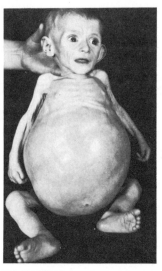

Fig. 414. Hirschsprung's disease, a very extreme neglected example.

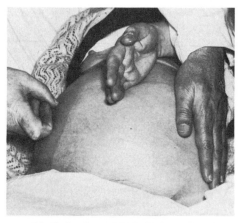

Fig. 415. Testing for a 'fluid thrill' (case of peritoneal carcinomatosis).

ASCITES

A general fullness of the abdomen may be due to: *F*at, *F*luid; *F*latus; *F*aeces; or *F*etus.

HARALD HIRSCHSPRUNG, 1830–1916, *Physician, Queen Louise Hospital for Children, Copenhagen.*

The latter, in the aggregate, is easily the commonest, but the patient usually supplies the diagnosis. Occasionally a woman near the menopause, or a mental defective, is unaware that she is pregnant. For varying reasons a woman may wish to conceal a pregnancy, so it is as well to cultivate a suspicious mind.

Fluid Thrill. The orthodox method of testing for ascites is shown in *Fig.* 415. An assistant places the edge of his hand firmly on the centre of the abdomen in order to damp down a fat thrill. The abdominal wall on one side is flicked, and the thrill is felt by the hand on the other side of the abdomen.

Shifting Dullness is a valuable sign when the quantity of fluid in the peritoneal cavity is comparatively small. Ask the patient to turn somewhat on to his left side. Wait for a minute in order to allow the fluid to gravitate. Commence percussion from the right side to the left, noting where the resonant area becomes dull and marking the spot on the abdominal wall. Then the patient is asked to turn slightly on to his right side, and after a reasonable interval, if shifting dullness is present, the dull area will have become resonant, and vice versa (*Fig.* 416). Remember that dilated coils of small intestine can also behave in this way in intestinal obstruction.

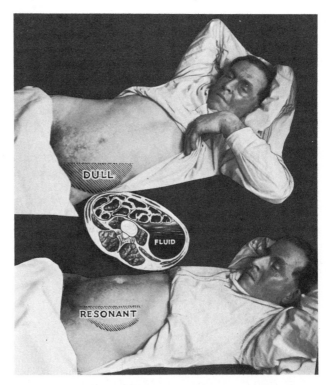

Fig. 416. Shifting dullness. The sign of free fluid in the peritoneal cavity.

'Dipping'. A special technique known as 'dipping' is required to palpate organs or tumours in cases of ascites. The pads of the fingers are placed on the abdomen, and then, by a quick push, the abdominal wall is depressed. An enlarged liver is often felt easily, and a tumour mass can usually be defined.

Having settled that ascites is present, unless the cause is known already, the clinician must set about elucidating it. In surgical practice the most common causes are carcinomatosis peritonei, portal hypertension and tuberculous peritonitis, but the overall commonest cause is congestive heart failure. In the last, engorgement of the veins of the neck is very often in evidence (*see* p. 17).

Still referring to cases where the cause of ascites is obscure, vaginal and/or rectal examination is most necessary. A pelvic neoplasm and occasionally tuberculous salpingitis may be discovered.

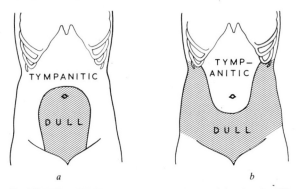

Fig. 417. Differential diagnosis between ovarian cyst (*a*) and ascites (*b*).

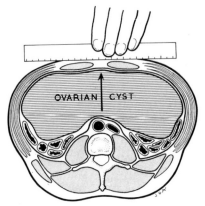

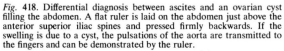

Fig. 418. Differential diagnosis between ascites and an ovarian cyst filling the abdomen. A flat ruler is laid on the abdomen just above the anterior superior iliac spines and pressed firmly backwards. If the swelling is due to a cyst, the pulsations of the aorta are transmitted to the fingers and can be demonstrated by the ruler.

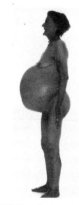

Fig. 419. Pseudomyxoma peritonei. A mucocele of the appendix had been removed two years previously.

Differential Diagnosis between an Extremely Large Ovarian Cyst and Ascites. After the bladder has been emptied by a catheter, the problem can be elucidated easily by percussion (*Fig.* 417). When the whole abdomen is filled by a cystic swelling, a rarity, this differential diagnosis becomes exceedingly difficult unless the method shown in *Fig.* 418 is applied. This phenomenon is not present in ascites (Blaxland).

Pseudomyxoma Peritonei. The patient presents with a massive enlargement of the abdomen (*Fig.* 419). A fluid thrill is present, but on attempting to tap the fluid, jelly-like material is obtained. Often the patient has already undergone an operation for removal of a pseudomucinous ovarian cyst or a mucocele of the appendix but sometimes the first intimation of the causative condition is the abdominal enlargement.

ATHELSTAN J. BLAXLAND, 1880–1963, *Surgeon, Norfolk and Norwich Hospital.*

Chapter 19

THE ABDOMINAL WALL, UMBILICUS AND GROIN

THE ABDOMINAL WALL

In the endeavour to elucidate the nature of a lump in the abdomen, the first step
is to exclude a swelling in the abdominal wall. A good method of rendering the
abdominal wall tense is:

Carnett's Test. The patient, who should be lying flat with no pillow, is asked to
extend both legs, and while keeping his knees stiff, to raise his feet from the bed.
This procedure renders the abdominal muscles tense. If the lump is intraperitoneal it disappears or if very large becomes less easily felt, but if situated *in* the
abdominal wall it persists (*Fig.* 420).

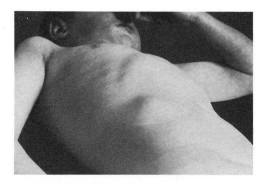

Fig. 420. A lump in the abdominal wall which
proved to be a cold abscess.

Infection of the Abdominal Wall can arise in any of its layers. The usual portal of
entry is a laparotomy wound.

Superficial Cellulitis. The earliest sign is that the skin stitches become embedded
in oedematous skin, and appear partially submerged. One or more days later the
pulse and temperature rise, and a cutaneous flush appears, extending for a
variable distance from the incision or the stitch holes. Palpation (*with a sterile
gloved hand*) will, as a rule, reveal that one area is more indurated than the rest.
Spreading Superficial Cellulitis usually signifies that intestinal leakage, especially
from the large intestine, is proceeding.

Postoperative Bacterial Gangrene. (*See* p. 33.)

Gas Gangrene of the Abdominal Wall is surprisingly rare. The presence of malodorous pus containing
gas bubbles is more likely to be due to a commencing faecal fistula than to gas gangrene. However,
when the skin takes on a bronze hue, the wound discharges bloodstained fluid with a 'mousy' odour,
and crepitation can be elicited, especially if the operation has been for a lesion of the large intestine,
the correct diagnosis is certainly gas gangrene.

'Pseudo-Gas Gangrene'. To those unfamiliar with the phenomenon, air entrapped in the subcutis
after laparotomy can be a source of anxiety, for around the incision—indeed, sometimes a
considerable distance from it—unmistakable crepitation can be elicited. The condition is entirely
innocuous and the air is soon absorbed.

Abscess of the Abdominal Wall. Unless it arises as a postoperative complication

JOHN B. CARNETT, 1876–1934, *Professor of Surgery, University of Pennsylvania, Philadelphia.*

by infection of a laparotomy incision, an abscess of the abdominal wall is, as a rule, an extension of an intraperitoneal abscess. A superficial abscess is diagnosed easily by fluctuation, and possibly by visible signs of inflammation. A subaponeurotic abscess can be distinguished from a localized collection of pus in the peritoneal cavity only by operation.

Tropical Pyomyositis is a suppurative condition of muscle which may affect the abdominal wall, particularly the posterior and lateral abdominal wall, in which case psoas spasm may be in evidence (*see* p. 315). Later a retroperitoneal mass may mimic appendix abscess (*see* p. 293). The anterior abdominal muscles are seldom affected but when they are, if Carnett's test is carried out, it will be appreciated that the inflammatory process is *in* the muscular layer. Look carefully for manifestations in the muscles of the extremities as the abscesses are often multiple. A single abscess may simulate a haematoma following trauma.

Is the Acutely Tender Lump in the Abdominal Wall? When called to see a patient with a tender lump situated in the medial part of the iliac fossa (often the right), to remember the following condition may one day bring its reward.

Rupture of the Rectus Abdominis Muscle and/or Tearing of the Inferior Epigastric Artery occurs usually during a bout of coughing or in pregnancy. Patients on anticoagulant therapy are also at risk. There is an extremely tender lump between the arcuate line and the pubic bone where the rectus ruptures. ————————————————→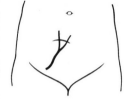

Effective tensing of the abdominal musculature causes the lump to become fixed, more obvious, and more painful. The difficulties of differentiating the condition from a strangulated Spigelian hernia (*see* p. 266) may be insuperable. Nevertheless, absence of vomiting favours the extraperitoneal lesion, while bruising of the overlying skin (infrequent during the first 24 hours) makes the diagnosis of haematoma certain.

Fatty Apron. A hanging sheet of fat below the umbilicus is almost the prerogative of the female sex in whom, in any case, obesity is much commoner (*see Fig.* 427). Failure to lift the apron in order to see what lies beneath may lead to diagnostic error (*Fig.* 421).

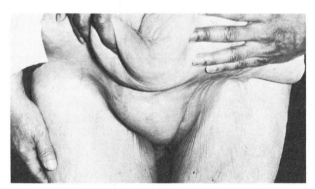

Fig. 421. Elevation of the fatty apron in this woman aged 73 revealed a right inguinal hernia, the cause of her obscure abdominal pain for which she had already had several radiological investigations performed.

Neoplasms of the Abdominal Wall are uncommon. *Desmoid Tumour, see* p. 28.

THE UMBILICUS

Every time an abdomen is examined the eyes of the clinician, almost instinctively, rest momentarily upon the umbilicus. How innumerable are the variations of this structure! Normally, placed almost equidistant along a line joining the tip of the xiphoid process with the top of the symphysis pubis (*Fig.* 422), the umbilicus is displaced upwards by a swelling arising from the pelvis (*Fig.* 423), or downwards by ascites (*Tanyol's sign*) (*Fig.* 424).

HASIB TANYOL, *Contemporary, Department of Medicine, Jefferson Medical College, Philadelphia.*

Exomphalos. The infant is born with a defect at the umbilicus, the protruding abdominal contents being covered only by a diaphanous membrane (*Fig.* 425). Through this transparent veil the viscera are exposed to view, as if exhibited in a show-case.

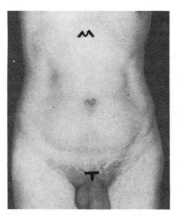

Fig. 422. The normal umbilicus is equidistant between the xiphisternum and the pubic symphysis.

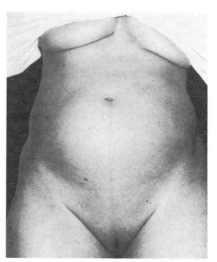

Fig. 423. In pregnancy and other tumours arising from the pelvis the umbilicus is displaced upwards. This patient proved to have an ovarian cyst.

Congenital Umbilical Hernia comes right through the centre of the umbilical scar (*Fig.* 426). At the neck of the sac one can feel a collar of fibrous tissue continuous with the linea alba (Browne). The condition is relatively much commoner in babies of African descent. The size varies from a simple failure of the umbilical ring to close completely, leaving a small defect large enough to admit the tip of the little finger with a protrusion of a small sac, to a fairly large opening admitting two or three fingers. In a doubtful case the method of seeking the hernia depicted in *Fig.* 462, p. 263, can be employed with advantage.

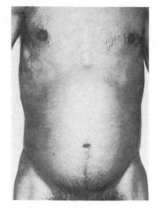

Fig. 424. In ascites the umbilicus is displaced downwards. Patient suffering from abdominal carcinomatosis.

Sir Denis Browne, 1892–1967, *Surgeon, Hospital for Sick Children, Great Ormond Street, London.*

Para-umbilical Hernia. There is no fibrous tissue collar. It should be noted that the so-called umbilical hernia of adults (seen most often in obese females) is a *para*-umbilical hernia (*Figs.* 427, 428) in which approximately half the fundus of the sac is covered by the umbilicus and the remainder by the skin of the abdomen immediately *above* it. The importance of this differential diagnosis is that a para-umbilical hernia does not become cured spontaneously.

If either an umbilical or a para-umbilical hernia should protrude and remain protruded, when the patient lies down an endeavour should be made to reduce it by gentle pressure. If the hernia has existed for any length of time, reduction is usually only partially successful, for omentum becomes adherent within the sac.

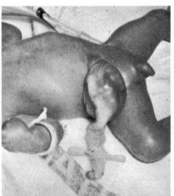 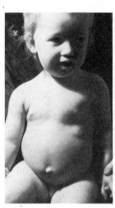 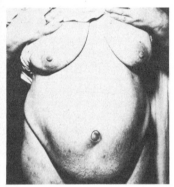

Fig. 425. Exomphalos.

Fig. 426. Congenital umbilical hernia. Spontaneous closure is almost invariable.

Fig. 427. Relatively small para-umbilical hernia occurring in a typical individual for this complaint. Note the 'fatty apron' (*see* p. 246).

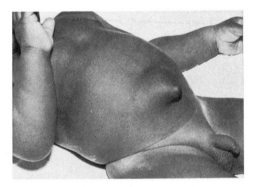

Fig. 428. Para-umbilical hernia in a West Indian baby. This variety will not close spontaneously.

Acquired Umbilical Hernia (as opposed to a para-umbilical hernia) is due to the umbilicus, which is a scar, giving way, and is always secondary to some increase in intra-abdominal tension. Therefore a search must be made for the cause—the commonest being ascites due to peritoneal carcinomatosis.

Unfolding of the Umbilicus. When the abdomen becomes distended the umbilicus tends partially to unfold. This is a helpful sign in early cases of intestinal obstruction or if there is doubt about the presence of ascitic fluid.

Omphalitis (Inflammation of the Umbilical Cord) is, as would be expected, far commoner in communities that do not practise aseptic severance of the umbilical cord, but it is not a rarity elsewhere. About the third or fourth day signs of inflammation appear at the cutaneous junction of the stump. Unchecked, the infection is liable to spread along the defunct hypogastric arteries (*Fig.* 429) or the incompletely obliterated umbilical vein, as a result of which, not infrequently, *an abscess of the abdominal wall* results. In such circumstances, digital pressure exerted first below (over the defunct hypogastric arteries) and, if negative, above the umbilicus will cause a bead of pus to exude from the umbilicus. Unless the abscess is drained *peritonitis* is a threatening complication. Infection along the umbilical vein can lead to *septicaemia*, in which event jaundice is an early sign (*see* p. 44). Tetanus (*see* p. 92) is a complication seen in primitive communities.

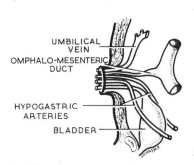

Fig. 429. Structures in the umbilicus that may remain patent or incompletely obliterated.

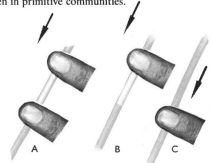

Fig. 430. Method of ascertaining the direction of blood flow in a vein. (A) Emptying the vein of blood. (B) The inferior finger removed; vein does not fill. (C) Inferior finger replaced, superior finger removed; vein fills, proving that the flow in this case is from above, downwards.

Congenital Umbilical Fistula. By exerting pressure below or above the umbilicus express and, if possible, collect some of the discharge, which may be urine (urachal fistula), faeces (patent omphalo-mesenteric duct), or mucus. Local infective dermatitis (*Fig.* 431) usually accompanies any umbilical fistula.

Acquired Umbilical Fistula. The umbilicus is a creek into which one of many fistulous streams can be diverted. For instance, gallstones have been discharged through the umbilicus; a discharging umbilicus has led to the discovery of a swab left in the peritoneal cavity at a previous operation; diverticulitis or colonic carcinoma have led to a faeculent umbilical discharge.

Umbilical Concretion, often black in colour, and composed of dirt and desquamated epithelium, is encountered from time to time, usually in elderly subjects. Symptomless for years, a time is reached when inflammation supervenes, and a discharge, often bloodstained, causes alarm.

Pilonidal Sinus of the Umbilicus. If hairs are seen protruding from the mouth of an umbilical sinus (*Fig.* 432), there should be no hesitation in making this diagnosis (*see* p. 274).

Enlargement of Veins around the Umbilicus (*see* pp. 18, 236).

The Differential Diagnosis between Enlarged Veins of the Abdominal Wall due to Portal Obstruction and those due to Inferior Vena Caval Obstruction. Below the umbilicus, the normal venous flow in the abdominal wall is downward; above it is upward.

In Portal Obstruction the direction of the flow is unchanged.

In Obstruction of the Inferior Vena Cava the flow below the umbilicus is reversed, because some of the blood is shunted through the superficial veins to the superior vena cava.

To determine the direction of the flow in a dilated vein: (1) Empty the vein as shown in *Fig.* 430 A; (2) Remove the lower finger (*Fig.* 430 B)—the vein remains collapsed if the flow is from above, downwards; (3) Replace the lower finger, and remove the upper finger (*Fig.* 430 C)—the vein fills if the flow is from above, downwards. (2) and (3) are reversed if the flow is from below, upwards.

SOME LESIONS OF THE UMBILICUS

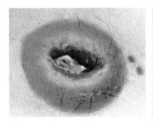

Fig. 431. Umbilical fistula, the discharge from which was ammoniacal. Note the local dermatitis.

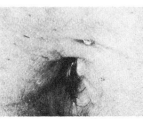

Fig. 432. Pilonidal sinus of the umbilicus.

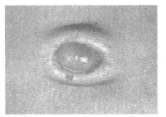

Fig. 433. Umbilical adenoma.

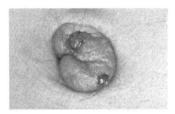

Fig. 434. Endometrioma of the umbilicus.

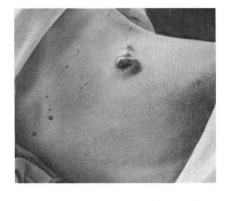

Fig 435. Secondary carcinomatous nodule at the umbilicus. The red spots near the costal margin are de Morgan's spots. (*See* p. 27.)

Umbilical Adenoma (Enteroteratoma). This clinical entity is most characteristic. It is a pedunculated (*Fig.* 433) raspberry-coloured mass. A similar, but somewhat paler, protuberance can arise from granulation tissue after separation of the umbilical cord (*umbilical granuloma*), and this disappears after two or three applications of a silver-nitrate stick. This treatment has no effect on the former.

Umbilical Endometrioma should be suspected when, in a woman between 25 and 50 years of age, there is a growth at the umbilicus simulating an umbilical adenoma. As in other situations, an endometrioma gives rise to periodic bleeding. On inquiry, in the case illustrated (*Fig.* 434), the patient said bleeding occurred from the umbilicus at each menstrual period.

Secondary Umbilical Carcinoma.

In advanced intra-abdominal carcinoma, more particularly carcinoma of the stomach, a neoplastic nodule can sometimes be seen (*Fig.* 435) or felt at the umbilicus.

Discoloration of the Umbilicus. Rarely, in certain acute abdominal conditions, the umbilicus and surrounding skin become discoloured. Cullen has observed a bluish tinge in cases of ruptured ectopic gestation (*Fig.* 436). Johnston noted a yellow tinge around the umbilicus in a woman with acute pancreatitis.

THOMAS S. CULLEN, 1869–1953, *Professor of Gynaecology, Johns Hopkins University, Baltimore.*
LLOYD B. JOHNSTON, 1894–1956, *Surgeon, Good Samaritan Hospital, Cincinnati.*

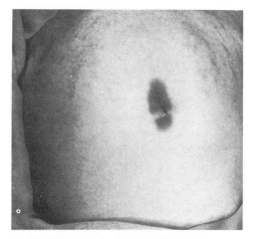

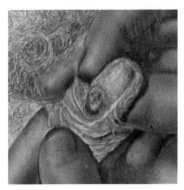

Fig. 437. This primary chancre, situated on the right side of the fraenum and hidden beneath the prepuce, was the cause of enlargement of the right inguinal lymph nodes.

Fig. 436. Cullen's sign in a late case of ectopic pregnancy. The umbilical 'black eye'.

THE GROIN

THE LYMPH NODES OF THE GROIN

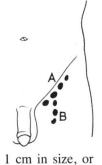

For clinical purposes there is no better division of the superficial inguinal lymph nodes than into an oblique set beneath and parallel to the inguinal ligament (A), and a longitudinal set overlying the femoral vessels (B) ──────────────→ These two groups should be palpated on each side. If any are found to be enlarged, seek the primary focus. Remember that in the male and the thin female the inguinal lymph nodes are normally palpable but no lymph node should be greater than 1 cm in size, or tender.

The leg, from the toes upwards, is inspected. Should no causative abnormality be found, the abdominal wall, buttocks, anus and the genitalia (*Figs.* 437–440) must be scrutinized for an infective lesion, because all these areas have lymphatic vessels draining into the groin. When the patient has a prepuce, it should be retracted fully, so as to expose the sulcus behind the corona. The region of the fraenum should be so displayed that no part of it is hidden from view (*Fig.* 437). This is an excellent opportunity to bring to the notice of those on the threshold of their life-study of human nature how often a patient suffering from venereal disease seemingly seeks to beguile his trusting clinician.

For instance, the silvery-haired, benevolent-looking possessor of the lesion displayed in *Fig.* 437 insistèd that a lump in the right groin (an enlarged inguinal lymph node) appeared as the result of a strain incurred during a cricket match!

Solitary Enlargement of Cloquet's Lymph Node (*see* p. 262).

ELUCIDATING THE CAUSE OF ENLARGED INGUINAL LYMPH NODES

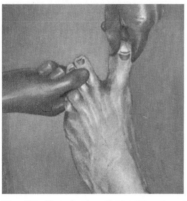

Fig. 438. Case 1. A patient with enlarged inguinal lymph nodes is presented. Scrutiny of the corresponding leg and foot reveals the focus of infection in the cleft between the first and second toes.

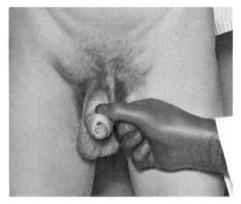

Fig. 439. Case 2. Beneath the prepuce, which cannot be retracted, a hard irregular swelling is rolled between the finger and thumb. A spot of blood appears. Carcinoma of the glans penis is the primary source of the stony hard inguinal lymph nodes seen on the right.

Fig. 440. Case 3. This patient says that while lifting at work he felt pain in the groin. With such a history, not unnaturally a hernia is suspected: instead, two enlarged, slightly tender inguinal lymph nodes are found. Nothing is discovered to account for these enlarged lymph nodes until the nates are separated. The patient denies that he has had even discomfort from these grossly inflamed anal skin tags.

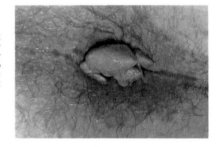

When no Primary Focus of Inguinal Adenitis can be found the clinician will do well to consider the possibility of the following conditions:

1. Cat-scratch Disease (*see* p. 34). The adenitis—completely antibiotic-resistant—progresses to suppuration and bubo.* The pus obtained from the latter is green, and characteristically sterile.

2. Lymphoma

3. Tuberculous Lymphadenitis. In the case of (2) and (3) the enlarged nodes exhibit the same characteristics of nodes elsewhere affected similarly (*see* pp. 140, 142). Biopsy is the only means of establishing a confident diagnosis.

4. Venereal Disease. *See* pp. 373–77.

---

* *Bubo*. Greek, βουβών = groin. An inflammatory swelling of a lymph node of the groin.

Abscess of the Groin. Any suppurating lymph node (particularly in children) can break down and lead to an abscess. This condition should not be confused with that depicted in *Fig.* 441 if the clinician remembers to examine the back.

Adenolymphocele of the Groin in Onchocerciasis.* The larva of *Onchocerca volvulus* are deposited subcutaneously, usually below the knee, by the bite of the intermediate host fly. They may migrate to the inguinal lymph nodes where they are arrested and set up an intense reaction which results in destruction of the elastic tissue in the overlying skin which hangs in folds (*Fig.* 442) and to the uninitiated may be mistaken for inguinal or femoral hernia. However there is no cough impulse.

Another manifestation is the result of the larvae migrating upwards until they reach a point where skin is adherent to underlying bone, notably at the greater trochanter. A rubbery hard nodule (*onchocercoma*) forms which consists of a tangled ball of worms surrounded by fibrous tissue.

This disease is found in Central Africa, Central and Northern South America and Arabia.

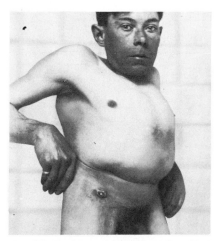

Fig. 441. An 'abscess in the groin' from Pott's disease via the psoas sheath. A psoas abscess opening into the groin.

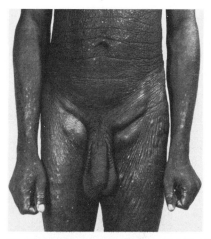

Fig. 442. Adenolymphocele of the groin in a Ugandan patient. The skin resembles Morocco leather.

PAIN IN THE GROIN

In clinical practice this is a common symptom. We are considering here the patient in whom a cause, e.g. enlarged lymph nodes, a groin hernia, is not obvious. Examine the hip joint (*see* Chapter 33) for osteoarthrosis or other disease. Re-examine carefully for a small unobtrusive femoral hernia which may be difficult to detect particularly in a fat person and also palpate carefully *above* the inguinal ligament for enlarged external iliac lymph nodes. An X-ray is necessary to detect a bone metastasis (*see* p. 425) or other bone disease not causing a palpable lump. Finally, it must be admitted, in some cases, no cause can be found. 'Muscle strain' is then the usual hypothetical diagnosis but it is to be hoped that, ultimately, some definite cause will be discovered just as, in the upper limb, cervical spondylosis and carpal tunnel syndrome have been found to be the cause of previously obscure symptoms (*see* Pain in the Upper Limb, p. 466).

---

* *Onchocerca.* Greek, ὄνχος = barb, κέεκος = tail. A genus of filarial worms.

Chapter 20

HERNIA

For practical purposes, hernia, which has been defined as the protrusion of a viscus, in part or in whole, through a normal or abnormal opening, is found only in relation to the abdomen. Exceptions are rare, e.g. lung hernia (*see* p. 189), muscle hernia (*see* p. 28). Apart from rare internal herniae which present with intestinal obstruction, a cause for which usually cannot be determined clinically, the diagnosis is obvious—a swelling is present which is easily reduced into the peritoneal cavity by pressure and which returns on invoking the aid of gravity by standing, or raising the intraperitoneal tension, particularly by coughing. However, the two varieties of inguinal hernia and femoral hernia comprise some 90 per cent of the total; groin herniae are sometimes difficult to detect and to differentiate one from the other.

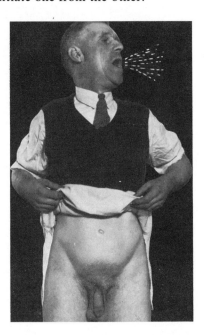

Fig. 443. Watching for a visible impulse on coughing. Note that the patient's head is turned to one side. A small left inguinal hernia has appeared as the patient coughs.

Irreducibility and Strangulation. A hernia which has *recently* become irreducible may have its blood supply jeopardized and there is no clinical test to differentiate these conditions with certainty. Pain and local tenderness over the hernia are points in favour of strangulation, but there are many exceptions either way. Intestinal obstruction (*see* p. 299) associated with an irreducible hernia suggests that there is a grave risk of strangulation and that an early operation is imperative.

Hernia as a Presenting Complaint of Patients with Increased Intra-abdominal Tension. Patients with increased intra-abdominal pressure, particularly those with ascites, sometimes present complaining of the recent appearance of a hernia. Do not fail to question the patient regarding frequency of micturition (enlarged prostate) (*see Fig.* 448 *b*) and make an examination of the whole abdomen in relevant cases.

INGUINAL AND FEMORAL HERNIA

Examination of a Patient for an Inguinal or a Femoral Hernia when there is no question of Strangulation. The patient, stripped below the waist, stands while the examiner sits.

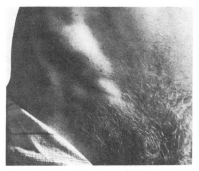

Fig. 444. Malgaigne's bulging on the right side.

Ascertaining the Presence of a Visible Impulse. An impulse is often better seen than felt. First adjust the patient. Almost certainly he will be leaning forward with his neck craning down to see what is about to be done. Tell him to keep his head erect, then (in order that you may avoid the salivary shower when he coughs) to turn his head to one side (*Fig.* 443). Observe carefully his abdominal musculature, and ask the patient to cough or blow his nose. Malgaigne's bulgings (*Fig.* 444) are normally seen in thin individuals. With the eyes glued on the external inguinal ring, request the patient to cough again. Observe whether there is an impulse. Ask him to cough once more, and compare with the ring of the opposite side. When neither a swelling nor an impulse can be seen, ask the patient to point to the place where he experienced pain or noticed a swelling.

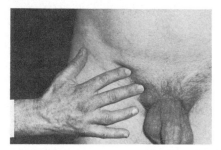
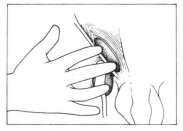

Fig. 445. Seeking a palpable impulse (right side) (Zieman's technique). The index finger lies over the indirect, the middle finger over the direct, and the ring finger over the femoral, site.

JOSEPH F. MALGAIGNE, 1806–1865, *Professor of Surgery, Paris.*
STEPHEN A. ZIEMAN, 1898–1973, *Surgeon, Providence Hospital, Mobile, Alabama.*

Ascertaining the Presence of a Palpable Impulse. With the patient still standing, the clinician rises and stands behind and somewhat to the right for the right side of the patient, and behind and somewhat to the left for the left side. In each instance employing the hand corresponding to the side to be examined, he places his index, middle, and ring fingers over the groin as shown in *Fig.* 445. While the fingers are maintained in these positions, the patient is instructed to hold the nose and blow (which in this instance is more effective than requesting him or her to cough). Should a hernia be present in any one of these sites, a peculiar gliding motion of the walls of an empty sac, or pushing sensation in the case of protrusion of a viscus into the sac, is felt beneath the relevant finger.

INDIRECT INGUINAL HERNIA

An indirect (oblique) inguinal hernia appears for the first time earlier in life than does a direct inguinal hernia. Indirect herniae which comprise over 80 per cent of inguinal herniae, occur frequently in children, and are not rare in women.

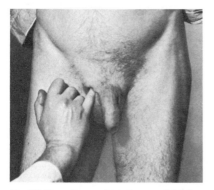

Fig. 446. Preparing to palpate the superficial ring. The skin of the scrotum is invaginated.

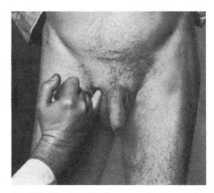

Fig. 447. The finger is then rotated so as to bring the finger-nail against the spermatic cord. The pulp will then be available to feel the superficial inguinal ring.

1. If there is no Obvious Lump. The signs described already, viz. the presence of a visible and/or a palpable impulse, are the main avenues of arriving at a diagnosis in a female. In the case of a *male*, resume the seated position and examine the hernial site in the following way:

Digital Palpation of the Hernial Orifice. Employing the right hand for the right side and the left for the left, invaginate the scrotum upon the little finger (*Fig.* 446); then rotate the finger so that the nail lies against the cord, and follow the spermatic cord upwards—this will lead the pulp of the finger, with its tactile sensibility, to the superficial inguinal ring (*Fig.* 447). If the finger is not introduced in this way, it is more than likely that the nail will abut against the ring, and the point of the examination will be missed. A normal ring feels like a triangular slit; it just admits the tip of the little finger. If more of the finger than this can be introduced it is unusual, but does not necessarily signify that an inguinal hernia is present. With the little finger thus placed, ask the patient to cough. A palpable expansile impulse confirms the diagnosis of an inguinal hernia.

2. If there is an Obvious Lump present (in both sexes). By grasping the swelling between the finger and thumb, ascertain whether it is possible to get above the swelling.

If it is possible to get above the swelling (*see Fig.* 449), manifestly the swelling is not issuing from the inguinal canal.

If it is not possible to get above the swelling, ascertain the relationship of the sac to, and its continuity with, the inguinal canal. Grasping the neck of the sac between the finger and thumb, ask the patient to cough, and note whether or not there is an impulse.

Method of Testing the Reducibility of an Inguinal Hernia. Instruct the patient to lie on an examining couch. In many instances, as soon as the patient is recumbent the hernia reduces itself. In others, the patient is able to reduce the hernia himself. If, on inquiry, the patient affirms this ability, by all means request him to carry out the manipulation. When a hernia has been irreducible for weeks or months, make no attempt to reduce it.

In the remaining cases the examiner effects reduction in the following way: flex the thigh, and in order to keep the pillars of the superficial inguinal ring relaxed, instruct the patient not to abduct the thigh. The digits of one hand surround the swelling and are used to form a funnel leading to the superficial inguinal ring, while those of the other hand grasp the swelling near the fundus. Gentle squeezing is carried out, with one hand alternating with the other. This is *taxis.** Forcible taxis is fraught with dangers. Contraindications to any form of taxis at any age are:

a. Intestinal obstruction.

b. Redness or oedema of the skin overlying the swelling (*see Fig.* 53, p. 26), either or both of which herald gangrene of the contents of the sac or (in the male) necrosis of the testis.

If Reducible, Method of Ascertaining the Contents of Sac

If the Hernia contains Omentum. In the first place it will give a doughy impression to the palpating fingers. But this is not so valuable as the second sign: the first part of the hernial contents will reduce easily, the last with difficulty (because of adhesions).

If the Hernia contains Intestine. The first part is difficult to reduce; the last part is reduced with ease, and returns to the general peritoneal cavity with a characteristic gurgle.

Examination of a Child for an Inguinal Hernia. Babies often have a roll of fat overlapping the groin so that a small inguinal hernia may be overlooked. To make visible a non-apparent existing hernia, often it is helpful to encourage a child to run about or, according to age, to bounce it up and down or to allow it to jump from the examination couch, or even, deliberately, to make it cry. Palpation of the superficial inguinal ring by invagination of the scrotum is impossible in infants and young children. Gentle palpation between the finger and thumb of the spermatic cord as it emerges from the superficial inguinal ring, and comparison with the cord of the opposite side, often reveals thickening due

---

* *Taxis.* Greek, τάξις = arrangement.

to the presence of a hernial sac, even when the contents thereof have been reduced completely.

Examine both inguinal regions carefully, as bilateral herniae occur quite frequently (15 per cent). At times it is impossible to confirm that a hernia is present, in which case a second examination should be arranged in a week's time or (better) when the lump appears. The greatest incidence of strangulated inguinal hernia in infancy and childhood is in the first year of life—most of them during the first three months. The ratio of boys to girls is 25:1.

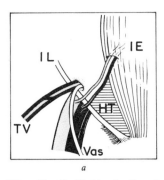
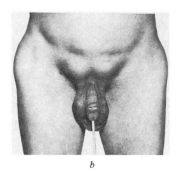

a   *b*

Fig. 448. *a*, Hesselbach's triangle, through which a direct inguinal hernia passes. Boundaries: inferior epigastric vessels, the inguinal ligament, and outer border of rectus sheath. TV, testicular vessels. (Right side viewed from within.) *b*, Bilateral direct inguinal hernia. The patient presented with acute retention of urine.

DIRECT INGUINAL HERNIA

A direct inguinal hernia does not come down the inguinal canal, but passes directly forwards through the inguinal (Hesselbach's) triangle (*Fig.* 448 *a*). While an indirect inguinal hernia may require considerable straining to manifest its presence, and definite pressure and manipulation to reduce it, a direct inguinal hernia appears as a globular swelling in close proximity to the tubercle of the os pubis on the slightest provocation, and reduces instantly on reclining because the wide mouth of the sac offers so little resistance to the entry of viscera. For the same reason, irreducibility and strangulation of a direct inguinal hernia are rare. Both indirect and direct inguinal herniae are often bilateral (*Fig.* 448 *b*). Usually a direct inguinal hernia is acquired, and it occurs in men over 40 years of age: it never occurs in children, and is relatively rare in women.

The Differential Diagnosis between Direct and Indirect Inguinal Hernia

1. On *inspection* of a direct hernia, ask the patient to cough; it is often apparent that the swelling is emerging straight through Hesselbach's triangle and not obliquely along the inguinal canal.

2. *The Sign of the Pubic Bone.* If on exploration by invagination of the scrotum a circular opening is revealed through which, apparently, the finger passes directly backwards into the abdomen instead of obliquely upwards and outwards, it is suspicious of a direct inguinal hernia. When, in addition, the edge of the external oblique can be felt superiorly and the pubic bone can be felt inferiorly, the evidence weighs heavily in favour of a direct hernia.

FRANZ K. HESSELBACH, 1759–1816, *Professor of Surgery, Würzburg, Germany.*

3. Finally, always examine the patient in the reclining position. On lying down, a direct hernia reduces itself instantly, and the bulge reappears with equal suddenness if the patient strains.

Differential Diagnosis between Inguinal Hernia and a Scrotal Swelling. *Is it possible to get above the swelling?* If, with the finger and thumb, one is able to get above the lump then obviously it cannot be a hernia (*Fig.* 449).

Confirmatory Test for Encysted Hydrocele of the Cord. Grasp the testis between finger and thumb and pull gently. When traction is made on the testis, if the swelling is a hydrocele of the cord it will move downwards with the cord (*Fig.* 450). For obvious reasons this test must be carried out with extreme care.

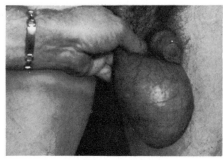

Fig. 449. Getting above the swelling.

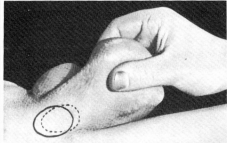

Fig. 450. When gentle traction is exerted on the testis a hydrocele of the cord moves with the testis.

Differential Diagnosis between an Inguinal Hernia and a Lipoma of the Cord. Sometimes it can be appreciated that a swelling is emerging from the inguinal canal which does not exhibit an impulse on coughing. However, the two often coexist and usually the diagnosis is not settled until the parts are displayed at operation.

Differential Diagnosis of an Inguinal Hernia in the Female. The hernia must be differentiated from other swellings of the labium majus.

A *reducible* hernia should offer no difficulty, although it may be overlooked if the patient is not examined in the standing position. On rare occasions, a psoas abscess points in the labium majus, and gives rise to a reducible swelling (*see* p. 253).

An *irreducible* hernia must be distinguished from:

A Hydrocele of the Canal of Nuck (*Fig.* 451). This is the commonest diagnostic problem. A hydrocele is smooth, fixed, fluctuant, and brilliantly translucent.

A Cyst of a Bartholin's Gland gives rise to a swelling (*see* p. 283) that is not usually translucent. It is confined to the labium majus, and does not extend up to the superficial inguinal ring and it is a simple matter to get above the swelling.

Differential Diagnosis in the Tropics between Inguinal and Femoral Hernia and Adenolymphocele of Onchocerciasis. *See* p. 253.

FEMORAL HERNIA

Femoral hernia is much less common than inguinal (1:5) and is more frequent in women (2:1).

ANTON NUCK, 1650–1692, *Anatomist, Leiden, Holland.*
CASPAR BARTHOLIN, THE YOUNGER, 1655–1738, *Professor of Medicine, Anatomy and Physics, Copenhagen.*

There is no Lump. As in the diagnosis of inguinal hernia, so in femoral, look and look again for the presence of a visible expansile impulse when the patient coughs. The bulge of a femoral hernia is below the inguinal ligament, and after a little practice the clinician will appreciate that this fleeting bulge is placed more laterally than that of an inguinal hernia. Confirm the presence of an expansile impulse by palpation, and note the relationship of the swelling to the tubercle of the os pubis.

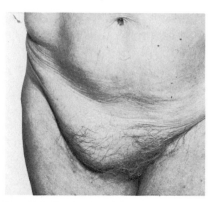

Fig. 451. Hydrocele of the right canal of Nuck. The swelling is irreducible, and brilliantly translucent.

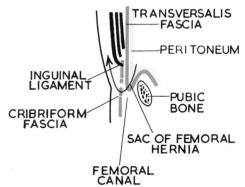

Fig. 452. Illustrating the path taken by a femoral hernia, and explaining the appearance of the fundus above the inguinal ligament, which sometimes occurs when a femoral hernia becomes irreducible.

There is a Lump. Three typical types of swelling are encountered; each is a stage in progressive protrusion of the femoral hernia along the path of the arrow, depicted in *Fig.* 452.

a. There is a rounded reducible swelling lying below the medial end of the inguinal ligament (*Fig.* 453 *b*).

b. The hernia, after passing through the narrow confines of the femoral canal, bulges into the femoral (Scarpa's) triangle. Usually this variety is irreducible (*Fig.* 454).

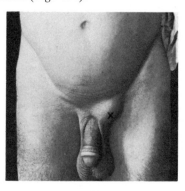

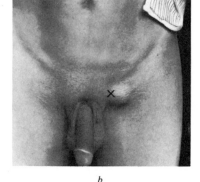

a   *b*

Fig. 453. *a*, Inguinal, and *b*, femoral herniae, compared. Note the relationship to the pubic tubercle (X). A small inguinal hernia lies medial to and above this landmark whereas a femoral hernia lies lateral and below.

ANTONIO SCARPA, 1747–1832, *Professor of Surgery, Modena, later Professor of Anatomy, Pavia, Italy.*

c. Further expansion in a downward direction being prevented by the blending of fasciae, the fundus mounts upward in front of the inguinal ligament and overlies the inguinal canal. By the time the contents have pursued so tortuous a course they are always irreducible.

Differential Diagnosis between Inguinal and Femoral Herniae. Determine the relationship of the lump or the cough impulse to the tubercle of the os pubis. A femoral hernia, even when it overlaps the inguinal ligament, must always lie to the outer side of this tubercle (*Fig.* 453 *b*). In fat individuals the landmark can be located by following up the tendon of the adductor longus to its attachment to the bone.

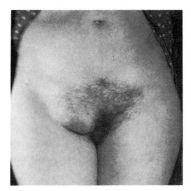

Fig. 454. Large irreducible femoral hernia.

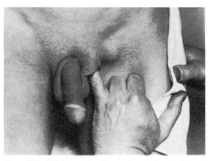

Fig. 455. Differential diagnosis of inguinal and femoral herniae. The little finger is in the inguinal canal, which is empty. The swelling, therefore, obviously cannot be an inguinal hernia.

If by the invagination test it is possible to demonstrate that the inguinal canal is empty, then obviously the swelling cannot be an inguinal hernia (*Fig.* 455). Inspection of the lump may prove a veritable trap, for the swelling caused by the hernia sometimes lies above the inguinal hernia; but even in these cases the knowing eye can often detect that the swelling is placed more laterally than it is with an inguinal hernia (*Fig.* 453).

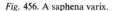

Fig. 456. A saphena varix.

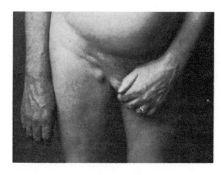

Try to reduce the swelling, applying extremely gentle pressure to the fundus with the thigh flexed and internally rotated. If unsuccessful, the clinician should not persist with taxis more than a moment or two, but recall the fact that *irreducibility is encountered ten times more frequently with a femoral hernia than with an inguinal hernia.*

Differential Diagnosis between a Small Reducible Femoral Hernia and a Saphena Varix (*Fig.* 456). Although both swellings give an impulse when the patient coughs, and both disappear visibly when the patient lies down, differentiation is fairly easy. Firstly in thin subjects a faint blue coloration of the varix is likely to be discernible in a good light. Usually a saphena varix feels softer than a femoral hernia. *Cruveilhier's Sign of Saphena Varix.* In the erect position, when the patient coughs or blows his nose, there is a tremor imparted to the palpating fingers as if a jet of water is entering and filling the pouch. Finally a saphena varix usually is associated with pronounced varicosity of the long saphenous vein and the Tap Sign (*see* p. 397) is positive.

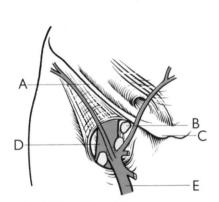

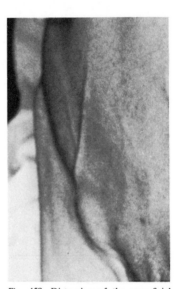

Fig. 457. The relations of the saphenous opening. A, Inguinal ligament; B, Cloquet's lymph node; C, Pubic spine; D, Femoral vein; E, Long saphenous vein.

Fig. 458. Distension of the superficial epigastric vein associated with an irreducible femoral hernia in a woman aged 77.

Differential Diagnosis between a Small Irreducible Femoral Hernia and an Enlarged Lymph Node in the Position of the Femoral Ring. This often proves a most perplexing problem, for when the lymph node in the femoral canal known as the 'lymph node of Cloquet' (*Fig.* 457) becomes enlarged, it simulates exactly an irreducible femoral hernia.

Search for a possible focus of infection. Examine the feet, legs, buttocks, perineum, anus and genitals for a new growth, boil, blister, or an abrasion. Most patients with an irreducible femoral hernia are old and many are thin. In these the sign noted by Gaur may be seen. Pressure by the hernial sac on the superficial epigastric and/or circumflex iliac veins causes distension of one or both of these veins on the side of the hernia (*Fig.* 458).

If these signs do not elucidate the problem, there are no physical signs that

JEAN CRUVEILHIER, 1791–1874, *Professor of Pathological Anatomy, Faculty of Medicine, Paris.*
JULES G. CLOQUET, 1790–1883, *Surgeon, Hôpital St. Louis, Paris.*
DURGA D. GAUR, *Contemporary Surgeon, Bombay Hospital, India.*

will.* The nature of the lump remains a matter of opinion that is best settled urgently in the operating theatre.

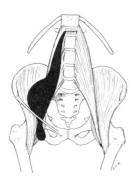

Fig. 459. A psoas abscess usually points in the femoral triangle *lateral* to the femoral artery. If this relationship is verified, the question of the swelling being a femoral hernia should not arise.

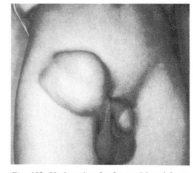

Fig. 460. Hydrocele of a femoral hernial sac, distinctly unusual in a male.

Differential Diagnosis between a Reducible Hernia and a Psoas Abscess pointing beneath the Inguinal Ligament. A cold abscess arising from tuberculous disease of the body of one of the lumbar vertebrae tracking along the psoas sheath to the insertion of the psoas major (*Fig.* 459) gives rise to a reducible, painless swelling. If the pulsations of the femoral artery can be felt it will be appreciated that the swelling is lateral to the artery. Examination of the back and (when the patient lies down) palpation of the corresponding iliac fossa clarifies the diagnosis and serves to remind the clinician that purely localized regional clinical examination sooner or later causes him to stumble, perhaps seriously.

Differential Diagnosis between an Irreducible Femoral Hernia and a Hydrocele of a Femoral Hernial Sac. A hydrocele of a femoral hernial sac (*Fig.* 460) is always brilliantly translucent.

EPIGASTRIC HERNIA

An epigastric hernia, also, and more explicitly, called a 'fatty hernia of the linea alba' (*Fig.* 461), can often be seen if the patient is spare and is placed in an oblique light.

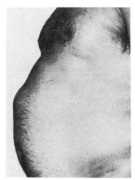

Fig. 461. Epigastric hernia visible only when the patient was examined standing up. He complained of symptoms suggesting a peptic ulcer.

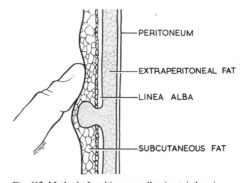

PERITONEUM

EXTRAPERITONEAL FAT

LINEA ALBA

SUBCUTANEOUS FAT

Fig. 462. Method of seeking a small epigastric hernia.

---

* An abdominal X-ray taken with the patient in the erect position showing fluid levels indicates that intestinal obstruction is present and that the swelling must be an irreducible femoral hernia.

Frequently, the smaller an epigastric hernia the greater the symptoms, which often simulate those of a chronic peptic ulcer. Many escape detection—but not if the following method is employed:

With the patient standing, exercising gentle pressure, draw the pulp of the index finger along the linea alba between the xiphoid process and the umbilicus. A small (they are often tiny) epigastric hernia will be palpable as a nodule (*Fig.* 462), occasionally reducible.

INCISIONAL HERNIA

The patient has had an abdominal operation and the hernia is usually obvious. Occasionally the test illustrated in *Fig.* 462 is of value when the possibility of a small incisional hernia through the anterior abdominal musculature is being considered. If there is still doubt, ask the patient to stand and re-examine him. A protrusion through the abdominal musculature, indiscernible when the patient was lying down, may become obvious.

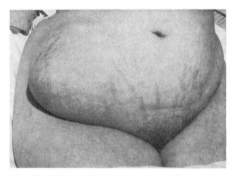

Fig. 463. Incisional hernia through a gridiron appendicectomy scar; dangerous variety.

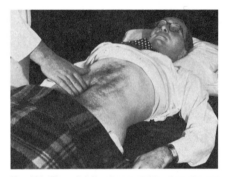

Fig. 464. The palpating fingers sinking into the gap resulting from a large incisional hernia.

With a moderate-sized or large incisional (ventral) hernia define the margins of the neck of the sac. The *dangerous* variety has a narrow neck (*Fig.* 463) which will only admit a finger or two, whereas with the *relatively safe* type on palpation, when the abdominal musculature is relaxed fully, the fingers discern a wide gap through which several fingers or the whole hand can sink (*Fig.* 464).

HIATUS (DIAPHRAGMATIC) HERNIA

Most sufferers from this condition are over 50 years of age; the fat are more frequent victims than the lean; there are no physical signs.

Pain is the dominant symptom. Its chief sites are shown in *Fig.* 465. It is not unusual for the patient to experience pain localized in more than one of these areas. What is extremely characteristic is that the pain is made worse by stooping, and sometimes by lying down.

Haematemesis. Serious haematemesis or melaena occurs in 10 per cent of cases.

The cause of the bleeding is peptic ulceration within the herniated portion of the stomach.

Perforation of such an ulcer is a rarity. So is the most important complication of external hernia, viz. strangulation, which complicates only the congenital and post-traumatic varieties in which a large opening may exist in the diaphragm. Respiratory movement of the left chest is restricted and bowel sounds may be heard in the chest. A radiograph is essential to establish the diagnosis.

When the hernia is large, occasional bouts of hiccup from irritation of the phrenic nerve occur. In a few patients agonizing attacks of substernal pain, simulating that of angina pectoris, are a leading symptom, in which event the diagnosis can be established only by normal electrocardiographs and positive radiological signs of hiatus hernia.

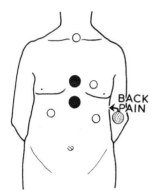

Fig. 465. Localization of pain in a hiatus hernia. Black circles, principal locations; outline circles, less common, or subsidiary, locations.

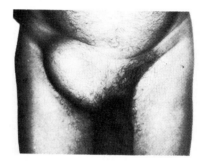

Fig. 466. A large Spigelian hernia.

Hiatus Hernia in Infants. The outstanding feature is effortless vomiting, often bloodstained, dating from shortly after birth and persisting. *See also* Cyanosis on Feeding a Newborn Infant, p. 196.

Hiatus hernia has become a fashionable diagnosis, and is demonstrated in about a third of patients submitted to a carefully carried out barium meal X-ray. The reader must therefore be vigilant lest an incidental, probably symptomless, hiatus hernia is accredited with the causation of symptoms due to another lesion. **Umbilical Hernia.** *See* p. 247.

SOME RARE HERNIAE

Obturator Hernia can be recognized only when it strangulates. It almost always occurs in thin females over 60 years of age. The symptoms are often obscure, for frequently the strangulation is of the Richter type.* The swelling is liable to be overlooked because the hernia is covered by the pectineus muscle, but a fullness (or even a lump) in the femoral triangle on one side is a suggestive sign. The lump lies below the pubic ramus, whereas a femoral hernia lies above. Usually the patient maintains the limb on the affected side in semi-flexion, and movements of the hip joint are limited by pain.

---

* *Richter's hernia* = strangulation of a portion only of the circumference of the intestine.

AUGUST G. RICHTER, 1742–1812, *Surgeon, Göttingen, Germany.*

Often the pain is referred along the obturator nerve to its genicular branch—the Howship–Romberg sign of pain in the knee. On vaginal examination sometimes the hernia can be felt as a tender swelling in the region of the obturator foramen.

Spigelian Hernia occurs through the linea semilunaris usually a few centimetres above the inguinal ligament (*Fig.* 466). Clinically it is difficult to differentiate from the following.

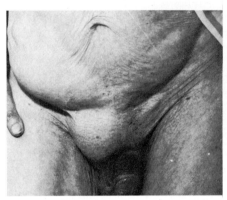 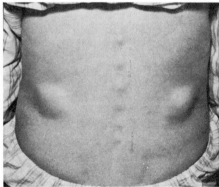

Fig. 467. Right interstitial hernia associated with in- *Fig.* 468. Bilateral lumbar herniae.
direct inguinal hernia.

Interstitial (Interparietal) Hernia. The sac passes between the layers of the abdominal wall in the region of the inguinal canal and is often associated with an inguinal hernia (*Fig.* 467). If the inguinal hernia can be reduced, a swelling is left which also reduces at or near the deep inguinal ring.

Lumbar Hernia (*Fig.* 468). This term does not include the hernia following an operation on the kidney, which is an incisional hernia.

JOHN HOWSHIP, 1781–1841, *Surgeon, Charing Cross Hospital, London.*
MORITZ H. ROMBERG, 1795–1873, *Director, University Polyclinic, Berlin.*
ADRIAAN VAN DER SPIEGEL, 1578–1625, *Professor of Anatomy, Padua.*

Chapter 21

RECTAL AND VAGINAL EXAMINATION

ANORECTAL EXAMINATION

Many times the omission of a rectal examination has been a cause of regret. 'If you don't put your finger in it, you put your foot in it.' In the acute abdominal case, 'It is more important to insert the finger into the lower end than to put the thermometer into the upper end of the alimentary tract' (Cope).

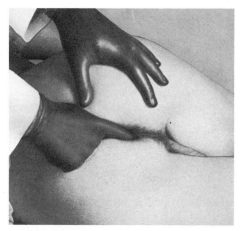

Fig. 469. Left lateral position.

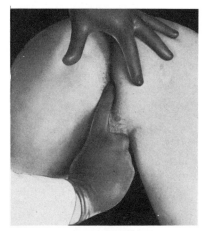

Fig. 470. Knee–elbow position.

Position of the Patient. The examination can be made in one of four positions, each having its advantages and special uses.

1. *The Left Lateral (Sims's) Position* (*Fig.* 469) is employed as a routine in women. It is also used as a standard procedure in the male in most clinics. Note that the upper (right) leg should be flexed while the lower (left) is semi-extended. The buttocks should project over the edge and the trunk should be *across* the couch or bed rather than parallel to its edge.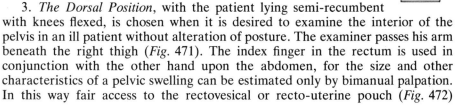

2. *The Knee–Elbow Position* (*Fig.* 470) is efficacious, particularly when the prostate and seminal vesicles are to be palpated.

3. *The Dorsal Position*, with the patient lying semi-recumbent with knees flexed, is chosen when it is desired to examine the interior of the pelvis in an ill patient without alteration of posture. The examiner passes his arm beneath the right thigh (*Fig.* 471). The index finger in the rectum is used in conjunction with the other hand upon the abdomen, for the size and other characteristics of a pelvic swelling can be estimated only by bimanual palpation. In this way fair access to the rectovesical or recto-uterine pouch (*Fig.* 472)

Sir Zachary Cope, 1881–1974, *Surgeon, St. Mary's Hospital, London.*
James Marion Sims, 1813–1883, *Founder and Surgeon, State Hospital for Women, New York City.*

(which in the circumstances mentioned is the main point of the examination) can be effected with minimum disturbance to the exhausted patient.

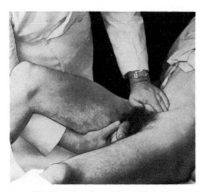

Fig. 471. The dorsal position. Method to be adopted when the patient is too ill to be subjected to much movement.

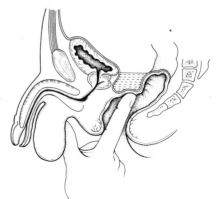

Fig. 472. Palpating the rectovesical pouch in a case of peritonitis In this instance there is a collection of pus, which imparts a softly cystic impression to the palpating finger. As a rule the swelling is exquisitely tender.

4. *The Lithotomy Position.* To make the examination in this position it is necessary to use an operating table. When a bimanual rectal (or vaginal) examination is made with the patient thus positioned (*Fig.* 473) the pelvic viscera become more accessible and a lesion high in the rectum is more likely to be felt. This is the best position, but it is not always available. Be that as it may, in almost all instances a rectal examination performed in one of the first three positions will give all the information that is required.

For the average clinician 10 cm is the probable limit of digital exploration.

Anatomical Structures felt by a Finger in the Rectum

1. *The Anal Groove (anal intermuscular depression).* Just inside the anal verge, a groove can be felt. This corresponds to the dividing line between the external and the internal haemorrhoidal plexus. It lies between the external and internal sphincter muscles.

2. *The Anorectal Ring* is situated at the junction of the anal canal (which, in the adult, is 2–3 cm in length) and the rectum. The posterior and lateral parts of the ring are felt easily, because of the sling-like arrangement of the puborectalis component of the levator ani muscle. The recognition of these muscular landmarks is of prime important in determining the location of an anorectal abscess (*see* p. 278) or a fistula-in-ano (*see* p. 273).

Above the anorectal ring the finger enters the spacious lower rectum.

3. *The Lowest Valve of Houston.* The ascending finger sometimes impinges on this soft fold of mucous membrane.

4. *The Sacral Promontory.* The lower part of the sacral promontory, as it curves forwards and upwards, can be felt, and in some individuals this can be employed as a point for orientation when palpating pelvic structures. The finger, moved laterally, can identify the *spine of the ischium.*

5. *The Prostate or the Cervix Uteri.* Sweeping the finger around the lateral

JOHN HOUSTON, 1802–1854, *Physician, City of Dublin Hospital, Ireland.*

wall until the pulp of the finger passes anteriorly, the prostate gland or the cervix uteri will come to lie beneath the finger.

a. The Prostate: Digital examination is considered on p. 356.

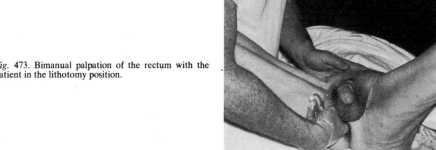

Fig. 473. Bimanual palpation of the rectum with the patient in the lithotomy position.

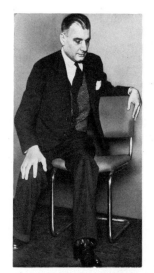

Fig. 474. Characteristic attitude of a patient with an acute anorectal condition awaiting his turn for a consultation.

b. The Cervix Uteri: The *pons asinorum**** of a rectal examination is the cervix which can be felt projecting through the anterior rectal wall. Even after considerable experience, its inconstant size and shape may, in a given case, cause momentary bewilderment. So great is the pitfall that, in making a rectal examination in the female, it should be the rule to find the cervix deliberately first, and take bearings from it.

Having mastered these theoretical considerations, the time is ripe to consider the practical applications of this frequently indispensable procedure, the when, the how, and the interpretation of which is a hallmark of clinical acumen.

Before commencing the description of the findings in various anorectal lesions, it is well to draw attention to the sitting posture (*Fig.* 474) adopted by many a patient with an acute anorectal condition, notably prolapsed haemorrhoids or a perianal abscess.

Anorectal Examination. Inspection must never be omitted. When a female is being examined disregard of this fundamental rule has many times led to a mistake, and the finger has been introduced into the wrong orifice. Furthermore, it often yields information of cardinal importance; for instance, rectal prolapse (*Fig.* 475), prolapsed internal haemorrhoids, and pruritus† ani (*Fig.* 476) can be diagnosed at sight. An external haemorrhoid (*Fig.* 477), or haemorrhoids, which are covered with skin, are at once apparent. In relevant cases look for the external orifice of a

---

* *Pons asinorum.* Latin = the bridge of asses. Euclid, Book I, Proposition V. A difficult problem for beginners.

† *Pruritus.* Latin, *prurire* = to itch.

SOME COMMON CONDITIONS REVEALED BY INSPECTION OF THE ANUS

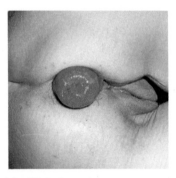

Fig. 475. Prolapse of the rectum—procidentia. The patient was typical for this condition, an aged female.

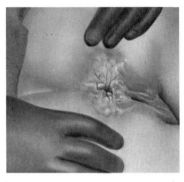

Fig. 476. Pruritus ani with cutaneous tags which are probably the cause of the irritation.

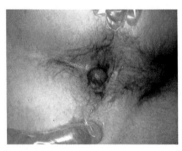

Fig. 477. 'Thrombotic pile' (syn. external haemorrhoid)—subcutaneous rupture of an anal venule.

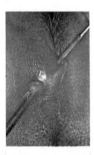

Fig. 478. Fistula-in-ano. A probe has been passed under anaesthesia prior to an operation.

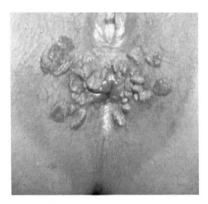

Fig. 479. Perianal warts.

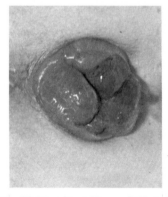

Fig. 480. Three internal haemorrhoids can be seen coming into view as the patient strains.

fistula-in-ano (*Fig.* 478) or the sentinel tag of a fissure (*see Fig.* 483). Perianal warts are very obvious (*Fig.* 479). Ask the patient to 'strain down', observe the relaxation of the external sphincter, and, in a normal person, the very slightest protrusion of mucosa. As the patient strains, internal haemorrhoids, which before were hidden from view, may now slowly protrude (*Fig.* 480). If the sphincter is tightly closed in spite of the patient 'straining down', be suspicious of a fissure-in-ano (*see* p. 273).

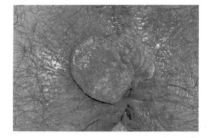

Fig. 481. Carcinoma of the anus.

Carcinoma of the Anus (*Fig.* 481) is often harboured by the patient for many months in the belief that it is a 'pile'. The swelling is firm in consistency, bleeds readily and cannot be reduced. The inguinal lymph nodes are usually involved at a late stage.

Melanoma of the anus presents as a bluish-black, soft mass, which is confused with a thrombotic pile but does not resolve spontaneously in 2 or 3 weeks as does the latter. As the melanoma ulcerates, its black colour is lost. The inguinal lymph nodes are involved early.

Technique of Rectal Palpation. At the present time disposable gloves (*see Fig.* 1, p. 2) are easily the most convenient as they are cheap and can be thrown away. Prior to the examination the gloved finger should be lubricated. At the end of the examination wipe the lubricant from the anus. If you omit to do this it is extremely uncomfortable for the patient when dressed.

Method of Introducing the Finger. One of the greatest factors in an efficient rectal palpation is that it should be a painless process. To a very large extent this can be achieved by correct technique. Always warn the patient what you are about to do. After you have placed him in the desired position, say: 'I am now going to examine the back passage. It will not hurt you. Open your mouth and breathe quietly in and out, and keep on breathing through your mouth.'

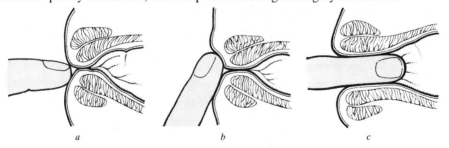

a   b   c

Fig. 482. Rectal examination. *a*, The wrong way of introducing the finger. *b*, The correct manner of commencing the examination: firm pressure is exerted until the sphincter is felt to relax. *c*, The finger has entered the anal canal and is about to enter the rectum.

Lay the pulp of the index finger flat upon the anal verge (*Fig.* 482), and exert firm pressure until the sphincter is felt to yield. Then, with a rotary movement, the finger is introduced *slowly*. If the rectum is found to be full of hard faeces, it will be wise to defer the examination (unless the case is urgent) and record this fact in your notes. In the absence of this stumbling block, when engaged in an examination of the rectum, unless there is some striking abnormality, it is well to have in mind a routine, a kind of formula, which will synchronize the brain and finger. Proceed in order, palpating and thinking all the time of what you are doing.

PALPATION OF THE RECTUM

In the Male
- Anterior wall
  1. Prostate, left lobe, right lobe
  2. Seminal vesicles, position of left vesicle, position of right vesicle
  3. Rectovesical pouch
- Left lateral wall
- Right lateral wall
- Superiorly, as far as can be reached
- Posteriorly { Hollow of sacrum / Coccyx

In the Female
- Cervix
- Recto-uterine pouch
- Left lateral wall
- Right lateral wall
- Superiorly, as far as can be reached
- Posteriorly { Hollow of sacrum / Coccyx

It is not unusual for the advancing finger to push a lesion of the rectum before it. Therefore, in its upward course, after the anorectal ring has been passed, endeavour to steer the fingertip clear of the rectal walls. Having reached the highest limit, flex the finger and withdraw it partially. Repeat the process at other cardinal points of the compass, for *a soft lesion of the rectal wall is more likely to be felt on the downward stroke of the finger than on its upward course.*

Having completed the routine palpation, look at your finger for blood, mucus, or pus: better still, wipe it on a gauze swab, which will show up the colour of the discharge.

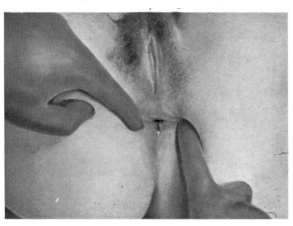

Fig. 483. Method of displaying a fissure-in-ano. The fissure is seen as a crevice lined by granulation tissue. The crevice has been well described as a canoe-shaped ulcer. In this case, at the distal end of the fissure a sentinel pile can be seen. In some instances, at the proximal end there is a hypertrophied anal papilla. The similarity to a Canadian canoe is then heightened.

DIGITAL FINDINGS IN VARIOUS ANORECTAL CONDITIONS

Fissure-in-ano. First let us consider a common condition where routine palpation must be halted. In fissure-in-ano the anal sphincter is in spasm; it is impossible to introduce the finger without causing pain. This is an occasion where rectal examination, as such, is contraindicated, but the anal canal must be inspected with especial care. With the pulps of the index fingers gently separate the folds of anal mucosa (*Fig.* 483) and look for the fissure, especially in the middle line posteriorly. A so-called 'sentinel'* pile is nothing more than a cutaneous tag which sometimes marks the distal extremity of the fissure.

Fissure-in-ano is not uncommon in children, and probably because the condition is not even thought of, let alone looked for, in a young child the diagnosis is frequently missed.

Fistula-in-ano is a track, lined by granulation tissue, resulting from an anorectal abscess that burst spontaneously, or was opened inadequately. If the opening is large enough for pus to escape, pain is not a symptom, and the principal complaint is that of a purulent discharge which causes local irritation and discomfort. Frequently there is a solitary external opening, usually situated within 4 cm of the anus, presenting a small elevation with granulation tissue pouting from the mouth of the opening (*see Fig.* 478).

Goodsall's Rule. Fistulae with an external opening in relation to the anterior half of the anus tend to be of the direct type; those with an external opening or openings in relation to the posterior half of the anus usually have curving tracks (due to outward deflexion of the pus around the sides of the puborectalis muscles) with the internal opening in the midline (*Fig.* 484), and may be of the horseshoe variety.

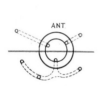

Fig. 484. Illustrating Goodsall's rule.

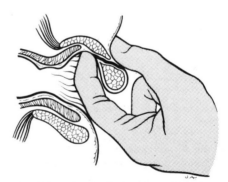

Fig. 485. Bidigital palpation for tracking the induration around a fistula-in-ano which feels like whip-cord.

Introduce a finger into the anal canal. Not infrequently the internal opening of the fistula can be felt as a small elevation about a centimetre from the anal verge. A common mistake is to search for an internal opening too high.

Probing a fistula-in-ano is often undertaken as part of the *clinical* examination. This has nothing to recommend it—even if the lightest pressure is used, it is easy to direct the probe through the lining granulation tissue, and not only to get a false impression of the direction of a tortuous fistula, but to complicate the

---

* Sentinel—because it metaphorically watches over the fissure.

DAVID H. GOODSALL, 1843–1906, *Surgeon, Metropolitan Hospital, London.*

situation by creating a side-track, and perhaps to initiate an exacerbation of the inflammatory process. Far better is it to rely on bidigital palpation combined with a clear mental picture of the relevant anorectal musculature. By inserting the index finger into the rectum, and then by utilizing the thumb of the same hand, all the tissues between the skin and the mucous membrane (*Fig.* 485), from the pelvic floor above to the anal verge below, can be palpated. Except in tuberculous fistulae, induration around a fistula can be recognized as a firm cord.

Special Types of Fistulae-in-ano

1. *Fistula associated with a Fissure.* In this instance pain (due to the fissure) is a leading symptom. The external orifice of the fistula frequently lurks beneath an overhanging sentinel pile. The internal orifice is in the fissure itself.

2. *Fistulae with Many External Orifices* suggest one of several diseases, each of which must be considered: regional ileitis, tuberculous proctitis, bilharziasis, lymphogranulomatous stricture of the rectum, colloid carcinoma.

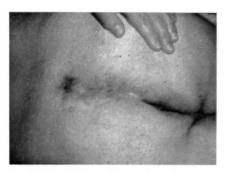

Fig. 486. Pilonidal sinus with several openings.

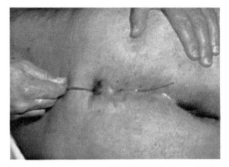

Fig. 487. Same case as *Fig.* 486. Under anaesthesia just prior to operation, a probe has been passed from one opening to emerge from another.

Pilonidal * Sinus. Some patients arrive at the out-patient department as 'fistula-in-ano'. Observe the opening of the sinus. It is situated in the middle line, over the coccyx, and is really quite a distance from the anus. Often multiple openings are present (*Figs.* 486, 487). Purulent fluid and sometimes loose hairs can often be expressed by pressure over the last segment of the sacrum. When the small mouth of the sinus becomes blocked, the contents become bottled up and a tender swelling is present which often lies to one or other side of the middle line. Patients often are dark, hairy men.

Pilonidal Sinus of the Umbilicus (*see* p. 249).
Barber's Pilonidal Sinus (*see* p. 475).

Internal Haemorrhoids. If neither engorged nor thrombosed, internal haemorrhoids are so soft that they cannot be felt with the finger. With suggestive symptoms, insertion of a proctoscope is necessary to confirm their presence.

Pruritus Ani. There is an intractable itching around the anus. Broadly speaking, there are two varieties—the moist and the dry. In the first there is usually a causative lesion, which includes an anal fissure, a fistula-in-ano, and prolapsed or external haemorrhoids; excessive ingestion of liquid paraffin can also produce a moist, irritable anus. A vaginal discharge, particularly one due to

---

* Pilonidal—because it contains a nest of hairs.

Trichomonas vaginalis, can cause irritation of the anus, as also (especially in young subjects) can threadworms (*Enterobius vermicularis*). When the anal skin shows some form of dermatitis which has a well-defined border, mycotic disease of the skin due to yeasts or fungi should be suspected. Culture of the mucopus taken from the region is necessary to establish the diagnosis in this instance.

Any of the foregoing produces in time lichenified pruritic skin around the anus (*see Fig.* 476).

Of the drier varieties without a demonstrable cause, consider the possibility of diabetes, lack of personal cleanliness, or excessive sweating.

Rectal Prolapse. *a. Prolapse of the Mucous Membrane* without haemorrhoids is uncommon in adults, but not particularly so in children. The protrusion is seldom more than 2 cm beyond the anal verge and, what is of prime importance, the mucous membrane is directly continuous with the perianal skin (*see Fig.* 520 *a*, p. 306). If the mucous membrane is allowed to protrude for any length of time it becomes eroded in places and bleeds, and tends to lose its pristine gloss. Prolapsed haemorrhoids are characterized by soft, sessile, deep-red *hillocks* on the mucous membrane (*Fig.* 480).

*b. Rectal Procidentia** is applied to a sliding hernia of all coats of the rectum, including a portion of the recto-uterine or rectovesical pouch. The condition is much commoner in women. It is diagnosed easily (1) because the protrusion is marked by circular folds in the mucous membrane (shown in *Fig.* 475), and (2) unlike prolapse of the mucous membrane, a sulcus exists between the protrusion and the perianal skin, enabling a finger to be passed in an upward direction between these two structures for a varying distance.

c. Sigmoidorectal Intussusception. In some individuals the distal sigmoid is extremely mobile and possesses a long mesentery, and from time to time intussusception occurs, which, if it fails to reduce itself spontaneously, protrudes at the anus. The appearance is similar to the above, but the examining finger inserted between the prolapse and the perianal skin, instead of coming to a full-stop at the bottom of a sulcus, passes *ad infinitum* into a bottomless pit (*see Fig.* 520, p. 306).

All varieties of rectal prolapse are favoured by a relaxed external sphincter. Should, however, the sphincter be capable of acting strongly and it goes into spasm after the protrusion has occurred, strangulation will result and gangrene of the prolapsed mass becomes possible, notably of the mucous membrane bearing internal haemorrhoids ('strangulated piles') (*Fig.* 488).

Sphincter Relaxation. Loss of sphincter tone can be demonstrated by digital traction on the sphincter when the finger is inserted into the anal canal and hooked above the anorectal ring. If, by this means, the sphincter can be made to gape so that the rectal lumen is displayed, a subnormal sphincter tone is certainly present.

Diminished tone, or absence of normal resistance to the entry of the finger into the anal canal, is due to damage to the sphincters, resulting from childbirth, a badly planned operation for fistula, congenital defects, disease of the spinal cord, and, most commonly, senility.

Carcinoma of the Rectum does occur in patients under 40 years of age, but, as might be expected, usually the sufferer is older. As the neoplasm can be felt digitally—in early cases as a plateau or as a nodule with an indurated base—it is incumbent upon the clinician to make a routine digital examination in every

---

* *Procidentia.* Latin = a prolapse, or falling down.

patient who complains of having passed blood per rectum, or in whom there has been a recent change in bowel habit. In this respect, as far as the general practitioner's responsibilities are concerned rectal examination reaches its zenith of importance. When the centre of the plaque or nodule ulcerates, a shallow depression will be felt, the edges of which are raised and everted (*Fig.* 489). This, combined with induration of the base of the ulcer, is a frequent and unmistakable finding. If one of the above findings is encountered, determine

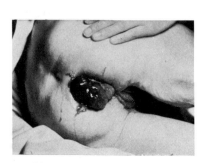

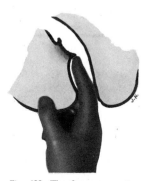

Fig. 488. Prolapsed internal haemorrhoids with strangulation. Three hours before admission the haemorrhoids came down, and could not be replaced.

Fig. 489. The finger encounters first the edge of a carcinomatous ulcer. When the ulcer is situated some distance from the anus, the floor of the ulcer may be out of reach.

whether it is possible to get above the growth. Next feel around the whole circumference of the bowel and decide the relationship of the neoplasm to the circumference. In this way one can ascertain whether the tumour is of the annular, tubular, ulcer, or cauliflower type. By trying to move the growth gently it is possible to discover whether it is fixed to the surrounding structures or tethered at any one point (e.g. to the sacrum). On withdrawing the finger, the glove is frequently bloodstained.

See also Bidigital Anovaginal Examination, p. 280.

Benign Tumours of the Rectum

Adenomatous Polyp occurs as a bright red, slightly lobulated, pedunculated tumour in the lower rectum. Nearly always advice is sought because of the passage of bright red blood, or bloodstained mucus, per rectum. If the pedicle is long enough, the adenoma appears at the anus during defaecation, causing pain and tenesmus.* On rectal examination sometimes it is possible to hook down the polyp with the examining finger (*Fig.* 490).

A Fibrous 'Polyp' at the anorectal junction is not uncommon in adults. This is not a neoplasm, but a result of either fibrosis of an internal haemorrhoid, or (as revealed by proctoscopy) more frequently a hypertrophied anal papilla.

A Villous Papilloma feels soft and velvety, or, where the fronds are lush, almost gelatinous. As a rule it covers a relatively large area of rectal mucosa and bleeds on being palpated.

---

* *Tenesmus.* Greek, τεινεσμός = straining, especially ineffectual and painful straining at stool.

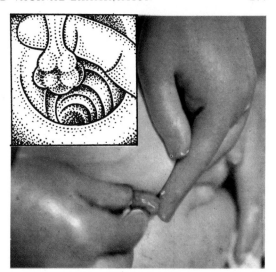

Fig. 490. An adenomatous rectal polyp showing (inset) the method of hooking it down.

Benign Stricture of the Rectum is encountered less frequently than an annular carcinoma except in regions where *lymphogranuloma inguinale* (*see* p. 376) is rife. Bear it in mind if the stricture is rubbery and tubular in character. Occasionally a narrow circular crescentic fold is felt 3 cm from the anal verge in a young person. This is a *congenital stricture* due to imperfect fusion of the hindgut with the proctodeum. A *fibrous stricture* in this neighbourhood in an adult is likely to be the result of an ill-performed operation for internal haemorrhoids, but it may result also from other conservative operations on the rectum or anal canal. When a supposed inflammatory stricture of the rectum bleeds on digital palpation, carcinoma should be suspected.

Senile Anal Stenosis. The external sphincter becomes fibrosed, and the entrance to the anal canal grasps the examining finger like a tight umbrella ring. Partial obstruction due to faecal impaction above the stricture is the usual reason for calling attention to the condition.

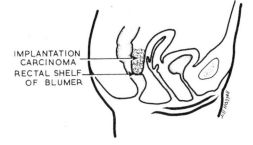

IMPLANTATION
CARCINOMA
RECTAL SHELF
OF BLUMER

Fig. 491. The rectal shelf of Blumer. In this case it is due to transcoelomic implantation of cancer cells from a carcinoma of the stomach to the rectovesical pouch.

The Rectal Shelf of Blumer is encountered on rectal examination performed (*a*) on account of rectal symptoms; (*b*) as a routine measure in cases of suspected carcinoma of the stomach. It is due to an extrarectal mass causing an indentation of the anterior wall of the rectum (*Fig.* 491) and can be distinguished from a stricture involving the mucous membrane of the rectum by the fact that it does not encircle the entire circumference, and often the mucous membrane can be made to move over the shelf. In the female, carcinoma of the stomach, being relatively uncommon, is not a frequent cause, and should transcoelomic implantation occur, cancer cells are more likely to alight on the

GEORGE BLUMER, 1858–1940, *Professor of Medicine, Yale University, New Haven, Connecticut.*

ovaries (*see* Krukenberg's Tumours, p. 228) than to pass into the recto-uterine pouch. However, a neoplastic shelf in this position occurs from time to time in late cases of carcinoma of the breast, by a path which is open to question. Any intra-abdominal cancer can be complicated by this condition, and even cancer of the bronchus.

'Frozen Pelvis.' Except perhaps posteriorly, the sensation imparted to the examining finger conveys to the mind the impression that all the pelvic viscera are set in a firm-to-hard solid medium, which indeed they are. Often this signifies extensive malignant disease usually originating in the pelvis, although on occasions it can result from pelvic cellulitis or colonic diverticulitis.

Ballooning of the Rectum suggests obstruction to the lumen higher up (e.g. at the pelvirectal junction). Once past the anorectal ring, the finger enters a voluminous space, and it has to be bent in this or that direction before the rectal wall is encountered. It is curious that the rectum *below* a constriction should be ballooned; possibly the phenomenon is due to interference with the neuromuscular mechanism. However, the sign is not of uniform reliability. For instance, it is found when the rectum is examined immediately after the administration of an enema, as then there still may be air or flatus distending the rectum. It is also seen with some instances of obstruction in the urinary tract and is then, presumably, reflex in origin.

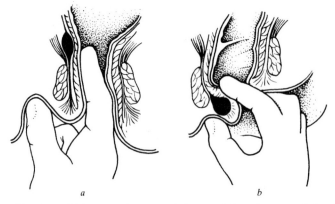

Fig. 492. *a*, Palpating a high intermuscular abscess: it is situated above the anorectal ring. *b*, Method of ascertaining the presence of a low intermuscular abscess—the most common variety of anorectal abscess.

Anorectal Abscess. *High Intermuscular Abscess* (10 per cent) is situated above the anorectal ring. Defaecation is agonizing, and the patient cannot sit in comfort: the temperature is moderately elevated. The diagnosis is made in the early stages by digital examination (*Fig. 492 a*) when an acutely tender, rounded lump is felt above the anorectal junction, generally posteriorly.

Low Intermuscular Abscess (80 per cent). The early diagnosis is made as shown in *Fig. 492 b*. Undiagnosed, or treated with antibiotics instead of by early incision, the abscess tracks to the subcutis of the perianal region, or invades the ischiorectal fossa.

Ischiorectal Abscess (6 per cent) gives rise to a tender brawny induration, palpable in the floor of the ischiorectal fossa as well as in the lateral wall of the anal canal of the corresponding side. Constitutional symptoms are severe unless masked by antibiotic therapy. In comparatively early cases there is no redness of the skin. Men are affected more often than women.

Abscess beneath the Anoderm (2 per cent) is felt as a tender elevation in the anal canal. It originates in the superficial portion of an anal gland. In the very great majority of the abscesses described above, infection originates in one of the deeper branches of such a gland.

Abscess beneath the Perianal Skin (Perianal Abscess) (*Fig.* 493) can arise through neglect of a low intermuscular abscess, or (in the middle line posteriorly) as the result of a sinus extending from a fissure-in-ano, in which case the abscess is situated in juxtaposition to a sentinel pile (*see Fig.* 483, p. 272). The only conditions with which such an anorectal abscess is likely to be confused are an abscess connected with a pilonidal sinus, an abscess of Cowper's gland (*see* p. 360), and an abscess of a Bartholin's gland (*see* p. 283).

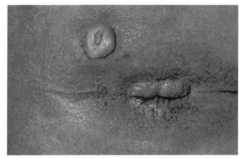

Fig. 493. Low intermuscular abscess. The commonest by far of anorectal abscess. If allowed to burst spontaneously, as has regrettably almost happened here, a fistula-in-ano results.

Perianal Cutaneous Amoebiasis should be borne in mind in the tropics. Spreading ulceration of the perianal skin is found with abscess cavities extending into the ischiorectal fossae. The patient is extremely toxic and the granulation tissue lining the ulcers and the abscesses abounds with *Entamoeba histolytica*.

Examination of a Case of Suspected Coccydynia. The index finger is introduced into the rectum in the usual way. It is then rotated so that the coccyx can be grasped between the finger and thumb (*see Fig.* 538, p. 330). Abnormal mobility and tenderness of the coccyx can be ascertained by this manœuvre. If the coccyx appears normal consider whether the pain is referred from a prolapsed lumbar intervertebral disc (*see* p. 208).

Massive Oedema of the Rectal Wall has been noted in volvulus of the pelvic colon. This is due to the inferior mesenteric vein becoming occluded by the torsion.

Is a Given Lump in the Wall of the Rectum or Outside It? Sometimes it is a difficult matter to decide whether a particular lump is arising from the wall of the rectum, or if it is outside the rectal wall. Pass the finger to one side of the lump and then slide it over the elevation. In this way one may be able to feel a continuity of the normal mucous membrane and to move the rectal wall on the lump—in which case the lump is outside the rectal wall.

Attention has been directed already to the character of the cervix uteri as felt through the anterior rectal wall. The student must also beware of a larger, domed, firm lump situated a little higher than the cervix uteri. On the downward stroke of the finger it becomes evident that the umbilicated bobbin (the cervix) is not present, or that the domed, firm lump felt previously has taken its place. That the lump is the fundus of a retroverted uterus (*Fig.* 494) becomes apparent on vaginal examination, for the cervix uteri, instead of pointing downward and backward, points downward and forward.

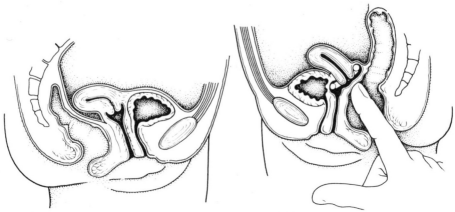

Fig. 494. Retroverted uterus felt on rectal examination.

Fig. 495. Make sure that a woman is not wearing a pessary before expressing an opinion on a lump that can be felt per rectum.

A Perplexing, and possibly an Embarrassing, Situation. A pessary or a tampon in the vagina can be felt per rectum (*Fig.* 495). It is astounding how often this seemingly obvious fact proves to be the cause of utter diagnostic confusion.

Rectal Examination as a Means of palpating the Pelvic Viscera. Bimanual recto-abdominal examination is an extremely valuable method of palpating the pelvic viscera. *In the male*, apart from permitting an examination of the prostate and seminal vesicles (*see* p. 356), its chief use is in deciding if a neoplasm of the bladder is of the infiltrating type (*see* p. 346). In individuals possessing a sigmoid mesocolon which is long enough to allow the bowel to dangle in the rectovesical pouch, a carcinoma situated near the middle of the pelvic colon or a mass connected with colonic diverticulitis is likely to be accessible. *In the female*, although it may be a little inferior to bimanual vaginal examination, bimanual rectoabdominal palpation is the only means available for palpating the internal organs of generation of female children and virgins of more mature years. *In a child* the whole of the pelvic viscera can be palpated with facility. In the female, in addition to the cervix uteri (*see* p. 285), typical, non-tender lumps lying outside the rectal wall that can be felt by digital examination of the rectum are the fundus of a retroverted uterus (*see above*), an ovarian cyst, a subserous fibroid of the uterus, and a swollen Fallopian tube.

By employing this method of examination, the detection of a pelvic abscess occupying the rectovesical pouch (*see Fig.* 511, p. 294) or the recto-uterine pouch is rendered a relatively simple matter, while a collection of blood in either of these situations imparts a softly cystic sensation to the examining finger. Both these swellings are tender.

Bidigital Anovaginal Examination. In a comparatively low-lying lesion of the anterior rectal or posterior vaginal wall in parous women much valuable information is obtained either by an index finger in the rectum and a thumb in the vagina, or by inserting the left index finger into the vagina and the right index finger into the rectum.

ANORECTAL EXAMINATION IN NEONATES AND INFANTS

Anorectal Anomaly. One infant in 4000 is born with an imperforate anus. Within

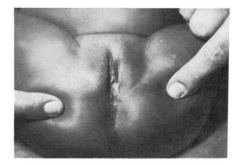

Fig. 496. Imperforate anus. High variety. An X-ray taken with the infant held upside down to demonstrate the level of gas in the blind-ending rectum is necessary to confirm the diagnosis. It is traditional, but unnecessary, to place a coin on the anal dimple while the X-ray is taken.

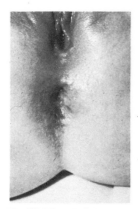
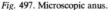

Fig. 497. Microscopic anus.

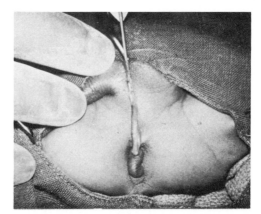

Fig. 498. Covered male anus. A fine probe demonstrates the fistula communicating with the anal canal.

an hour of birth, usually it is apparent that there is no normal anal orifice, or that meconium is being discharged from an abnormal exit. Sometimes these obvious facts are overlooked for two or three days, by which time the infant is in the throes of intestinal obstruction.

High Variety (Rectal Agenesis) (*Fig.* 496). The rectum ends blindly well up in the pelvis 2 cm or more proximal to the anal dimple. To settle the important question as to whether the case before us belongs to this category, or to one of the less serious varieties, while the child cries, the perineum must be watched, palpated, and, if necessary, probed. In the male the external urinary meatus and the urine are inspected for meconium (*recto-urethral fistula*). In the female the labia are separated with a view to finding a vaginal discharge of meconium or an imperforate hymen bulging with dark meconium behind it (*rectovaginal fistula*).

A Simple Septum is rare. If the anal dimple bulges when the child cries, and particularly if the anal membrane is dark because of meconium abutting against it, it is certain that the case is one of a simple septum.

Microscopic Anus is so minute (*Fig.* 497) that only an occasional speck of meconium reveals its presence ('fly speck'—Browne).
Stenosis at the Junction of the Hind-gut with the Proctoderm is discovered only by rectal examination.

SIR DENIS BROWNE, 1892–1967, *Surgeon, Hospital for Sick Children, Great Ormond Street, London.*

Vaginal Ectopic Anus. The anus opens by a comparatively small hole into the vagina, so that faeces are passed per vaginam. Usually the opening is in the lower third. 'Shot-gun' perineum is merely a variation of the normal in which the anus and vagina lie much closer together than usual.

Covered Female Anus results from excessive fusion of the genital folds.

Covered Male Anus. (*Fig.* 498.) No anal orifice can be seen, but there is a thin blue line running forward from the anal dimple. The orifice of this subcutaneous sinus discharges meconium on to the perineum.

Examination of the Rectum of a Neonate. The little finger should always be employed for this purpose as the index finger is too large and may inflict damage. In *Fig.* 499 the little finger has entered the anus of an infant a few days old, and the findings are those of Hirschsprung's disease (*see* p. 242).

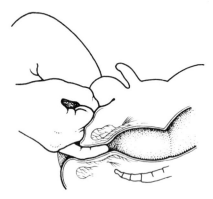

Fig. 499. Rectal examination in a neonate, employing the little finger. Findings in a case of Hirschsprung's disease.

Rectal Examination in Infancy. After the age of three months (retarded premature infants excepted) the infant's anus can be entered by the index finger, and because of the relatively small size of the pelvis an astoundingly wide vista lies within range, and even structures in the lower half of the abdominal cavity can be palpated. Rectal examination under two years of age rarely, if ever, is of any help in elucidating tenderness because of crying, and serves only in the identification of a palpable lump.

Intussusception (*see* p. 305).

VAGINAL EXAMINATION

'Never insult the vagina by examining the rectum first' is an old axiom, which can be retained provided it does not convey to the clinician the impression that, having completed a vaginal examination, he is entitled to proceed with a rectal examination using the same glove. Some infections, including gonorrhoea, are conveyed from the vagina to the rectum in this manner. Actually it is immaterial which of these examinations is done first; the important point is to *change the glove*.

Vaginal examination is dealt with so thoroughly by the gynaecological department that only a comparatively brief reference to this important method will be made. Vaginal examination as it concerns clinical surgery is portrayed here.

Position. In the consulting room the left lateral position (*see* p. 267) is usually utilized. If it is desired to scrutinize the urethral orifice the dorsal position (*see* p. 267) is better. In gynaecological practice it is wise to re-examine the patient bimanually in the lithotomy position after the bladder has been emptied with a catheter, before embarking on an operation. This examination is conveniently carried out under anaesthesia.

Technique. The hands are washed thoroughly. The right hand should be gloved and its index and middle fingers lubricated. After inspecting the external genitalia, the labia are separated by the thumb and the forefinger of the left hand. The index finger is introduced into the vagina, followed, in women who have borne children, by the middle finger. First the cervix is located, and its characteristics are noted. The anterior, posterior and lateral fornices are palpated in turn.

The Female Urethra is discussed on p. 346.

The Vulva. All those lesions that are found on the penis (*see* pp. 354, 374)—a primary chancre, the primary lesion of lymphogranuloma inguinale, granuloma inguinale, chancroid, herpes, leucoplakia and carcinoma—also occur on the labia or the margin of the introitus. Papillomata acuminata are often more luxuriant than those occurring on the penis, and in Africans they sometimes assume enormous proportions. A sebaceous cyst (or cysts) is relatively common.

Pruritus vulvae produces the same symptoms and effects on the labia as pruritus ani does on the anus. The investigations are similar (*see* p. 274) bearing in mind that a vaginal discharge (*see below*) is often the cause.

The following conditions are analogous with imperforate anus but are unlikely to be detected in infancy as they are symptomless:

Absent Vagina: Imperforate Hymen (*see below*): *Adherent Labia Minora*—non-separation of the labia mimics the first two and in practice is commoner than both combined.

Palpation of Bartholin's (Greater Vestibular) Glands. While a fully formed abscess of a Bartholin's gland is obvious (*Fig.* 500), nevertheless considerable enlargements of this gland (due, usually, to a retention cyst, but rarely to an adenocarcinoma) can be missed unless they are searched for correctly. Palpate the posterior part of the labia majora between the finger and thumb (*Fig.* 501). The gland lies more deeply and more posteriorly than one would expect.

The Vaginal Outlet (the introitus) is inspected and the presence or absence of the hymen is noted. The virginal hymen has a small sharp-edged opening that usually admits only the fingertip, but sometimes allows one finger to enter. In rare instances the hymen is imperforate, and after puberty it is seen to be bulging and purple from retained blood behind it. A slight bluish tinge of the introitus suggests early pregnancy.

A Vaginal Discharge is more likely to be present in patients with a roomy introitus than those with an intact hymen. Normally a variable amount of white curdy mucus is found. A bloodstained discharge can be due to menstruation, an impending or recent abortion, an ectopic pregnancy, or to uterine carcinoma. A profuse whitish or purulent discharge denotes salpingitis, endometritis, cervicitis or, most commonly, vaginitis. *Trichomonas vaginalis* infestation causes a profuse watery pale yellow, sometimes frothy, discharge with intense pruritus. Especially in a virgin and during pregnancy, thrush (*Candida albicans*) leads to a thick

---

CASPAR BARTHOLIN (*Secundus*), 1655–1738, *Professor of Medicine, Anatomy, and Physics, Copenhagen.*

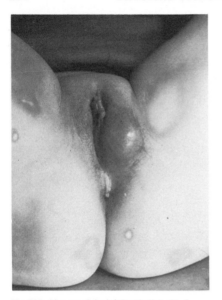

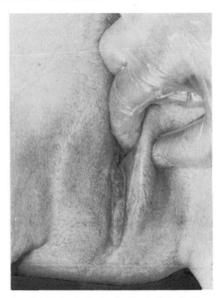

Fig. 500. Abscess of the left Bartholin's gland.

Fig. 501. Method of palpating Bartholin's gland.

cheesy discharge which is particularly excoriating. In gonorrhoea the discharge is purulent.

Testing the Supporting Musculature. At this juncture, ask the patient with an ample introitus to 'strain down'. If present, a *cystocele* (descent of the bladder through the anterior vaginal musculature (*Fig.* 502)) or a *rectocele* (descent of the rectum through the posterior vaginal musculature) becomes apparent. With the latter, the musculature of the perineum is tested by bidigital anovaginal examination (*see* p. 280). When the pelvic diaphragm and the ligaments supporting the uterus are defective, as a result of straining, the cervix appears at the introitus and becomes extruded for a varying distance (*procidentia*).

Unless it is known that the bladder is empty, ask the patient to cough several times. When the sphincter urethrae is not fully competent, urine will be spilled from the bladder by these expulsive efforts (*stress incontinence*) (*see also* p. 347).

Bimanual Palpation.* The lubricated finger or fingers of the right hand are passed into, and are kept high in the vagina, while the left hand presses downwards and backwards above the pubic symphysis (*Fig.* 503). The size and other characteristics of the uterus can be ascertained by this method. In particular a decision should be reached at the outset of the examination whether it is in its normal anteverted position or is retroverted (*see Fig.* 494). Normal ovaries may be felt in a thin patient. Normal uterine (Fallopian) tubes are not palpable. The size and other characteristics of a pelvic swelling, whether or not it is attached to the uterus, whether it is cystic or solid, fixed or free, regular or irregular, can be ascertained by skilful bimanual palpation.

In general, resistance or swelling anterior to the cervix denotes an affection

---

* Bimanual palpation of the pelvis was introduced by Puzos in the eighteenth century.

Nicolas Puzos, 1686–1753, *Army surgeon, afterwards Professor of Midwifery in the Royal Academy of Surgery, Paris.*

of the bladder or pelvic connective tissue, while posteriorly anything abnormal is in the recto-uterine pouch.

The Cervix. While a torn cervix or the gross irregularity produced by an established carcinoma of the cervix can be detected by digital examination, it would be idle to dwell on these findings when the cervix is displayed so readily to direct inspection by the passage of a vaginal speculum—a procedure that is beyond the scope of this work.

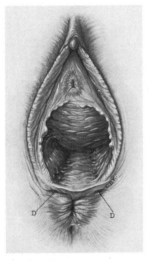

Fig. 502. Cystocele caused by a bygone birth injury. There is also an inconspicuous rectocele, but the entire perineal body has been torn through and the dimples (D) mark the ends of the separated sphincter ani.

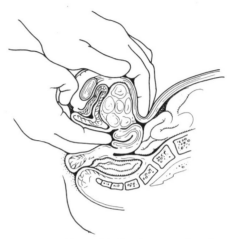

Fig. 503. The bimanual findings in a case of a solitary fibromyoma of the uterus.

Fibromyoma (Fibroid). The characteristic findings are a painless, insensitive enlargement of the uterus which is nodular, hard and movable. Usually fibroids are multiple and vary in size; sometimes one or more is immense. A solitary fibroid (*Fig.* 503) which has degenerated and become soft and perhaps cystic is often difficult to distinguish from normal pregnancy or an ovarian cyst.

Ovarian Cyst is usually unilateral, and may become so large as to fill the abdomen, when the differential diagnosis must be made from ascites (*see* p. 244). In the ordinary course of events the cyst is distinguished from other swellings by its rotundity and free mobility. In the case of a large cyst, a second small cyst is often found at operation on the opposite side. It is unusual to be able to make a clinical diagnosis of bilateral ovarian cysts and, indeed, the distinction is academic.

Endometriosis is more difficult to diagnose. The patient is usually between 25 and 40 years of age. The characteristic findings are in the adnexae. The ovaries are enlarged, fixed, and at least somewhat tender. The uterus may be slightly enlarged by the disease. When right-sided, the condition is occasionally mistaken for an appendix abscess. Endometriosis also occurs rarely in the wall of the bladder and the rectosigmoid, when it gives rise to signs of neoplasm of those organs.

Carcinoma of the Uterus

Carcinoma of the Corpus Uteri. In most parts of the world carcinoma of the body of the uterus is less common than that of the cervix. It tends to occur after the menopause and is thus a common cause of postmenopausal bleeding.

While carcinoma of the cervix soon produces a foul discharge, in carcinoma of the body of the uterus usually the discharge remains non-odorous and serosanguineous. The uterus is inclined to be bulky, but in early cases there are no pathognomonic signs on bimanual palpation. The diagnosis rests on microscopical examination of the products of curettage.

Carcinoma of the Cervix Uteri occurs commonly before the menopause. Post-coital bleeding is suggestive. The most important signs are that vaginal examination invokes bleeding, and there is induration and irregularity of the cervix. Later, parametrial invasion gives a characteristic feel as though the cervix were embedded in plaster-of-Paris.

Vaginal Examination in Acute Abdominal Conditions (*see* pp. 317–9).

Venereal Disease (*see* pp. 373–7)

Chapter 22

ACUTE ABDOMINAL CONDITIONS

'Happy is he who has no serious consequences of his erroneous diagnosis to regret.'—
Marsh.

Physical signs and their interpretation reach a high pinnacle of importance in the diagnosis of acute abdominal disease. Frequently an urgent and all-important decision has to be reached by their aid alone. For this reason no other section of this book rivals this in responsibility. Descriptions of the methods of taking the history in varying circumstances, and the vast amount of helpful information that frequently is garnered thereby, are beyond our scope. At this point it should be stressed that in cases of doubt, which are numerous, repeated examination at hourly intervals often solves the problem.

Radiographs are helpful in many instances but are of no value unless there is a sufficient degree of intestinal obstruction to produce contrasting collections of gas and fluid in loops of bowel on taking a film with the patient in the erect position (fluid levels), or sufficient free gas in the peritoneal cavity to show up as a translucency under the diaphragm. In many inflammatory conditions such radiographic abnormalities are only seen at a late stage. On the other hand in infancy an abdominal radiograph is essential for reasonably early diagnosis of intestinal obstruction.

When called upon to examine the abdomen of a patient who has been placed in the sitting posture, unless there is some contra-indication, have him placed, for the time being, flat, with one pillow beneath his head. It is impossible to examine the abdomen thoroughly unless the patient is recumbent.

PRELIMINARY INFORMATION

Before embarking on the method of eliciting, and the interpretation of, physical signs connected with individual acute intraperitoneal lesions, some signs applicable to any intraperitoneal inflammatory condition, and especially to one in which the parietal peritoneum is implicated, will be explained.

Is the Abdominal Rigidity Involuntary or Voluntary?
Voluntary contraction of the abdominal musculature (due to fear, resentment at being examined, exposure of the naked abdomen to a cold atmosphere, or laying on of a hand less warm than the patient's skin) has to be distinguished from:
Involuntary reflex rigidity due to inflammation of the peritoneum.

Patience in the examination of the patient (usually a child) together with experience and perhaps repeated examination can enable differentiation. Even so, the most experienced of clinicians make mistakes. If in doubt it is wise to have the patient admitted to hospital where a rising pulse rate over a period of several hours indicates the necessity for laparotomy.

In deciding the momentous question, 'Is this an acute abdominal condition?' there are four signs that may prove helpful in a general way:

The Pointing Test. Ask the patient to point to the site of the pain. If this proves to be the site of localized tenderness it is also almost certainly the site of the diseased viscus. An important application is in acute appendicitis.

Frederick H. Marsh, 1839–1915, *Surgeon, St. Bartholomew's Hospital, London.*

The Cough Test. Ask the patient to cough. If pain is felt in the abdomen it suggests an inflammatory process at the site of the pain. A patient with inflammation of the pleura will state that the action causes pain in the chest.

Rebound Tenderness (Release Sign; Blumberg's Sign). Having palpated the suspected area as deeply as circumstances allow, the palpating hand is withdrawn suddenly and completely. As a result of this abrupt removal of the pressure that was applied slowly and gently, but with increasing firmness, the stretched abdominal musculature springs back into place, viz. ⎯⎯⎯⎯⎯⎯⎯⎯⎯⎯⎯⎯⎯⎯⎯⎯⎯⎯⎯⎯⎯⟶ carrying with it attached peritoneum which, if inflamed, causes the patient to wince, or in many instances to cry out in pain (*Fig.* 504). This sign is employed directly over any part of the abdomen suspected of harbouring an inflamed focus when there is *doubt* about the presence of early peritonitis. *It is quite unnecessary with undoubted involuntary rigidity.*

Blumberg himself pressed in the *left* iliac fossa, and if the patient complained of pain in the lower abdomen (he did not specify any particular part of the lower abdomen) he concluded that his provisional diagnosis of acute appendicitis was confirmed.

The Bed-shaking Test (Bapat). If still in doubt whether early peritonitis is present go to the foot of the bed and shake it. This will cause pain at the site of the inflammation if such be present.

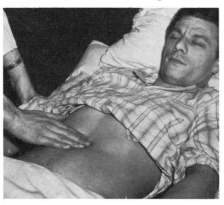 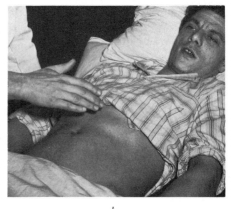

a   *b*

Fig. 504. *a*, Exert deep pressure at the site of pain. *b*, Remove the hand suddenly. If the test is positive the patient winces or cries out.

ACUTE APPENDICITIS *

Should the student feel that undue prominence is given here to the diagnosis of this condition he is reminded that, in most parts of the world, it is the commonest cause of the 'acute abdomen'.

Take the pulse and temperature. These show but little alteration in the early stages. Usually an acceleration of the pulse rate signifies the onset of peritonitis.

---

* Although the vermiform appendix had previously been removed from hernial sacs the first abdominal appendicectomy was probably performed by R. Lawson Tait, in 1880. However Reginald Fitz first described acute appendicitis accurately in 1886 and McBurney (*see* footnote, p. 289) advanced the art of diagnosis sufficiently to remove the first unruptured appendix in 1889.

Morir Blumberg, 1873–1955. *General practitioner-surgeon in Berlin.*
S. D. Bapat, *General practitioner, Bombay.*
R. Lawson Tait, 1845–99. *Birmingham surgeon.*
Reginald H. Fitz, 1843–1913. *Professor of Pathology, Harvard University.*

The pain of acute appendicitis seldom commences in the right iliac fossa. Ask the patient where the pain *began*; usually he places a finger near the umbilicus (*Fig.* 505 *a*). Now ask where the pain is *now*; the pointing finger passes to the right iliac fossa (*Fig.* 505 *b*). The pointing test, when positive, is of the greatest possible diagnostic significance.

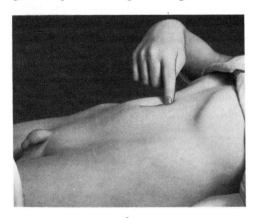
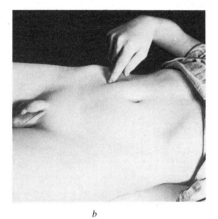

a   *b*

Fig. 505. The pointing test in appendicitis. *a*, The answer to the question, 'Where did the pain begin?'—He is pointing to the umbilicus.† *b*, The answer to the question, 'Where is the pain now?'

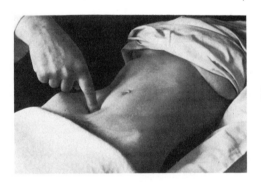

Fig. 506. Fingertip pressure over McBurney's point in a child.

Inspection. Unless an acutely inflamed obstructed appendix has perforated, and diffusing peritonitis has ensued, no alteration in the contour of the abdomen can be expected.

Palpation. Commence palpation diagonally opposite the point where pain is or was experienced, viz. lay the hand upon the left hypochondrium. Next palpate the right hypochondrium, then the left iliac fossa, leaving the right iliac fossa until last. In typical cases localized rigidity and tenderness can be demonstrated in the right iliac fossa so convincingly that no doubt remains in the mind of the

---

* Pain evoked by high intraluminar pressure in any part of the midgut is referred to the umbilicus. Wilkie showed that acute appendicitis is commonly obstructive in type, the obstruction being due to a faecolith blocking the lumen.

SIR DAVID WILKIE, 1882–1938, *Professor of Surgery, University of Edinburgh.*
CHARLES MCBURNEY, 1845–1913, *Surgeon, Roosevelt Hospital, New York. Described a point 'very exactly between an inch and a half and two inches from the anterior superior spinous process of the ilium on a straight line drawn from that process to the umbilicus'.*

clinician as to their presence. *This is the most important point in the diagnosis of acute appendicitis: all other signs are subsidiary.*
Rebound Tenderness. In the event of doubt in diagnosis a small area in the right iliac fossa will show a positive response.

When the diagnosis is still in doubt two further physical signs can be sought:
McBurney's Sign. Fingertip pressure is made over McBurney's point (*Fig.* 506), which, if the sign is positive, registers the maximum abdominal tenderness. This sign is sometimes useful in very early or subacute cases of appendicitis.

Rovsing's Sign. Even pressure is exerted over the descending colon. If, when the left iliac fossa is pressed, pain is appreciated in the right iliac fossa, the case is probably one of acute appendicitis. This sign appears to be due to the shift of coils of ileum to the right impinging on an inflamed focus in the right iliac fossa. When taken into consideration with other evidence, a positive Rovsing's sign is contributory evidence of acute appendicitis.

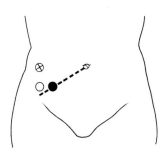

Fig. 507. ● = McBurney's point. ○ = point of maximum tenderness in retrocaecal appendicitis. ⊗ = point of tenderness in maldescent of the caecum, which may be as high as the level of the umbilicus.

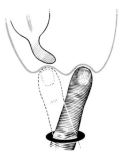

Fig. 508. Differential rectal palpation.

Signs in Retrocaecal Appendicitis. The organ may be entirely retroperitoneal. Rigidity is inclined to be ill-defined anteriorly, but sometimes it is present in the lateral or posterior aspect of the abdominal wall. Do not therefore confine attention to the front of the abdomen, but examine the right flank and the posterior aspect of the abdominal wall, as far as the lateral border of the sacrospinalis muscle. To do so, the patient must roll towards the left side. Tenderness, as opposed to rigidity, will, in many instances, be most in evidence just medial to the anterior superior iliac spine (*Fig.* 507). In cases of high retrocaecal appendicitis the greatest tenderness is in the same plane, but higher—even as high as the level of the umbilicus.
Rectal Examination is essential for every patient with suspected appendicitis with the exception of a young child in whom the examination causes such distress as to make it worthless. The technique is detailed in Chapter 21. Proceed as follows: Palpate the left side of the rectovesical pouch or, in the female, the recto-uterine pouch; then palpate the right side (*Fig.* 508). If there is any doubt as to the relative tenderness, repeat the process, asking the patient, 'Is there any difference in the two sides?' In early cases of pelvic appendicitis the discovery of tenderness on the right is often crucial in the diagnosis. In later cases the finding of a tender lump or cystic swelling (pelvic abscess), when perhaps there

THORKILD ROVSING, 1862–1937, *Professor of Surgery, Copenhagen.*

are few signs on abdominal examination, brings home the almost indispensable necessity for rectal examination.

Atypical Acute Appendicitis is the most difficult of all intra-abdominal emergencies to diagnose. About one out of four cases is atypical. This high proportion is due to: (i) the variability in the length of the appendix (sometimes the terminal portion alone is diseased); (ii) the inconstant position of the organ; (iii) the fact that the disease can occur in infants, the aged, and in pregnant women.

For the real case of doubt and difficulty there are yet two signs that sometimes prove helpful, for they disclose the presence of an inflamed deeply placed appendix lying in contact with the psoas or the obturator muscle respectively.

The Psoas Test. When an inflamed focus lies in contact with the psoas muscle, to relieve the pain the patient often flexes the corresponding thigh. A lesser degree of psoas spasm is ascertained in the following way: With the patient lying on the left side, *hyperextend* the right hip joint. If the psoas muscle is in a state of irritation, this manœuvre causes pain.

The Obturator Test. Flex the right thigh, rotate the hip joint internally. This puts the obturator internus on the stretch. An inflamed appendix in contact with and adherent to this muscle will be irritated by this movement; pain will be experienced in the hypogastrium (Cope).

Acute Appendicitis during Pregnancy. The enlarging uterus causes upward displacement of the caecum thus rendering the pain higher and more lateral than usual, and the area of maximum tenderness is not only displaced likewise, but protected by the uterus and more difficult to demonstrate.

Shifting Tenderness. Having located the most tender spot, mark it on the skin. Now request the patient to turn on the left side and wait for a full minute. Should the tenderness be uterine in origin (concealed accidental haemorrhage; necrobiosis of a uterine fibroid) it will shift with the uterus, whereas in appendicitis the position will remain constant (Alders).

Needless to say, no pregnant woman should have an operation for suspected appendicitis without first having the urine examined microscopically for pus cells.

Acute Appendicitis in the Elderly. In those who have a lax abdominal wall, or those with an overwhelming toxic infection, rigidity is often very slight or even absent. The peculiar danger in the aged is that an atherosclerotic appendicular artery probably favours rapid gangrene of an inflamed obstructed appendix. The distension due to peritonitis leads the clinician to a conclusion that intestinal obstruction is present, an enema is given, the bowels may act as a result, and further delay follows.

Nevertheless acute-on-chronic intestinal obstruction due to colonic carcinoma is also frequent at this time of life and in these cases the brunt of the obstruction is often borne by the caecum (*see* p. 302). Therefore, palpate the whole course of the colon and explore the rectum digitally for the presence of a lump (a carcinoma). If in doubt ask for an erect abdominal X-ray and look for the tell-tale fluid levels indicative of small bowel obstruction.

Acute Appendicitis in Infancy and Childhood

a. In Infancy. Certain vagaries of the clinical picture occur, the four earliest signs at this time of life being pyrexia, abdominal pain, vomiting and local tenderness. Any of these may predominate, any may be absent, any may be associated with another which is uncommon in the early stage in older patients, namely, diarrhoea (Bunton). In a baby the temperature rises precipitously with the onset of an infection, and early considerable pyrexia is present in over 50 per cent of

Sɪʀ Zᴀᴄʜᴀʀʏ Cᴏᴘᴇ, 1881–1974. *Surgeon, St. Mary's Hospital, London.*
Nɪᴄʜᴏʟᴀs Aʟᴅᴇʀs, *Contemporary Emeritus Obstetrician and Gynaecologist, Bournemouth and E. Dorset Hospital Group.*
Gᴇᴏʀɢᴇ L. Bᴜɴᴛᴏɴ, *Contemporary Surgeon, University College Hospital, London.*

cases. The administration of an antibiotic masks the pyrexia and the increased pulse rate more quickly and more certainly than in those of more mature years. Screaming attacks of abdominal pain are usual and call for examination (often repeated examinations) of the abdomen beneath the bedclothes (*see Fig.* 519, p. 305) during the intervals. Always entertain the *possibility* of acute appendicitis *together with* a respiratory infection, gastro-enteritis, or one of the exanthemata. *b. In Childhood.* Screaming children, too young to cooperate in the search for physical signs, sometimes can be placated by the following expedient. The abdomen is palpated with the child's own hand (*Fig.* 509). When the point of maximum tenderness is approached, the child pulls its hand away, and commences crying. This simple method, if carried out patiently, will often succeed in elucidating the area of maximum tenderness when other methods are inconclusive (Grainger). If there is doubt even after this, sedate the child and re-examine when he has fallen asleep. If there is an area of local tenderness due to peritonitis assuredly the child will wake when this area is palpated.

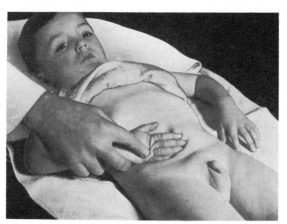

Fig. 509. Palpating the abdomen with the child's own hand.

THE DIFFERENTIAL DIAGNOSIS OF ACUTE APPENDICITIS

'If vomiting or distinct nausea precedes pain, the case is not one of appendicitis.'—
Murphy.

Manifestly it is impossible here to discuss this subject at length, and it suffices to urge that the right lung, right kidney and the pelvic organs in the female be examined. In children consider *non-specific mesenteric adenitis* (*see* p. 315).

The Right Lung. The differentiation between referred abdominal pain attending the diaphragmatic inflammation of pleuropneumonia and peritonitis is a highly responsible one, for obviously to administer an anaesthetic to a patient with pneumonia is, to say the least, undesirable. Such pain can be accompanied by some rigidity, but the absence of rebound tenderness will demonstrate that the peritoneum is not tender, therefore not inflamed, and therefore not the primary source of the abdominal pain. A patient with abdominal pain, not obviously colicky (*see* p. 300) and unaccompanied by tenderness, anywhere in the abdomen, or by tenderness within the pelvis as elicited by rectal examination, can, with confidence, be kept under observation for two or three hours without fear that an urgent surgical emergency is being overlooked.

The Thoracic Compression Test. When it is difficult to decide whether a young child has acute appendicitis or basal lung involvement, compression of the lower thorax from side to side elicits obvious distress when the lesion is above the diaphragm, whereas in appendicitis it has no effect (Dott).

The Right Kidney and Ureter. Perhaps the most confusing differential diagnosis is between acute appendicitis and ureteric colic resulting from a stone in the right ureter (*see* p. 340). To remove the normal appendix of a patient who is suffering from a stone in the right ureter is disconcerting, but relatively harmless. To reverse the mistake, and attribute the pain of an acutely inflamed appendix lying in contact with the right ureter to 'pyelitis' or to ureteric colic is an extremely serious error. Woe betide a patient who has blood or pus cells in the urine because of ureteritis secondary to an inflamed appendix lying in contact with the right ureter. *If localized tenderness persists in the right iliac fossa and a diagnosis of stone in the ureter cannot be confirmed by radiography it is safer to remove the appendix.*

The Pelvic Organs in the Female. *Acute Salpingitis,* although still a condition requiring diagnostic vigilance when accounting for pelvic peritonitis in women of child-bearing age, is less frequently encountered than formerly. This is due to the greatly improved control of gonorrhoea by antibiotics. As emphasized on p. 318, tenderness in salpingitis is commonly bilateral.

Other conditions also liable to be mistaken for appendicitis are ruptured lutein cyst (*see* p. 317), ruptured ectopic gestation (*see* p. 316), and twisted right ovarian cyst (*see* p. 317). All these require surgical treatment and, particularly in women, if there is doubt about the diagnosis, an operation incision should be utilized which is capable of extension to deal with a pelvic abnormality if necessary.

APPENDIX MASS

The patient gives a history consistent with acute appendicitis but several days have elapsed since the onset of the illness. On abdominal examination a mass is found in the right iliac fossa.

Palpate the lump gently. It is very helpful to mark out the limits of the mass with a skin pencil, particularly if the case is to be treated conservatively. The general signs are watched by keeping an hourly pulse and 4-hourly temperature-chart. The local signs can be kept under observation by noting the increase or decrease of the limits of the lump (*Fig.* 510).

Pelvic Appendix Mass. Rectal examination is essential to ascertain whether the abscess is invading the pelvis (*Fig.* 511). Note that acute diarrhoea, accompanied by the passage of mucus, in a patient who has not had dysentery or ulcerative colitis, is suggestive of a pelvic abscess.

POST-APPENDICECTOMY PYREXIA

One is called to see a patient some days or even weeks after an operation for acute appendicitis or appendix mass (or, for that matter, any other abdominal operation) because his condition is unsatisfactory; the temperature is swinging

NORMAN M. DOTT, 1897–1976, *Professor of Neurosurgery, University of Edinburgh.*

and the pulse is elevated—signs that foretell the pocketing of pus. Proceed as follows:

1. Examine the wound and the adjacent abdominal wall for an abscess.
2. Consider the possibility of a pelvic abscess (*see above*).
3. Palpate the left iliac fossa for an abscess in this situation.
4. Examine the loin for a perinephric abscess (*see* p. 344).
5. Look at the legs to exclude the possibility of phlebitis.
6. Examine the sclerae for an icteric tinge and the liver for enlargement. Also inquire if the patient has had rigors—signs that denote pylephlebitis.
7. Examine the lungs—pneumonia, atelectasis, or pulmonary embolus (*see* pp. 192–5).
8. Examine the urine for pus (pyelonephritis) and, in the tropics, the faeces for blood and pus (dysentery).
9. Examine the blood for malaria parasites if the patient has visited the tropics.
10. Lastly, concentrate diagnostic endeavour upon the possibility of a subdiaphragmatic abscess (*see* p. 313).

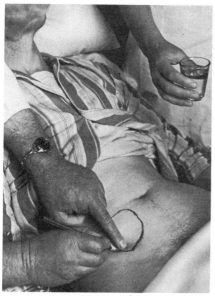

Fig. 510. Appendix abscess. Method of marking out the periphery of the lump with a skin pencil.

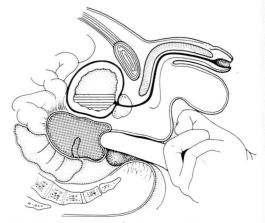

Fig. 511. The rectal findings in an appendix abscess invading the pelvis.

ACUTE COLONIC DIVERTICULITIS

Ninety-five per cent of colonic diverticula giving rise to symptoms are situated in the pelvic colon.

Uncomplicated Acute Diverticulitis. Typically the pain commences in the hypogastrium and passes to the *left* iliac fossa, where the maximum tenderness is situated. This makes the differential diagnosis from appendicitis simple. Nevertheless, the condition presents in many guises. For instance, when an inflamed diverticulum is situated in a loop of colon lying in the pelvis, tenderness is elicited mainly by pelvic examination, and the differentiation between acute pelvic appendicitis and acute diverticulitis is not apparent until laparotomy has been performed.

Acute Free Perforation of an inflamed colonic diverticulum is not uncommon. The signs are those of a very rapid, diffusing peritonitis, and most of the patients have no premonitory symptoms of colonic diverticulitis.

Localized Peridiverticular Abscess is a common complication of acute diverticulitis. When an inflamed diverticulum situated within the mesocolon bursts, the pus will be confined, at any rate for some time, between the layers of the mesocolon. In these circumstances the mesocolon becomes greatly thickened, the bowel angulated, and oedema resulting from pressure on lymphatics and blood vessels is liable to result in incomplete intestinal obstruction. When a slow perforation is not thus confined, it gives rise to a peridiverticular abscess walled in by greater omentum and coils of small intestine and sometimes a tender mass can be palpated in the left iliac fossa but it may be obscured by overlying rigidity.

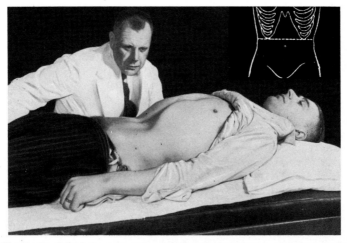

Fig. 512. Watching for abdominal movement on respiration. The patient is placed between the light and the examiner. In this instance retraction of the epigastrium is apparent.

PERFORATED PEPTIC ULCER

Pulse. *For the first six hours the pulse rate is often practically unaltered.* The gravity of the prognosis varies directly with the pulse rate; the great majority of patients diagnosed and treated correctly recover while the pulse is still under 100 beats per minute. As the pulse rate rises the outlook becomes gloomier.

Temperature. The temperature is likely to be subnormal owing to shock. There are few exceptions to this rule.

Inspection. *Retraction of the Epigastrium.* In an early case, especially if the subject is a spare, muscular man, this is a characteristic sign (*Fig.* 512). If well-marked, when viewed laterally, the appearance is as if an invisible rope was constricting the abdomen at the level indicated in *Fig.* 512 (inset) due to

muscular contraction of the diaphragm and anterior abdominal wall (Willan).
As time passes this sign is lost.

Carefully inspect the abdomen for respiratory movement. The patient should
be placed between the light and the examiner. In perforated ulcer the abdominal
muscles are held so rigidly that respiration is almost entirely of the thoracic type.
The respirations are often of a peculiar grunting character.

'Point to the place where it hurts you now.' Often the patient indicates that the
whole abdomen is painful.

'Point to the place where the pain started.' Quite frequently there is a finger
pointing to the epigastrium.

Palpation. The abdomen is now palpated systematically, commencing in the left
iliac fossa. *Board-like rigidity* is characteristic, and the cardinal sign of the
condition. With the onset of diffusing peritonitis and consequent distension,
rigidity (and to a great extent the agonizing pain) passes off to a varying degree.

Percussion. The absence of liver dullness in the midaxillary line is very fair
evidence of gas in the peritoneal cavity. As a rule it is only in late cases of
perforation that sufficient gas collects to give a tympanitic note. However, when
sought for carefully, this sign proves helpful in making the diagnosis.

It is possible to be deceived by overlying emphysema of the lung. If in doubt
on clinical grounds (which is unusual) a radiograph with the patient erect will
confirm a crescent of translucency beneath the right cupola of the diaphragm.

Rectal Examination. When the patient is in great pain, rectal examination should
be undertaken in the dorsal position. Sometimes tenderness can be detected in
the rectovesical pouch (*see Fig. 511*).

Reflexes. Test the knee jerks and the reaction of the pupils to light if definite rigidity is absent. A
gastric crisis of tabes dorsalis is now a rarity and perforated peptic ulcer is more likely than a crisis
in patients with tabes dorsalis.

Perforated Gastric Ulcer. The diagnosis is seldom really difficult. Diaphragmatic
pleurisy and coronary thrombosis (*see* p. 319) are most likely to be confused.
The clinician who is unaware of the three entities mentioned under the heading
of Abdominal Aortic Catastrophes on p. 320 is likely to mistake these, admittedly
uncommon conditions, for a perforated gastric ulcer.

Special Features of Perforated Duodenal Ulcer. Perforated duodenal ulcer is
considerably more common than perforated gastric ulcer, and while, as a rule,
the physical signs to which each gives rise are identical, in the case of perforated
duodenal ulcer there is one diagnostic pitfall—the phenomenon of the right
paracolic gutter. When a duodenal ulcer perforates, the ascending colon may
act as a watershed and direct the escaping fluid to the right iliac fossa (*Fig. 513*).
Thus, as judged by the extent of abdominal rigidity, the differential diagnosis
between a perforated duodenal ulcer and perforated appendicitis can become
difficult. It is true that in the former the rigidity tends to be more extensive and
the maximum tenderness is found to be higher than would be expected in
appendicitis, but it is sometimes a problem to decide which organ is at fault. In
this connection Rovsing's sign (*see* p. 290) is of assistance.

Perforated Duodenal Ulcer sealed by Omentum. This is well worth bearing in
mind. The patient can move about surprisingly well; indeed, he may walk to
hospital. Rigidity is variable depending on the amount of leakage, but confined

ROBERT J. WILLAN, 1878–1955, *Professor of Surgery, University of Durham, Newcastle upon Tyne.*

to the epigastrium and right hypochondrium (*Fig.* 514) and soon disappears if oral intake is stopped and an intravenous infusion started.

Fig. 513. Fluid tracking down the right paracolic gutter, which explains how the symptoms and signs of a perforated duodenal ulcer can be referred to the right iliac fossa.

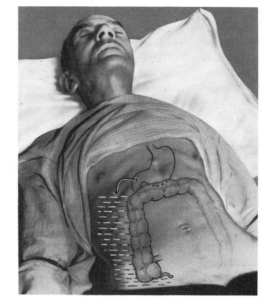

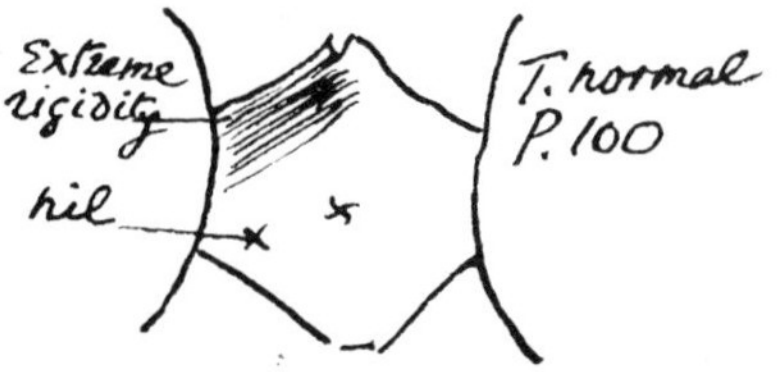

Fig. 514. Physical signs recorded in a case of perforated duodenal ulcer sealed by omentum, known colloquially as 'dry perforation'.

MASSIVE HAEMORRHAGE FROM A PEPTIC ULCER WITH OR WITHOUT HAEMATEMESIS

When the loss of blood is great enough to produce signs of hypotension or necessitate the administration of 1500 ml or more of blood in 24 hours, by convention the haemorrhage is said to be massive.

First visit: The patient should lie flat in bed with only one pillow beneath the head, and be kept warm, but not heated artificially in any way. Take the pulse rate and the blood pressure. These data as compared with those at a future examination are often more valuable than laboratory reports. Inquire whether the patient has ingested aspirin recently; this can cause bleeding from the normal gastric mucosa in susceptible persons. Come to a conclusion concerning the patient's pallor (if present) in the facies, the conjunctiva of a lower lid, and the fingernails—these are the best guides. Examine the tongue for dryness. Then examine the abdomen. Palpate gently for tenderness and rigidity to exclude a concomitant perforation. Deep palpation for a lump in the epigastrium should be eschewed at this early stage. Always disturb a partially exsanguinated patient as little as possible. None the less, Troisier's Sign (*see* p. 140) should be sought from in front. Also exclude portal hypertension by examining for spider naevi, palmar erythema, and an enlarged liver and spleen.

Rectal examination is of fundamental importance. If faeces are present the all-important question is, 'Is the faecal matter blended with recognizable blood, or are the faeces tarry?' If the latter, enquire if the patient is taking an iron preparation by mouth.

Second visit: Once the patient has had one hour's rest, with blood transfusion, the pulse rate is a reliable guide. Signs that bleeding has seriously depleted the blood volume, and is probably progressing, are beads of perspiration on the forehead, cool clammy hands, and increasing anaemic pallor, though the last is sometimes difficult to perceive in artificial light. Quickening of the quarter-hourly pulse rate is the best single sign of progressive or renewed bleeding. A gastric aspiration tube should be *in situ*, and the nature of the aspirate is valuable direct evidence.

Should the rate of respiration increase *pari passu* with the pulse, the cause is more likely to be cardiac failure or bronchopneumonia, particularly if increasing pallor is not in evidence.

A probable source of severe melaena in childhood and in youth (up to the age of about 16) is a peptic ulcer in the vicinity of a Meckel's diverticulum. Often the blood passed per rectum is bright red; it is unmixed with mucus.

ACUTE CHOLECYSTITIS

The onset is often sudden and the pain is usually severe. After a variable period (usually 2 to 3 hours) biliary colic is superseded by dull, throbbing pain localized in the right hypochondrium. Nausea, retching and vomiting, together with belching of a large quantity of gas, a rise in temperature, and an elevated pulse rate, are characteristic. Examination of a patient with an acute inflammation of the gallbladder does not differ from that for chronic inflammation (*see* p. 229). Tenderness and rigidity can be elicited in the right hypochondrium, and Murphy's sign (*see* p. 230) is present. Jaundice occurs in about 25 per cent of cases. Charcot's triad is due to infection of pent-up bile in the common bile duct (cholangitis) and consists of pain, jaundice and rigors, the latter being due to septicaemia. A palpable swelling in the region of the gallbladder—indisputable evidence that the organ is wrapped in protective greater omentum—often becomes recognizable at some time in the clinical course, but often not when most required to clinch the diagnosis, for overlying rigidity renders the mass impalpable. Often the diagnosis presents no particular difficulty; sometimes, right-sided pyelonephritis must be excluded. The conditions most difficult to differentiate is a sealed-off perforation (*see* p. 296) or a myocardial infarct (*see* p. 319) or the following:

Sudden Tender Enlargement of the Liver in Congestive Cardiac Failure. The temperature is normal and the patient is manifestly short of breath. The fact that the liver is uniformly enlarged may be masked by overlying rigidity. The essential clue is that the external jugular veins are engorged (*see Fig.* 32, p. 17).

ACUTE PANCREATITIS

Acute pancreatitis can occur at almost any age, but is unusual before the thirtieth year and rare in childhood. In some parts of the world, notably the USA, alcoholism is an important factor.

Pain. This condition competes with perforated peptic ulcer in producing the most severe of all abdominal pains which is constant more often than colicky and gradually increases in agonizing severity. The pain is centred in the epigastrium

Johann Friedrich Meckel (the Younger), 1781–1833, *Professor of Anatomy and Surgery, Halle, Germany.*
Jean-Martin Charcot, 1825–93, *Physician, Hôpital Salpêtrière, Paris.*

and it tends to radiate to the back or to the left loin. In order to gain some measure of relief, often the patient sits up and leans forward ———————————————→ 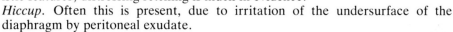 or lies on the side in the knee–chest position.

Vomiting usually follows the pain, but it has no characteristic features; distressing retching is much in evidence.

Hiccup. Often this is present, due to irritation of the undersurface of the diaphragm by peritoneal exudate.

Pulse. The pulse rate is nearly always quickened from the commencement of the acute pancreatitis.

Temperature is at first subnormal. Seldom during the first 24 hours does it rise much above normal.

Shock. Some degrees of shock is present in 25 per cent of cases: only in very severe or untreated cases is it pronounced and long-lasting.

Cyanosis. In its most severe forms acute pancreatitis is accompanied by slight cyanosis of the lips.

Jaundice. Slight jaundice is often evident in natural light.

Abdominal Examination. *Rigidity*: The absence of general rigidity, or at any rate the absence of board-like rigidity, is a sign of considerable importance. As with almost every dogmatic statement relating to clinical matters, there are exceptions.

Tenderness and rebound tenderness are present in the central region of the upper abdomen and are usually most pronounced just above the umbilicus. When acute pancreatitis is suspected the left costovertebral angle should be palpated for tenderness due to inflammation of the tail of the pancreas.

Differential Diagnosis. Acute pancreatitis is most frequently mistaken for a perforated peptic ulcer. Nearly as often, biliary colic is diagnosed. Myocardial infarction also is to be reckoned with when the attack is very sudden and severe, and pallor, sweating, low blood pressure and oliguria dominate the picture.

An incontestable diagnosis of acute pancreatitis is essential, because it is now agreed that laparotomy should not be performed for this condition. The diagnosis should thus be confirmed by a scientific method or methods, if facilities exist. *The serum-amylase level* is the pillar upon which rests the diagnosis. A considerable rise is good corroborative, but not absolute, evidence.

Later Manifestations. *Ileus*: After 12 hours, peristalsis diminishes and unless it is prevented by gastrointestinal aspiration, abdominal distension supervenes.

A Tender Mass in the Epigastrium due to fluid in the lesser sac (pseudopancreatic cyst) can occasionally (1 in 30 cases) be felt from the fourth to sixth days.

Skin Discoloration has been reported in the left flank and also around the umbilicus in a few late cases.

ACUTE INTESTINAL OBSTRUCTION

Whether it be of the strangulating or the non-strangulating variety, the mortality from acute intestinal obstruction rises with each passing hour from the onset of symptoms. Consequently early diagnosis remains a great responsibility. Often it can be made without radiological assistance which, although desirable, is not essential except in cases of doubt.

ACUTE OBSTRUCTION OF THE SMALL INTESTINE

This is more difficult to diagnose in its comparatively early stages than similar obstruction of the large intestine.

Pain. When the obstruction lies in the jejunum or high in the ileum, the characteristic bouts of intestinal colic, each waxing in intensity to an agonizing zenith and then waning, occur at intervals of 3–5 minutes. In obstruction of the terminal ileum the intervals are longer-lasting—6–10 minutes.

Vomiting. Retrograde peristalsis causes the stomach to eject whatever food or fluid it contains; this is followed by the contents of the duodenum, which are predominantly bile. Later the contents of the small intestine above the site of the obstruction are expelled with gradual lessening force as the antiperistaltic waves grow weaker. Inspect the vomitus as described on p. 19. Only after three or more days of virtually complete intestinal obstruction does the vomit become faeculent.

Dehydration. Obstruction of the jejunum or high in the ileum results in a tremendous loss of water and electrolytes. Conversely, obstruction of the terminal ileum is associated with relatively little loss of fluid and salts, for most of the secretions of the alimentary canal are resorbed for at least·two or three days after the onset of obstruction situated in this region. It therefore follows that signs of dehydration are slow to develop in obstruction of the terminal ileum, whereas in obstruction of the jejunum they become obvious, and often overwhelming, in 48 hours.

Constipation. The absence of a history of recent constipation in no way excludes a diagnosis of obstruction of the small intestine. For instance, if the patient had his bowels open in the morning and the symptoms commenced in the afternoon, it would be necessary to wait for at least 24 hours for constipation to be a significant sign. Moreover, the rule that constipation is present in intestinal obstruction is broken in mesenteric vascular occlusion (*see* p. 308), Richter's hernia, and a pelvic abscess associated with obstruction by adhesions—all of which are liable to produce an irritative diarrhoea.

The Tongue. In late untreated obstruction it is brown, furred and dry.

Abdominal Examination. In a suspected case of acute intestinal obstruction, the first duty should be to *examine the hernial sites, inguinal, femoral and umbilical.* This axiom is an old one, but one that can still bear much repetition. An umbilical hernia can hardly be missed; an irreducible inguinal hernia usually is obvious; it is the small unobtrusive femoral hernia that is the stumbling-block, the frequency with which such a hernia, often of the Richter type, being overlooked is astonishing. Usually the patient is an old lady. Occasionally the attending doctor has seen and felt the lump, but has considered it to be an enlarged lymph node. Far more frequently, pandering to the false modesty of his patient, he has failed to draw down the bedclothes far enough. With proper exposure (*Fig.* 515), almost invariably the tell-tale lump is perfectly evident, the exception being extreme obesity.

Inspection. In the early stages obstruction of the small intestine rarely shows more than perhaps a suggestive fullness. Ladder patterns are very characteristic (*Fig.* 516) but are not commonly seen, and, for that matter, should not be, for their presence indicates a late diagnosis. Visible peristalsis more often requires

---

AUGUST G. RICHTER, 1742–1812, *Surgeon, Göttingen, Germany. In 1777 described strangulation of a portion only of the gut wall.*

patient watchfulness. Sit down beside the bed and watch the abdomen. Sometimes gentle flicking of the abdominal wall will initiate visible peristalsis.

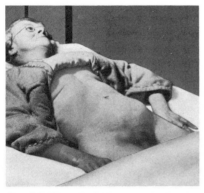

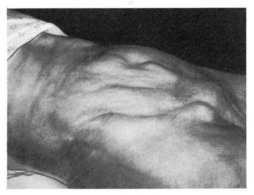

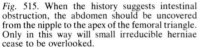

Fig. 515. When the history suggests intestinal obstruction, the abdomen should be uncovered from the nipple to the apex of the femoral triangle. Only in this way will small irreducible herniae cease to be overlooked.

Fig. 516. Visible peristalsis, showing the characteristic ladder pattern. Case of irreducible right femoral hernia, which can be seen also.

Palpation occasionally reveals a lump, such as an intussusception, a neoplasm of the small intestine, an intra-abdominal abscess to which small intestine is adherent, or, exceptionally, a coil of distended intestine entrapped by a band or in an internal hernia. Even when peristalsis is not visible, it may be palpable. If the hand is kept flat upon the abdomen the underlying coil may be felt to harden and soften alternately, much like a pregnant uterus (Burgess).

Rebound tenderness (*see* p. 288) in a localized area suggests that the obstructed bowel has lost its blood supply (i.e. it is strangulated).

Percussion usually is inconclusive except that a resonant note is obtained all over, indicative of gaseous distension of the bowel.

Auscultation. All the time we have been watching, percussing and palpating the abdomen, we should at the same time have been listening—for borborygmi. Now comes the time for unhurried abdominal auscultation. Again sit beside the right side of the patient's abdomen. Apply the cup of the stethoscope to the abdominal wall just below and to the right of the umbilicus. When the case is one of acute obstruction of the small intestine in its comparatively early stages, it will not be long before the clinician will hear gurgling sounds. These characteristic sounds commence at a low pitch and, in the course of 30 seconds, rise to higher-pitched tinkles, the pitch becoming higher as intraluminal tension rises. *The coexistence of intestinal colic and borborygmi answering to this description establishes the diagnosis of obstruction of the small intestine in more than 9 out of 10 cases.*

A *Succussion Splash* (*see* p. 227) heard with the stethoscope is confirmatory evidence that there is a distended loop or loops of bowel containing fluid.

Rectal Examination. In cases of obstruction of the small intestine digital examination of the rectum usually reveals no abnormality. Occasionally it is possible to make out a distended coil of small intestine in the pelvis. It is also

ARTHUR H. BURGESS, 1864–1948, *Surgeon, Manchester Royal Infirmary.*

possible that the lump caused by an intussusception, a neoplasm of the small intestine, or a gallstone obstructing the small intestine may be felt.

ACUTE OBSTRUCTION OF THE LARGE INTESTINE

In many parts of the world acute obstruction of the large intestine is, almost exclusively, the result of a carcinoma of the colon or of the rectum. The minority of remaining cases is due to chronic diverticulitis or, in the case of the rectum, to faecal impaction. Such obstruction is, more correctly speaking, acute-on-chronic obstruction. Only in those dwelling in, or hailing from, Eastern Europe, Peru, Scandinavia, Ghana and some parts of India is obstruction from these causes rivalled in frequency by volvulus of the pelvic colon (*see* p. 307), which gives rise to very acute, as opposed to acute-on-chronic, intestinal obstruction. In Iran volvulus of the pelvic colon, caecum and small bowel make up nearly half of all intestinal obstructions (Saidi). In Nigeria the commonest cause of intestinal obstruction at all ages (apart from external hernia) is idiopathic intussusception.

Before detailing the peculiar features of acute-on-chronic obstruction of the large intestine it is essential to dwell for a moment on the ileocaecal valve, which is a sphincter (Chesterman). When occlusion of any part of the large intestine occurs its behaviour determines the clinical course, and therefore the physical signs, of the obstruction. There are three possibilities, each present in approximately a third of cases (*Fig.* 517).

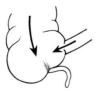 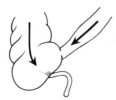 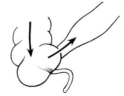

| Fig. 517a. | Fig. 517b. | Fig. 517c. |

Type 1 (*Fig.* 517*a*). *The Valve retains its Normal Function,* i.e. it prevents reflux into the ileum but its periodic relaxation synchronizes with each peristaltic wave of the ileum. This allows the contents of the small intestine to pass into the large intestine and causes a comparatively rapid and great increase of intraluminal pressure within the colon, and particularly within the caecum. The distension is confined to the large intestine above the site of the obstruction, and is so excessive that it sometimes imperils the blood supply of the caecal wall and terminates in gangrene.

Type 2 (*Fig.* 517*b*). *The Valve remains Contracted.* Increasing distension of the large intestine proceeds at a moderate pace, while signs of obstruction of the ileum, due to its inability to pass its contents onwards, commence a few hours after the onset. By the time the patient presents, more often than not the signs are those of combined large and small gut obstruction.

Type 3 (*Fig* 517*c*). *The Valve relaxes and remains Incompetent.* Reflux from the large into the small intestine permits the former to decompress itself into the latter. As a result, signs of acute intestinal obstruction are long-delayed, and when they do become apparent they are virtually indistinguishable from those of obstruction of the ileum. Only in this type of large-gut intestinal obstruction is ballooning of the caecum absent.

For these reasons, in acute large bowel obstruction the clinician must expect a varying picture. However, in general it can be stated that obstruction of the large intestine commences less abruptly than that of the small intestine, and in the acute-on-chronic variety it is always preceded by increasing constipation

Farrokh Saidi, *Contemporary Surgeon, Tehran, Iran.*
Judson T. Chesterman, *Contemporary Thoracic Surgeon, City General Hospital, Sheffield.*

over several, if not many, days. When the acute stage has been reached, the intervals between the bouts of the colicky pain and hyperperistalsis are longer and less rhythmical than when the obstruction is situated in the small intestine. Vomiting is delayed for days. Thus, unless the acute obstruction has been allowed to persist until a very advanced stage, or complications have set in, the patient neither looks nor feels ill. The distension is mainly gaseous.

Abdominal Examination. *Inspection.* Except in Type 3, there is early abdominal distension which fills the flanks. In Type 1 and Type 2, wherever the obstruction may be, the brunt will be seen at the caecum, which occasionally can be seen momentarily rising with each wave of peristalsis, like a small balloon, so that particular attention should be paid to the right iliac fossa.

Palpation. The main objective is to seek the presence of a lump in the course of the colon, but as it is an annular carcinoma, as opposed to a large mass, that usually gives rise to obstruction, we are seldom thus favoured because of the concomitant distension. The incidence of obstruction in the right half of the colon is five times less than that in the left half.

Percussion. Hyper-resonance, particularly over the caecum, is a *sine qua non*.

Rectal Examination is imperative, carcinoma of the rectum being an occasional cause of acute large-intestine obstruction. Sometimes a mass of inspissated faeces causing impaction will be felt, its identification becoming indisputable if the mass can be indented by the finger. The apex of an intussusception initiated by the presence of a circumscribed benign or malignant neoplasm of the colon is an infrequent, but welcome, finding—welcome because, even if it should prove to be a carcinoma, the neoplasm that intussuscepts is assuredly at an early stage of its development. Ballooning of the rectum is a not infrequent, but unreliable, sign of obstruction beyond the finger. If the rectum is completely empty, it is at least suggestive of higher obstruction.

Other Methods of Examination. In doubtful cases an *enema* should be given, but it should be remembered that it is the second enema which yields the more useful information. By absolute constipation is meant that after the *second* enema no faeces and, above all, no flatus is passed.

If in doubt and radiographic facilities are lacking take a *tape measure* and place it round the abdomen at the level of the umbilicus. Note the measurement. Leave it in place behind the patient, and measure again in 2 hours. This accurate measurement of the girth is more reliable than an impression as to whether distension is greater than at a previous examination.

Before leaving the subject of intestinal obstruction it is necessary to warn the reader to keep a sharp look-out for *uraemia*, which on occasions simulates intestinal obstruction closely (*see* p. 309).

SPECIAL VARIETIES OF INTESTINAL OBSTRUCTION

Intestinal Obstruction in the Newborn. During the first 36 hours of life 90 per cent of babies vomit amniotic fluid, vaginal secretions and blood, swallowed respectively before and during birth. When a newborn baby continues to vomit repeatedly there are only three explanations—intracranial haemorrhage, severe infection and intestinal obstruction. As a rule, the first two show such special characteristics that their identification is assured; exceptions are a subdural haematoma (*see* p.66) and meningitis, especially that due to *E. coli*.

The Vomiting of Intestinal Obstruction. Should the vomitus become bile-stained (green*) it is safe to assume that the cause of vomiting is intestinal obstruction.
Abdominal Distension. Minor degrees are difficult to perceive because of the normal protuberance of an infant's abdomen. Pronounced fullness at birth suggests intestinal obstruction arising in utero, but there are other causes, notably a distended bladder due to urethral obstruction, congenital cystic kidneys, fetal ascites and meconium peritonitis. In all except the last, a considerable part or most of the abdomen is dull to percussion. When tympanitic distension is present at birth, and dilated veins are seen coursing over the abdominal wall (*Fig.* 518), the case is almost certain to be one of meconium ileus (inspissated meconium blocking the ileum—a condition due to fibrocystic disease of the pancreas). Distension due to congenital atresia of the intestine does not appear until six or more hours after birth, and is for the most part the result of the swallowing of air.

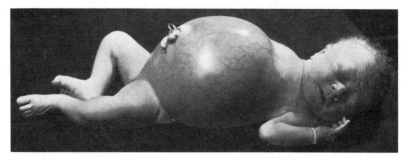

Fig. 518. Meconium ileus. The superficial dilated veins and the shiny appearance of the skin are characteristic.

Failure to pass Meconium is an important corroborative sign of neonatal intestinal obstruction. Nevertheless, during the first three days of life its passage is not inconsistent with a diagnosis of intestinal obstruction; indeed, 40 per cent of infants suffering from intestinal atresia pass meconium stools.
Rectal Examination. Imperforate anus is discussed on p. 280. In other varieties of intestinal obstruction the anal canal and distal rectum are often narrowed, and withdrawal of the finger is seldom followed by the passage of meconium, as is usual in neonates.
General Appearance. Normally the neonate lives on its own resources until the maternal flow of real milk is established, and it is this fact that accounts for the seeming lustiness of a neonate with intestinal obstruction during the first 48 hours of life—a misleading fact that encourages procrastination in making the diagnosis. Only in the strangulating obstruction of volvulus of the midgut is this misleading paradox absent, for dehydration and electrolyte depletion occur rapidly because of the copious vomiting of bile and pancreatic and gastric secretions.
Sudden Deterioration of the Infant usually coincides with commencing gangrene of the intestine; the chemical imbalance resulting therefrom causes instability of

---

* In the newborn yellow coloration of the vomitus derives from carotene present in colostrum and is not abnormal.

the respiratory centre and early exodus from collapse of the lungs or weakening of the cough reflex, which invites inhalation of gastric contents, and inevitable pneumonia.

Although intestinal obstruction in the newborn is often remediable by early operation, frequently the condition remains undiagnosed for several days. Therefore greater effort should be made to recognize the signs set out above and to resort immediately to *plain radiography of the abdomen* to help in confirming the diagnosis before the infant becomes enfeebled.

When confronted with a neonate who exhibits some of the signs of intestinal obstruction consider the following possibilities:

Congenital Atresia of the Oesophagus. *See* p. 195.

Infantile Pyloric Stenosis (*see* p. 228) is rare before the third week of life. There is no bile in the vomit.

Hirschsprung's Disease. *See* p. 241.

Examination of an Infant for an Intussusception.* The age incidence has altered, probably due to earlier weaning. Cases are now seen as early as two months and up to two years but most occur in the first year of life.

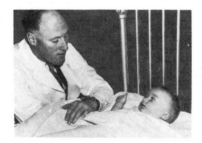

Fig. 519. Examination of the abdomen of an infant for an intussusception. Palpation under the bedclothes between the spasms. The clinician must be seated.

Almost invariably the nurse will start to pull down the bedclothes in order to expose the child's abdomen. Request her not to do so. If the child is asleep, so much the better, but we are rarely so favoured. Take a chair and sit beside the bed—wait, and warm the right hand. Slip the warm hand under the bedclothes, place it upon the abdomen, and go on waiting until the child stops crying (*Fig.* 519). One cannot expect to feel an intra-abdominal swelling when the child is screaming; its abdominal muscles are contracted rigidly. When the crying has ceased—palpate. Pay particular attention to the right hypochondrium. Sometimes the swelling will be felt to harden as a wave of peristalsis commences, and the diagnosis is certain. In the splenic region the lump may pass beneath the costal margin, thus eluding the examiner ⟶

During the whole time palpation has been in progress, the clinician should be observing the patient's face intently. When crying has ceased, the colour of the cheeks is noted: is the child paler than it should be? In this connection, bear in mind that a child suffering from intussusception never smiles, and in cases of more than 6 hours' duration signs of dehydration (*see* p. 45) appear.

---

* *Intussusception.* Latin, *intus* = within + *suscipere* = to receive. The receiving of one part within another.

One important piece of information to be gleaned from the face is, is the baby undergoing spasms of colic? If the abdominal muscles harden simultaneously with a fleeting expression of pain as a prelude to an attack of crying, there can be no doubt: the little patient *is* experiencing colic.

Pyrexia. In most patients the temperature becomes somewhat elevated during the first 24 hours. A clinician unfamiliar with the condition might interpret the pyrexia to indicate an infection rather than an intussusception, but severe colic and pallor, with intervals of quietude, contrast with the continual whimpering and flushing of the face of a baby with upper respiratory infection.

The '*Signe de Dance*' a feeling of emptiness in the right iliac fossa—is not of much help, seldom being ascertainable in these small patients except, possibly, when under an anaesthetic preparatory to an operation.

Rectal Examination. If the lump is low enough in the colon, it will be felt. The apex of an intussusception feels exactly like a cervix uteri. Look at the examining finger afterwards—a 'red-currant jelly' exudate is pathognomonic (*see Fig. 36, p. 20*). Ask to see the baby's soiled napkin and scrutinize the discharge.

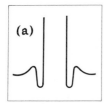 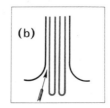

Fig. 520. The differential diagnosis between (a) rectal prolapse and (b) intussusception protruding from the anus. In rectal prolapse the projecting mucosa will be felt continuous with the perianal skin, whereas in intussusception the finger passes *ad infinitum* into the depths of the sulcus.

Intussusception protruding from the Anus. This is now a rarity except in areas remote from medical facilities. The differential diagnosis between prolapse of the rectum and intussusception causes perplexity, for in both there is a large rosette of congested mucosa presenting externally. The problem is solved as shown in *Fig. 520*.

Intussusception in Adolescence is usually caused by an inverted Meckel's diverticulum. Peutz–Jeghers syndrome (*see* p. 109) is worthy of exclusion.

Acute Intussusception in Adults. Unless the apex of the intussusception appears at the anus, or can be felt per rectum, the correct diagnosis rarely is made before operation. The key physical sign is a sausage-shaped lump that can be felt to harden beneath the palpating fingers; a lump that is felt at one time, but not at another. In its fully developed state the intussusception gives rise to strangulating obstruction.

Intussusception and Purpura. Sometimes in older children and adults the symptoms of intussusception (intestinal colic and the passage of bloodstained mucus) are closely mimicked by purpura with intestinal symptoms; indeed, occasionally an intussusception results from the protrusion caused by a submucosal haemorrhage occurring in this condition. At first sight, especially in an artificial light, the characteristic multiple small petechial* haemorrhages in the skin have been mistaken for fleabites. If the whole body is examined, larger ecchymoses† or definite bruises may be found, especially on the buttocks (*Fig. 521*) and the ear lobules.

In such cases the abdomen should be palpated for the presence of a lump, and the left hypochondrium examined for enlargement of the spleen. In only a quarter of cases of thrombocyto-

---

* *Petechia.* Latin= a spot.
† *Ecchymosis.* Greek, ἐκ = out + χυμός = juice. Skin discoloration due to extravasation of blood.

JEAN B. H. DANCE, 1797–1832, *Physician, Hôpital Cochin, Paris.*

paenic purpura (the most common variety to give rise to intestinal symptoms) is the spleen enlarged to the extent of being palpable.

Hess's Tourniquet Test. This is performed by applying the cuff of a sphygmomanometer to an arm, and after taking the blood pressure, inflating the cuff to register a pressure midway between that of the systolic and diastolic pressures, for 5 minutes after which the cubital fossa is examined for petechiae. If more than twenty are present in a 3-cm diameter circle (*Fig.* 522) the test is positive, indicating excessive capillary fragility—*the abnormality in all the purpuras.*

Gallstone Ileus. Obturation* of the small intestine by a gallstone is perhaps the most elusive form of intestinal obstruction. Usually the subjects are elderly, and the obstruction in the early stage is of an intermittent character. The possibility of this supremely remediable condition should be before us in every doubtful case of obstruction occurring in the evening of life.

An abdominal radiograph may show the stone; alternatively, the bile passages may be outlined by gas which has entered via the fistula between the gallbladder and bowel.

Food Bolus Obstruction. As with gallstone ileus the obstruction tends to be intermittent. Clues to the correct diagnosis are firstly that the patient has had an operation which includes some form of gastro-enterostomy or pyloroplasty, and secondly has recently ingested vegetable matter (commonly orange-pith) which has been improperly chewed, the patient often being edentulous.

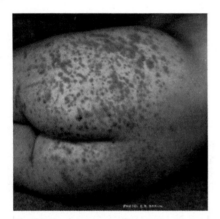

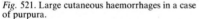

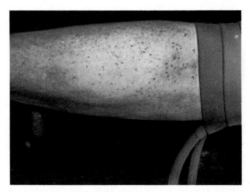

Fig. 521. Large cutaneous haemorrhages in a case of purpura.

Fig. 522. Tourniquet test for purpura—a positive reaction.

Volvulus of the Sigmoid Colon. Middle-aged or elderly males are the usual victims. There is often a history of attacks of abdominal pain with constipation, followed by watery stools and copious evacuation of flatus. These attacks are due to twists that undergo spontaneous rectification. As a rule, the onset is sudden, and is characterized by severe abdominal pain, usually coming on while the patient is straining at stool. In no other conditions does extreme abdominal distension come on so quickly (*Fig.* 523). In a matter of six hours the whole abdomen becomes distended. Hiccup and retching occur early; vomiting is late. Constipation is absolute, but an enema may be returned bloodstained. As mentioned on p. 279, occasionally the rectal wall is felt to be oedematous.

---

* *Obturation.* Latin, *obturore* = to stop up. Intestinal obstruction due to an object within the bowel lumen.

ALFRED F. HESS, 1875–1933, *Clinical Professor of Pediatrics, New York University.*

Volvulus of the Caecum. For this to occur the caecum must have a mesentery which often serves the whole of the small intestine as well as the right half of the colon. Consequently, do not expect the ballooned obstructed caecum necessarily to occupy the right iliac fossa. Typically a tense, palpable, resonant swelling occupies a central position and sometimes becomes visible during a spasm of colic, being thrown into relief by a concavity in the right iliac fossa.

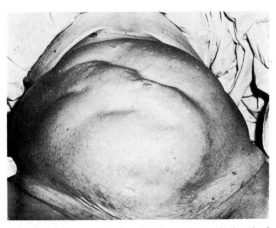

Fig. 523. In volvulus of the sigmoid colon, owing to the length of the mesentery, the swelling is seen first in the right iliac fossa.

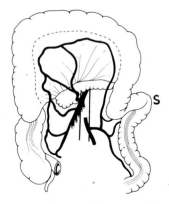

Fig. 524. The marginal artery of Drummond. The transverse colon has been elevated to demonstrate its mesentery. S = splenic flexure of colon.

CONDITIONS SIMULATING ACUTE INTESTINAL OBSTRUCTION

Mesenteric Vascular Occlusion. The signs are those of intestinal strangulation but seldom those of intestinal obstruction. After a variable length of time (hours–days), signs of diffuse peritonitis monopolize the entire picture.

Mesenteric *arterial* occlusion occurs suddenly.

Shock is pronounced in the early stages.

Pain is colicky at first but after about an hour it becomes unrelenting. The pain appears too severe to be reconciled with the moderate signs exhibited on abdominal examination: in this respect mesenteric arterial occlusion resembles acute pancreatitis.

Vomiting is so oft-repeated that it occasions great distress. Gastric intubation having been carried out, the aspirate continues to be copious and soon changes from 'pure bile' to more faeculent-appearing fluid.

Haematemesis and/or Melaena occurs in about a third of cases.

ABDOMINAL EXAMINATION. *Rigidity* is circumscribed: it is confined to that part of the abdominal wall overlying the infarcted area.

Tenderness on palpation and rebound tenderness are also confined to the above-named area, which is usually centred just above the umbilicus.

An Indefinite Lump is found in a few cases. If present, it is likely to react to gravity when the patient is placed on the side, i.e. it shifts towards the flank.

Should a patient with the above symptoms and several, or all, of the above signs be known to be suffering from mitral stenosis or auricular fibrillation, or be an elderly patient with pipe-stem arteries and cardiac impairment, the provisional diagnosis of mesenteric arterial occlusion should follow but the condition sometimes occurs spontaneously in healthy individuals.

Mesenteric *venous* occlusion is a somewhat different type of lesion; it occurs over many hours or even days. Usually it follows intra-abdominal infection or results from portal hypertension. When infarction becomes massive the signs become indistinguishable from those of mesenteric arterial occlusion. A diagnostic enema often produces a stool containing much dark blood.

Ischaemic Colitis. In contradistinction to the above the degree of arterial blockage (which occurs in middle-aged or elderly patients who usually suffer from associated vascular disease) does not frequently cause frank gangrene and the bowel usually recovers, sometimes with stricture formation. The occluded vessel is the marginal artery of Drummond (*Fig.* 524) which is narrowest at the splenic flexure, the segment of bowel predominantly affected.

Clinically there is incomplete intestinal obstruction (due to narrowing of the oedematous bowel), with rectal bleeding and tenderness in the left abdomen due to localized peritonitis. In *acute* colonic diverticulitis (*see* p. 294) bleeding is a rarity, a fact which may enable differentiation from ischaemic colitis which is much less frequently encountered.

Pseudo-intestinal Obstruction. A patient presents with extravagant abdominal distension and has not passed faeces or flatus for several days. It seems obvious that he is suffering from advanced intestinal obstruction but rectal examination reveals some faeces, and as the patient is old and decrepit an erect abdominal X-ray is ordered to confirm the presence of fluid levels. Surprisingly these are few or absent, the distension being largely confined to the colon. Reconsider the situation carefully. Respiratory embarrassment due to elevation of the diaphragm by the distended colon is common—an unusual feature with organic intestinal obstruction. Laparotomy, in many cases, has shown distended colon without organic obstruction, and is best avoided. On occasion the caecum ruptures from extreme distension and tenderness on palpation in the right iliac fossa makes laparotomy essential. Otherwise treatment should be conservative although an urgent barium enema X-ray may prove necessary to confirm that there is no obstructing colonic carcinoma.

Uraemic Ileus. Abdominal distension, hiccup and vomiting are frequent accompaniments of advanced uraemia, and uraemic ileus is not infrequently mistaken for intestinal obstruction. Both intestinal obstruction and uraemia can give rise to oliguria. Uraemia from chronic renal failure can mimic intestinal obstruction in two ways. In the first place intense vomiting of sudden onset sometimes occurs in uraemia and it simulates the vomiting of obstruction of the small intestine. If the patient is very thin, normal peristalsis is visible and the resemblance to intestinal obstruction is heightened. Secondly, uraemia often is accompanied by unmistakable abdominal distension due to paralytic ileus, and in view of the fact that most examples of obstruction of the large intestine occur in elderly patients, among whom renal insufficiency is not uncommon, the possible presence of uraemic ileus must be kept in mind.

When the signs are due to uraemia there may be a uriniferous smell in the breath; infrequently an enlarged kidney or kidneys can be palpated—in cases due to congenital cystic kidneys there is seldom difficulty in this direction. In uraemia the urine is likely to be, but is not necessarily, loaded with albumin. Furthermore, there is no evidence of increased peristaltic activity as recognized by abdominal auscultation, nor evidence of mechanical obstruction on a plain erect radiograph of the abdomen, but there is *considerable* elevation of the blood urea.

HAMILTON DRUMMOND, 1882–1925, *Surgeon, Royal Victoria Infirmary, Newcastle upon Tyne.*

ACUTE MANIFESTATIONS OF REGIONAL ILEITIS

Acute Terminal Ileitis is now known to be, not a manifestation of Crohn's disease, but an entirely different self-limiting condition due to infection with the organism of pseudo-tuberculosis (*Yersinia pseudotuberculosis*). The symptoms and signs resemble those of acute appendicitis closely and the diagnosis can only be made at laparotomy.

Acute Episodes in the Course of Chronic Regional Ileitis (Crohn's Disease)

a. The patient presents with pain in the right iliac fossa and a tender mass can be felt in that region, and frequently by pelvic examination also. If there is a history extending over months or years of intestinal colic accompanied by diarrhoea remember the possibility of Crohn's disease. Should he be suffering from an anal fissure, fistula, ulcer, or oedematous skin tags, this distinctly strengthens the tentative diagnosis; so does a normal or nearly normal temperature. As in the case of an appendix abscess, the next step is to mark out accurately on the skin the periphery of the lump. In a relatively young patient should the appendix have been removed previously, and/or should he appear anaemic, a tentative diagnosis of regional ileitis can be made.

Treated expectantly, unlike most appendix abscesses, the lump does not resolve, but neither do lumps due to carcinoma nor those due to actinomycosis or tuberculosis. The difficult differential diagnosis between these four conditions requires for its elucidation radiological and laboratory aid and sometimes elective (as opposed to early) laparotomy.

b. The patient is admitted with acute intestinal obstruction. Unless he is known to suffer from Crohn's disease there is no means of diagnosing the cause of the obstruction before laparotomy.

DIFFUSE PERITONITIS

When the clinician sees for the first time a patient in whom bacterial peritonitis is already diffuse, the diagnosis is sometimes difficult, for the signs resemble those of late intestinal obstruction. Even when a diagnosis of diffuse peritonitis has been made, the problem is only half solved, for it is highly desirable to know the site of origin of the peritonitis.

Helpful in arriving at a diagnosis of diffuse peritonitis is the fact that the patient prefers to lie with his knees drawn up. Should the presence of abdominal tenderness be doubtful, as it is when the patient is highly toxic, a useful manœuvre is to press the anterior surface of the upper part of the thigh of the patient, who will generally agree that there is no tenderness there. The pressure is continued upwards. If, when the inguinal ligament has been crossed, the patient suddenly complains of tenderness, it is proof that peritoneal irritation is present.

Meconium Peritonitis is a sterile chemical peritonitis in which, usually the perforation becomes sealed during intra-uterine life. Should it still be patent at the time of birth, to the chemical peritonitis is added bacterial peritonitis soon after the first feed. The signs resemble those of intestinal obstruction, but distension is more in evidence than vomiting. When bacterial peritonitis has supervened, oedema of the abdominal wall is an additional characteristic sign.

Pneumococcal Peritonitis now a rarity, may occur primarily, or as a complication of pneumonia. The signs closely resemble acute appendicitis with pelvic peritonitis, the only distinguishing features being:

BURRILL B. CROHN, *Contemporary Professor Emeritus of Medicine, Mount Sinai Hospital, New York, first described this disease in* 1932.

1. The type of individual. Usually a poorly nourished female child.

2. Considerable meteorism is often an early feature. Should an inguinal hernia be present, the sac is likely to be distended, but the contents are reduced easily.

3. Even in the primary variety; a tinge of cyanosis often is discernible and the alae nasi may move as actively as in pneumonia; often herpes on a lip or a nostril is present.

4. After 24–48 hours profuse diarrhoea, occasionally bloodstained, is characteristic. Increased frequency of micturition also is often present. Both are due to pelvic peritonitis.

Primary Streptococcal Peritonitis is also rare. Apart from (3) above the physical signs are identical with those of pneumococcal peritonitis. In both varieties the diagnosis must be confirmed by finding no other cause at laparotomy.

Peritonitis following Parturition or Abortion. Rigidity seldom is much in evidence; this, at any rate in part, is due to the stretched state of the abdominal musculature. The lochia may be offensive, but not necessarily so. Diarrhoea is common, due to a pelvic abscess which may be detected on rectal examination.

Postoperative Peritonitis. It is hard to decide whether the signs are due to paralytic ileus following operative trauma, or to infection. Rigidity, one of the mainstays of the recognition of other forms of peritonitis, frequently is non-existent. Tenderness, though present, is likely to be attributed to the recent laparotomy wound. More likely than not a narcotic has been administered and this masks the signs, indefinite as they are. Absence of bowel sounds, distension (which is slight in fulminating cases), and the bile-stained gastric aspirate will almost certainly be thought to be due to paralytic ileus rather than to postoperative peritonitis. There is often evidence of postoperative atelectasis (*see* p. 193), which may be thought to account for the rise in pulse rate and temperature.

A steadily increasing pulse rate and perhaps an undue sharpness of the intellect with some excitability are signs that give an astute clinician a lead in this extremely important (and if undetected early, very fatal) catastrophe. Often after some hours the Hippocratic facies (*see Fig.* 162, p. 90) becomes manifest.

OTHER CONDITIONS COMPLICATING AN OPERATION

Paralytic Ileus.* A certain amount of distension and flatulence are only too frequent after abdominal operations; such symptoms are due to intestinal paresis. Paralytic ileus can be looked upon as a more advanced, and much more serious, stage of intestinal paresis—a stage in which there is widespread inhibition of the peristaltic wave.

Obstructive symptoms commencing *within three days after operation* are usually due to paralytic ileus: true postoperative intestinal obstruction usually comes on *between the sixth and tenth postoperative days.* As a rule, paralytic ileus sets in rapidly and the physical signs to which it gives rise are as follows:

No pain is experienced but sometimes the patient complains of discomfort due to distension. He is usually unapprehensive, indeed quite oblivious of the fact that a serious complication is at hand.

Thirst is the leading symptom unless the patient is receiving adequate parenteral fluid. If the patient is allowed to satisfy it, the fluid ingested is regurgitated effortlessly.

The Pulse rate rises almost *pari passu* with the degree of the distension.

---

* *Ileus.*—In the majority of cases the condition commences in the ileum—hence the name.

ABDOMINAL EXAMINATION. *Inspection.* Early cases show distension most apparent below the umbilicus. Soon the whole abdomen becomes involved, by which time breathing is mainly of the costal type, and because the excursions of the diaphragm are rendered less deep, the respiratory rate is increased.

Palpation. There is complete absence of rigidity; slight tenderness is present, even well away from the area of a recent abdominal incision.

Percussion. Usually the whole abdomen is tympanitic.

Auscultation is of overriding importance. One often sees the stethoscope applied here and there to the surface of the abdomen for a matter of seconds; this is useless when the important diagnosis of paralytic ileus is at stake. Exhort those in attendance to make every effort to keep quiet and to command anyone in the vicinity to do likewise. Be seated. Apply the cup of the stethoscope firmly to the skin just below and to the right of the umbilicus, and keep it absolutely still, if necessary for 3 full minutes—a more exacting undertaking than might be imagined. If there is a gurgle within any part of the peritoneal cavity, assuredly it will be heard at this central 'listening post'. In paralytic ileus the clinician must expect to hear, not the hissing, turbulent, rumbling sounds associated with the colic of intestinal obstruction, but an ominous silence, broken only by the 'lub, dub' of the patient's heart beats, transmitted, presumably, to the abdomen via the overdistended intestinal coils (Patel), broken also by succussion splashes if the patient moves, and by very occasional weak tinkles.

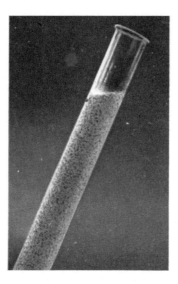

Fig. 525. Acute dilatation of the stomach. If a specimen of the vomit is placed in a test tube and held in a strong light, its characteristic colour will become evident and myriads of small particles may be discerned suspended in the fluid.

Measurement of abdominal girth with a tape measure (*see* p. 303) every 12 hours is useful in assessing progress.

Acute Dilatation of the Stomach comes on very suddenly, usually after operations, but sometimes after trauma; for instance, it may arise as a complication of fracture of the femur or spine. Typically the patient vomits—usually a very large amount—and soon exhibits signs of shock. He continues to vomit enormous quantities; one wonders where it has all come from. The character of the vomit should suggest the diagnosis. The very large quantity of brownish-black fluid, which may be likened to the storm water of a peat-laden stream, is pathognomonic (*Fig. 525*).

MANUBHAI D. PATEL, *Contemporary Surgeon, Shree Sayaji General Hospital, Baroda, India.*

Early Diagnosis. The day should have passed when sudden attention is focused on the patient because he brings up an enormous quantity of the characteristic fluid. In many instances the clinician is summoned to the bedside because there is something amiss. The pulse is rising. The patient need not look gravely ill. He is not in any pain, but he usually says that he feels uncomfortable. It is of paramount importance to realize that vomiting occurs relatively late. At this stage the patient does not necessarily experience even nausea, but an occasional hiccup is not uncommon. The output of urine is invariably scanty, although during the first few hours this fact cannot be gauged with accuracy. Careful observation of the upper abdomen may show slight fullness.

Occasionally when the abdomen is examined a dilated stomach can be made out, but as the greater curvature may be so low as to be hidden in the pelvis, usually a general fullness is all that can be seen. Succussion splash (*see* p. 227) can be elicited. If the condition is even suspected a gastric aspiration tube should be passed and the contents of the stomach aspirated. The use of intravenous drips for supplying fluid postoperatively together with the prohibition of early drinking has greatly reduced the incidence of this complication (and of paralytic ileus).

Subdiaphragmatic (Subphrenic) Abscess

Aetiology. Nearly all subdiaphragmatic abscesses follow a known intraperitoneal lesion but occasionally the abscess follows a condition which has subsided without an operation. The commonest causes are:

1. Perforated peptic ulcer	25 per cent
2. Following abdominal trauma	15 per cent
3. Following operations on biliary tract	10 per cent
4. Following operations on stomach	10 per cent
5. Following operations on colon	10 per cent
6. Acute appendicitis	5 per cent

Other causes constitute a miscellaneous collection of intraperitoneal inflammatory lesions, on the relative frequency of which it is unprofitable to linger.

Diagnosis. The majority of patients feel and look ill. In addition to pain, they complain of anorexia and nausea. The complexion is frequently muddy. 'Signs of pus somewhere, signs of pus nowhere else, signs of pus *there*' was Barnard's aphorism regarding subdiaphragmatic abscess, and a truly marvellous compendium of the situation it is. Having excluded pus in other situations (*see* p. 293), have regard to the following:

The Temperature* nearly always fluctuates between 38 and 39 °C or more. In a few cases it alternates, remaining lower, but rarely normal, for a few days, and then rising again. Most exceptionally the patient is apyrexial.

Rigors are uncommon, and usually occur in patients with concomitant pylephlebitis or a liver abscess.

The Pulse rate is likely to be raised more than expected from the temperature.

The Respiratory rate is usually raised and corresponds to the extent and nature of the thoracic complications.

Pain is not a prominent feature but when present it is usually felt on the side of the lesion. It is often localized in the hypochondrium, although nearly as frequently it is experienced in the lower part of the thorax of the corresponding side. Occasionally the pain is located in the lumbar region. Referred pain in the corresponding shoulder is not infrequent, but special inquiries must be made concerning it.

Jaundice is most unusual in subdiaphragmatic abscess. When it is present it is nearly always due to coexisting obstruction to the common bile duct by a calculus, or to suppurative pylephlebitis.

---

* To some extent this important sign is masked by antibiotic therapy.

HAROLD L. BARNARD, 1868–1908, *Surgeon, The London Hospital.*

Hiccup is occasional.

Abdominal Signs. In postoperative cases, when the primary lesion was situated in the right upper quadrant of the abdomen, there is nearly always a purulent discharge from the wound. In cases of a right posterior abscess (the commonest situation) there is often tenderness over the 11th intercostal space. To elicit this satisfactorily the patient must be turned on to his face. When the abscess is left-sided and anterior, there is usually tenderness and sometimes a swelling in the position shown in *Fig.* 526.

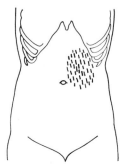 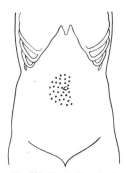

Fig. 526. Sketch of the tenderness and fullness in a case of left anterior sub-phrenic abscess.

Fig. 527. Usual site of pain in acute non-specific lymphadenitis. Note the large area and compare it with the relatively circumscribed area of acute appendicitis (*see Fig.* 505 *a*, p. 289).

Thoracic Signs. Just as in acute osteomyelitis there is a sympathetic arthritis of the near-by joint, so in subdiaphragmatic abscess there is a concomitant basal pleurisy or pleuropneumonia. It must, therefore, be clearly understood that *signs of atelectasis at the base of the lung favour, rather than hinder, the diagnosis of subphrenic abscess.*

Percussion. When gas is present, percussion may yield the classic four areas of altered resonance, which are, from below upwards: (1) Dull—due to liver; (2) Resonant—due to gas* in the abscess; (3) Dull—due to collapsed lung or pleural effusion; (4) Resonant—the normal lung resonance. Unfortunately it is not usual to find this picture.

In any patient in whom there is a reasonable suspicion of the presence of a subdiaphragmatic abscess X-ray screening of diaphragmatic movement should be carried out. Usually the affected diaphragm does not move fully.

Ultimately diagnosis must rest with an exploratory procedure, usually after a period of antibiotic therapy and observation.

Pylephlebitis (Portal Pyaemia). In the early stages this is difficult to differentiate from subdiaphragmatic abscess. Both arise as a complication of inflammatory conditions of organs draining their venous blood into the portal system, and both give rise to a swinging temperature.

In pylephlebitis the patient soon develops a slightly jaundiced tinge. Rigors are usual. When the liver is examined it will be found to be enlarged and often tender. As a rule, pylephlebitis becomes manifest a few days *after* (it may have been present before) the inflammatory focus which gave rise to it has been removed. When there is no known focus of infection the rectum should be examined for thrombosed inflamed haemorrhoids, which, however, are a most unusual cause of this condition.

---

* This gas, when demonstrated radiologically, provides confirmatory evidence.

If the patient (with antibiotic help) can combat the onslaught of this often fatal disease, one or more liver abscesses may form. The signs then do not differ from those of an amoebic liver abscess (*see* p. 321).

ABDOMINAL AND PELVIC LYMPHADENITIS AS A CAUSE OF ACUTE ABDOMINAL SYMPTOMS

Acute Non-specific Mesenteric Lymphadenitis is, in the first decade of life, as common as acute appendicitis. The incidence falls abruptly after the age of 6 years; beyond 15 years the diagnosis should not be entertained.

Pain. There are spasms of abdominal colic, usually referred to the umbilicus, with intervals of freedom that never appertain in obstructive appendicitis.

Vomiting. As a rule vomiting occurs at the very outset of the attack, and synchronizes with the onset of abdominal pain—in this it differs from acute appendicitis, in which pain precedes vomiting.

Temperature averages 38° C but it varies, as it does in acute appendicitis.

Pulse rate is slightly increased. It is never unaltered, as is the case in some examples of acute obstructive appendicitis in the early stages.

ABDOMINAL EXAMINATION. *Inspection.* When asked to do so, the child maps a relatively wide inconstant area rather more medial and higher than in appendicitis (*Fig.* 527) to indicate the site of the pain. With the passing hours the site of the pain remains constant; cf. the shift of pain in appendicitis (*see* p. 289).

Palpation. True rigidity is not present. The tensing of the abdominal musculature is due to muscular resistance. If the child's attention is diverted, the resistance ceases. This does not occur in appendicitis. Having broken through the muscular resistance, and exercising gentleness and patience, endeavour, by deeper and deeper palpation just below and to the right of the umbilicus, to feel the enlarged lymph nodes. In about 25 per cent of cases one or more nodes can be imprisoned between the palpating fingers and the promontory of the sacrum as discrete, mobile lumps, each the size of a grape, that slither beneath the fingers.

Rebound tenderness is not present or, at the most, only very slight pain is elicited.

Klein's Sign of Shifting Tenderness. After laying the patient on the left side for a few minutes the maximum site of tenderness moves to the left of the original site. Even if positive, this does not rule out the possibility of acute Meckelian diverticulitis, a rarity.

RECTAL EXAMINATION is almost invariably entirely normal.

The differential diagnosis between acute non-specific mesenteric lymphadenitis and acute appendicitis is sometimes quite straightforward: at other times it is extremely difficult. Helpful signs are that in the former there is frequently an antecedent respiratory infection, and at times the disease is mildly epidemic, and in about half the cases the face shows a malar flush, with or without circumoral pallor. In doubtful instances several hours observation (preferably in hospital) resolves the matter. In acute appendicitis localized tenderness in the region of McBurney's point becomes obvious in this time.

Suppurating Deep Iliac Lymph Nodes are a diagnostic Waterloo. Often psoas spasm is in evidence; the thigh is flexed. ⟶
This, combined with pain and tenderness in the *right* iliac fossa, leads to a diagnosis of appendicitis, while on either side purulent arthritis of the hip joint or osteomyelitis of the upper end of the femur may be suspected. Sometimes the superficial inguinal lymph nodes are palpably enlarged,

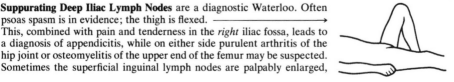

WILLIAM KLEIN, 1881–1970, *Surgeon, Morrisania City Hospital, New York.*

but this is by no means part and parcel of this clinical entity. Hip-joint diseases can be eliminated by putting the joint through the routine movements, when it will be found that all with, perhaps, the exception of full extension (psoas spasm) are unimpaired, provided they are elicited cautiously. Deep pressure over the upper end of the femur does not cause pain. On inspection a fullness may be perceived above the inguinal ligament. However, whether visible or not, *the* characteristic sign is a firm, tender palpable lump tending to occupy a position rather nearer the anterior superior iliac spine than the tubercle of the pubis.

The differential diagnosis from an appendix abscess can be extremely difficult. The whole of the lower limb, commencing with the toes and the clefts between the toes, must be scrutinized for a focus of infection. Remember to look at the heel and the back of the limb, as well as the more accessible parts (e.g. the perianal region). The finding of such a focus in the shape of a scratch or a sore is very significant and is found in about three-quarters of cases.

In the tropics filarial infestation and tropical pyomyositis are causes of psoas spasm.

Similar signs are seen in haemophiliacs (*see* p. 322) with retroperitoneal haematomata.

ACUTE INTRA-ABDOMINAL CONDITIONS PECULIAR TO THE FEMALE

Ectopic Gestation is the most common cause of intraperitoneal haemorrhage. The condition terminates abruptly in one of two ways and consequently the symptoms come on suddenly: (1) The ovum is aborted through the abdominal ostium of the Fallopian (uterine) tube; (2) The Fallopian tube or the broad ligament in which the ovum is situated ruptures. In the latter, which is less common, the bleeding into the peritoneal cavity is violent, and produces signs of internal haemorrhage so severe and sudden that they approach the classic picture (*see* p. 43). In tubal abortion there is a series of smaller bleedings, each accompanied by a recrudescence of pain, and often a *feeling* (in only a fifth of cases does the patient actually faint) of faintness, which tends to pass off as the vasomotor system adjusts the blood pressure. The physical signs will vary greatly according to the stage at which the patient is examined.

It will be assumed that the patient has had two or three attacks of pain, that the lower intra-abdominal viscera are bathed in blood, but the signs of shock are not yet in evidence.

Pain is often sharp and stabbing; as a rule the pain is situated in the pelvis, frequently it radiates to the rectum—the so-called 'lavatory' sign.

Pulse–Temperature Ratio. An increased pulse rate with a normal or slightly subnormal temperature is characteristic. Seldom is the pulse rate below 80 beats per minute. Should the haemorrhage cease spontaneously, in an hour or more, the temperature becomes slightly elevated.

Shoulder Pain usually does not come on until the haemorrhage is considerable and it occurs in about 30 per cent of cases. It may be referred to one or both shoulders and may be complained of only after the foot of the bed has been raised (to combat the shock).

ABDOMINAL EXAMINATION. *Inspection*. Slight distension often is in evidence. It is due to meteorism, which comes on early when there is blood in the peritoneal cavity. The abdomen moves well with respiration.

On a few occasions a blue discoloration of the umbilicus has been noted: this is a most exceptional phenomenon, but it should be looked for in passing (Cullen's sign, *see* p. 250).

Palpation. There is absence of rigidity during the first few hours, but invariably deep tenderness is present in one or both hypogastric areas (*Fig.* 528). The rebound sign will be positive on the affected side at an early stage.

GABRIELLO FALLOPIO, 1523–1562, *Professor of Anatomy, Surgery, and Botany, Padua, Italy.*

Percussion. Shifting dullness should be sought (*see* p. 243). If sufficient fluid blood is in the peritoneal cavity the sign will be positive.

VAGINAL EXAMINATION. Vaginal bleeding is usual; this is sometimes darker and thicker than the normal menstrual flow ('prune juice blood'). As the patient is pregnant the cervix feels softer than normal: gentle tilting of the cervix causes pain—a most valuable sign. All the fornices are tender, and this is of considerable importance, as in inflammatory conditions tenderness is present only in the posterior and one or both of the lateral fornices (Connell).

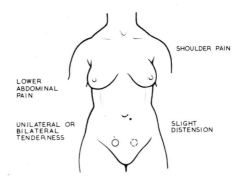

Fig. 528. The symptoms and signs of ectopic pregnancy. Only when a clinician becomes ectopic-minded are cases of tubal abortion and tubal rupture likely to be diagnosed early. Of cardinal significance, the history of a missed period is too often lacking to be a sheet anchor.

SHOULDER PAIN

LOWER ABDOMINAL PAIN

UNILATERAL OR BILATERAL TENDERNESS

SLIGHT DISTENSION

The patient should be questioned about the dates of her monthly periods. The history of a missed period is of the greatest possible significance, but it is by no means always obtainable.

If 'ruptured ectopic' is doubtful a rising pulse rate and a falling blood pressure are points in favour of the diagnosis. Quarter-hourly readings are advisable.

Ruptured Lutein Cyst. The patient is an unmarried, or young married, woman. The pain occurs half-way between two menstrual periods ('mittelschmerz'*). Particularly when right-sided, a ruptured lutein cyst is extremely difficult to differentiate from acute appendicitis. Unlike the latter, the pain *commences* in the iliac fossa and tends to decrease in a matter of a few hours. In exceptional cases intraperitoneal haemorrhage is considerable, and the signs simulate those of ectopic gestation.

Twisted Ovarian Cyst. A very sudden onset of abdominal pain, followed by attacks of lower abdominal pain of a colicky nature recurring at frequent intervals, together with repeated vomiting, is the usual history. If a lump is present (*Fig.* 529), the diagnosis is tolerably simple. Overlying rigidity tends to mask the lump, which, if small, is situated entirely within the pelvis.

Before examining the patient bimanually, either per vaginam or per rectum according to circumstances, always have the bladder emptied by a catheter.

Torsion or Degeneration of a Uterine Fibroid. The symptoms and clinical findings are similar to the above; the finding of an obviously enlarged fibroid uterus on vaginal examination is suggestive but remember that fibroids may be coincidental with other causes of the acute abdomen.

Acute Salpingitis. Often the illness commences at the time of menstruation, or during the first week after abortion or delivery. The salient points in the diagnosis of acute salpingitis are as follows: (1) A vaginal discharge whether of recent onset or an exacerbation of a long-standing discharge is frequent but not

---

* *Mittelschmerz.* German, *mittel* = middle + *schmerz* = pain.

JAMES S. M. CONNELL, 1889–1960, *Gynaecologist, Midland Hospital, Birmingham.*

invariable; (2) The pain of acute salpingitis *commences* in the iliac fossa, not in the epigastrium or around the umbilicus as in appendicitis; (3) Usually the temperature is higher than that commonly found in acute appendicitis, but this should not bias the diagnostician unduly; (4) Dysuria is a frequent symptom—

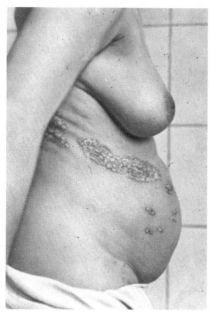

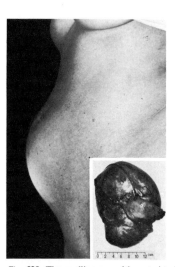

Fig. 529. The swelling caused by a twisted ovarian cyst (right side). Inset, the specimen removed at an emergency operation.

Fig. 530. Eruption of herpes zoster, lower thoracic spinal nerves. Two days previously the patient had been admitted to hospital with a diagnosis of cholecystitis.

scalding micturition with increased frequency is suggestive; (5) Although there are exceptions, abdominal rigidity is not much in evidence; (6) Maximum tenderness is fairly constantly low down, i.e. just above the inguinal ligament; frequently it is bilateral; ⟶ (7) Rebound tenderness is often positive in one or both of these areas. If only positive on the right side, pelvic appendicitis is not excluded.

VAGINAL EXAMINATION. The uterus will be found to be somewhat fixed and movement of it causes extreme pain. When the infection occurred during the puerperium or following abortion the uterus will be found to be enlarged. In cases following abortion the cervix is softer than normal. It is only with the subsidence of the acute stage that the unilateral or bilateral thickened, swollen tubal mass can be distinguished.

Tubo-ovarian Abscess. In spite of the fact that the use of antibiotics has resulted in decrease in the incidence and severity of pelvic inflammation, cases still occur quite frequently. It is met with during the reproductive period. Pyrexia is a feature. The patient complains of pain on the side of the abscess. In about 50 per cent the condition is bilateral. Intraperitoneal rupture is a complication to be borne in mind. When right-sided rupture is impending or actual the condition is difficult to differentiate from pelvic appendicitis. A previous vaginal discharge is suggestive of tubo-ovarian abscess. When rupture occurs, there is severe pain in the lower abdomen, often followed by rigors, and less frequently by vomiting. The degree of accompanying shock is proportional to the amount of pus liberated.

SOME EXTRA-ABDOMINAL CONDITIONS MIMICKING ACUTE INTRA-ABDOMINAL DISEASE

In the course of the preceding demonstrations on acute intra-abdominal conditions the reader's attention has been directed to several extra-abdominal conditions that mimic 'the acute abdomen'. Others simulating acute abdominal conditions are:

Coronary Occlusion. Myocardial infarction often causes upper abdominal pain. Men are more susceptible than women: usually the victim is past 40 years of age. The onset is sudden and the pain severe: it is located in the lower sternal region and radiates to the epigastrium. Cardiac pain often radiates to both shoulders and down the left arm. The patient is apprehensive and moves about in bed, which is in contrast to one who is stricken with an acute intra-abdominal catastrophe. Pain of gallbladder origin is most often confused with cardiac pain, be it angina pectoris or that due to coronary occlusion; a factor that heightens the difficulty is that occasionally gallstones give rise to reflex precordial pain identical with that produced by coronary thrombosis.

Cyanosis. Like ultra-acute pancreatitis, the patient may have a cyanotic tinge, but, unlike acute pancreatitis, the patient suffering from coronary occlusion is often dyspnoeic.

Observe the Veins of the Neck. In cardiac failure they are distended or at least full.

The Electrocardiogram usually shows characteristic changes.

Diaphragmatic Pleurisy (including Bornholm* Disease). When there are no physical signs to be found on examination of the thorax, as may happen in diaphragmatic pleurisy, the differentiation between it and upper abdominal surgical conditions, e.g. cholecystitis, sealed-off perforation of a peptic ulcer, becomes exceedingly difficult in the absence of X-ray facilities. Helpful signs are as follows:

    1. In suspected pleuropneumonia with abdominal pain ask the patient to cough—if the pleura is inflamed this will cause pain in the chest.

    2. In referred abdominal pain due to the diaphragmatic inflammation of pneumonia, abdominal rebound tenderness is absent.

Herpes Zoster. When the pain radiates *from* the back along one or more spinal nerves of the lower thoracic segments *to* the midline anteriorly, herpes zoster should spring to mind.

    The pain, which on the right side has been mistaken for that of acute

---

* Named from the Danish island, Bornholm.

cholecystitis, is rather severe and usually it is unremitting: it precedes the skin eruption (*Fig.* 530) by several days. It is in the preherpetic stage of herpes zoster that confusion with visceral disease occurs. The following are the most helpful differentiating signs:

1. *Skin hyperaesthesia* occurs along the whole course of the affected nerve or nerves.

2. *Herpes zoster* usually follows a respiratory infection, the constitutional symptoms are mild, and rarely does the temperature reach 38 °C.

3. *Rebound tenderness* is absent.

Spinal Extradural Abscess (*see* p. 221) is a considerably rarer condition in which root pain mimics abdominal disease.

ABDOMINAL AORTIC CATASTROPHES

A patient, usually a middle-aged or elderly male, presents in extremely severe abdominal or lower chest pain, and markedly shocked. Apart from the relatively common occurring conditions, namely, perforated peptic ulcer, coronary thrombosis and acute pancreatitis, there are three uncommon possibilities, the differential diagnosis of which is important, as surgical treatment is feasible. Of these the first is most often encountered, the second is uncommon, and the third, *spontaneous rupture of the oesophagus* (*see* p. 196), is rare.

Ruptured or Leaking Aortic Aneurysm. In passing, it should be noted that, with the disappearance of the ravages of untreated syphilis, the abdominal aorta has become easily the commonest site of aneurysm. Before rupture, the aneurysm (which is almost invariably situated below the renal arteries) is found as a pulsating epigastric swelling occupying the midline but extending rather more to the left. The patient is usually hypertensive, but when leakage starts the blood pressure falls catastrophically. He is also manifestly anaemic and complains of severe central abdominal pain radiating through to the back.

Abdominal Signs. If leakage has been slight the aneurysm is still palpable. As leakage gives way to frank rupture variable rigidity is found, usually more marked on the left side. A mass (blood clot) in the left iliac fossa resembles that found with a pericolic abscess due to diverticulitis (*see* p. 294).

Arterial Pulses in the Lower Limbs (*see* p. 379) are reduced or absent if the rupture has diverted most of the blood flow through the aorta into the retroperitoneal and peritoneal spaces.

Aortic Dissecting Aneurysm. A severe degree of hypertension (of which the patient or a relative may be aware) initiates the dissection which usually commences in the aortic arch. The pain, which is excruciating, thus commences in the retrosternal region, radiates between the shoulders, and spreads into the upper abdomen as the dissection proceeds downwards.

The *signs of shock* are apparent but the blood pressure may lie within normal limits, which is low for the particular hypertensive patient.

Abdominal signs are absent until the aneurysm ruptures into the retroperitoneal space with the patient's demise within a few minutes.

Anuria is a sign that the dissection has spread to involve the renal arteries.

Arterial Pulses in all Four Limbs. Owing to partial blockage of the main branches of the aorta by the dissection, the blood pressures (as measured by a sphygmomanometer) in the right and left arms differ. Similarly, the femoral pulses may be unequal. A unique sign is that, if observed over a period of an hour or two, these differences alter as the limit of the dissection advances. Ultimately complete blockage of the arterial blood supply of one or more limbs is caused, the condition simulating an embolus (*see* p. 385) in this respect.

THE ACUTE ABDOMEN IN THE TROPICS

A knowledge of endemic disease is necessary as the tropical diseases found in any particular area vary widely. In addition, non-tropical conditions differ inexplicably in their frequency, e.g. the high incidence of intussusception in Nigeria, and of volvulus of the sigmoid colon in Ghana and Uganda (*see* p. 302).

Amoebic Liver Abscess is a complication of amoebic dysentery. It should be noted especially that as amoebiasis occurs in all parts of the world, it is not essential for a sufferer from this condition to live, or have lived, in a tropical or a subtropical zone, although such residence so greatly favours a tentative diagnosis as to warrant the term 'tropical abscess of the liver'. Adult males are the usual sufferers.

Pain in the liver area is dull and constant, worsened by alcohol and also so much increased by jarring that while walking or riding in a vehicle the patient supports the right side with the hands when he expects a jar or vibration. When present this sign is highly characteristic.

Pyrexia and *Rigors* with profuse sweating at night are the rule.

Other signs are depicted in *Fig.* 531. Radiography, sigmoidoscopy, radio-isotope liver scan and aspiration of the contents of the abscess (chocolate-coloured pus) are required to establish the diagnosis.

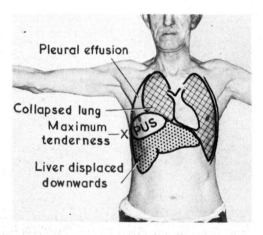

Fig. 531. Physical signs of an amoebic liver abscess (most common site depicted). Basu notes that the right lower intercostal spaces may bulge and sometimes exhibit pitting oedema (due to the underlying abscess) and also that an abscess in the right lobe may present as a mass in the region of the gallbladder. An abscess of the left lobe may cause an epigastric swelling.

The patient may not come under observation until soon after the abscess has ruptured (*a*) into the peritoneal cavity (acute peritonitis with board-like rigidity), (*b*) into the pleural cavity (empyema), or more happily, (*c*) into the lung (chocolate-like pus expectorated), or (*d*) into the intestine.

Amoeboma (an inflammatory mass due to an amoebic granuloma) may occur in the caecum simulating an appendix abscess, or in the rectum where it is liable to be mistaken for a carcinoma. The response of both to metronidazole is so rapid as to constitute a therapeutic test.

The Typhoid Abdomen. It may, or may not, be known that the patient is suffering from typhoid fever. When perforation of the small bowel occurs the poor general condition of the patient usually modifies the course of the resultant peritonitis so that the condition resembles that of postoperative peritonitis (*see* p. 311) rather than that of acute peritonitis due to flooding of the peritoneal cavity in perforated peptic ulcer (*see* p. 295).

Intestinal Obstruction due to Worms. Obturation by a mass of worms may, particularly in children, cause incomplete intestinal obstruction. An abdominal mass corresponding to the obturating bolus of worms may be palpable. If this condition is suspected, the stools and the vomitus (if any) should be examined for the usual cause, *Ascaris lumbricoides*. If found, remember that the abdominal pain may be due to peritonitis, the worms having penetrated the intestinal wall, and look for signs of this (*see* p. 310).

AJIT K. BASU, *Contemporary Emeritus Professor of Surgery, Institute of Post-Graduate Medical Education, and Research, Calcutta.*

Rupture of an Enlarged Spleen due to Tropical Disease. The enlarged spleen in the tropics is more friable than usual and rupture (*see* p. 324) is common. Delayed rupture in particular is relatively frequent.

Oriental Cholangiohepatitis (*see* p. 231).

Tropical Pyomyositis (*see* p. 246).

ABDOMINAL CRISES OF MEDICAL CONDITIONS

If the patient appears to be in acute abdominal pain, but the four preliminary signs mentioned on pp. 287–8 are lacking (particularly the rebound sign), the conditions mentioned in this section must be considered.

Diabetic Crisis. Abdominal pain sometimes occurs when coma is impending. Thus if routine examination or the urine shows ketones and sugar, the diabetes should be treated urgently. If the pain is not relieved thereby, or if the pain is typical of an acute abdominal condition, remember that it is much commoner to come across an 'acute abdomen' in a diabetic than a crisis. However, in the former circumstances, valuable time has not been wasted; it is necessary to control the diabetes before an operation is undertaken.

Porphyria. The abdominal crises, which are characterized by violent intestinal colic with constipation, are liable to be precipitated by the administration of barbiturates, oestrogens or sulphonamides, to which there is an idiosyncrasy. The abdomen is distended, rigidity being absent. On examining the left hypochondrium, the spleen is occasionally found to be enlarged. The correct diagnosis is made when a specimen of urine left over-night is noted to have become a characteristic amber colour (*see* Fig. 547, p. 336). There are conclusive laboratory tests for porphyrinuria.

Hyperlipidaemia. Attacks of abdominal pain, often left-sided and sometimes associated with a raised serum amylase (*see* p. 299), occur in sufferers from this group of diseases which are often familial. Clues are that the patient may show arcus senilis (*see* p. 5) and/or xanthomatosis (*see* p. 71). Turbidity of the blood plasma due to an excess of fat globules supports the diagnosis but confirmatory laboratory tests are necessary.

Malaria. In the tropics, or in persons who have resided or passed through the tropics or subtropics, abdominal cramps with diarrhoea and vomiting may be due to malaria, or pain in the left upper abdomen may be due to destruction of red blood cells by the spleen which is often, but not always, palpably enlarged. Examination of a blood smear for the parasite is essential.

Sickle-cell Anaemia. West Indians and others of African descent are liable to similar episodes of destruction of the abnormal red cells in the spleen (which may be enlarged in children) or blockage of mesenteric blood vessels with abdominal pain. Painless haematuria may be the presenting symptom. Leg ulceration (*see* p. 528) or dactylitis (*see* p. 483), if present, is a clue. Blood examination again will suggest the diagnosis. In the tropics an unnecessary operation on a patient with this disease is almost as foolhardy as such an operation in the following condition.

Haemophilia. The male patient who states, or whose parents state, that he is a haemophiliac and is complaining of abdominal pain should be regarded as suffering from a retroperitoneal haematoma unless there is extremely strong clinical and ancillary evidence to the contrary. To operate unnecessarily on a haemophiliac is the height of surgical folly and the decision to open the abdomen should not be made by the person for whom this book is intended. Suffice it to state here that the advice of a haematologist must be sought and an estimation of the anti-haemophilic globulin in the blood obtained.

Lead Colic (*see* p. 117)

Acholuric Jaundice (*see* p. 232)

Tabetic Crisis (*see* p. 296)

THE ABDOMINAL MALINGERER

We are not concerned here with the patient (usually female) who complains of chronic abdominal pain which, although vaguely reminiscent of one or more of the conditions discussed in Chapter 18 (Non-acute Abdominal Conditions), on careful investigation proves to have nothing detectably wrong. Many in this category are relieved of their pain by a negative investigation, and those who are not might well be termed 'neurotic' provided the clinician is absolutely certain that no disease is present. The problem is not urgent in contradistinction to the following category which occurs almost invariably in males.

Münchausen's Syndrome. For a clinician to jump to a conclusion that the patient before him is suffering from this because there are several scars on the abdomen and the symptoms are out of proportion to the physical signs, is so dangerous that it would be far better if he had never read about it. The hoaxer who exhibits Münchausen's syndrome is sometimes skilful, but he can never reproduce the sounds of turbulent peristalsis: nor can he produce fluid levels on an erect radiograph of his abdomen. There are three varieties of Münchausen's syndrome (Asher): the abdominal type, the bleeding type, and the type who specializes in faints, fits and palsies. Thus two out of three of these psychopathic malingerers are likely to cross the surgeon's path.

Often the patient says that he is on a long journey to explain his presence at a hospital not in the vicinity of his normal abode (Angell). This hinders the clinician in ascertaining the details of previous operations. Another characteristic is a tendency to quarrel with the hospital staff.

BARON HIERONYMUS K. F. VON MÜNCHAUSEN, 1720–1797, *a German officer who fought with the Russians against the Turks and returned to tell tall stories that were recorded in book form.*
RICHARD ASHER, 1912–1969, *Physician, Central Middlesex Hospital, London.*
JAMES C. ANGELL, *Contemporary Urologist, Ashford Hospital, Middlesex.*

Chapter 23

ABDOMINAL AND PELVIC INJURIES

Under this heading 'closed' injuries, as opposed to wounds, will be considered, although it may be mentioned in passing that correct diagnosis with a penetrating wound of the trunk can only be attained by thorough exploration in the operating theatre. Cursory stitching of the skin in the casualty department leads, on occasion, to serious errors. When a patient has sustained an injury to the trunk, often there is little external bruising to guide the clinician. The problem is to decide as quickly as possible whether the patient has sustained an intra-abdominal lesion. This is often difficult, particularly when shock is severe. In such circumstances the correct procedure is to treat the shock and to examine and re-examine the patient at frequent intervals.

Bear in mind that acute abdominal pain and rigidity can be due to irritation of the lower intercostal nerves by fractured ribs. It is essential therefore to examine the thorax carefully, not only for the presence of a fractured rib or ribs, but for thoracic complications arising therefrom. A lacerated lung causing a pneumothorax or a haemopneumothorax can produce symptoms that simulate closely those of a serious intra-abdominal lesion. Another pitfall is an unsuspected lesion of the spinal cord which may cause the most excruciating pain.

In this mechanized era, if a patient has sustained a head injury—particularly if that injury is the result of a road accident—it is of fundamental importance to search for evidence of injury elsewhere. In particular the thorax, abdomen and pelvis must be examined. Especially with an unconscious patient, one such negative examination must not lull the clinician into thinking that he has done his duty in this respect. The patient must be re-examined when he has regained consciousness.

TRAUMATIC HAEMOPERITONEUM

Under modern conditions with fluid and blood replacement progressive bleeding into the peritoneal cavity may lead to obvious abdominal swelling: non-infected blood is not extremely irritant to the peritoneum.

RUPTURE OF THE NORMAL SPLEEN

This, the most common injury caused by non-penetrating violence to the abdominal wall, can be divided advantageously into three groups: (1) The patient rapidly bleeds to death; (2) Initial shock—recovery from shock—signs of ruptured spleen; (3) The signs of an intra-abdominal disaster are delayed for more than 24 hours.

1. The Patient succumbs rapidly. A comparatively rare result unless there are associated injuries. Complete avulsion of the spleen from its pedicle is most likely to give rise to this catastrophe.

2. Shock—Immediate Signs of Rupture. This is by far the largest group—more than three-quarters of all cases belong to it. It is not always possible to state precisely which organ is damaged, but in the majority the physical signs point clearly to the spleen as the site of injury.

GENERAL SIGNS. As a rule the patient is pale.

Pulse Rate. In early cases the pulse may not rise above 90 beats a minute. The reason is that the initial shock and the moderate haemorrhage from the spleen cause a temporary fall in blood pressure, and during this time adequate clotting occurs to control the haemorrhage temporarily. Thus by the time the patient is first seen there may be little in the general appearance to arouse a suspicion of the true nature of the injury. The local signs therefore become correspondingly important.

LOCAL SIGNS. In cases where the spleen is the only viscus injured, the pain is variable, tenderness slight but constant, the abdomen is soft, and bowel sounds are present. If a rib or ribs are fractured, pain is increased.

Rigidity is present in more than half the total. Usually it is most pronounced over the left upper abdomen.

Local Tenderness is found very constantly in the same region.

Meteorism commences to appear about three or four hours after the accident; it is due to paralytic ileus (*see* p. 311).

Shifting Dullness in the flanks (*see* p. 243) is present fairly regularly.

Referred Pain to the Shoulder is a very valuable sign, and should be inquired for specially in cases of abdominal injury (Kehr's sign). When rupture of the spleen (or of the liver) is suspected and other signs are doubtful, the patient should be asked to lie flat in bed on the back; then the foot of the bed is raised 0·5 m. Wait for 10 minutes. If the peritoneal cavity contains liquid blood it will gravitate towards the diaphragm, and frequently the patient complains of pain in one or other shoulder—usually the left. An obvious but useful way of distinguishing referred pain from that due to a shoulder injury is that in the referred type the pain is made no worse by movement of the joint or pressure over the site.

3. The Delayed Type of Case. Following the accident, there is a period of comparative freedom from symptoms, which often is extremely deceptive. A navvy, aged 40, was hit in the upper abdomen by a pole. He fainted, but soon recovered sufficiently to walk to hospital, where he was examined and told to report the next day. On the morrow he felt better, and stayed at home. Five days later he was brought in with well-marked signs of internal haemorrhage, having collapsed at home a few hours before admission. Recovery followed splenectomy.

Delay of serious bleeding may be explained in three ways: (1) The great omentum, performing its well-known constabulary duties, shuts off that portion of the general peritoneal cavity in the immediate vicinity of the spleen; (2) A bloody coagulum temporarily seals the rent; (3) A subcapsular haematoma forms, and later bursts. It is probable that each of these three factors, at one time or another, temporarily arrests serious haemorrhage.

RUPTURED LIVER

The force of a blow necessary to rupture the liver is greater than that necessary to rupture the spleen, consequently associated injuries are more common and make the diagnosis more difficult. Nevertheless, the salient physical signs are, in most respects, similar to those of a ruptured spleen. There are also three comparable types: (1) The patient rapidly succumbs; (2) Shock, recovery, more shock, signs of internal haemorrhage; (3) Delayed rupture.

HANS KEHR, 1862–1916, *Professor of Surgery, Halberstadt, Saxony.*

The right lobe is involved five times more frequently than the left. Often one or more of the lower ribs on the right side and/or the transverse processes of the first two lumbar vertebrae are fractured. If the local signs point to a right-sided lesion there is no particular difficulty in differentiating a ruptured liver from a ruptured spleen. When the rupture is in the central part of the liver, some bleeding occurs into the large radicles of the biliary tree so that liquid blood is carried along the bile passages into the duodenum, and the patient may vomit blood.

LACERATION OF THE MESENTERY

Haemorrhage from the mesentery is likely to be brisk, and if the tear is parallel to the gut the blood supply to the intestine in the immediate vicinity of the tear is endangered. There are signs of a haemoperitoneum without any pointers to the liver or to the spleen. Early meteorism from bruising of the intestinal wall suggests that it is the intestine that is ruptured.

INJURIES WITHOUT MASSIVE INTERNAL HAEMORRHAGE

These are just as dangerous as those belonging to the group giving rise to internal haemorrhage; indeed, without early diagnosis and laparotomy the patient's chance of survival is negligible, for blood transfusion alone cannot help.

RUPTURED INTESTINE

With small intestinal injury, for several hours following the accident, in many cases, there is no radiographic evidence of free subdiaphragmatic gas in the peritoneal cavity. Therefore do not rely on X-rays; repeated clinical examination remains the diagnostic sheet-anchor.

Pointing Test is a sign of great value in ruptured intestine. Ask the patient to point with one finger to where the pain is most acute or where it started. The patient may locate accurately the site of the perforation.

London's Sign. The presence of 'pattern' bruising of the skin (i.e. an imprint of the clothing is noted on the skin) indicates that a crushing force has been applied sufficient to rupture the bowel against the vertebral column. This sign is a strong indication to carry out a laparotomy.

Local Tenderness is often the key to the site of the rupture. When a patient has been struck upon the abdomen and tenderness on pressure, and especially rebound tenderness, can be evoked in one special area, even in the absence of all other signs, if the tenderness persists for an hour the abdomen should be explored.

Remember that the blow may be, and often is, a comparatively trivial one. The disparity between the force of the blow on the abdomen and the serious nature of the intra-abdominal injury is greatest in cases of rupture of the intestine. The intestine is likely to rupture at a point where the blow impinges it against the vertebral column; consequently the relatively fixed first and last 0·5 m of the small intestine are the most frequent sites for traumatic rupture. Early diagnosis is of paramount importance. The time interval between the perforation and the development of peritonitis depends on the size of the rupture, on the character

PETER S. LONDON, *Contemporary Surgeon, The Accident Hospital, Birmingham.*

of the intestinal contents, and on whether the perforation occurs into the free peritoneal cavity. In cases where there is a tear of the jejunum large enough to admit a finger, the rigidity simulates that of an early perforated peptic ulcer.

The Association of Inguinal Hernia and Traumatic Rupture of the Intestine. There is an important relationship between an uncontrolled inguinal hernia (usually on the right side) and traumatic rupture of the intestine. A portion of small intestine lying within an inguinal hernial sac can be ruptured by *direct* force applied to the hernia or, what is even more important to know, as pointed out by Aird, rupture of the intestine can be caused by *indirect* violence (*Fig.* 532), in which event laparotomy, and not exploration of the hernia, must be carried out as soon as possible.

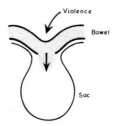

Fig. 532. Remote external violence causes rupture of small bowel at the point where it abuts against the unyielding neck of the hernial sac.

RUPTURE OF THE LARGE INTESTINE

Can be intra- or extraperitoneal. For obvious reasons, rupture of the large intestine, especially the intraperitoneal variety, is very lethal: fortunately it is comparatively rare. Very occasionally serious symptoms are delayed in the following way: the colon is bruised by the trauma, and slowly necrosis of the thin colonic wall occurs: suddenly the gangrenous portion perforates.

Seat-belt Injury of the Colon. The victim of a car accident appears to have been spared serious injury by his seat belt. However, the colon may have suffered a shearing injury causing ischaemia so that symptoms and signs of peritonitis are delayed, perhaps for as long as several days. Concomitant injuries include crush fractures of vertebrae and rib and pelvic fractures.

Extraperitoneal Rupture of the Duodenum. The signs are often particularly misleading. After the initial shock has passed off, there is sometimes an interval of comparative freedom from symptoms. Then, usually following a meal or a drink, sudden pain, frequently situated in the lower thoracic and upper lumbar regions posteriorly, commences, and repeated vomiting occurs. Pain in the testes, particularly the right testis, due to extraperitoneal irritation of their nerve supply, is sometimes present. If performed, the serum-amylase test will show a high reading. When the diagnosis is missed, and operation is not performed, or when the rupture is overlooked at laparotomy, extreme toxaemia supervenes. Should the patient survive, signs similar to those of a perinephric abscess (*see* p. 344) develop, incision of which is followed by a duodenal fistula.

Rupture of the Pancreas is a rare accident which is not infrequently accompanied by damage to other organs, particularly the spleen, duodenum, or jejunum. When the pancreas alone is injured, signs of a serious intra-abdominal injury are often lacking for some hours after recovery from the initial shock; then, owing to extravasation of pancreatic ferments, epigastric pain and repeated vomiting set in. Again a raised serum amylase is good evidence of this injury. A pseudopancreatic cyst (*see* p. 238) may be the first intimation of the injury.

Rupture of the Diaphragm. Most ruptures are on the left side of the diaphragm: the stomach and other hollow viscera then pass into the thorax so that abnormalities of percussion and auscultation are elicited on the left side of the thorax. Occasionally bowel sounds heard through the chest wall help to suggest the diagnosis, which is frequently overlooked.

INJURIES TO THE KIDNEY AND URETER

Renal injuries can be divided into slight, severe and critical.

Slight injuries comprise those where the parenchyma is damaged without

IAN AIRD, 1905–1962, *Professor of Surgery, Post-graduate Medical School, London.*

rupture of the capsule or extension of the laceration into the renal pelvis or a calix. Severe injuries are those where the capsule is broken and/or disruption into the renal pelvis or calices has occurred. An injury is termed 'critical' when the vessels of the renal pedicle are torn or the kidney is shattered.

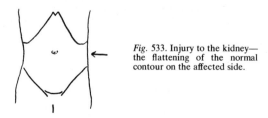

Fig. 533. Injury to the kidney— the flattening of the normal contour on the affected side.

The absence of superficial bruising counts for nothing; it is present in only a small proportion of cases. The same may be said of the classic 'swelling in the loin' when the posterior aspect of the patient is inspected. Of greater general utility, as an early sign, is a flattening of the normal contour of the affected side when viewed from the front, provided the patient is spare (*Fig.* 533). Rigidity of the anterior abdominal wall on the affected side is present constantly in cases of ruptured kidney. Owing to the greater mobility of the kidney in females, as well as to the somewhat more sheltered life of women, and possibly to the protection afforded by the wearing of corsets, the relative incidence of injuries in adult men and women is 10:1.

Haematuria. This cardinal sign of a damaged kidney may not make its first appearance until some hours after the accident. In quite a large proportion of cases the urine voided soon after the accident is clear. The second sample, however, shows blood and urine intimately mixed.

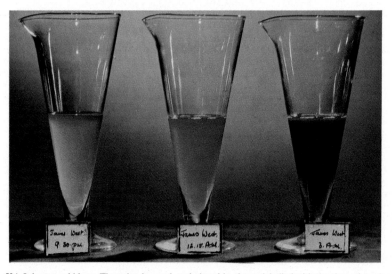

Fig. 534. Injury to a kidney. The urine is saved, and placed in glasses labelled with the time of passing. In this way one sample of urine may be compared with a later specimen, and an estimation can be formed as to whether the bleeding is progressive or not.

In all cases the urine should be saved and placed in glasses bearing a label indicating the time of voiding (*Fig.* 534). It is then possible to compare one sample of urine with a later specimen, and thus to estimate whether the bleeding is progressive. If, after the initial examination, it is decided that no immediate operation is necessary, the patient is made as comfortable as possible, shock is treated (if necessary), arrangements are made for the pulse to be recorded quarter-hourly, for an intravenous pyelogram to be carried out, if possible, and the clinician revisits the patient as often as the gravity of the case demands.

Rarely, macroscopic haematuria ceases within a few hours; this, of course, is likely when the injury is trivial. Nevertheless, one must not jump to this conclusion, for cessation of haematuria occurs also when the ureter becomes occluded by blood clot. Haematuria is entirely absent in renal injuries only when the renal pelvis is avulsed from its ureter, a rarity.

Delayed Rupture. Sudden profuse haematuria may occur (usually between the third and the fifth days) in a patient who appeared to be progressing favourably. The determining factor is probably some movement which dislodges a clot in the renal pelvis (*haematurie tardive*, Tuffier).

Residual Haematuria may be the cause of some anxiety after nephrectomy has been performed for ruptured kidney. Postoperatively bloodstained urine continues to be passed and one wonders whether the remaining kidney is injured also. The explanation is that urine becomes stained by washing over clots that are present in the bladder. Doubtless this is also the explanation of cases of prolonged haematuria following renal injury.

Clot Colic. Two different clinical conditions are included under this heading:

1. *Ureteric colic* is not very common, and when present usually occurs within 48 hours of the accident. The passage of clots down the ureter gives rise to pain radiating from the loin to the groin less severe than that produced by a calculus.

2. *Bladder colic* is much more frequent. It occurs generally between the third and fifth days after the accident, and is due to the passage of blood clot from the bladder. The pain is considerable, and is referred to the glans penis in males.

Meteorism. In many cases of severe renal injury abdominal distension comes on within 36 hours of the accident, and may give rise to difficulty in precise diagnosis. On rectal examination ballooning (*see* p. 278) is found, suggesting that this phenomenon is reflex in origin.

Perinephric Haematoma should be suspected if there is even a slight flattening of the normal contour of the loin (*see Fig.* 533). Rarely is abdominal relaxation sufficient to permit accurate palpation of the renal region, although when perirenal bleeding is extensive, a mass can be felt in spite of the overlying rigidity. In patients treated expectantly, a haematoma exceptionally causes a bulging in the loin. More often the blood tracks retroperitoneally to the iliac fossa, where a swelling is felt. On occasion the extravasated blood follows the course of the spermatic artery and gives rise to a thickening of the spermatic cord and to swelling and ecchymosis of the scrotum of the same side after a day or two.

Dual Rupture of the Spleen and Left Kidney. A variable degree of shock is present in all but very slight injuries to the kidney. When shock is profound, and fails to respond quickly to the treatment, if there is no more obvious injury to account for it, a concomitant intraperitoneal lesion should be suspected, and the commonest dual lesion is rupture of the spleen and the left kidney.

THEODORE TUFFIER, 1857–1929, *Professor of Surgery, University of Paris.*

FRACTURE OF THE PELVIS

Clinically there are two varieties: firstly the isolated fracture without damage to the urinary organs and relatively little blood loss; secondly, a double fracture with marked displacement of the pelvic bones due to shattering of the pelvic ring. Blood loss is severe, leading to shock, and injury to the bladder or urethra is possible and, with severe disruptions, likely. With the latter, also look for evidence of sciatic-nerve injury (*see* p. 412).

When a fracture is present transverse compression (*Fig.* 535) and distraction (*Fig.* 536) of the pelvis are likely to produce acute pain. The genitocrural fold is explored by following the bony margin of the ischiopubic ramus (*Fig.* 537).

A rectal examination may yield valuable information, particularly in cases of fracture of the coccyx. *Fig.* 538 shows the technique of examining for this fracture.

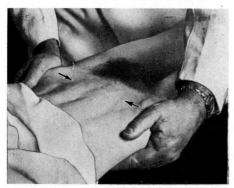

Fig. 535. Compression.

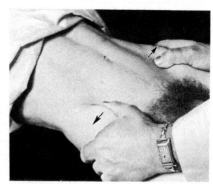

Fig. 536. Distraction.

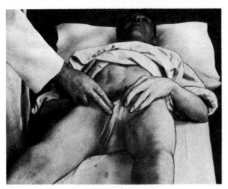

Fig. 537. Palpating the ischiopubic ramus.

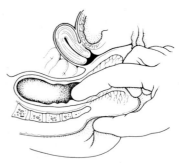

Fig. 538. Examining for a fractured coccyx.

RUPTURED BLADDER AND URETHRA

The prelude to the examination of an injury of the trunk should be an inquiry whether the patient has passed urine since the accident. For obvious reasons the importance of the rule reaches its zenith in injuries to the pelvis. Rupture of the bladder can be intraperitoneal, extraperitoneal, or both.

By reason of the ever-increasing number of road accidents, cases of fractured pelvis complicated by rupture of the bladder have become more common. Of these, the rupture is extraperitoneal in 80 per cent of cases. Conversely, as a result of increased sobriety, cases of intraperitoneal rupture of the bladder due to a blow upon the abdomen have become less common. Intraperitoneal rupture of the bladder is more likely to occur in an inebriated person for two reasons: (1) The victim is off his guard, and consequently the abdominal musculature is not braced to receive the blow; (2) The bladder is likely to be full.

Intraperitoneal Rupture of the Bladder. There is sudden agonizing pain in the hypogastrium, often accompanied by severe shock and perhaps syncope. However, in a few minutes the pain lessens—so much so that sometimes the patient resumes his occupation—but the abdomen soon distends because of paresis of intestinal coils bathed in urine (*Fig.* 539). Following the accident the patient usually has no desire to micturate. On examination a varying degree of abdominal distension is present. In spite of the fact that the patient has not passed urine since the accident, the bladder is not distended. There is tenderness in the hypogastrium. Abdominal auscultation discloses an absence of, or greatly decreased, intestinal sounds. If the amount of urine in the peritoneal cavity is considerable, shifting dullness can be elicited. Rectal examination often reveals a tender bulging in the rectovesical pouch. When the urine is sterile, symptoms and signs of peritonitis are delayed for several hours.

Should the patient not be seen until 24 hours after the accident, signs of diffuse peritonitis make the differential diagnosis from rupture of some other hollow viscus impossible, unless no urine has been passed since the accident.

Extraperitoneal Rupture of the Bladder. The signs are identical with those of intrapelvic rupture of the urethra (*see below*).

Intrapelvic Rupture of the Urethra. Usually signs of a fractured pelvis are evident and shock is pronounced, for, in addition to a fractured pelvis, about half the patients will be found to have sustained other fractures; but this does not complete the list of major concomitant lesions. One must always be alert to the possibility of an additional intraperitoneal lesion. The patient has not passed urine since the accident, and the escape of blood via the meatus is a common occurrence. In intrapelvic rupture, as opposed to rupture of the bulbous urethra, there is no perineal swelling, but ecchymoses may be visible. On examining the abdomen tenderness above the pubes is always present. As a rule, a swelling can be felt in the hypogastrium. Extravasation into the pelvic fascia occurs early and, curiously, it usually proceeds more on one side than on the other (*Fig.* 540). Unless the rounded dome of the bladder can be palpated distinctly from the rest of the swelling (the extravasation), it is impossible to arrive at a differential diagnosis between extraperitoneal rupture of the bladder and intrapelvic rupture of the urethra by abdominal examination alone. Not infrequently, the key to the situation lies in a *rectal examination*. If, on introducing a finger into the rectum, the prostate cannot be felt, but in its position there is an indefinite doughy swelling (blood and urine) (*Fig.* 541), or if the prostate is felt, but is displaced upwards, then the diagnosis of a complete intrapelvic rupture of the urethra is certain (Vermooten's sign)—unfortunately this is not present regularly.

When, clinically, a ruptured urethra or bladder is suspected, further investigation, notably an attempt to pass a catheter, must be carried out in the

Vincent Vermooten, 1897–1969, *Professor of Urology, University of Texas, S.W. Medical School, Dallas.*

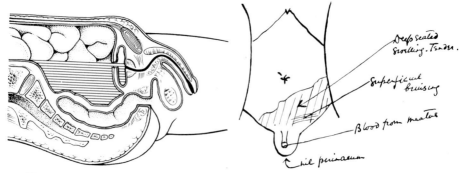

Fig. 539. Intraperitoneal rupture of the bladder.

Fig. 540. The physical signs recorded in a case of intrapelvic rupture of the urethra complicating a fractured pelvis. There was pain on compressing the iliac crests.

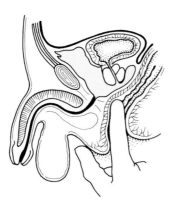

Fig. 541. In intrapelvic rupture of the urethra the puboprostatic ligaments are torn and the prostate becomes displaced posteriorly. In its place the palpating finger encounters a soft mass (blood clot).

Fig. 542. Rupture of the bulbous urethra after a fall astride on to a beam. The haematoma in the perineum is plainly visible. Blood is trickling out of the meatus. At operation the urethra was found completely divided.

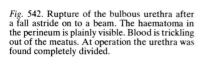
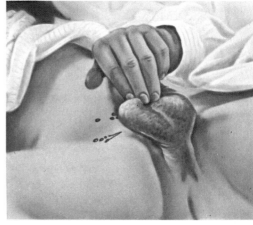

operating theatre, where sterility can be ensured and an operation follow immediately. When incomplete intrapelvic rupture of the urethra has occurred a catheter may pass into the bladder. In cases of complete intrapelvic rupture the catheter does not enter the bladder and urine does not drain freely.

Extrapelvic Rupture of the Urethra. This accident is almost always the result of a fall astride. *Fig* 542 shows a patient who had sustained a complete rupture of the bulbous urethra three hours before the photograph was taken. There is an obvious haematoma in the perineum. The external urinary meatus was examined and showed a few drops of bright red blood escaping. The bladder was percussed, and it was found to be moderately distended, for, in order to prevent superficial extravasation of urine (*see below*), the patient, before being sent to hospital, was rightly warned *not even to try* to pass urine.

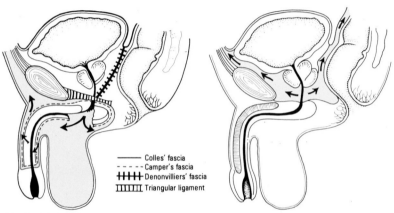

```
——— Colles' fascia
- - - - - Camper's fascia
╫╫╫ Denonvilliers' fascia
ШШШ Triangular ligament
```

Fig. 543. The fascial planes concerned in superficial extravasation of urine. The fusion of Colles' fascia with the anterior layer of the triangular ligament prevents extravasated urine from passing backwards beyond the middle perineal point.

Fig. 544. Deep extravasation of urine following intrapelvic rupture of the urethra.

EXTRAVASATION OF URINE

Superficial (Subcutaneous) Extravasation will òccur into the substance of the penis if Camper's fascia is intact. When, as is more usual, Camper's (syn. Buck's) fascia* is torn or eroded, diffusion occurs superficial to this fascia, but beneath Colles' fascia, distending the perineum to the midperineal point, the scrotum, and the penis. Unrelieved, the extravasation or cellulitis that accompanies it passes up the abdominal wall beneath Scarpa's fascia, which is continuous with Colles' fascia (*Fig.* 543). In many cases superficial extravasation arises as a complication of periurethral abscess (*see Fig.* 585, p. 357), which in turn is the result of a urethral stricture. Traumatic rupture of the bulbous urethra accounts for some instances, while the unskilled passage of instruments such as sounds, catheters, or a cystoscope is the cause in others.

---

* This fascia is known as 'Camper's fascia' in Europe, and as 'Buck's fascia' in the USA.

CHARLES P. DENONVILLIERS, 1808–72, *Surgeon, Paris.*
PETER CAMPER, 1722–1789, *Professor of Medicine, Anatomy, Surgery, and Botany, Gröningen, Holland.*
GURDON BUCK, 1807–1877, *Surgeon, New York Hospital.*
ANTONIO SCARPA, 1747–1832, *Professor of Surgery, Modena, and Professor of Anatomy, Pavia, Italy.*
ABRAHAM COLLES, 1773–1843, *Professor of Anatomy and Surgery, Dublin.*

The extravasated urine cannot pass: (1) Behind the midperineal point, because of the fusion of Colles' fascia (deep layer of the superficial perineal fascia) with the anterior layer of the triangular ligament (*Fig.* 543); (2) Into the thighs, for Scarpa's fascia (deep layer of the superficial fascia of the anterior abdominal wall) blends with the fascia lata just distal to the inguinal ligament; (3) Into the inguinal canal, because of the intercolumnar fibres and fascia of the external oblique.

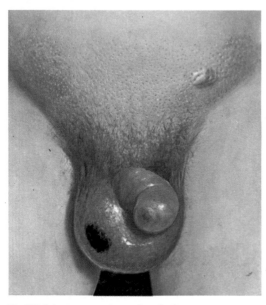

Fig. 545. Subcutaneous extravasation of urine.

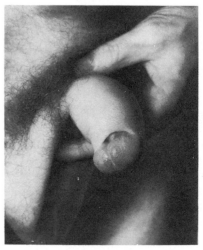

Fig. 546. Obvious oedema of the prepuce with palpable scrotal oedema. The patient was admitted as a case of extravasation of urine. Examination of the perineum showed no peri-urethral abscess or induration of a stricture. This aroused suspicion. Examination of the ankles revealed pitting on pressure. The cause of the oedema was congestive cardiac failure (*see* p. 10).

It therefore must pass: (1) Into the scrotum; (2) Into the subcutaneous tissues of the penis; (3) Up the abdominal wall in the subcutaneous planes (*Fig.* 545).

Superficial extravasation may be simulated very closely by oedema complicating a failing heart (*Fig.* 546).

Deep Extravasation of Urine takes place into planes of deep pelvic fascia (*Fig.* 544). It occurs in intrapelvic rupture of the urethra and extraperitoneal rupture or perforation of the bladder (*see* p. 331).

Chapter 24

CLINICAL EXAMINATION OF THE URINARY ORGANS

Diagnosis of urinary disease is largely a matter for special investigation. With intelligent use of the cystoscope, the urethroscope, X-rays (including arteriography), ultrasonography and biochemistry, clinical methods are comparatively unimportant. Often the principal object of the preliminary clinical examination is to suggest the exact form that special investigations will take, and to exclude disease of other organs. Be that as it may, careful inspection of recently voided urine when a patient is first seen is often of inestimable value.

The clinician should develop a routine of examining the urinary organs, starting with the kidneys and extending systematically downwards to the external urinary meatus. Some prefer to conduct the examination in a reverse manner.

HAEMATURIA

When the bleeding proves transitory, sometimes, sad to relate, instead of a full urological investigation being arranged, the patient is seen wending his way homewards carrying a supply of antibiotics. It is fervently requested that the reader of this book will never permit his clinical conscience to subscribe to this trouble-saving course that may well seal his patient's doom.

Often, by the time the patient arrives for the consultation, the bleeding has ceased. Not infrequently he brings with him a bottle of bloodstained urine. For a woman to collect a specimen is more difficult. Pour the urine into a glass and observe if the specimen contains any sediment or clots. When it seems probable that the bleeding is still in progress, it is more valuable to obtain a fresh specimen, and with a male, watch him pass urine. Is the blood integrally mixed with the urine? Is it bright red? Is there more or is there less blood in the terminal portion of the specimen? Such are the data the clinician should collect.

If blood is mixed with the whole specimen of urine it is possible for the lesion to be in the bladder, but much more often it is in a kidney. On the other hand, if the bleeding occurs either at the beginning or at the end of micturition, the source is much more likely to be in the bladder, especially in its neck, or in the prostate. Nevertheless, the elucidation of the cause is a problem in which cystoscopy combined with radiography has so minimized the importance of physical signs as to render the findings so obtained little better than a tentative hypothesis.

In the tropics haematuria often complicates *schistosomiasis*, being typically terminal, i.e. blood is noticed in the last few drops of urine.

INSPECTION OF THE URINE OTHER THAN FOR HAEMATURIA

Time was when the colour, the clearness or cloudiness, and the quantity of urine passed in the twenty-four hours—all still supremely important—were the only methods* of examining the urine known to clinicians. The following physical observations remain of steadfast value.

A Midstream Specimen of Urine should be inspected before being dispatched for bacteriological examination. If there is a sediment, it may be due to phosphates or to pus—add a few drops of acetic acid to the specimen: if the sediment disappears, it is due to phosphates. A description of other chemical tests is beyond the scope of this work.

Bile in the Urine. Bile pigments give the urine a greenish-brown colour with a yellow or brown foam when the container is shaken. On standing, bile-stained urine may assume a greenish hue (oxidation of bilirubin into biliverdin).

Porphyria. As a rule, the urine of patients suffering from porphyria is orange-coloured (which is often dismissed as 'concentrated'). On exposure for a few hours the top of the specimen (where it is exposed to the air) becomes amber-coloured (*Fig.* 547).

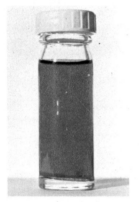 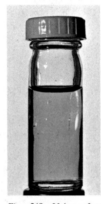 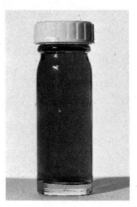

Fig. 547. Colour of urine, after standing overnight, in porphyria.

Fig. 548. Urine after ingestion of a patent medicine containing methylene blue.

Fig. 549. 'Beeturia'. The urine is the colour of cherry brandy.

Change of Colour due to Drugs. Cascara, senna and rhubarb tend to render the urine brown. Salicylic acid renders it reddish-yellow. Rifampicin (used in the modern chemotherapy of tuberculosis) commonly colours it purple. Methylene blue (a constituent of some patent medicines) produces a greenish colour. The patient whose urine is shown in *Fig.* 548 had lumbar pain, for which he took 'backache pills'. On passing green urine he hurried to hospital in an agitated state, believing that his kidneys were grossly diseased. Investigation showed no abnormality, and physiotherapy cured his lumbago.

'Beeturia'. Clinical acumen is never superfluous, for example, when beetroot is in season. The shade of red given by urine containing blood certainly varies very greatly, but it never resembles the cherry brandy-like hue of *betacyanuria* (the correct term) which is present in some 10 per cent of the populace (*Fig.* 549).

Chyluria. The urine is milky-white from the fat globules of the chyle. Chyluria occurs as the result of obstruction to the thoracic duct or the cisterna chyli, gross dilatation of lymphatic vessels, and

---

* Thomas Willis first drew attention to the sweet taste of diabetic urine.

THOMAS WILLIS, 1621–1675, *Physician in Oxford, later London. Discovered the arterial circle in the skull.*

rupture of a distended lymphatic vessel into some part of the urinary tract. Obstruction of a main duct can occur from a neoplasm pressing upon it, or from tuberculous mesenteric lymphadenitis pressing upon the cisterna, but by far the most common cause is occlusion of lymphatic vessels by *Wuchereria bancrofti.* Therefore inquire if the patient has resided in a tropical or subtropical zone, and look for evidence of filariasis by examining the scrotum or the labia majora (*Fig.* 550) for solid oedema.

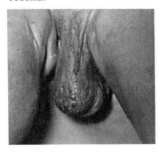

Fig. 550. Solid oedema of the left labium majus (elephantiasis). As the patient had suffered from lymphogranuloma inguinale (note the scar) as well as filariasis, it is problematical which was the cause of the lymphatic obstruction.

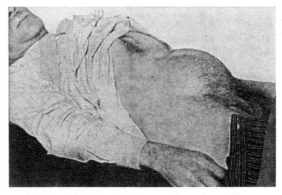

Fig. 551. Acute retention. Bladder extending to the umbilicus.

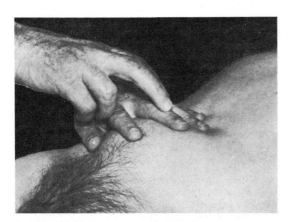

Fig. 552. Percussing the bladder. The patient was aged 70 and presented with chronic retention of urine which, on investigation, proved to be due to carcinoma of the prostate.

ACUTE RETENTION OF URINE

Distension of the Bladder. The distended bladder can be seen in the subject illustrated in *Fig.* 551 as a rounded swelling arising out of the pelvis. When the full bladder is either not full enough, or the abdominal wall is too well covered to permit the swelling thus produced to be seen, it can be felt and percussed. This should be carried out from above downwards—that is, from the resonant area to the dull (*Fig.* 552).

Cause of the Retention. *In the male* the meatus should be examined for atresia or a urethral discharge; the perineum observed for signs of periurethral abscess. Palpation along the course of the urethra, particularly in the neighbourhood of the penoscrotal junction, may reveal the induration of a stricture; rarely an

JOSEPH BANCROFT, 1836–1894, *Surgeon, Brisbane General Hospital, Brisbane.*

impacted urethral calculus can be felt. The prostate should next be palpated by rectal examination (*see* p. 357). It should be recalled that benign prostatic enlargement is easily the commonest cause of retention of urine, and with a full bladder it may not be possible to appreciate the exact size of the prostate. On the other hand, if the retention is caused by carcinoma of the prostate (*see* p. 359), the typical hardness of the gland can be detected usually, even with a full bladder. Where the cause is not evident the integrity of the central nervous system should be investigated. It used to be taught that testing the knee jerks and the reaction of the pupils suffices as a means of detecting organic disease of the central nervous system affecting the reflex arc of micturation. With the virtual disappearance of tabes dorsalis this is no longer true. It is better to test the ankle jerks and the cutaneous sensation in the perineum—two simple measures that supply this essential information (Gibbon).

For practical clinical purposes recall Shakespeare's 'Seven Ages of Man' from *As You Like It*.

Jacques   All the world's a stage,
And all the men and women merely players:
They have their exits and their entrances:
And one man in his time plays many parts,
His acts being seven ages. At first the infant,
Mewling and puking in the nurse's arms.
And then the whining schoolboy, with his satchel,
And shining morning face, creeping like snail
Unwillingly to school. And then the lover,
Sighing like furnace, with a woeful ballad
Made to his mistress' eyebrow. Then a soldier,
Full of strange oaths, and bearded like the pard,
Jealous in honour, sudden and quick in quarrel,
Seeking the bubble reputation
Even in the cannon's mouth. And then the justice,
In fair round belly with good capon lin'd,
With eyes severe, and beard of formal cut,
Full of wise saws and modern instances;
And so he plays his part. The sixth age shifts
Into the lean and slipper'd pantaloon,
With spectacles on nose and pouch on side;
His youthful hose well sav'd a world too wide
For his shrunk shank; and his big manly voice,
Turning again towards childish treble, pipes
And whistles in his sound. Last scene of all,
That ends this strange eventful history,
Is second childishness, and mere oblivion—
Sans teeth, sans eyes, sans taste, sans everything.

Apply these to the case of acute retention of urine in the *male*:

1. 'The infant, mewling and puking in the nurse's arms.' The cause of his retention is a posterior urethral valve.

2. 'The whining schoolboy, with his satchel' probably has an enlarged bladder neck (Marion's disease), but obturation by a stone should be suspected in areas where bladder calculi are still common.

3. 'The lover, sighing like furnace' is likely to be a case of retention following acute urethritis.

NORMAN O. K. GIBBON, *Contemporary, Director Liverpool Regional Urological Centre, Liverpool.*
JEAN MARION, 1869–1960, *Professor of Urology, Faculty of Medicine, Paris.*

4. 'The soldier, full of strange oaths' almost certainly has a urethral stricture.

5. 'The justice, in fair round belly with good capon lin'd' is most probably a case of benign enlargement of the prostate.*

6. When 'the sixth age shifts into the lean and slipper'd pantaloon', carcinoma of the prostate becomes relatively more frequent.*

7. During the last age 'that ends this strange eventful history' carcinoma is even more likely although cases of benign enlargement still occur.*

In the *female*, acute retention is comparatively uncommon except post-operatively and postpartum. Apart from these, pelvic masses connected with the reproductive organs, bladder neck and urethral obstruction and neurological causes in that order should be sought. The time-honoured hysteria is rare but does occur.

Postoperative Retention of Urine—a common condition in both sexes—can be due to any of the causes listed but more often the patient cannot micturate lying down. Others have a 'bashful bladder'; they cannot pass urine when another person is in the immediate vicinity.

SUPPRESSION OF URINE

The importance of the tongue as an indicator of efficient renal excretion has been discussed on p. 8.

Prerenal Anuria occurs from any cause that reduces the blood pressure below that where filtration from the glomeruli ceases. A common cause is shock, and if after restoration of the blood pressure to a more satisfactory level the patient does not pass urine, he should be catheterized to ascertain if urine is being excreted.

Renal Anuria. Urine excretion becomes ineffective from damage or destruction of renal epithelium. The causes are numerous and among those of particular surgical importance are incompatible blood transfusion, the crush syndrome, concealed uterine haemorrhage, and as a terminal event in congenital cystic kidneys. In this variety of anuria there is gradually increasing oliguria,† and the oliguric phase lasts about ten to twelve days. Unless the condition is reversible and diuresis sets in during the second week, or is treated, clinical deterioration follows. Usually vomiting commences; abdominal distension is seldom absent. With prolonged oliguria somnolence may progress to stupor, mild delirium, or coma. Convulsions in oliguria nearly always signify excessive administration of water and sodium.

Postrenal Anuria. The most common cause is blockage by calculus in both ureters or in the ureter of a sole functioning kidney (*calculous anuria*). Another cause is accidental ligation of both ureters during hysterectomy, or occlusion by a carcinoma of the cervix uteri. As a rule the anuria, which is rarely complete, commences suddenly during an attack of ureteric colic, and for the first five or six days the patient often feels comparatively well. However, unrelieved, the tongue becomes coated and the patient constipated, and eventually drowsy.

---

* Retention of urine (acute and chronic) in men after middle age is due to adenomatous enlargement of the prostate in 85 per cent, carcinoma in 10 per cent and prostatic fibrosis in 5 per cent.

† Oliguria is an excretion of less than 300 ml of urine in 24 hours.

Dryness of the tongue, meteorism, vomiting and coma usher in the end, death occurring after about eight or ten days. In the last stages the temperature is often subnormal, and muscular twitchings are common. On abdominal palpation, provided overlying rigidity permits, one kidney is found to be enlarged and tender, and that kidney is the last to be obstructed. The bladder is empty; the urine is exceedingly scanty and probably bloodstained.

CLINICAL EXAMINATION OF THE KIDNEYS

In order to be precise and accurate, it is best to discard the term 'renal colic' and speak of 'renal pain' and 'ureteric colic'.

Renal Pain is usually a dull ache situated mainly in the costovertebral angle, but also in the upper and outer quadrant of the abdomen. Often the patient indicates the site of this pain in the manner shown in *Fig.* 553. Renal pain is not strictly lumbar.

RENAL PAIN AND URETERIC COLIC

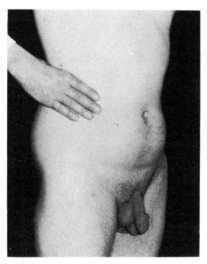

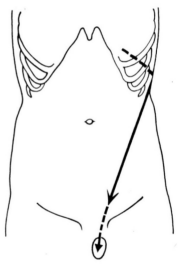

Fig. 553. A usual position of the hand of a patient who is showing where he experiences renal pain.

Fig. 554. The pointing test in ureteric colic. The patient will map out the direction of the pain as passing from the loin to the groin.

Ureteric Colic is usually characteristic—the pain passes from the loin to the groin, and in the male frequently this radiation is prolonged to the testis, which becomes retracted. The patient can often map the course accurately (*Fig.* 554).

During, or soon after, an attack the pulse and temperature are normal. Palpation will reveal in the corresponding loin and iliac fossa some tenderness and guarding, but no true rigidity. In the highly important differentiation of ureteric colic from appendicitis and intestinal colic, the rebound test (*see* p. 288) is of signal value *between* the attacks of colic. In ureteric colic the discomfort of deep palpation is relieved when the examining hand is released. In appendicitis deep palpation causes fairly severe pain which is *accentuated* on releasing the hand.

This leaves intestinal colic to be differentiated from ureteric colic. The unilateral distribution of the pain in ureteric colic and the frequent deep tenderness along the line of the ureter (*see* p. 345) or over the kidney (*see below*) will more often than not soon establish the colic as ureteric. In a few cases meteorism and ballooning of the rectum (*see* p. 278) lead to confusion. However, in ureteric colic the patient continues to pass flatus. If there is real doubt a radiograph of the abdomen should resolve it (calculus or fluid levels seen).

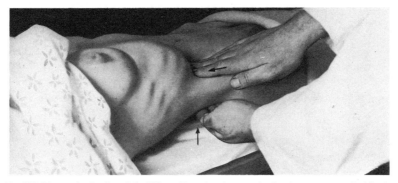

Fig. 555. Bimanual palpation of the kidney. Note that the posterior hand presses upward while the fingers of the anterior hand are directed cephalad and downward, and then slid in the reverse direction.

Recurrent Renal or Ureteric Calculi. Palpate the thyroid gland for the possible presence of a parathyroid tumour, although for such a tumour to be large enough to be felt is most exceptional. Hyperparathyroidism, which 'causes the patient to pass his skeleton in his urine', results in a great increase in the elimination of calcium in the urine. Repeated estimation of the serum calcium, and, in late cases, radiographs to display bone decalcification, are required to make the diagnosis. This condition as a cause of urinary calculi is much less common than imperfect drainage of the renal pelvis or incomplete emptying of the bladder plus urinary infection.

Palpation of the Kidneys. The patient should lie on his back. The value of the examination is enhanced by placing a pillow beneath the knees, and often it is advisable to have the patient rolled slightly towards the side that is being examined.

There are several variations in technique. Probably the best is the bimanual method, which is illustrated in *Fig.* 555. After the hands have been adjusted nicely in position, and the maximum amount of relaxation of the patient's musculature has been ensured, he is asked to take a deep breath. The pulps of the fingers of the two hands are approximated as *expiration* is in progress. The second method is shown in *Fig.* 556. It is possible to endeavour to palpate both kidneys at one and the same time by this method, which is of service only in thin subjects and children. In cases of difficulty, it is valuable to examine the kidney with the patient lying upon the sound side (*Fig.* 557).

In a thin adult with poorly developed abdominal musculature the lower pole of the right kidney sometimes is palpable as a firm, smooth, somewhat rounded structure that descends with respiration. The normal left kidney is impalpable unless the patient is unusually thin.

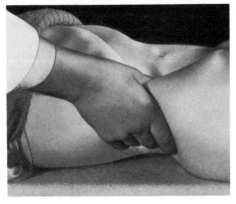

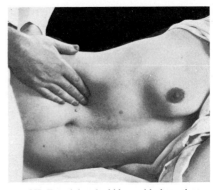

Fig. 557. Examining the kidney with the patient on the sound side. A useful method of examining and determining the nature of a lump that *may* be the kidney.

Fig. 556. Another method of palpating the kidney.

The Renal Angle Test (Murphy's 'Kidney Punch'). The patient sits up and folds his arms in front of him. The thumb is then placed under the 12th rib, and short, jabbing movements are made (*Fig*. 558). At first the movements are very gentle, but if pain is not experienced their strength is increased. This sign is of great value in determining deep-seated tenderness.

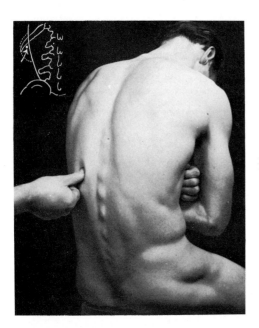

Fig. 558. The renal angle test (Murphy's 'kidney punch'). The thumb is placed under the 12th rib and to the lateral side of the sacrospinalis muscle, and sharp jabbing movements are made.

A Renal Swelling. An enlarged kidney, from any cause, possesses these characteristics: (1) It lies in the loin, or can be moved into the loin; (2) Usually it maintains its original reniform shape; (3) It moves on respiration; (4) There is a band of colonic resonance anteriorly; (5) It is dull posteriorly.

JOHN B. MURPHY, 1857–1916, *Surgeon, Mercy Hospital, Chicago.*

This classic picture will seldom be seen in its entirety, e.g. it is frequently impossible to demonstrate the band of colonic resonance.

Neoplasms of the kidney tend to enlarge anteriorly (*see Fig.* 560) while large abscesses and hydronephroses sometimes produce considerable posterior projection.

Differential Diagnosis between an Enlarged Left Kidney and an Enlarged Spleen. This not unusual error can be obviated by the following means:

1. If a sharp anterior border and/or a notch is felt, it is the spleen.

2. Unless it is extremely adherent to surrounding structures, which is unusual, an enlarged kidney gives the sign of ballottement (*see* p. 13).

3. The spleen enlarges inferiorly and medially, i.e. towards the right iliac fossa. Usually the kidney enlarges medially and posteriorly.

4. If dullness of the palpable swelling is continuous with the normal splenic dullness, it is the spleen.

In doubtful cases radiographic demonstration of the kidney is necessary.

Congenital Cystic Kidneys. When both kidneys are much enlarged and *irregular*, congenital cystic kidneys should be thought of, particularly if the symptoms are few. Haematuria due to spontaneous rupture of one or more of the cysts, pain due to intracystic tension or to the supervention of infection or calculus formation, or symptoms of renal insufficiency eventually cause the patient to seek advice. Infrequently the condition is mainly unilateral, when the diagnosis from a neoplasm becomes impossible without radiological investigation.

Renal Ectopia as a Cause of an Abdominal Lump. A misplaced kidney can give rise to an abdominal swelling, and almost always there is considerable perplexity concerning its nature. First, there is crossed ectopia, which results in both kidneys lying fused one above the other. The renal mass is palpable, and sometimes it is a little tender. Next there is the more common low position of a kidney with a short ureter. Such a kidney, which sometimes is the only kidney, lies in the iliac fossa or in the pelvis. In either of these situations it gives rise to a lump, and because a misplaced kidney is frequently the seat of ascending infection, the lump to which it gives rise is acutely tender and consequently usually is mistaken for an appendix abscess, diverticulitis, or a twisted ovarian cyst.

The Association of Malformation of the Ears and Congenital Renal Abnormalities. Malformed ears, particularly if asymmetrical, are quite commonly associated with congenital malformations of the urinary tract such as double ureter, hydronephrosis and horseshoe kidney. The deformity of the pinna is a bat-ear or a crumpled pinna somewhat like that of the Collins–Franceschetti syndrome (*see Fig.* 150, p. 80).

NEOPLASMS OF THE KIDNEY

A. Nephroblastoma (Wilms's Tumour) ranks second only to retroperitoneal neuroblastoma (of the adrenal gland) as the most common malignant tumour of childhood. In two-thirds of the cases there is a swelling (*Fig.* 559) discovered, as a rule, by the mother when bathing or dressing the child. In one-third painless haematuria is the presenting sign. In a few, the first symptoms are those of metastases in the lungs, unlike adrenal neuroblastoma which metastasizes predominantly to bone.

An advanced nephroblastoma often spreads across the midline as the example illustrated in *Fig.* 559 has done, but a neuroblastoma almost invariably remains on the side on which it originated.

B. Adenocarcinoma (Grawitz's Tumour) is the most common variety of renal malignant disease in adult life. By far the most frequent sign is painless,

MAX WILMS, 1867–1918, *Professor of Surgery, Heidelberg.*
PAUL A. GRAWITZ, 1850–1932, *Professor of Pathology, Greifswald, Germany.*

profuse, intermittent haematuria. Radiographic investigation should be made before a mass (*Fig.* 560) becomes palpable (pyelography, arteriography sometimes).

Less common ways of presentation are symptoms arising from a metastatic deposit, the primary neoplasm being quite silent. The commonest situation for such a deposit is a long bone, and it sometimes requires a biopsy to determine the nature of the neoplasm. A spontaneous fracture from this cause, or a persistent cough or haemoptysis from metastases in the lungs, also occurs. Another, but more unusual, symptom is persistent dull pain without haematuria. The development of an acute varicocele is a rare first manifestation (*see* p. 370) as is obstruction to the inferior vena cava (*see* p. 18). Lastly, there is a type in which intermittent pyrexia is the only sign, there being no associated infection.

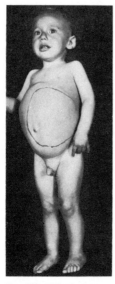

Fig. 559. Wilms's tumour (nephroblastoma) is the second most frequent cause of abdominal enlargement due to a solid unilateral intra-abdominal tumour in childhood.

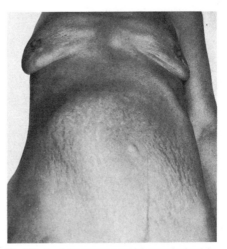

Fig. 560. An abdominal mass which arose in the right loin and was associated with long-standing haematuria. Pyelography confirmed a Grawitz's tumour. Seldom is a patient first seen at such a late stage.

PERINEPHRIC ABSCESS

The diagnosis of perinephric abscess rests almost entirely on the clinical examination, and it is necessary to bear the condition constantly in mind when one is investigating pyrexia of unknown origin. Too often the diagnosis is delayed unduly because the patient's *back* has never been examined (*Fig.* 561).

Inspection. First examine the patient in the sitting posture. The area immediately beneath the last rib and lateral to the sacrospinalis muscle is scrutinized; it is compared with the opposite side and the merest fullness is often the indication of a large collection of deep-seated pus. Scoliosis of the lumbar spine with concavity towards the affected side is almost a constant sign, even in early cases.

When an abscess is related to the lower pole of the kidney, a swelling in the renal area may be present early but when, as is more usual, it is related to the upper pole or the posterior surface of the kidney, the mass is imperceptible, even in well-advanced cases, because the rigid lower part of the costal cage renders it inaccessible.

Palpation. The renal angle test (*see* p. 342) is now applied. In cases where diagnosis is still in doubt, pillows should be removed, and the patient instructed to lie prone and quite straight. On the sound side the fingers can be dipped deeply towards the kidney; on the affected side, muscular resistance prevents this.

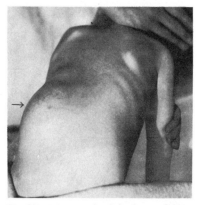

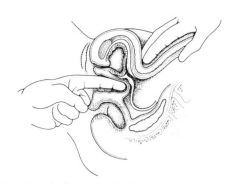

Fig. 561. A large perinephric abscess. Seldom is a swelling like this apparent. It is to direct attention as to where to look for the faintest semblance of a fullness that this illustration is included.

Fig. 562. Palpating a stone in the ureter via the vagina. A thickened tuberculous ureter also can be detected by this procedure.

THE URETER

Ureteric Calculus. Only if a scar in the right iliac fossa proclaims that the appendix has already been removed can the clinician be absolutely certain that acute pain in that situation is not due to acute appendicitis.

For the differentiation of ureteric colic from acute appendicitis and intestinal colic *see* p. 340.

Plain radiographs often show an opacity which *could* be a stone in a ureter, but pyelography (either intravenous or retrograde) is frequently necessary to be absolutely certain. Without this investigation the diagnosis of ureteric calculus from non-acute abdominal conditions is difficult, and sometimes impossible.

Transabdominal Palpation of the Ureter is of service in detecting a grossly thickened tuberculous ureter in a thin patient, and also for eliciting ureteric tenderness. The technique is that of deep abdominal palpation (*see* p. 225 and *Fig.* 396), but in this instance stand on the same side as the ureter to be examined and place the hands flat upon the abdomen over the line of the ureter.

Vaginal Palpation of the Ureter. The index finger is passed into the vagina and into the lateral fornix upwards and outwards until its pulp reaches the highest point it can touch; it is then carried downwards and inwards. Sometimes a large ureteric calculus just above the bladder can be felt bimanually (*Fig.* 562); a thickened tuberculous ureter can occasionally be discerned.

THE BLADDER

Never express an opinion on a swelling rising out of the pelvis until the bladder has been emptied by a catheter (*see* p. 227).

Acute Retention of Urine (*see* p. 337).

Retention with Overflow. The patient makes but little or no complaint of pain or dysuria but dribbles urine constantly. The swelling arising out of the pelvis is wont to be mistaken for some other condition. This error is more frequent when the contour of the bladder is unorthodox (*Fig.* 563, inset).

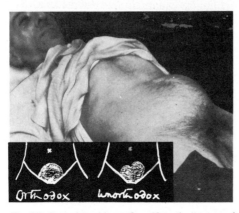

Fig. 563. Retention with overflow. Note the contour of the dome of the over-full bladder well to the left of the midline in this instance. The patient made no complaint of pain or difficulty of micturition.

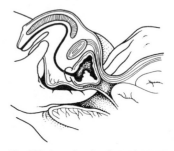

Fig. 564. Assessing the size and extent of a carcinoma of the bladder, under general anaesthesia. The bladder must be completely empty.

An empty bladder cannot be felt; it must extend above the pubic symphysis before it can be palpated. In infancy and childhood the bladder contains relatively little urine before it becomes palpable. That the swelling in question *is* the bladder is suggested by the fact that steady pressure upon it will evoke a desire to micturate or increase the dribbling in retention with overflow.

Diverticulum of the Bladder. Occasionally a large vesical diverticulum surrounded by inflammatory thickening can be recognized by deep palpation above the pubes or per rectum.

Carcinoma of the Bladder. It is only when a neoplasm of the bladder is very advanced that it becomes palpable by ordinary methods: on the other hand, bimanual palpation (*Fig.* 564), especially when performed under the relaxation afforded by anaesthesia, is of diagnostic assistance in assessing the extent of a vesical neoplasm, the presence of which has been ascertained by cystoscopy.

Carcinoma of the Bladder complicating Schistosomiasis (notably in Egypt). A mass is often palpable which consists of neoplasm plus a thickened bladder wall. This does not necessarily, in these circumstances, indicate an advanced growth.

Palpation of the Bladder per Rectum. So unusual is it for affections of the bladder, other than retention of urine and carcinoma, to provide any physical signs, that it is sometimes forgotten that a large stone in the bladder can be felt per rectum. In cases of prostatic enlargement it is useful to examine the base of the bladder per rectum *soon after the patient has passed urine.* By careful palpation a rough idea will be obtained of the amount of residual urine present.

Ectopia Vesicae. In this the bladder mucosa (*Fig.* 565), with the ureteric orifices discharging urine, can be seen.

THE FEMALE URETHRA

For the examination of the female urethra the dorsal position, with the thighs abducted, is desirable; indeed, it is almost essential. When the labia are separated

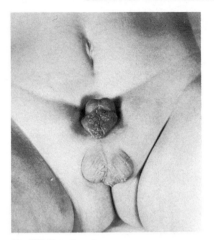

Fig. 565. Ectopia vesicae.

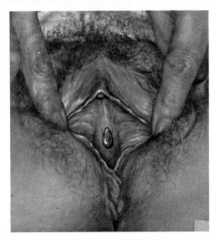

Fig. 566. Urethral caruncle: the so-called 'raspberry' tumour.

preparatory to vaginal examination (*see* p. 282) the eyes of the trained observer are directed first to the urethral orifice.

Urethral Caruncle is at once apparent as a small, pouting, granulomatous mass about the size of a pea (*Fig.* 566). With a probe, it can be determined that the protrusion arises from a broad pedicle attached to the posterior urethral wall. The mass is exquisitely tender and bleeds readily.

Carcinoma of the Urethra, although rare, occurs twice as frequently in the female as in the male. A visible protrusion that bleeds easily is the commonest manifestation. The final differential diagnosis between this and the above condition is histological, but a 'caruncle' of larger size than usual (*Fig.* 567), and one of any dimensions with induration, should be diagnosed provisionally as carcinoma. Palpate the inguinal lymph nodes, enlargement of any of which, in the absence of infection, makes the diagnosis of carcinoma almost certain.

Prolapse of the Urethra. Prolapse of the posterior urethral margin occurs in many women past the menopause, and becomes apparent when the patient is asked to strain. When the patient suffers from urethrotrigonitis, which causes straining at micturition, the prolapse becomes progressively larger. With partial prolapse the orifice is eccentric; when complete it is central.

Urethritis. The urethra can be palpated through the anterior vaginal wall; the meatus should first be swabbed. In cases of gonorrhoea sometimes pus can be milked from the urethra in this way (*Fig.* 568). In urethritis from any cause, gentle pressure of the anterior urethra against the symphysis causes pain. This sign of urethral tenderness is most reliable, and explains the fact that the chief complaint of many women with this condition is dyspareunia.

Stress Incontinence. The patient, usually multiparous, cannot control the escape of urine while coughing, laughing, or when the opportunity to empty a full bladder is not available immediately. That stress incontinence is present can be demonstrated by examining the urethral orifice while the patient has a (at least moderately) full bladder and requesting her to cough. When the urethral sphincter is not fully competent urine escapes at each expulsive effort.

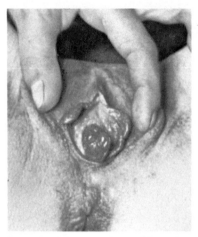

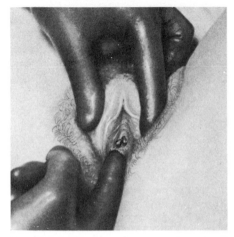

Fig. 567. Papilliferous carcinoma of the urethra.

Fig. 568. Palpating the urethra through the vagina. In relevant cases pus can be milked from the urethra and expressed from Skene's tubules, which are shown exuding pus in this case.

Pass a finger into the vagina and seek the pubococcygeus muscle, the main controlling sphincter of the urethra. When the development, integrity and tone of this muscle are normal it can be felt as a broad muscular band 1 cm proximal to the introitus, i.e. just proximal to the pubic rami. Ask the patient to contract her muscles 'as though trying to hold her water'. In stress incontinence the contractions of pubococcygeus are weak and the vagina beyond is commodious.

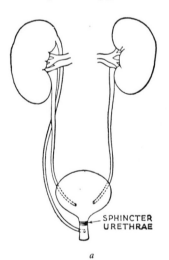

SPHINCTER
URETHRAE

a

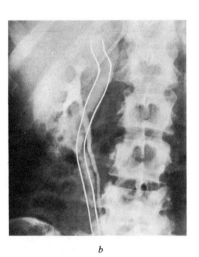

b

Fig. 569. *a*, Showing how an accessory ureter opening in an ectopic position below the urethral sphincter can cause intractable urinary incontinence in a female. *b*, Intravenous pyelogram showing a dilated ectopic ureter arising from the poorly functioning upper pole of the right kidney in a patient with urinary incontinence. Cured by upper pole nephrectomy.

ALEXANDER J. C. SKENE, 1838–1900, *Surgeon, Long Island College Hospital.*

Intractable Urinary Incontinence. Apart from one with spinal dysraphism (*see* p. 199), any girl or woman who has dribbled for as long as she can remember, despite the fact that she has a normal desire to void, and indeed does urinate, has an ectopic ureteric orifice (*Fig.* 569). The demonstration of this orifice is often extremely difficult. If the renal tissue drained by the ectopic ureter is sufficiently active to concentrate the dye, the diagnosis can be established by giving an intravenous injection of indigocarmine, and placing one swab in the vestibule and another in the vagina. The swab coloured blue signifies the position of the ectopic orifice.

Urethral Diverticulum (urethrocele) is commoner in women than in men. As the diverticulum enlarges in size, inability to pass all the urine at one time, or dribbling after micturition, occurs. On digital examination the swelling can be felt on the anterior vaginal wall in the line of the urethra, and when it is compressed, urine, usually obviously purulent, is expressed.

Chapter 25

THE MALE GENERATIVE ORGANS: VENEREAL DISEASE

While the patient is getting ready for the examination behind a screen or in a side-room (he should at least strip from the waist down), he is requested to micturate into a glass. If, however, there is a history of a urethral discharge, he should be asked to micturate after the meatus has been inspected (*see* p. 351).

The patient should be recumbent, so that in due course the groins, the perineum and the abdomen can be examined. Then a rectal examination is undertaken. Finally, for a thorough examination of the testes, the patient must stand (*see* p. 362).

EXAMINATION OF THE PENIS

The chief of a number of abnormalities and diseases that are encountered will now be discussed briefly.

Phimosis. This term should not be applied loosely; it is necessary to distinguish between *redundancy of the prepuce* and true *phimosis.** Only if the foreskin cannot be retracted because its orifice is stenosed, is phimosis present. The prepuce normally may be adherent to the glans penis during the first three years of life, and there is no need to separate the adhesions, for this is not true phimosis. Phimosis can also be acquired, usually in the elderly, as the result of cicatricial contraction following long-standing chronic balanoposthitis.†

When the prepuce is present ask the adult patient to retract it; that this is a wise preliminary step to an examination of the urogenital organs is shown by a perusal of the legends of *Figs.* 570 and 571. When the foreskin is not adherent to the glans the situation shown in *Fig.* 572 becomes a possibility.

Because phimosis prevents any prospect of the glans being cleansed, it leads to retention of smegma and chronic balanoposthitis. Thus it may well be the cause of chronic irritation that leads to carcinoma of the penis (*see* p. 354).

Paraphimosis. It is remarkable that paraphimosis, especially when it has been present for several days, is overlooked so often because the clinician mistakenly assumes that the uncircumcised patient with his exposed glans imprisoned outside a tight prepuce is in fact circumcised. Obviously the first thing to do is to ask the patient if he has been circumcised. It is amazing how often some seemingly intelligent men do not appear to know. With paraphimosis, if the skin of the penis is drawn towards the pubis, and the area behind the corona scrutinized, oedema limited abruptly by a constricting band (*Fig.* 573) can be seen. This leaves no doubt as to the diagnosis.

Reverting to the general examination of the penis and to the original request for the patient to retract his foreskin:

---

* *Phimosis.* Greek, φίμωσις = a stopping-up; a closure.
† *Balanitis.* Greek, βάλανος = an acorn, the glans penis + ιτις = inflammation.
  Posthitis. Greek, πόσθη = prepuce + ιτις = inflammation.

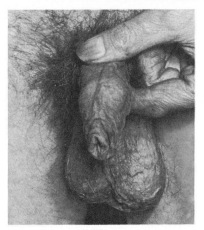

Fig. 570. **Case I.** The patient is a man of 71, complaining of great difficulty in micturition. In this illustration the patient's redundant foreskin, which shows nothing unusual, is seen.

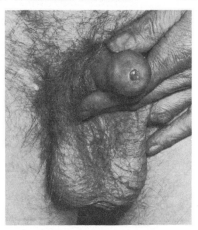

Fig. 571. When an attempt is made to retract the prepuce it is evident at once that the patient has a most extreme phimosis—the orifice in his foreskin is no larger than that which could be made by a large pin. Circumcision cured the condition completely.

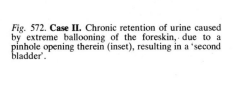
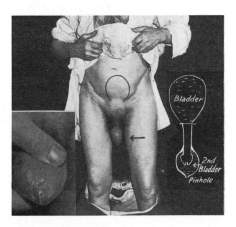

Fig. 572. **Case II.** Chronic retention of urine caused by extreme ballooning of the foreskin, due to a pinhole opening therein (inset), resulting in a 'second bladder'.

The Prepuce can be retracted.
When a discharge is present, observe whether it comes from the interior of the preputial sac or whether it issues from the urethra. A subpreputial discharge, which frequently is confused with a urethral discharge, may be due to one of several causes, notably chancre, chancroid, balanoposthitis, or a carcinoma.

Examination of the External Urinary Meatus
Pinhole meatus is often overlooked, both in infants and those of more mature years. *Fig.* 574 shows the method of testing whether the orifice is adequate.

Infection of Morgagni's Follicles. These are a pair of follicles that open laterally just behind the lips of the urethra. Often they become infected in urethritis, and then their mouths are more obvious, and perhaps pus can be seen exuding therefrom (*Fig.* 575). Frequently they are overlooked for want of inspecting the meatus in the manner shown in *Fig.* 574.

Infection of Tyson's Glands. These are bilateral sebaceous glands, which produce smegma, situated on either side of the fraenum and communicating, not with the urethra, but with the preputial sac. An infected gland (usually in gonorrhoea) gives rise to a firm, tender swelling (sometimes bilateral) on the under-surface of the glans penis, just lateral to the fraenum.

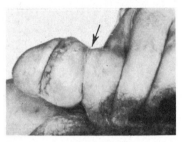

Fig. 573. Paraphimosis. The constricting band is often inconspicuous until the skin of the shaft of the penis has been put on the stretch.

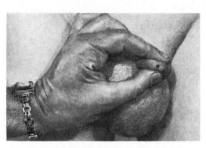

Fig. 574. Is the meatus adequate? By compressing the tip of the penis between a finger and thumb anteroposteriorly the lips of the meatus are opened, and it can be observed at once whether the orifice is stenosed.

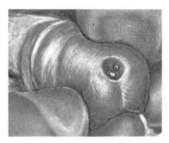

Fig. 575. Pus exuding from the right follicle of Morgagni.

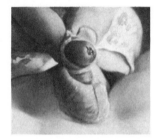

Fig. 576. Meatal ulcer with scab formation. The scab occludes the external urinary meatus.

Meatal Ulcer of infant boys is a clinical entity that is rarely found in the uncircumcised. It occasionally occurs after circumcision (a good argument against indiscriminate use of this operation), although eighteen months may elapse between the operation and the onset of symptoms. It probably is due in the first place to abrasion of the delicate unprotected mucosa by napkins, and is characterized by alternating open ulceration and scabbing of the meatus (*Fig. 576*), giving rise respectively to a drop of bright red blood on the diaper and attacks of screaming from temporary retention of urine. More often than not, on close examination the anteroposterior diameter of the external urinary meatus is shorter than normal. Untreated, cicatricial contracture of the meatus— in other words, an acquired pinhole meatus—is liable to ensue.

CONGENITAL ABNORMALITIES

Hypospadias is the most common congenital malformation of the urethra; it occurs once in every 350 males. The external urinary meatus is situated at some point upon the under-surface of the penis, or in the perineum. (*a*) *Glandular,*

EDWARD TYSON, 1649–1708, *Professor of Anatomy, Royal College of Surgeons of England.*

the opening being situated in the glans, but below the normal location, generally at a point where the fraenum (which is absent) is normally attached. A blind depression marks the normal site of the meatus. This is by far the most common variety. (*b*) *Penile*: The opening is situated at some point on the under-surface of the penis between the glans and the penoscrotal junction (*Fig.* 577). (*c*) *Perineal*: This is least common, the opening being situated about 3 cm in front of the anus. The scrotum is cleft and the testes, if descended, usually are small. In all varieties the penis curves downwards (*chordee**) but this is minimal in (*a*).

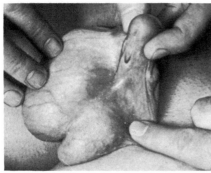

Fig. 577. Penile hypospadias. In this case the urinary meatus is situated half-way down the penis.

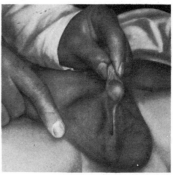

Fig. 578. Male pseudohermaphrodite. The patient was brought up as a girl until the age of 20, when the urge to become a male became manifest.

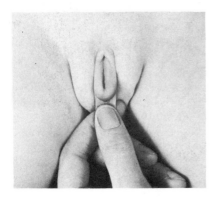

Fig. 579. Epispadias.

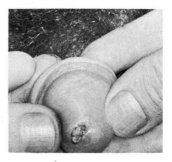

Fig. 580. Urethral papilloma protruding from the external urinary meatus.

A Male Pseudohermaphrodite (X–Y female) is a person with intra-abdominal testes, perineal hypospadias, and cleft scrotum, the latter being mistaken for labia majora (*Fig.* 578). Sometimes there is a short vagina. If in doubt have a histological examination performed on epithelial cells obtained by scraping the buccal mucosa and chromosome analysis to determine whether the patient is, in fact, male or female.

Epispadias is very uncommon. The urethra lies above the corpora cavernosa and opens at some point on the dorsal surface of the penis (*Fig.* 579). In epispadias totalis the malformation is accompanied

---

* *Chordee.* French, cordée = a cord.

by incontinence of urine, and frequently is associated with ectopia vesicae (*see* p. 346). The penis curves upwards.

Urethral Papilloma. From time to time a solitary papilloma springs from the fossa navicularis and protrudes from the external urinary meatus (*Fig.* 580). The typical symptom of papilloma of the urethra is slight haematuria immediately preceding micturition.

Venereal Warts (Papillomata Acuminata*) are the most common benign neoplasms of the penis. They occur in both the uncircumcised and the circumcised, and are most luxuriant in the coronal sulcus (*Fig.* 581). As a rule, these papillomata are moist, and are attended by an evil-smelling serous discharge.

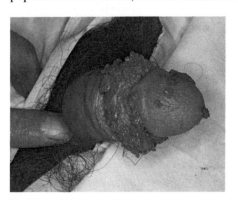

Fig. 581. Papillomata acuminata.

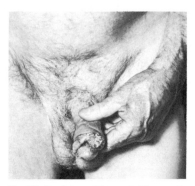

Fig. 582. Carcinoma of the penis. The growth, now ulcerative and indurated, probably commenced as a papilliferous neoplasm.

Carcinoma of the Penis. The incidence of carcinoma of the penis is particularly high among Hindus (who do not practise circumcision), Chinese, and the inhabitants of Malaya, but it is by no means uncommon in those of European descent. In addition to chronic balanitis, leucoplakia of the glans (precisely similar to the well-known condition on the tongue) is a precursor. It is almost unknown in Jews who practise circumcision shortly after birth and relatively rare in Moslems who undergo the operation at puberty.

Other rarer, but definitely precarcinomatous, conditions are Paget's disease of the penis (similar to Paget's disease of the nipple, *see* p. 165) and Queyrat's erythroplasia. The latter is a bright red, shiny lesion, velvety to touch, accompanied by a copious serous exudate, usually occurring in a single area and situated in the coronal sulcus: there is no induration.

When the prepuce is retractable the patient may present with a carcinoma of the penis at a fairly early stage. There are two forms of the disease, papilliferous and ulcerative (*Fig.* 582), and each is diagnosed by the induration of the base of the lesion. Should induration be doubtful, biopsy is essential. More often the foreskin cannot be retracted, and the neoplasm remains symptomless until it produces an evil-smelling discharge, which later becomes bloodstained. In such cases, unless there is considerable oedema produced by the concomitant balanoposthitis, the neoplasm can be felt through the foreskin. The reader is exhorted not to jump to a conclusion that the cause of the discharge is a venereal disease, even though the patient be comparatively young (carcinoma of the penis

---

* *Acuminatus.* Latin = sharp-pointed.

SIR JAMES PAGET, 1814–1899, *Surgeon, St. Bartholomew's Hospital, London.*
LOUIS QUEYRAT, 1856–1933, *Physician, Hôpital Cochin, Paris.*

is not unusual below the age of 40 years, particularly in coloured races). If in doubt the proper course is to slit the foreskin on the dorsum under anaesthesia, and thus expose what lies beneath.

Palpation of the Inguinal Lymph Nodes. In every case of an inflammatory, or a suspected neoplastic, lesion of the penis the inguinal lymph nodes must be palpated. Often they are found to be enlarged, but unless the nodes are stony hard, reserve judgement as to the cause of the enlargement, for in 50 per cent of cases of carcinoma of the penis the enlargement of the nodes is inflammatory, and not due to metastases.

Sebaceous Cysts in the skin of the shaft of the penis are uncommon. When one becomes subacutely infected, it offers a diagnostic problem. Before rupture, it can simulate a bubonulus.* After indolent rupture, like Cock's 'peculiar' tumour (*see* p. 53), it can resemble a carcinoma.

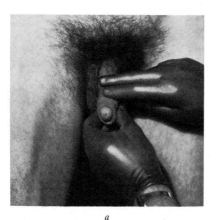
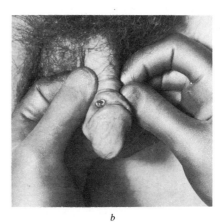

a   *b*

Fig. 583. *a*, Palpation of the dorsum of the shaft of the penis reveals an indurated subcutaneous cord. *b*, On retracting the prepuce a typical Hunterian chancre is displayed. Case of thrombosis of the dorsal vein.

Thrombosis of the Dorsal Vein of the Penis gives rise to a physical sign that is absolutely characteristic. On palpation (*Fig.* 583 *a*), in the subcutaneous tissues of the middle line of the dorsum of the penis there is what feels like a 'pipe cleaner', as a patient graphically described it. Retraction of the prepuce, if present, usually reveals the cause of the thrombosis at once (*Fig.* 583 *b*).

Priapism. The penis remains persistently erect and is painful. Most often the erection is due to idiopathic thrombosis occurring in the corpora cavernosa; less frequently it is associated with leukaemia or sickle-cell anaemia. Secondary malignant deposits in the corpora cavernosa or the pelvis account for a small proportion of cases. In another, completely different, category are cases due to spinal injury or disease. There is unlikely to be any difficulty in associating a spinal injury with priapism, but when organic disease of the central nervous system is the cause, often a full neurological examination is required to elucidate it.

Induratio Penis Plastica (Peyronie's Disease) is uncommon. Lateral curvature of the erect penis is the only symptom, except in the early stages, when pain on erection is experienced. A localized, painless induration about half-way down the dependent part of one or both corpora cavernosa, but never in the corpus spongiosum, is pathognomonic of the condition. When the area is rolled between the finger and thumb the impression gained is that the spongy tissue has been converted into soft cartilage. The cause is unknown.

---

* *Bubonulus.* Latin = a small bubo. Occurs in the course of a lymphatic vessel, especially of the penis. Is a manifestation of lymphogranuloma inguinale (*see* p. 376).

FRANÇOIS DE LA PEYRONIE, 1678–1747, *Surgeon to Louis XV, and Founder of the Royal Academy of Surgery, Paris. Mainly due to him, Paris became a great surgical centre in the eighteenth century.*

Palpation of the Floor of the Male Urethra, from the glans to the triangular ligament (*Fig.* 584), often yields valuable information, for instance:

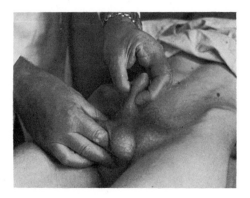

Fig. 584. Palpating the floor of the urethra. This should be done systematically from the external urinary meatus to the triangular ligament. Note that in order to palpate the deep urethra it is necessary to invaginate the scrotum.

A Urethral Stricture can sometimes be felt from without, and a favourite site is the penoscrotal junction.

Carcinoma of the Urethra. This rarely complicates a long-standing urethral stricture but can occur *de novo.* As a rule the only symptom is a profuse urethral discharge, which later becomes bloodstained. When, in addition, there is considerable localized induration in the floor of the urethra, and because a urethral discharge is so unusual in cases of inflammatory stricture, carcinoma of the urethra should spring to mind. If, as it is hoped, this deduction is made the clinician will forthwith palpate the inguinal lymph nodes—often these are implicated early by metastases.

Urethral Diverticulum (Urethral Pouch). The pouch can be seen on the under-surface of the penis, and if it is not obvious it usually can be made apparent when the patient interrupts the urinary stream by pinching the glans. On palpation, a soft swelling will be felt in the midline, and on compressing it, urine, sometimes purulent, issues from the external urinary meatus.

Penile Periurethral Abscess. A rounded, pea-like swelling under the skin, attached to the urethral floor situated about the middle of the penile urethra, is characteristic of a closed abscess of a paraurethral (Littre's) gland. Later it becomes tender and fluctuant.

THE MALE PERINEUM

The male perineum, being hidden by the scrotum, is liable to escape scrutiny unless the practice is made of examining this region with the patient in the spread-eagle position and the scrotum elevated. Conditions in which cardinal diagnostic assistance is derived from displacing the scrotum upwards are depicted in *Figs.* 585–588, and a fifth illustrated in *Fig.* 542, p. 332.

Referring to *bulbous periurethral abscess*, in only 50 per cent of cases does it occur behind a urethral stricture. In its most acute form it gives rise to spreading cellulitis along the planes described for superficial extravasation of urine (*see Fig.* 543, p. 333).

Examination of the bulbo-urethral (Cowper's) glands is described on p. 360.

THE PROSTATE AND ITS ADNEXA

As a prelude to palpation of the prostate, the patient is asked to empty his bladder. When possible the act of micturition should be watched, for loss of projectile power is significant. It is inadvisable to examine the prostate before a general examination of the abdomen has been conducted at which special

ALEXIS LITTRE, 1658–1725, *Surgeon and Anatomist, Paris; spelt his name without an accent.*

SOME CONDITIONS REVEALED BY INSPECTING THE MALE PERINEUM

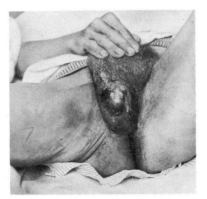

Fig. 585. Bulbous periurethral abscess.

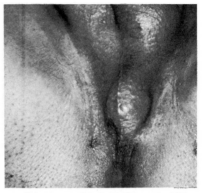

Fig. 586. Abscess of the left bulbo-urethral (Cowper's) gland.

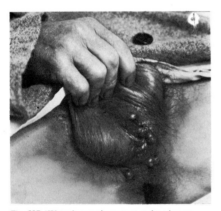

Fig. 587. 'Watering-can' scrotum and perineum. Case of neglected stricture of the urethra.

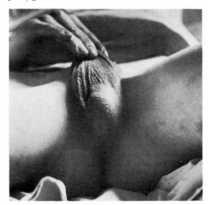

Fig. 588. Perineal testis.

attention should be paid to the bladder, for if by palpation and percussion it is found to be distended in spite of urination, not only is that discovery of cardinal importance, but it also foretells that the rectal findings on the state of the prostate are likely to be unreliable (*see* p. 338).

Routine examination of the prostate is performed best with the patient in the knee–elbow position (*Fig.* 589). The finger, well lubricated, is introduced slowly in the manner described on p. 272.

Visualizing the Parts to be palpated. It is essential to have a clear conception of the relationship to the palpating finger of structures about the prostate, and to know what can be felt normally. The prostate feels firm and elastic, and this is in sharp contrast with adjacent tissues. Each of its ovoid lateral lobes, which are separated by a median furrow, is about the size of the distal segment of the thumb. They project posteriorly but very slightly.

Passing the finger *downwards* along this median furrow, immediately after the prostate has been traversed, the finger impinges upon a soft area—here lies the membranous urethra. On each side of the midline at this point are situated the bulbourethral (Cowper's) glands. Sliding the finger *upwards* along the furrow, a little to each side of the superior limit of the prostate lie the seminal vesicles within reach of the finger. A normal vesicle cannot be felt. Between the vesicle and the lateral lobe of the prostate of each side there is a sulcus which is traversed by the lymphatics leaving the prostate. These anatomical facts must be understood clearly and *Fig.* 590 visualized before diagnosis of the abnormal is attempted.

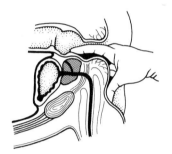

Fig. 589. Palpation of the prostate with the patient in the knee–elbow position. Each lateral lobe is palpated, paying particular attention to its consistency.

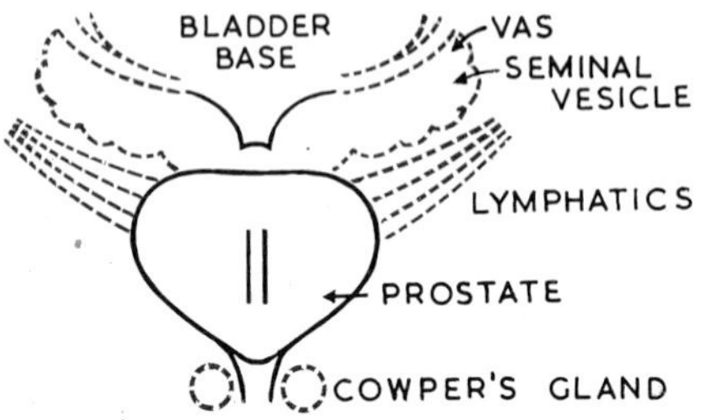

Fig. 590. The parts in *black* are felt normally, those in *red* only when they are diseased. (*After Thomson-Walker.*)

Before expressing an opinion on the size of the prostate, it is necessary to be certain that the bladder is empty. Especially in the case of acute retention of urine the posterior surface of the full bladder can be mistaken for a large prostate. Affections of the prostate, translated into terms of palpation, can be described as follows:
Prostatitis. *Acute*. Palpation must be very gentle. An enlarged, swollen, tense but slightly oedematous, tender, hot prostate is diagnostic of acute prostatitis. Sometimes acute prostatitis is associated with acute seminal vesiculitis. If an abscess* or abscesses have formed they will be detected as areas of softening.
Chronic. Chronic prostatitis is not common. It can follow acute prostatitis, or be chronic from the commencement. Diagnosis is often uncertain and it is not always easy to decide if the patient's symptoms are due to the prostatic infection. The gland may be slightly enlarged or normal in size. Similarly, tenderness may be slight or absent. Frequently the prostate is somewhat nodular, with occasional boggy spots. Clinical differentiation from carcinoma may prove difficult. Microscopical examination of the fluid expressed by prostatic massage (*see* p. 360) for pus cells is the only reliable method of demonstrating the infection.
Tuberculous Prostatitis. Almost always one, and sometimes both, seminal vesicles are implicated. Both these structures are hard, irregular and can be best described as 'craggy'. The vas deferens is nearly always involved (*see* p. 368).
Benign (Adenomatous) Enlargement of the Prostate. In benign enlargement affecting the lateral lobes, increase in their size is evident. They are smooth, convex and typically elastic, but because all grades of fibro-adenosis occur, the fibrous element may give a firm consistency. In all cases the rectal wall can be

---

* The fact that rectal or perineal pain persists after antibiotic treatment of acute prostatitis suggests that an abscess has formed, particularly in a diabetic.

Sɪʀ Jᴏʜɴ Tʜᴏᴍsᴏɴ-Wᴀʟᴋᴇʀ, 1870–1937, *Urologist, St. Peter's Hospital, London.*

made to move over the prostate. While as a rule some
degree of enlargement is apparent to the examining finger,
it must be realized that the enlargement is frequently
mainly, and sometimes entirely, confined to the middle
lobe, viz. ————————————————————————→

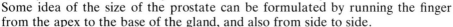

The palpating finger should pass over the entire gland.
It will note the presence of the median groove, which may,
or may not, be distorted by bosselations in its vicinity.
Some idea of the size of the prostate can be formulated by running the finger
from the apex to the base of the gland, and also from side to side.

Carcinoma of the Prostate. The chief obstacle to early diagnosis is the absence
of symptoms and the chief hope of early recognition is the routine examination
of the prostate in men over 45 years of age who present for life assurance, or for
conditions not referable to the prostate. Another difficulty is that when the
carcinoma commences deep in the lateral lobes, or in the middle lobe, it cannot
be felt per rectum. In an average case, however, the carcinoma commences in
the posterior part of the gland near the surface, and can
be recognized as a rounded area of induration beneath the
capsule, viz.————————————————————————→

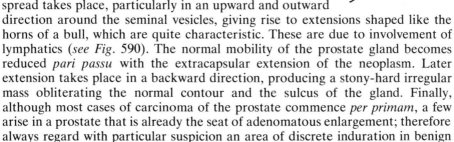

contrasting in consistency with that of the normal prostate.
As it increases in size, the nodule acquires stony hardness.
Somewhat later the vertical median groove between the
lateral lobes (*see Fig.* 590) becomes obliterated. Further
spread takes place, particularly in an upward and outward
direction around the seminal vesicles, giving rise to extensions shaped like the
horns of a bull, which are quite characteristic. These are due to involvement of
lymphatics (*see Fig.* 590). The normal mobility of the prostate gland becomes
reduced *pari passu* with the extracapsular extension of the neoplasm. Later
extension takes place in a backward direction, producing a stony-hard irregular
mass obliterating the normal contour and the sulcus of the gland. Finally,
although most cases of carcinoma of the prostate commence *per primam*, a few
arise in a prostate that is already the seat of adenomatous enlargement; therefore
always regard with particular suspicion an area of discrete induration in benign
enlargement of the gland.

Contracture of the Bladder Neck (Fibrous Prostate). The prostate is either
normal in size or, more usually, smaller. The gland is distinctly harder than
usual, but its shape is preserved and its contour smooth; the latter serves to
differentiate the condition from carcinoma, but when the gland is stony hard
laboratory tests and biopsy are required to eliminate a scirrhous carcinoma.

Prostatic Calculi. When these small stones are near enough the periphery to be
detected by palpation, they are so embedded in the fibrous stroma as to simulate
the irregular hardness of a carcinoma. Very occasionally the stones are
comparatively free, and they impart to the palpating finger an impression
described so aptly by Erichsen as of 'beads in a bag'.

Bimanual Palpation of the Prostate. Where the diagnosis is not certain, bimanual
palpation of the prostate (*see Fig.* 473, p. 269) in the lithotomy position is a
valuable procedure. In a thin subject with the bladder completely empty, an
intravesical lobe sometimes can be felt. When pressure is exerted on the apex of

Sɪʀ Jᴏʜɴ E. Eʀɪᴄʜsᴇɴ, 1818–1896, *Surgeon, University College Hospital, London.*

the prostate by the finger in the rectum, it will be found that a gland which is the seat of benign enlargement possesses a limited degree of mobility. Fixity of a carcinomatous prostate becomes most evident by this manœuvre. Residual urine in a post-prostatic pouch can sometimes be felt as a soft swelling above the prostate. Good access to the seminal vesicles is also afforded. It is usual to carry out this examination in conjunction with cystoscopy under general anaesthesia.

Examination of the Seminal Vesicles. There is probably no method of physical examination that is more dependent upon the clinician's physical attributes, for if he is endowed with a long finger, these structures can be palpated per rectum readily. Usually the knee–elbow position is adopted for the examination of the seminal vesicles particularly when a specimen of their contents is required.

A seminal vesicle may be enlarged or fibrous as a result of chronic inflammation, which usually is non-gonococcal in origin, by which is meant that the infection is an extension of non-specific urethritis or a mixed infection. A *tuberculous* vesicle gives to the palpating finger a very characteristic sensation, which is best described as 'craggy'.

Palpation of the Bulbo-urethral (Cowper's) Glands. Cowperitis, both acute and chronic, is often mistaken for prostatitis or vesiculitis. The diagnosis is often missed for lack of a simple examination. On passing the forefinger into the rectum and placing the thumb first on one side and then on the other of the median raphe of the perineum the bulbo-urethral glands can be palpated (*Fig.* 591). In acute cases the least pressure causes excruciating pain—in chronic cases the enlarged gland can be felt. It varies in size from 0·5 to 2 cm, is hard, and feels not unlike a malignant lymph node.

Prostatic Massage as a Test of Prostatitis or Seminal Vesiculitis. The prostate and seminal vesicles are massaged as shown in *Fig.* 589, the patient being in the knee-elbow position. Slow, firm downward strokes with the pressure applied evenly are employed, after which the contents of the penile urethra are milked down. The external urinary meatus is examined for a bead of the fluid thus expressed and the macroscopical characters of the bead noted, after which microscopical and bacteriological examination are arranged.

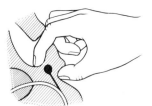

Fig. 591. Bidigital palpation of the bulbo-urethral glands. The index finger is placed in the rectum, and the thumb in the perineum to one side of the middle line. An enlarged gland can be felt between the finger and thumb.

THE SCROTUM

Soft Pitting Oedema of the scrotum is seen in decompensating cardiac cases (*see* p. 334) and in chronic nephritis.

Extravasation of Urine (*see* p. 333) *and Spreading Cellulitis* (*Fig.* 592), sometimes arising from a bulbous periurethral abscess (*see Fig.* 585) but in young boys often idiopathic (*Idiopathic Scrotal Oedema*), each give rise to scrotal oedema of a more solid variety than the foregoing. Owing to the extreme laxity of the scrotum, subcutaneous cellulitis thereof is relatively painless, although it is tender.

Following Retropubic Prostatectomy. Oedema of the scrotum is an uncommon complication, and is due to thrombosis of the pelvic veins.

Subcutaneous Emphysema of the Scrotum (*see* p. 16 and *Fig.* 343, p. 183).

WILLIAM COWPER, 1666–1709, *London Surgeon who published anatomical works in a sumptuous fashion.*

Idiopathic Gangrene of the Scrotum (Fournier's Gangrene). The three cardinal characteristics of this distinctly rare disease are: (*a*) Sudden appearance of scrotal inflammation in the midst of apparently good health; (*b*) Rapid onset of gangrene (*Fig.* 593); and (*c*) Total absence of any of the usual causes of gangrene. The condition commences as an acute inflammatory oedema of the scrotum, and is followed in a matter of hours or days by sloughing gangrene. Although usually idiopathic, the urine should always be tested for sugar.

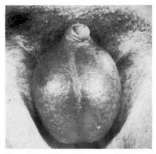

Fig. 592. Subcutaneous cellulitis of the scrotum.

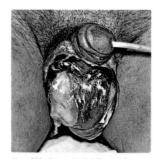

Fig. 593. Fournier's idiopathic gangrene of the scrotum.

Fig. 594. Squamous carcinoma of the scrotum. The groin lymph nodes on the left side were involved.

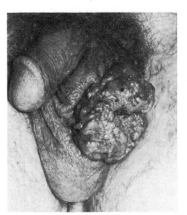

Non-filiarial Elephantiasis can occur following bilateral extirpation of inguinal lymph nodes, and as a result of extensive metastases in, or from, fibrosis following inflammation of these nodes.

Tropical Elephantiasis is caused by the infestation of the relevant lymphatics by *Wuchereria bancrofti*, which is transmitted by mosquito bites. The larva of this parasite can only be found in the peripheral blood at night, or when the patient is asleep, be it night or day. Secondary hydroceles are a usual accompaniment of tropical elephantiasis.

In the above two conditions the skin of the penis is involved also.

Carcinoma. The great majority of carcinomata of the scrotum (*Fig.* 594) occur in workers in pitch, tar, or bitumen,* or those whose occupation occasions shale

---

* In days gone by carcinoma of the scrotum was so common in chimney-sweeps that the disease was known as 'chimney-sweep's cancer'.

JEAN A. FOURNIER, 1832–1914, *Venereologist and Dermatologist, St. Louis Hospital, Paris.*
JOSEPH BANCROFT, 1836–1894, *Surgeon, Brisbane General Hospital, Australia.*

mineral oil coming into contact with the scrotum, e.g. cotton mule-spinners. It takes up to twenty-five years for the carcinoma to become manifest as a result of exposure to these carcinogens. Therefore always question the patient about his previous employment. In doubtful cases biopsy should be undertaken.

Sebaceous Cysts occur rather frequently in the scrotum. Often they are small and multiple. Should one large cyst suppurate it emits a peculiarly obnoxious odour. Sometimes a suppurating cyst is mistaken for a carcinoma.

Intertrigo (chafing) is frequently to be found on opposing surfaces of the scrotum and the thigh in obese men.

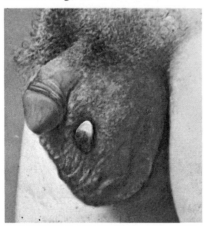

Fig. 595. Gumma of testis commencing to ulcerate.

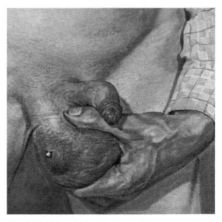

Fig. 596. Skin of the scrotum adherent posteriorly where a sinus has developed. Case of tuberculous epididymitis.

EXAMINATION OF THE TESTIS

The patient should stand in a good light before the seated clinician. In this position the left testis usually hangs fractionally lower.*

To commence with, ascertain if the scrotum is anchored at any point to the underlying testis. Should it be thus tethered anteriorly, it is slight contributory evidence of gumma (*Fig.* 595); if posteriorly, of tuberculosis (*Fig.* 596); whilst a new growth may invade any portion of the overlying skin, the anterolateral aspect being the site of election. By the time the scrotum is implicated visibly, underlying testicular disease is far advanced.

Palpation. In order to carry out a thorough examination of the testis, it is useful to palpate its constituent parts in a definite order (*Fig.* 597).

1. Palpate the body and compare it with the unaffected side.

2. While doing this, bear in mind the relationship of the tunica vaginalis. It is blended intimately with the anterior surface of the body.

3. Palpate the epididymis, body, globus major (head) and globus minor (tail).

4. Palpate the spermatic cord up to the external abdominal ring. The technique has been described accurately by Lockwood: 'Pass the index finger under the neck of the scrotum, pinch the thumb down upon it, and slip the

---

* In transposition of the viscera the right testis hangs lower, a useful clinical clue (Birch).

C. ALLAN BIRCH, *Contemporary Physician Emeritus, Chase Farm Hospital, Enfield, Middlesex.*
CHARLES B. LOCKWOOD, 1856–1914, *Surgeon, St. Bartholomew's Hospital, London.*

constituents of the scrotum through your fingers from within outwards. You ought to feel the vas, which is like hard whipcord. You will feel a number of other small cords and strings and fibres, which you cannot define. You may possibly be able to feel the nerves of the cord, more especially the genitofemoral and branches of the ilioinguinal, but I think the fibres which you feel are probably the fibres of the cremaster muscle. Unless you feel these things clearly and accurately, you are not feeling a normal spermatic cord.'

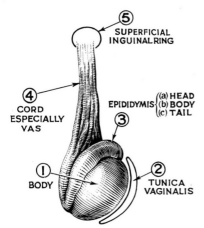

Fig. 597. Order in which the constituent parts of the testis are palpated.

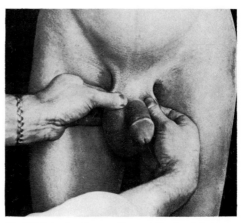

Fig. 598. Palpating the vasa. Compare the size of the vas on each side.

Testing for a Minor Degree of Thickening of the Vas. Using both hands, both vasa should be palpated simultaneously, and as these whipcord-like structures pass through the fingers, their relative sizes are estimated (*Fig.* 598).

Test for Translucency. Anyone who is in close touch with clinical surgery will have seen cases where the diagnosis has been vitiated by failure to carry out the test for translucency, or by carrying it out inefficiently. In the case of an intrascrotal swelling the first essential is to make the swelling tense by grasping the neck of the scrotum between the fingers and thumb. A pocket torch is applied to the distal side of the swelling and most hydroceles and cysts of the epididymis can be diagnosed irrefutably at once because of their translucency (*see Fig.* 606). There are cases in which the sign is doubtful, especially in sunlight. To go to the trouble of pulling down a window blind or to take the patient to a dark room frequently diminishes doubt. On transillumination of a large, tense hydrocele the relationship of the testis to the cyst, indeterminable by palpation, becomes apparent as a dark oval shadow, usually situated *behind* the illuminated cyst. Transillumination is *the* sign in the diagnosis of hydrocele.

The fallacies of efficient transillumination in the diagnosis of hydrocele are few. Obviously, if the walls are thick or calcareous the sign will be negative. Another possible error is in the case of a young child, particularly an infant (a vaginal hydrocele is common in the male newborn baby). At this time of life, if small intestine distended with gas is present in the sac of an inguinal hernia, so gossamer-like is the wall of gas-containing gut that the swelling to which it gives rise is likely to be translucent. However, usually an inguinal hernia in an infant is reducible, while a vaginal hydrocele is not.

Testicular Sensation. When the normal testis is squeezed gently between the finger and thumb the patient experiences a peculiar 'sickening pain'. This sign is mentioned only to condemn it; apart from the pain it occasions, it is dangerous, at least on theoretical grounds, if the enlarged testis is neoplastic, for malignant cells may be squeezed into the venous or lymphatic circulation. Syphilitic orchitis, in which testicular sensation is lost, is now rare, and in any case can be confirmed with a blood test.

Examination of the Regional Lymph Nodes. The lymphatic drainage of the testis passes up the spermatic cord and follows the spermatic artery to the para-aortic nodes just below the origin of the renal arteries. It should be noted that the lymphatic vessels of the testis have no connection either with the inguinal lymph nodes or with the contralateral channels in the pelvis. It therefore follows that when the testis is the seat of an advanced neoplasm, secondary deposits are to be expected above the level of the umbilicus, i.e. enlarged para-aortic lymph nodes may be palpable in the epigastrium. The supraclavicular lymph nodes are occasionally implicated (*see* p. 140).

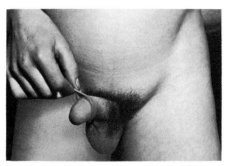

Fig. 599. Imperfectly descended testis at the left superficial inguinal ring.

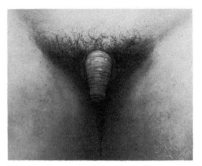

Fig. 600. Cryptorchid* at puberty. The scrotum is empty, contracted, and barely perceptible.

IMPERFECTLY † DESCENDED TESTIS

A maldescended testis is one that cannot be made to touch the bottom of the scrotum.

a. In Adolescents and Adults. Certainly most patients with an imperfectly descended testis have a superadded inguinal hernia, but it should not require the peculiar talents of a Sherlock Holmes to detect that there is but a solitary testis in the scrotum. Nevertheless, over and over again the swelling produced by a testis lodged near the superficial inguinal ring (*Fig.* 599) has been diagnosed as an inguinal hernia without the location of the testis being questioned.

On the other hand, when both testes fail to reach their normal destination and the patient is approaching, or has attained, years of maturity, the fact that the scrotum is empty and undeveloped (*Fig.* 600) is too arresting to escape notice.

When seeking a retained testis a light touch over the upper part of the inguinal canal, especially when the patient is examined in the upright position, sometimes reveals a mobile tell-tale ovoid lump which up to that time had defied definition.

b. In Juvenile Patients. In infancy imperfect descent of the testis, bilateral more

---

* A cryptorchid is a male whose testes are hidden from view and impalpable, i.e. they are situated retroperitoneally above the level of the deep inguinal ring.

† An undescended testis, strictly speaking, is one which has not moved from the place in which it had its origin, i.e. just below the kidney. Testes in this position are exceedingly rare.

often than unilateral, is common. At birth Scorer found it in 2·7 per cent of full-term babies but in no less than 20 per cent of premature infants. During the first 3 months of life the testes fail to descend spontaneously in only a few of the babies mentioned above who are born with maldescent, so that the overall figure is only 8 per 1000 births (0·8 per cent). For these reasons the clinician's concern is centred on those above 3 months after which further descent does not occur (Scorer). At this juncture it is essential to stress that numerous children are believed to be suffering from 'undescended' testes when the only abnormality present, if abnormality it can be called, is a retractile testis or testes.

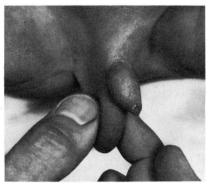

Fig. 601. Retractile testis (*right*) manœuvred from obscurity to the bottom of the scrotum.

Retractile Testes. In infant boys intermittent contraction of the cremaster muscle pulls the testis into the inguinal canal. These can be segregated from imperfectly descended ones by correct technique, but in refractory children more than one examination may be required.

The examination should be conducted in a warm room, with warm hands. First of all scrutinize the scrotum: when the scrotal skin of the affected side is smaller than the normal side, it is probable that that half of the scrotum never contained a testis. The pulps of the index and middle fingers are placed over and below the region of the deep inguinal ring. Exerting moderate, even pressure, the fingers are drawn downwards in the line of the inguinal canal. In this way a testis of the retractile type will be thrust into the neck of the scrotum, where the awaiting finger and thumb of the other hand will be ready to grasp it. By this manoeuvre the retractile testis can be made to touch the bottom of the scrotum (*Fig.* 601). In difficult cases the 'chair test' (Orr) should be tried: the young patient is asked to sit on a chair and hug his knees to his chest————————————————————————————→

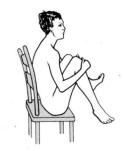

Pressure thus directed on to the inguinal canal causes a retractile testis to descend into the scrotum.

Ectopic Testis. This condition, although given undue attention in surgical texts is, in fact, rare. If the scrotum on one or both sides is empty and an imperfectly descended testis is not found in the inguinal canal, look for an ectopic testis in the perineum (*see Fig.* 588), at the root of the penis, and in the femoral triangle. It is permissible to test gently for testicular sensation (*see* p. 363) if such a swelling is found.

CHARLES G. SCORER, *Contemporary Surgeon, Hillingdon Hospital, London.*
LOUIS ORR, 1899–1961, *Urologist, Orlando, Florida.*

THE DIFFERENTIAL DIAGNOSIS OF INTRASCROTAL SWELLINGS

Of all organs, the testis, separated as it is from the examining fingers by little more than a covering of loose skin, is the most accessible. Consequently, one would suppose the diagnosis of intrascrotal swellings to be a comparatively simple matter. On the contrary some testicular swellings are most difficult to diagnose with confidence. However, many are misdiagnosed, not because of inherent difficulties, but because of slipshod methods of examination, or illogical interpretation of the physical signs elicited.

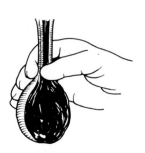

Fig. 602. As shown, it is possible to get above an intrascrotal swelling when that swelling arises from the testicular apparatus.

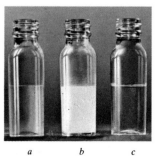

a   *b*   *c*

Fig. 603. *a*, The fluid withdrawn from a vaginal hydrocele resembles normal urine; *b*, That from a spermatocele is like barley water because of the spermatozoa present; *c*, That from a cyst of the epididymis is crystal-clear, like water.

Traps for the Unwary

a. Because there is a swelling within the scrotum, it does not signify that it arises in connection with the testicular mechanism. The first question should always be, 'Can I get above the swelling?' (*Fig.* 602).

b. A secondary hydrocele may mask underlying testicular disease. If doubt exists as to the condition of the underlying parts, it is advisable to aspirate the fluid there and then, and to palpate the unmasked organ. The fluid withdrawn from a cyst connected with the testis throws considerable light on the diagnosis (*Fig.* 603).

c. About 1 man in every 14 has an anteversion,* by which is meant that the epididymis is in front instead of behind. Unless the possibility of this anatomical variation is recognized, the physical signs elicited are difficult to interpret and much confusion caused.

TRANSLUCENT SWELLINGS

Determine the relation of the translucent swelling to the testis. Sometimes the dark shadow of the body of the testis can be seen contrasted against the brilliantly illuminated area. Another reliable method that is often possible is to identify the testis by palpation. A **vaginal hydrocele**† lies in front and to a variable degree above the body of the testis (*Fig.* 604, **1**).

---

* Findings based on the examination of 850 army recruits by Waddy.

† This is so called in the British Commonwealth because it originates in the tunica vaginalis. In the USA it is known as a 'scrotal hydrocele'—also a good term.

SIDNEY H. WADDY, 1894–1956, *General Practitioner, Huddersfield.*

Cyst of the Epididymis and Spermatocele (*Fig.* 604, **2**) are usually encountered in middle-aged men and are indistinguishable clinically before the contained fluid is aspirated (*Fig.* 603). Both conditions are often bilateral although unequal in size and the patient may have noticed a swelling on one side only. Often the swelling is small as compared with a hydrocele, but there are occasions when it is as large. The cyst is (unless anteversion is present) situated above and behind the body of the testis and when small, tends to slip about; therefore it should be grasped firmly between the finger and thumb to stretch the overlying scrotum tightly over it (*Fig.* 605). A pocket torch is then applied behind the cyst, which is illuminated most effectively (*Fig.* 606).

THE DIFFERENTIAL DIAGNOSIS OF TESTICULAR SWELLINGS

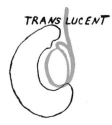

1. Vaginal hydrocele, often found to be bilateral.

2. Cyst of the epididymis or spermatocele. Swelling tense. Often somewhat lobulated. May be in any part of the epididymis.

3. Cyst of the hydatid of Morgagni perched on the upper and anterior surface of the testis.

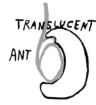

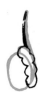

4. In anteversion a vaginal hydrocele simulates a cyst of the epididymis. Largely an academic problem.

5. Epididymo-orchitis. Epididymis enlarged and tender. Vas may be thickened.

6. Tuberculous epididymo-orchitis. Epididymis craggy. Vas considerably thickened.

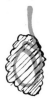

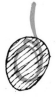

7. An advanced neoplasm. Body of the testis enlarged and irregular. Epididymis cannot be felt. Old clotted haematocele gives rise to same signs.

8. Early neoplasm. Any painless nodule in the body or even in the epididymis should be displayed to the light of day.

9. Syphilis of the testis. Smooth, painless enlargement of the body. Gumma shows a degree of irregularity.

Fig. 604. If, on the simple outline shown in *Fig.* 2, p. 3, the physical signs elicited are recorded, a reasoned diagnosis will be probable. Diagrams accompanying the notes of 9 patients with various scrotal swellings.

Cyst of an Appendix of the Testis is a separate clinical entity. It forms a small globular swelling at the superior pole of the testis (*Fig.* 604, **3**) usually unilateral. The cyst is liable to undergo axial rotation (*see Fig.* 615, p. 373).

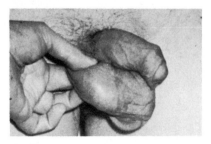

Fig. 605. Cyst of the epididymis. With the scrotum stretched over it, the cyst is fixed between finger and thumb.

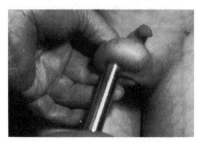

Fig. 606. Transillumination from behind. A cyst of the epididymis will be found to be brilliantly translucent.

Congenital Hydrocele can occur only when the processus vaginalis communicates with the peritoneal cavity and the orifice is too small to allow the development of an inguinal hernia. When the scrotum is elevated (i.e. at night) the fluid in the pouch gravitates into the peritoneal cavity, usually slowly, but it returns to the sac when the erect posture is resumed. The presence of a congenital hydrocele in an adult signifies that there is an excess of serous fluid in the peritoneal cavity with all that this implies (*see* Ascites, p. 242).

NON-TRANSLUCENT SWELLINGS

Acute Epididymo-orchitis. This is much the commonest form of inflammatory disease of the scrotal contents; it is unsafe to diagnose acute epididymo-orchitis at any age when there is no urethral discharge and no pus to be found when the urine is examined. In cases of acute epididymo-orchitis, usually it is possible to distinguish the enlarged epididymis from the body of the testis. In cases of torsion of the testis (*see* p. 371) it is unusual to be able to palpate the two structures separately. Reverting to the more usual acute epididymo-orchitis note that the scrotal contents are acutely tender and often greatly enlarged, the skin is diffusely reddened, and urinary *symptoms* are not invariably present.

Acute Epididymo-orchitis of Mumps develops in about a fifth of male sufferers, as a rule when the parotid inflammation is subsiding. The testis becomes swollen and painful. Especially in infants, epididymo-orchitis of mumps can occur without parotitis.

Tuberculous Epididymo-orchitis. Except in the rare acute forms, the comparative absence of tenderness helps to differentiate tuberculosis from other forms of epididymitis. When the condition is fully established physical signs are characteristic (*Fig.* 604, **6**). Normally the testis can be moved freely within its coverings, particularly in an upward and downward direction. This movement is often restricted in tuberculosis. If suppuration ensues, scrotal skin involvement soon occurs, usually at the back of the scrotum (*see Fig.* 596), but anteriorly with anteversion (*Fig.* 607).

Irrespective of whether genital tuberculosis presents in the epididymis or in the prostate and seminal vesicles, there is a well-marked thickening of the vas deferens most in evidence near the epididymis. Beading and irregular nodularity of the vas are not pathognomonic of tuberculosis; sometimes it occurs in non-tuberculous infections.

Rectal Examination is essential if tuberculous epididymo-orchitis is suspected. Involvement of the seminal vesicle (*see* p. 360) is strong confirmatory evidence.

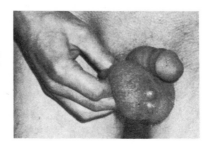

Fig. 607. Abscesses of the anterior wall of the scrotum secondary to tuberculous epididymo-orchitis with right anteversion.

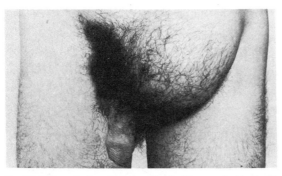
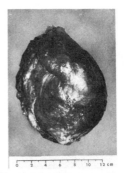

Fig. 608. This gradually enlarging swelling had been noticed by the 22-year-old patient for eighteen months. The left testis was absent from the scrotum. The histological diagnosis of the excised tumour (*right*) was 'teratoma of the testis'. Maldescended testes are many times more liable to malignancy than fully descended testes.

Malignant Disease. Painless enlargement of the testis is the presenting sign in 75 per cent of patients, and in 15 per cent only is the initial symptom pain in the organ. A further clinically helpful statistic is that 95 per cent occur between 20 and 45 years of age. The most frequent starting-point of the growth is the lower part of the body of the testis. When there is just a hardness of the body of the testis or an unexplained nodule (*Fig.* 604, **8**), even if that nodule is in the epididymis, an exploratory operation should be carried out. Should this course be followed the clinician will, from time to time, suffer humiliation, for an old clotted haematocele (*Fig.* 604, **7**), an atypical tuberculous lesion, or even a gumma of the testis will be removed unnecessarily. With reasonable clinical acumen such mistakes, if one can call them mistakes, are few and are relatively unimportant.

The Sign of the Vas helps in the differential diagnosis between a testicular neoplasm and an inflammatory lesion which causes the vas to become considerably thickened; in neoplasms it remains normal in all respects. This sign refers to the vas deferens, and not to the spermatic cord which with a neoplasm of the testis remains normal for a considerable time, but as the neoplasm becomes larger, and therefore heavier, the cord becomes bulkier due to hypertrophy of the cremaster muscle and engorgement of the veins of the pampiniform plexus.

Secondary hydrocele occurs with 1 in 10 testicular neoplasms: it is entirely justifiable to aspirate the hydrocele so as to enable proper palpation of the testis.

Rectal Examination reveals no abnormality in the prostate or seminal vesicles.

Metastases. See p. 364. A chest X-ray is essential.

The Association of Maldescent of the Testis and Malignancy (Fig. 608).

Old Clotted Haematocele. Some patients presenting with an old clotted haematocele can recall neither a history of trauma to the testis nor of pain in the organ. An old clotted haematocele simulates a neoplasm of the testis closely. The differential diagnosis usually depends on the length of the history; a swelling present unaltered for some years cannot be a neoplasm.

Syphilis of the testis, in most communities now a rarity because of the effective treatment of syphilis in its early stages, is encountered in three forms:

Orchitis of Congenital Syphilis. Should an untreated congenital syphilitic boy be fortunate enough— if he can ever be called fortunate—to reach puberty, certain ills befall him. He tends to become *lame* because of Clutton's joints, *deaf* because of neurolabyrinthitis, *blind* because of interstitial keratitis, and *impotent* because of diffuse fibrosis and atrophy of the testes due to an attack of bilateral interstitial orchitis. Usually this occurs in infancy causing 'pigeon-egg testes'.

Tertiary Interstitial Orchitis. When the condition is full established, the testis is rounded, densely hard, and completely movable in its scrotal covering (*Fig.* 604, **9**). What better name could be given to it than the 'billiard-ball' testis?

Gumma. In its early stages gives rise to signs much the same as those of neoplasm of the testis. A positive serological test for syphilis is, of course, most suggestive, but it should be remembered that it is possible for malignant disease to appear in a syphilitic patient.

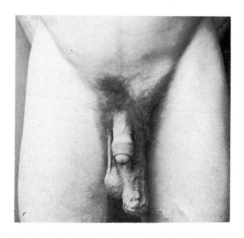

Fig. 609. Varicocele. The left testis hangs much lower than the right. The patient also has a left inguinal hernia.

Varicocele. The enlarged veins of the pampiniform plexus are so obvious that it is unlikely that a varicocele (*Fig.* 609) will be confused with any other condition. A varicocele is nearly always left-sided. On light palpation the impression conveyed has been well likened to that of feeling a bag of worms.

After the examination in the erect position is concluded, the patient should lie down; when the testis is elevated the veins will empty. In cases of long standing, due to a minor degree of atrophy, the body of the testis of the affected side will be found to be somewhat smaller and distinctly softer than that of its fellow.

Varicocele as a Cause of Subfertility. That oligospermia is a frequent accompaniment of a varicocele is fully substantiated, possibly because the increased blood flow raises the intrascrotal temperature to the detriment of both testes, possibly due to the fact that so often a patient with a varicocele wears a jock-strap, or other support, and so conserves intrascrotal heat.

Secondary Varicocele. Much academic attention has been paid to a rapidly oncoming varicocele as a sign of malignant disease of the kidney. This sign occurs only in 0·04 per cent of cases of malignant neoplasm of the kidney (Riches). In those cases in which it is present there is, as a rule, an easily palpable renal tumour so the sign is virtually valueless.

Atrophy of the Testis. Commencing atrophy must be distinguished from under-development. Usually atrophy is unilateral. In partial atrophy the testis is smaller and softer than normal, as is found typically in long-standing cases of varicocele. Complete atrophy of the testis occurs: (1) Following infarction consequent upon torsion; probably this is the commonest cause. (2) Following epididymo-orchitis of mumps. (3) Following operation for: (*a*) inguinal hernia (especially in infants); (*b*) for varicocele; (*c*) orchiopexy. In this instance it must be assumed that the spermatic artery was damaged at the operation. The findings on palpation of a case of complete atrophy of the testis following herniotomy in early life are ⟶ Bilateral incomplete atrophy occurs frequently in leprosy and hepatic cirrhosis, and always after oestrogen therapy for carcinoma of the prostate.

TORSION OF THE TESTIS (SPERMATIC CORD)

Should a boy or young man complain of sudden, intense pain in the inguinal region and of vomiting, and upon examination the testis on that side is found to be enlarged and tender, torsion of the testis should be the *first* thing to cross the clinician's mind. In early cases the spermatic cord will be found thickened, and on occasion twists in the cord can be felt distinctly. Regarding the direction of the torsion, a simple rule, almost invariably correct (Sparks) is that the twist is *away* from the midline, i.e. clockwise on the right, anti-clockwise on the left (*Fig.* 610), owing to the direction of the fibres of the cremaster muscle.

There are, however, on numerous occasions, departures from this classic picture. In the first place quite frequently the onset is not sudden, and instead there is a dull ache of gradually increasing intensity in the hypogastrium in the region of the deep inguinal ring, or even in the loin (Smith). Secondly, it is not rare for torsion of the testis to occur in infancy, and even at birth, and, except for screaming, there is little to call attention to the condition until the corresponding half of the scrotum becomes reddened by inflammation. Torsion of the testis remains unrivalled among surgical emergencies for the frequency with which it is misdiagnosed.

Broadly speaking, all cases fall into one of two categories:

1. Torsion occurring in an Imperfectly Descended Testis is almost impossible to distinguish clinically from a strangulated inguinal hernia. All that is required of the clinician is to note the absence of the testis in the scrotum of the affected side, and arrange that the painful swelling of the inguinal canal be operated on as soon as possible. An indecisive preoperative diagnosis of '? torsion of an imperfectly descended testis', '? strangulated inguinal hernia' is wise.

Sir Eric Riches, *Contemporary Emeritus Surgeon and Urologist, Middlesex Hospital, London.*
John P. Sparks, *Contemporary Medical Officer, Rugby School, Rugby.*
Kenneth H. Smith, *Contemporary Surgeon, Caernarvon and Anglesey Hospital, North Wales.*

2. Torsion occurring in a Completely Descended Testis. This must be distinguished particularly from acute epididymo-orchitis. To add to the difficulty, in addition to the fact that the local signs of inflammation may simulate exactly those of acute epididymo-orchitis (*Fig.* 611), the temperature is consistently raised. Because so often the patient is a boy between the ages of 10 and 18 it is reasonable to expect the clinician, before pronouncing the diagnosis of epididymo-orchitis, to reason thus: Here is a boy who has no history of dysuria, no signs of a urethral discharge, no pus to be found when the urine is examined: there have been no cases of mumps at his school or in the district: no swelling or tenderness of the prostate is detected on rectal examination, and the seminal vesicles are impalpable. Why on earth should he be suffering from a *bacterial inflammation* of the testis?

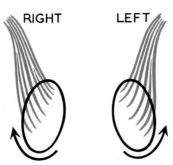

Fig. 610. Showing the direction of the twist in torsion of the testes; the fibres of cremaster muscle are shown in brown.

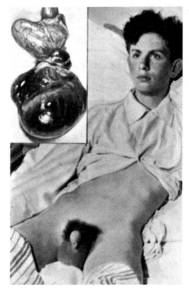

Fig. 611. Torsion of the left testis of 24 hours' duration in a boy aged 15. The inflamed acutely tender testis and scrotum simulate acute epididymo-orchitis exactly.

Confirmatory Signs of Torsion of the Testis

1. The affected testis *lies higher than its fellow* (*Fig.* 612) as a result of the twisting of the spermatic cord or because of spasm of the cremaster muscle. This sign is especially valuable on the left side.

2. *Angell's Sign.* The development anomaly allowing of torsion, namely the presence of a mesentery between the testis and the epididymis, is almost invariably bilateral. If the patient is examined *standing*, the *opposite* testis will be found to lie horizontally instead of in the normal vertical (*Fig.* 613). The sign is usually obscured on the affected side.

3. In cases of epididymo-orchitis sometimes it is possible to distinguish the enlarged epididymis from the body of the testis. In cases of torsion it is unusual to be able to palpate these two structures separately.

Another infrequent difficulty is when the sac is small, very tense, and situated in the upper part of the inguinal canal, a strangulated inguinal hernia causing compression of the veins of the spermatic cord with swelling and tenderness of

JAMES C. ANGELL, *Contemporary Urologist, Ashford Hospital, Middlesex.*

the testis (*Fig.* 614) mimics torsion of a completely descended testis. As an early operation is imperative the distinction is academic.

Torsion of an Appendage of the Testis. The appendage to undergo axial rotation is usually the hydatid of Morgagni (*Fig.* 615). Again the signs lead the unwary to diagnose acute epididymo-orchitis. The temperature is slightly elevated, and, as might be expected, other symptoms and signs are milder, although the scrotal oedema, and later redness, is out of proportion to the minute lesion. A reliable rule of thumb is: if the patient is able to walk to seek advice, he has a torsion of an appendage of the testis, whereas in torsion of the spermatic cord, the symptoms are such that the clinician is summoned to the bedside.

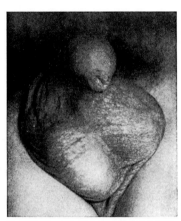

Fig. 612. Upward retraction of the left testis in a case of torsion of the testis of 3 hours' duration.

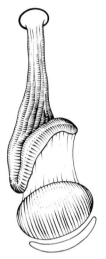

Fig. 613. The testis is found to lie horizontally (cf. *Fig.* 597) on the opposite side to a torsion.

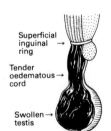

Superficial inguinal → ring

Tender oedematous → cord

Swollen → testis

Fig. 614. Explanation of how a small strangulated hernia may cause testicular symptoms by pressure on the cord.

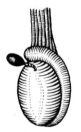

Fig. 615. Torsion of the hydatid of Morgagni.

EXAMINATION FOR SUSPECTED VENEREAL DISEASE

Inquire first as to the date of the last sexual exposure. A knowledge of the duration of the incubation period is helpful in the differential diagnosis. It is essential to wear gloves. *In the male* first inspect the external genitalia. An

GIOVANNI B. MORGAGNI, 1682–1771, *Professor of Medicine and Anatomy, Padua.*

external sore may be obvious, or a dorsal lymphangitis may be discerned—hot and tender in gonorrhoea and chancroid, painless and indolent in syphilis. Next, as the prepuce (if present) is retracted, attention is focused on ascertaining whether a discharge (a frequent presenting symptom) issues from the preputial sac or from the external urinary meatus. After, if necessary, cleansing the sub-preputial area with cotton-wool moistened with saline solution, the glans penis is inspected carefully for the presence of a sore; then the lips of the meatus are separated, so that a meatal chancre is not overlooked. In all cases in either sex, if a sore or ulcer is present some of the discharge must be examined for a causative organism. The urethra is now milked gently in a downward direction to bring any discharge to the meatus.

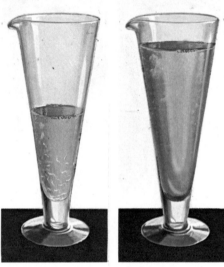

Fig. 616. The two-glass test. The patient is instructed to pass some urine into the first glass, the rest into the second. The first specimen shows mucopus and prostatic threads, while the second specimen is clear. Presumptive diagnosis—urethritis.

Thomson-Walker's Two-glass Test will demonstrate if the urethra is the seat of infection, for in the first glass there will be turbidity or threads, or both, while in the second glass there will be non-turbid urine without debris (*Fig.* 616). When the bladder is involved in the inflammation, mucopus will be present in both glasses. The presence of prostatic threads, which is excellent evidence of prostatitis, is likely to be shown unmistakably if the test is undertaken after prostatic massage (*see* p. 360).

In the female. See Vaginal Examination, p. 282. Frequently the patient is not seen until the inguinal lymph nodes are involved (*see* p. 376).

Primary (Hunterian) Chancre usually appears 3–5 weeks after inoculation. Commencing as a papule, in the span of a few days it becomes a painless ulcer, characterized by induration that causes it to feel like a button. Examples of penile chancres are illustrated on pp. 37, 251, and 355. A urethral chancre occurs on the lips of, or just inside, the external urinary meatus. The discharge to which it gives rise is often mistaken for that of a urethritis. Even if untreated a chancre heals in 3–8 weeks leaving a papery thin scar.

Gonorrhoea. The incubation period is usually from 4 to 7 days. The outstanding symptom is a urethral discharge,* usually accompanied by burning pain on

---

* In passive male homosexuals a rectal discharge may be the only clinical finding.

Sir John Thomson-Walker, 1870–1937, *Surgeon, St. Peter's Hospital, London.*
John Hunter, *See footnote* p. 37.

micturition in the early stage. The urinary meatus is somewhat red and swollen. At the onset the discharge is thin and almost colourless, but after an interval it becomes creamy in consistency (*Fig.* 617) and yellowish-green in colour. If the initial anterior urethritis spreads to the posterior urethra, the pain on micturition becomes severe, increased frequency and urgency of micturition are much in evidence, and the urine is turbid, containing threads and sometimes bloodstained debris. In severe cases painful nocturnal erections, occasionally accompanied by *chordee* (*see* p. 353), complicate the situation.

Chronic gonorrhoea is painless unless symptoms of chronic prostatovesiculitis supervene; in many cases a thin drop of discharge observed at the external urinary meatus on rising, before the patient micturates, is the only sign. This sign, although invariably present, is not pathognomonic of gonorrhoea, for it occurs in other varieties of chronic urethritis, and is spoken of as *gleet*.*

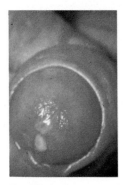

Fig. 617. Acute gonococcal urethritis.

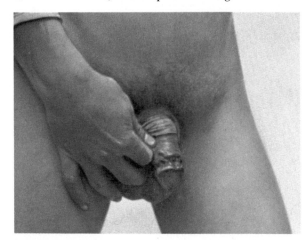

Fig. 618. Chancroid (soft sore) with suppurating left-sided inguinal nodes (bubo).

Non-specific Urethritis has become much more common with the decline in the incidence of gonorrhoea, resulting from relative control of that disease by antibiotics. The incubation period is from 2 to 3 weeks. The discharge is more watery than that of gonorrhoea, and it contains much mucus. In non-specific urethritis unusual organisms (*chlamydiae* and *mycoplasmas*) can often be isolated by special methods. A small proportion (1–2 per cent) develop Reiter's Disease (*see* p. 439).

Chancroid (due to infection with *Haemophilus ducreyi*) appears 3–6 days after inoculation, and is characterized by a painful non-indurated ulcer which becomes somewhat irregular in outline. It is common in the tropics. As a rule the ulcer, which is extremely tender, becomes duplicated or multiple (*Fig.* 618) by auto-inoculation. The complete absence of induration led to the term 'soft sore'. When situated beneath the prepuce, very often it causes the prepuce to become oedematous, and sometimes a foreskin, formerly retractable, becomes irretractable. In such cases ulcerative destruction is wont to proceed apace, and to become secondarily infected (phagedena†).

---

* *Gleet*. Old French, *glete* = litharge; oxide of lead.
† *Phagedena*. Greek, φαγεῖν = to eat.

AUGUSTO DUCREY, 1860–1940, *Professor of Dermatology, Pisa, Italy.*

Lymphogranuloma Venereum (Inguinale) (Tropical Bubo) is a virus-borne venereal disease that in white people sometimes causes considerable constitutional symptoms. The disease, as its synonym implies, is rife in tropical and subtropical climes; it is also much in evidence in the Southern States of the USA. It is by no means a rarity among European seafarers, and in recent years (due to an influx of West Indian immigrants) has become a condition that no clinician in the great cities of the British Isles can afford to disregard. The incubation period is from 7 to 15 days. The primary lesion on the glans penis, or in the vagina, or on the cervix is rather like herpes, and of fleeting duration. The diagnosis must be confirmed by special skin or blood tests.

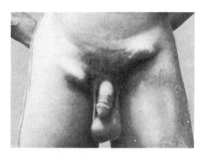

Fig. 619. Lymphogranuloma inguinale.

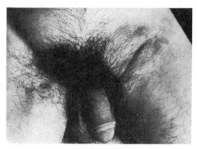

Fig. 620. The sign of the groove.

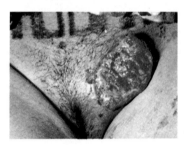

Fig. 621. Granuloma inguinale.

Granuloma Inguinale (Granuloma Venereum). Do not confuse *granuloma* inguinale with *lymphogranuloma* inguinale. Although, like lymphogranuloma inguinale, granuloma inguinale is a venereal disease, endemic in warm climates, that can be brought by natives of those countries and transmitted to inhabitants of temperate climates, it is an entirely different infection, due to a bacillus, the *Donovania granulomatis*, demonstrable in the lesion which affects predominantly the inguinal, genital, perineal, and peri-anal regions. The incubation period is from 10 to 40 days. Commencing as a painless vesicle, it soon develops into an ulcer or a mass of exuberant granulation tissue (*Fig.* 621). Pain and tenderness are singularly absent unless secondary infection occurs. The lesion progresses slowly by peripheral extension, and also by satellites due to auto-infection. It should be noted particularly that, although the inguinal region is often involved, the inguinal lymph nodes are not implicated until late, and then only if secondary infection supervenes.

Examination of the Regional Lymph Nodes. In either sex the significant findings are:

In syphilis in only 50 per cent of cases the inguinal lymph nodes become palpable three to five days after the appearance of the chancre—that is, rather later than in other venereal diseases. The enlargement, like most syphilitic manifestations, is unobtrusive; the nodes are painless, non-tender, elastic, and (in the absence of secondary infection) freely movable under the skin. The whole group of nodes from the saphenous opening upward, and those along the inferior border of the inguinal ligament, are usually involved bilaterally and symmetrically.

CHARLES DONOVAN, 1863–1951, *Lieutenant-Colonel, Indian Medical Service.*

In gonorrhoea in only 15 per cent are the nodes on both sides moderately enlarged and slightly tender.

In non-specific urethritis, as in all abacterial infections, lymphadenitis is absent, but should pyogenic bacterial infection become superadded, inguinal adenitis is likely to supervene.

In chancroid considerable tender enlargement of the inguinal lymph nodes occurs early and frequently suppuration follows (*see Fig.* 618). Constitutional symptoms are more pronounced than with the lymphadenitis of other venereal diseases.

In lymphogranuloma inguinale a lymph node enlarges in one groin, or, in a quarter of cases, in both groins (*Fig.* 619). The infection spreads to other nodes, and often the external iliac group becomes involved. In this event the fold of the groin is not obliterated and a sulcus separates the supra-inguinal from the infra-inguinal lymph nodes—the sign of the groove (*Fig.* 620). Soon periadenitis occurs, the mass increases in size, and the overlying skin (in white races) becomes purple. Untreated, the lymphadenopathy proceeds to liquefy, and the mass breaks down and discharges thick white pus. The resulting sinus persists for months or years. In the late stages elephantiasis (*see* p. 399) and rectal stricture (*see* p. 277) are liable to occur.

Chapter 26

THE CIRCULATION IN THE EXTREMITIES

THE ARTERIES

Atherosclerosis is a degenerative condition affecting chiefly the large and medium-sized arteries. The pathological process, 'atheroma'*, is confined to the *intima*. The abdominal aorta and the iliac and femoral arteries are the common sites, with occasionally the tibial vessels involved. The arteries of the heart and brain are frequently affected but those of the upper extremities nearly always escape severe involvement. There are no physical signs of this disease. Its presence can be surmised only by its chief complication—arterial thrombosis, i.e. complete blockage.

Arteriosclerosis. With advancing age calcification of the *media* always occurs. 'As old as his arteries' is an everyday expression. The arteries feel hard and can be visualized readily in a radiograph. Clinically, the state of the temporal artery is often a guide to the presence of this common development, but the radial, brachial and femoral arteries should also be palpated. Arteriosclerosis by itself does not cause arterial blockage, but atherosclerosis often coexists.

Intermittent Claudication.† Only arterial insufficiency produces *on walking* the phenomenon of (*a*) pain in the leg (especially in the calf but sometimes in the thigh or buttock or instep) increasing steadily until the patient is compelled to stop; (*b*) relief of that pain by rest. Should he resume his journey on foot, this sequence is repeated, and he is compelled to halt at exactly the same distance (*claudication distance*) as before. Thus he progresses in stages to his journey's end, or until he decides on an alternative method of transportation. Almost invariably this symptom is caused by blockage of a segment of a main artery. The collateral circulation provides enough blood for the relevant muscles at rest, but not during activity. An atheromatous plaque is the commonest precursor of the causative arterial thrombosis; consequently the arteries need not necessarily feel 'pipe-stemmed', or even thickened.

Nearly all patients with intermittent claudication have impalpable pulses below the femoral on the affected side or sides.

Rest Pain in obliterative vascular disease of the lower extremity is of much graver significance than intermittent claudication; gangrene is never far away. Usually the pain is felt in the foot and is worse at night when the foot becomes warm beneath the bedclothes which increases the oxygen requirements. The patient endeavours to seek relief by hanging the leg or legs out of the side of the bed. Standing on a cold floor is another expedient. So insufferable does the pain become that not infrequently the patient elects to sleep in a chair. With rest

---

* *Atheroma.* Greek, ἀθήρη=porridge+ὦμα=tumour. The fatty degeneration resembles porridge in appearance. First noted on post-mortem by Leonardo da Vinci.

† *Claudication.* Latin, *claudicare*=to limp.

LEONARDO DA VINCI, 1452–1519, Florentine artist, inventor and anatomist. Predicted the submarine, the parachute, the tank and the ability of man to fly.

pain, trophic ulcer (*see* p. 414) of the ischaemic foot is a frequent precursor of gangrene.

Feeling the Pulses of the Lower Extremities. A knowledge of how to feel the pulses is an indispensable accomplishment not only in cases of intermittent claudication and rest pain, but in suspected arterial disease and in threatened or established gangrene of a toe or toes. The student is advised to practise feeling the pedal pulses (*Fig.* 622) in normal persons. When in doubt whether a pulse in the distal part of the lower extremity is really being felt, or whether the examiner's own arterial beat is being appreciated by the finger pulp, simultaneously palpate the patient's radial pulse; if the latter synchronizes with the doubtful pulse, it must be the patient's.

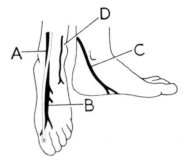

Fig. 622. Points for seeking the pulsation of (a) the anterior tibial; (b) the dorsalis pedis; (c) the posterior tibial; and (d) the peroneal arteries.

The Dorsalis Pedis Artery. The toes are grasped lightly in the left hand so as to steady the foot. The fingers of the right hand are slid along the groove between first and second metatarsal bones, upwards towards the ankle, the pulps of the fingers being directed slightly towards the first metatarsal bone. Usually the pulse is felt just lateral to the tendon of the extensor hallucis longus at the proximal end of the groove (*Fig.* 623). In 10 per cent of persons the artery is congenitally absent from its usual position, and therefore lack of its pulsation is valueless unless corroborated by other signs of obliterative arterial disease.

The Posterior Tibial Artery is accessible about halfway between the back of the medial malleolus and the medial border of the tendo Achillis, especially when the foot is dorsiflexed and inverted (*Fig.* 624). Sometimes it is difficult to feel, and absolute reliance cannot be placed upon the absence of its pulsation.

When neither of these pulses can be discerned, arterial pulsation should be sought in the region of the ankle-joint, namely:

The Anterior Tibial Artery becomes superficial just above the level of the ankle joint, and it can be felt midway between the two malleoli (*Fig.* 622).

The Peroneal Artery replaces the anterior tibial artery in 5 per cent of cases (Cohen). It should be sought 1 cm medial to the lateral malleolus (*Fig.* 622).

Intermittent Claudication with Foot Pulses Present. The history is strongly suggestive, but to one's surprise the dorsalis pedis and posterior tibial pulses (or one of these) are easily felt. Ask the patient to exercise by walking or running sufficiently to bring on the pain. Prompt re-examination will show that the foot pulses have disappeared if the pain is truly that of intermittent claudication (De Weese). The explanation is that a major artery is partially or completely blocked but there is a good enough collateral circulation for pulsations to reach the foot. Exercise increases the oxygen requirements of the muscles sufficiently to by-pass the blood reaching the foot arteries, the pulsations of which become impalpable.

SOLLY M. COHEN, *Contemporary Emeritus Surgeon, Medway and Gravesend Group Hospitals, Kent.*
JAMES A. DE WEESE, *Contemporary Professor of Cardiothoracic Surgery, School of Medicine, Rochester, New York.*

FEELING THE PULSES OF THE LOWER EXTREMITY

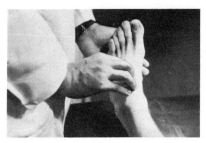

Fig. 623. Feeling the dorsalis pedis pulse.

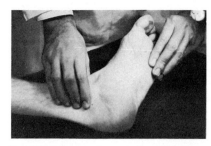

Fig. 624. Palpating the posterior tibial pulse behind the medial malleolus.

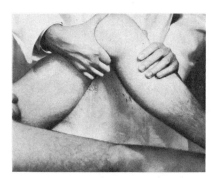

Fig. 625. Palpating the popliteal pulse: Method I. (*See Fig.* 834, p. 517, for Method II.)

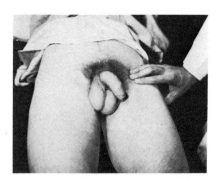

Fig. 626. Feeling the femoral pulse.

The Popliteal Artery, which lies deeply in the midline, can be sought by flexing the knee to a right-angle and palpating very deeply (*Fig.* 625). Commence somewhat medially and bring the fingertips transversely across the line of the artery. Should it not be possible to locate the artery in this way (and in fat persons its identification is difficult) the prone position, with the knee flexed, is used to palpate the space (*see Fig.* 834, p. 517). In cases where it is necessary for the patient to turn face downwards, it is convenient to palpate the femoral artery before making a renewed search for the popliteal artery.

The Crossed Leg Test for Popliteal Pulsation (Fuchsig). This test, and for that matter routine palpation of the popliteal artery, is unnecessary if one or more foot pulses are present, for the latter could not be felt if the popliteal artery were blocked. It is performed with the patient seated (*Fig.* 627). When a person sits with the legs crossed oscillatory movements of the foot occur synchronously with the pulse if the popliteal artery is patent. It is important to continue to take the history or otherwise interest the patient in order that his attention is distracted from the legs. While so doing carefully observe the foot for oscillations.

The Femoral Artery is not always easy to feel in a well-covered individual. Palpate rather deeply (*Fig.* 626) below the inguinal ligament, midway between the anterior superior iliac spine and the symphysis pubis. Absence of this pulse indicates that the external or common iliac artery is occluded; if both pulses are impalpable it suggests that the abdominal aorta is occluded.

PAUL FUCHSIG, 1908–1977, *Professor of Surgery, Vienna University.*

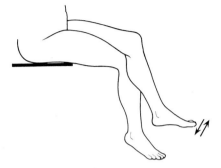

Fig. 627. Movements of the foot of the crossed leg when the popliteal artery is patent.

Buerger's Postural Test is an easily performed, practical clinical test applicable to *any variety* of fairly advanced occlusive arterial disease of the lower extremities, and is not, as is sometimes thought, peculiar to sufferers from Buerger's disease. It should be carried out in broad daylight. The patient lies on

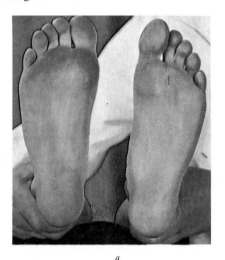

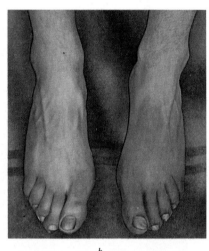

a　　　　　　　　　　　　　　　　　*b*

Fig. 628. Buerger's postural test. *a*, Pallor of the involved foot in the elevated position; *b*, Cyanosis of the same foot in the dependent position.

his back, and lifts both legs high, keeping the knees straight. The legs are supported by the examiner, while the patient flexes and extends his ankles and toes to the point of mild fatigue. When there is a defective arterial blood supply to the limb, the sole of the foot assumes a cadaveric pallor and prominent veins on the dorsum of the foot become empty and 'guttered'. The feet are lowered, and the patient adopts a sitting posture. In two or three minutes a ruddy, cyanotic hue spreads over the affected foot (*Fig.* 628). This sequence signifies that a major lower-limb artery is occluded.

LEO BUERGER, 1879–1943, *Professor of Urology, Polyclinic Medical School, New York.*

SPECIAL VARIETIES OF PERIPHERAL OCCLUSIVE VASCULAR DISEASE—
EARLY SIGNS

Thrombo-angiitis Obliterans (Buerger's Disease) is of such rarity that some observers doubt its existence as an entity separate from atherosclerosis. However, Szilagy encountered 22 undoubted cases in 1400 examples of peripheral vascular disease (1·5 per cent). Also, it is relatively common in Japan (Ishikawa), where it composes a third of cases of arterial disease, and in Indonesia. It gives rise to symptoms before the age of 30 and is peculiar to men; in women it is virtually unknown. The patient is always a very heavy smoker and the inevitable progress can be halted only by the cessation of smoking—almost a therapeutic test.

Arteries. Signs of arterial insufficiency usually appear first in the lower extremities, but sooner or later the arms suffer also. Intermittent claudication in the feet, and similar cramp-like pains in the hands, is often a leading symptom. Sometimes the examiner will notice coldness and colour changes in both upper extremities. The distal pulses are diminished or absent, although the arteries (as judged by more proximal pulses) remain soft. Usually the episodic nature of the disease allows an adequate collateral circulation to develop in response to each successive block, but it may strike with appalling rapidity, and all four limbs may be lost in a short time.

Veins. Superficial migratory thrombophlebitis, often commencing in the veins of the feet and frequently associated with fungus infection of the interdigital clefts, occurs in the majority and may precede or accompany the arterial manifestations of the disease.

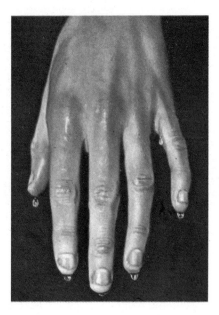

Fig. 629. Raynaud's disease: spasm induced by the patient (aged 30) dipping her hands in ice-cold water. She complained of coldness of the hands only since the previous winter. The other hand was only slightly affected when she was first seen.

Acrocyanosis (Hereditary Cold Extremities) is a common complaint of varying severity, commencing in youth, due to intermittent spasm of the small peripheral arteries initiated by cold. There is *persistent* cyanotic discoloration of the hands when exposed to cold. Often the palms of the hands are moist at a comfortable room temperature. It usually occurs in women but is not as rare in men as is the following condition. The feet are similarly affected usually, which, together with its mildness and non-progressive nature, serves to differentiate it from Raynaud's disease.

Raynaud's Disease is comparatively rare. It occurs mainly in women, and commences between the ages of 25 and 45 years as a unilateral affection; in its

EMERICK SZILAGY, *Contemporary Professor of Cardiovascular Disease, University of Michigan Medical School, Ann Arbor.*
KOICHI ISHIKAWA, *Contemporary Professor Emeritus of Surgery, University of Tokyo.*
MAURICE RAYNAUD, 1834–1881, *Physician, Hôpital Lariboisière, Paris.*

earliest stages it is indistinguishable from acrocyanosis. In a matter of a few months the attacks become more frequent, bilateral, and last longer. Often the tip of one or more fingers remains numb and cold long after the rest of the digits have regained an adequate circulation. Rarely is the thumb affected.

To diagnose Raynaud's disease the typical spasms, of which there are three phases, must be observed. In the first the digits become paroxysmally ashen white; in the second, blue, and in the last reddened with painful reactive hyperaemia. To provoke the causative arteriospasm ask the patient to put one hand (the comparatively normal one) into cold water. This may initiate an attack (*Fig.* 629).

As the disease progresses atrophy of the terminal pulp of the finger or fingers most affected occurs. This gives the finger or fingers a tapering effect, viz. ———→ The nails are often ridged and brittle and paronychia is 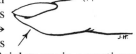 common. In advanced cases small areas of painful superficial necrosis, sometimes preceded by cutaneous calcification, are wont to occur on the fingertips. Occasionally gangrene involves a more substantial portion of a finger.

In cases of many years' standing, other signs should be sought: (*a*) scleroderma—the skin of the hands (*Fig.* 630), especially of the fingers, and of the face (*Fig.* 631), becomes atrophic; similar changes in the oesophagus cause dysphagia: (*b*) telangiectases occurring over the face, hands, and forearms.

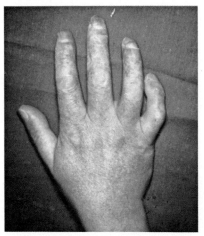

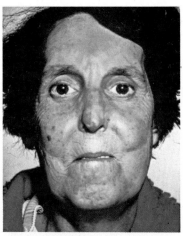

Fig. 630. The hand in long-standing scleroderma.

Fig. 631. Mask-like facies in scleroderma. The atrophic skin becomes bound down particularly over the bones of the nose and cheek.

Raynaud's Phenomenon in Men. (*a*) Vibrating tools, notably pneumatic drills, pneumatic hammers, and certain tools used in the shoe trade cause a condition similar to that described already. At first the attacks come on only in the man's leisure hours. In the patient who has used a pneumatic hammer, usually the left hand is the first to become implicated, the index finger being most affected. In half the cases the condition remains entirely unilateral and, when well-established, attacks in bed at night are a noteworthy feature. Rarely does the condition progress to a stage of cramps, pain, trophic changes, or gangrene, but even when diagnosed early and the patient is forbidden to use vibrating tools, symptoms recur for years. (*b*) Digital atherosclerosis (*see* p. 378) is the usual cause when vibrating tools are not implicated. (*c*) Buerger's disease (*see* p. 382).

Erythromelalgia (Erythralgia) may be *primary* (aetiology unknown and very rare) or *secondary*. It is characterized by attacks of severe burning pain and rubor (which must be distinguished from the rubor of ischaemia, *see Fig.* 628) in the *feet*, seldom in the hands. So great is the sensation of heat that the patient puts the feet out of bed or immerses them in cold water. Seen during an attack, the feet are flushed, the veins prominent, the skin temperature slightly raised and the surface of the skin is so hyperaesthetic that the slightest touch is resented. The secondary type is not uncommon in obliterative vascular disease when sepsis is present, is seen with erythrocyanosis frigida (*see* p. 382), polycythaemia, gout and also after frost-bite.

PERIPHERAL ARTERIAL THROMBOSIS

Arterial thrombosis is a common complication of atherosclerosis (*see* p. 378). Ordinarily a slow process, it can occur in an acute form (*see* p. 385).

Thrombosis of the Femoral or the Popliteal Artery. The leading symptom is intermittent claudication. The popliteal and foot pulses are not palpable. Buerger's test (*see* p. 381) may be positive. Wasting of the calf muscles is often evident. The thrombosis slowly extends downwards into the smaller distal vessels over a period of months and years and ultimately the collateral circulation is insufficient to prevent gangrene, at first of the toes, later extending up the foot.

Thrombosis of the Smaller Arteries of the Leg. The popliteal pulse remains palpable, but the pulses at the ankle are absent. As one would expect, the signs are confined to the foot. There is intermittent claudication with pain in the instep, constant bluish-red discoloration and coldness of the toes, extending for a variable distance on to the foot; in many instances ulceration or gangrene of a portion of the discoloured area follows. Some patients in this group have claudication in the calf, which in the presence of a popliteal pulse must be attributed to obstruction to the muscular branches of the main vessel.

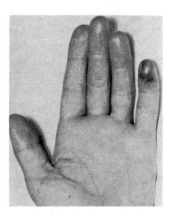

Fig. 632. The extent of gangrene in a patient with arteriographically proved thrombosis of the brachial artery.

Thrombosis of the Bifurcation of the Aorta (Leriche's Syndrome). Thrombosis always starts in an iliac artery and is generally observed in an individual in the prime of life. It is progressive, ultimately producing a complete bilateral occlusion of the iliac arteries and lower part of the abdominal aorta up to the renal arteries. Intermittent claudication, mainly in the thigh or buttock, develops in one or both lower limbs. Sufferers from early aortic or iliac arterial occlusion with pain situated in the buttocks due to diminished blood supply of the sciatic nerve are frequently referred to the orthopaedic department with a diagnosis of 'sciatica'. There is easily appreciated coldness in one limb, and later in both limbs. Wasting of the buttocks and the muscles of one, and later the other, leg occurs in half the cases. In the male there is always diminishing, and later complete disappearance of, penile erection. Undoubtedly the most important sign is loss of pulsation of the femoral artery,

RENÉ LERICHE, 1879–1956, *Professor of Medicine at the Collège de France, Paris—the highest professional honour in France.*

first on one side and then on the other. In thin subjects vigorous pulsation can be felt in the abdominal aorta above the block.

Intermittent Claudication in a Young Person. A young adult (usually male) presents with this symptom but with no evidence of Buerger's disease or other cause for arterial obstruction. In the affected limb the femoral pulse is easily palpable but no pulses are felt distal to this. The possible causes can only be detected by arteriography and an exploratory operation:

1. Popliteal artery entrapment due to an abnormal origin of the gastrocnemius muscle.
2. Cyst formation in the media of the popliteal artery causing occlusion of the lumen.

Thrombosis of a Major Artery of the Upper Extremity is uncommon. As a rule the collateral circulation is sufficient to spare the limb although pain on working with the arm, the equivalent of intermittent claudication, may result; exceptionally, limited gangrene of the fingertips follows (*Fig.* 632).

Thrombosis of the axillary artery following the use of an axillary crutch for many years has occurred and also in patients with chronic bronchitis, probably as a result of contusion of the subclavian artery over the first rib during a severe bout of coughing.

The Pulseless Disease of Takayasu (Aortic Arch Syndrome). No pulse can be felt in one or both arms or the corresponding side or sides of the neck and temples due to progressive occlusion of the arterial trunks arising from the aortic arch. In the West it is due to atherosclerosis but it also occurs in young women in the Far East (arteritis) and because of its slow development (giving opportunity for a collateral circulation to open up) it remains unnoticed for some time. It is characterized by attacks of fainting on turning the head suddenly, or on arising from the supine to a sitting posture, atrophy of the face, headaches, cataracts, optic nerve atrophy without papilloedema (occlusion of the carotid arteries), and weakness and paraesthesia of the upper extremities (occlusion of the brachial arteries). Untreated, death from hemiplegia or convulsions is the usual termination.

Arterial Obstruction in the Neck. *See* p. 148.

SUDDEN OCCLUSION OF A MAJOR PERIPHERAL ARTERY

'*A totally inexcusable tendency to conservatism in the management of acute embolic limb ischaemia still persists as indeed it does in the treatment of suspected major arterial injury.*'— Eastcott

Sudden occlusion of a major peripheral artery can be due to (*a*) acute arterial thrombosis, (*b*) arterial embolus, (*c*) trauma.

Acute Arterial Thrombosis. The most common site is the lower end of the femoral artery, where the artery leaves the subsartorial canal to enter the popliteal space. *At this site acute thrombosis is more frequent than peripheral embolism.* Each produces acute ischaemia with signs so similar that occasionally a differential diagnosis is impossible. When faced with this problem a golden rule is—*the absence of a cardiac lesion is strong evidence in favour of primary thrombosis.*

Commonly, acute thrombosis arises in an artery considerably narrowed by arterial disease. In this event the collateral circulation is established already, and the extent of the ischaemia is limited correspondingly. Moreover, with acute-on-chronic arterial thrombosis *the patient will almost certainly give a history of intermittent claudication.*

Peripheral Arterial Embolism.* The past history and an examination of the heart are of overriding importance. In half of the cases the patient suffers from auricular fibrillation. Most of the remainder have suffered recently from cardiac infarction. The embolus originates from a clot in the left auricle or ventricle or,

---

* *Embolism.* Greek, ἐν = in+βάλλειν = to throw. Material foreign to the bloodstream.

Mikito Takayasu, 1860–1938, *Professor of Ophthalmology, Medical College, Kanazawa, Japan.*
Harry H. G. Eastcott, *Contemporary Surgeon, St. Mary's Hospital, London.*

in a small minority, detachment from an atheromatous plaque in the aorta.

Shock is singularly absent (cf. Phlegmasia Cerulea Dolens, p. 392).

Pain in the limb is the initial symptom in 95 per cent. Numbness and weakness are present also, and in 5 per cent precede the pain. Classically the pain is abrupt and excruciating, but in a third it comes on more gradually.

Colour Changes are limited to the more distal part of the limb, the ischaemic portion of which assumes a cadaveric pallor, described as 'waxy'. An hour or more later the area becomes cyanosed distally, and mottled more proximally. Raising the limb decreases the cyanosis and 'gutters' (empties) any prominent vein.

Pulses are absent distal to the impaction.

Local Temperature. It is not long before the ischaemic area of the affected limb becomes appreciably colder than that of the opposite side.

Other Signs. Calf tenderness or pain on dorsiflexion of the foot (*see* p. 390) is often present in an otherwise anaesthetic limb. Soon after the occlusion the involved muscle is flaccid, but within a few hours it becomes turgid. About this time the foot assumes the position of plantar flexion, shown in *Fig.* 633.

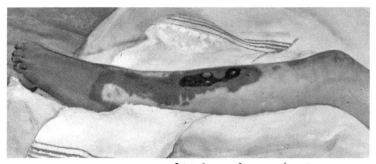

Fig. 633. Too late to save the limb! An embolus became lodged in the common femoral artery 48 hours before the patient's admission to hospital. The patient is a young woman with mitral stenosis.

Site of Impaction. As a rule, the embolus becomes arrested in the lower half of the body at or just below the site of bifurcation of a major artery (*Fig.* 634). Less frequently it lodges in an artery of the upper extremity (10 per cent).

It is not usually difficult to ascertain where the embolus has lodged. The best guide is the absence of pulses below the embolus and the level of coldness. Thus lowered skin temperature is usually found as follows:

Aortic bifurcation embolism—both limbs below the groins.

Common iliac embolism—one limb below the groin.

Common femoral embolism—below the knee.

Popliteal embolism—the foot.

The Auscultation Test. Temporarily occlude the femoral (or brachial) artery at the root of the limb with the pressure of a sphygmomanometer cuff. A stethoscope is applied at various points along the course of the artery, from above downwards. After the pressure is released the booming of the returning arterial flow (as in taking the blood pressure) will be heard until the site of the embolus is reached, when there is an abrupt cessation of sound (Last).

RAYMOND J. LAST, *Contemporary Visiting Professor of Anatomy, University of California, Los Angeles*.

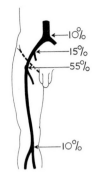

Fig. 634. Sites and frequency of impaction of emboli in the lower limb.

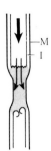

Fig. 635. The explanation of so-called 'traumatic arterial spasm'. The media (M) remains intact but the intima (I) ruptures. In effect the artery has been transected as there is no flow through the narrowed segment. Between the intimal ends clot may collect.

Arterial Trauma. Arterial insufficiency following a closed injury of an extremity may be due to several conditions:

1. Injury to a major artery by a bone fragment.

2. Pressure on a major artery by an angulated bone end.

3. Intimal rupture of a major artery due to a fracture or dislocation (*Fig.* 635).

4. Occlusion of the artery by a haematoma enlarging beneath the unyielding deep fascia. In haemophilia relatively minor trauma may cause this.

These complicate, notably, the following fractures and dislocations (approximate order of frequency):

Supracondylar (including displaced epiphysis in children) or shaft of humerus.

Dislocated shoulder.

Supracondylar (including displaced epiphysis) or shaft of femur.

Dislocated elbow.

Dislocated knee.

Examine carefully for loss of pulsations and coldness of the extremities, particularly with the above injuries. *See also* Volkmann's Ischaemia, p. 479.

In young patients with hemiplegia after trauma be on the look-out for arterial thrombosis consequent on intimal rupture as a result of direct trauma to the internal carotid artery by sudden hyperextension and lateral flexion of the neck. Arteriography is necessary to confirm that the cause is not an ordinary stroke (Rowbotham).

GANGRENE OF THE EXTREMITIES

Gangrene Threatened. In the comparatively early painful stage the ischaemic foot (or finger) is nearly always pink, the skin being atrophic as though it were stretched tightly over underlying structures (Oakley).

Local Temperature. The skin feels cooler than on the normal side.

Pulses. The pulses of the affected foot are usually absent.

Hair on the Digits as a Guide to the Severity of Ischaemia. Most normal persons have hair on their toes. The hairs of the toes are shorter and fewer in women than in men, and there is a sharp reduction in number after the age of 50 years. Patients with peripheral arterial occlusion with severe ischaemia have fewer hairs on the toes on the more affected side. This sign is only of value if the blood supply of the opposite foot is good.

Established Gangrene. A patient with gangrene of a portion of an extremity (*Fig.* 636) is presented. We wish to know the probable cause, and to ascertain

GEORGE F. ROWBOTHAM, 1899–1975, *Neurosurgeon, Royal Victoria Infirmary, Newcastle upon Tyne*.
WILFRID G. OAKLEY, *Contemporary Emeritus Physician, Diabetic Department, King's College Hospital, London*.

the condition of the circulation above the gangrenous area. Inspect the limb. Decide if the process is infected (moist) or 'dry'.

Lay the hand upon the surface of the skin above the gangrenous area and observe whether it is colder than it should be.

Most cases of gangrene are due to atherosclerosis often associated with diabetes. Therefore proceed at once to test the urine for sugar. Also observe the toes for the typical deformity associated with diabetic neuropathy (*see Fig.* 676, p. 414).

The Diabetic Foot. It is often difficult to decide whether a foot lesion in a diabetic is due to ischaemia, neuropathy or both. Eastcott notes that *painful* necrosis in a cold foot is due to ischaemia; *painless* necrosis at a pressure area is due to neuropathy. With either, superadded infection may cause a warm pink foot.

Having palpated the arteries of the upper extremity, return to the affected limb and palpate its arteries (*see* p. 379) and compare with the opposite side.

If the clinician is puzzled as to the cause of the local death, it is profitable to ask oneself a few questions:

Is it Frostbite? (*Fig.* 637). On one occasion during summer a case of gangrene of two fingers presented in a man who described himself as a meat porter. A further inquiry brought to light the fact that he spent his working days in a refrigerator!

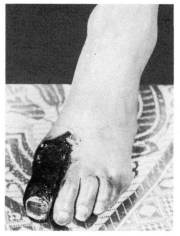

Fig. 636. Atherosclerotic gangrene showing a well-defined line of demarcation.

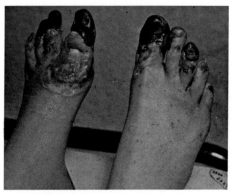

Fig. 637. Gangrene developing after frostbite in a Kentish farm labourer during a severe frost.

Is it Thrombo-angiitis Obliterans? (*See* p. 382.) The gangrene is usually moist.
Is it Raynaud's Disease? (*See* p. 382.)

Gas Gangrene. In civil life this is comparatively rare. Usually it is a complication of a compound fracture, but is not infrequent after surgical removal of gangrenous bowel in a hernial sac and after septic abortions and delivery. Clostridial organisms rarely become pathogenic unless they enter previously damaged tissues.

Early Diagnosis. Pain is frequently the first indication of something amiss. An anxious look and a rising pulse (out of proportion to the temperature) increase the suspicion and call for inspection of the wound. The characteristic odour has been described on p. 39. Examination of the wound shows a surrounding area of red, brawny swelling. Gas gangrene spreads along the muscle planes. Crepitus is sought in the manner described on p. 15, both above and below the wound; sometimes it is elicited some distance away, but unless it is abetted by other signs of clostridial infection, this is insufficient evidence of gas gangrene—the alarm that crepitus due to air entrapment in the tissues sometimes occasions has already been referred to on p. 245.

The most frequent sites for this infection are the adductor region of the lower limb and the buttocks. In the upper limb the subscapular region is the most common site.

Later General Signs that suggest possible clostridial septicaemia include an alert sensorium with irritability, dyspnoea and tachycardia out of proportion to the pyrexia.

Non-clostridial Gas Gangrene in Diabetics. A great variety of pathogenic bacteria may be associated with the presence of gas in the tissues of a gangrenous extremity in a diabetic (Wagner). The patient may appear very ill because of uncontrolled diabetes, but true clostridial infection is a rarity, an important factor in deciding on the need for, and the level of, an amputation.

THE VEINS

VENOUS THROMBOSIS

Phlebothrombosis can be superficial or deep. 'Silent' deep phlebothrombosis constitutes one of the most important diagnostic problems of the day, the paramount importance of which lies in early detection, the better to avoid the dreaded sequence, deep phlebothrombosis→pulmonary embolism. Despite such measures as 'early rising' in the postoperative period and the control of infections by antibiotics, postoperative phlebothrombosis shows no evidence of decline—rather the contrary, possibly due to the increasing age and infirmity of patients deemed fit for operations.

Phlebothrombosis Decubiti. Undoubtedly the early detection of clotting in the deep veins of the leg is proportional to the diligence of the search. Ideally, every patient mainly or entirely confined to bed, i.e. medical cases, and all those who have undergone an operation recently, deserve a routine daily examination of the legs. Except in particularly well-staffed institutions, this is a counsel of perfection. It is therefore most desirable to know which patients are most likely to suffer this complication. The answer is: those more than 40 years of age; obese patients; those with otherwise unexplained pyrexia; those with organic heart disease; and those who have undergone an abdominal operation, particularly prostatectomy or cholecystectomy, nailing of fractured neck of the femur, and also, curiously, patients who have undergone an operation for cataract.

Before commencing a routine search for the discovery of 'silent' deep phlebothrombosis remember that dislodgement of clot by rough manipulation is an ever-present danger. Therefore be gentle and do not hurry. The degree of pressure necessary to elicit tenderness is not great.

Have the bedclothes turned up (not down) to display the whole of both extremities.

WILLIAM WAGNER, *Contemporary Surgeon, Rancho los Amigos Hospital, Downey, California.*

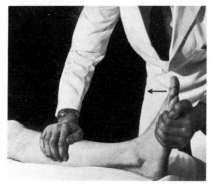

Fig. 638. Dorsiflexion of the foot to ascertain if this causes pain in the calf.

1. *Observe the Limbs* (*a*) for inequality of girth (which is unlikely to be present in early cases); (*b*) pay particular attention to the relative prominence of the veins of the dorsum of the foot and look for visible (not varicose) veins coursing over the upper third of the tibia on the affected side, useful signs of thrombosis of the popliteal vein.

2. *Palpate the Instep*, and follow this up by finger-stroking around the sulcus beneath the medial malleolus and by testing the ankle for pitting oedema.

3. *Dorsiflex the Foot* (*Fig.* 638). This exerts slight traction on the posterior tibial vein, which, if involved, causes pain in the calf (Homans' sign). In women accustomed to wearing high-heeled shoes, with in consequence a short tendo Achillis, a false positive result is not unusual.

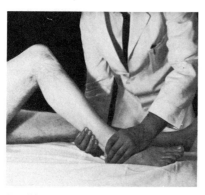

Fig. 639. Seeking tenderness of the calf muscles, beginning near the tendo Achillis.

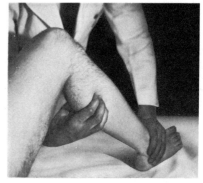

Fig. 640. Method of ascertaining tenderness or fullness of the soleus muscle.

4. *Examine the Calves*. Request the patient to draw up the knee and lie quietly, keeping the leg in that position. Commencing near the tendo Achillis (*Fig.* 639) grasp the calf, and while retracting it from the tibia, squeeze it gently. Proceed in this way in an upward direction until the main muscle belly is reached (*Fig.* 640) to ascertain whether the soleus is tender, for carefully performed necropsies on patients who have been in bed for more than a week before death show a high incidence of thrombosis of the veins of the soleus muscle. Next alter

JOHN HOMANS, 1877–1954, *Professor of Clinical Surgery, Harvard University, Boston*.

the grip on the calf, so as to be able to compress the main muscle belly forwards. Tenderness elicited in this way suggests strongly phlebothrombosis of the posterior tibial vein. Comparative palpation of the bellies of both calf muscles is valuable.

5. *Palpate the Popliteal Space* for tenderness. Now ask the patient to let down his legs, so that they rest on the bed comfortably.

6. *Seeking Tenderness in the Thigh.* Place the tip of the index finger over the saphenous opening (for surface marking, *see Fig.* 457, p. 262) and draw the finger ⟶ downwards along the course of the femoral (not the long saphenous) vein.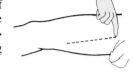

7. *Ascertaining the Presence of Very Early Oedema.* Pinch up a small portion of skin. In very early oedema there is a resistance that is not present on the normal side, owing to thickening of the dermis and subcutaneous tissues (Rose).

8. *Comparative Mensuration.* Lastly, if there is any question that one leg is swollen, comparative measurements at identical points on the calf and thigh (*see* p. 491) will settle the question.

The Crescent Sign in Calf Haematoma. The detection of deep phlebothrombosis has become so important in the prevention of pulmonary embolism that a sign described by Tibbutt and Gunning in patients with calf tenderness, thought to be due to phlebothrombosis but later proved to be caused by haemorrhage into the calf muscles, becomes important. In the former anticoagulant therapy is indicated, in the latter it is strongly contraindicated. The blood in the calf tends to gravitate downwards and can be seen as an area of crescentic bruising at the medial or the lateral malleolus, or both (*Fig.* 641).

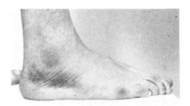

Fig. 641. The 'crescent sign'.

Phlegmasia Alba Dolens* (White Leg; Milk Leg) results from iliofemoral phlebothrombosis. Very seldom it occurs spontaneously: nearly always it arises after immobilization in bed following an operation or childbirth. There is also an appreciable incidence among patients confined to bed with medical as opposed to surgical illnesses. Obstetricians have reported cases occurring during late pregnancy, as opposed to during the puerperium.

The process often commences in the veins of the soleus muscles, and the thrombosis proceeds in an upward direction. Many cases seem to arise without those premonitory signs referred to in the section on Phlebothrombosis Decubiti, and in these clotting commencing at a valve of the femoral vein or in the pelvic veins is the cause.

---

* *Phlegmasia alba dolens*—painful white leg; *Phlegmasia cerulea dolens*—painful blue leg. (Literally, painful white/blue *inflammation*.) Eighteenth century accoucheurs believed the former to be due to excess milk being directed to the legs!

SIDNEY S. ROSE, *Contemporary Surgeon, University Hospital of South Manchester*.
DAVID A. TIBBUTT, *Contemporary Physician, Worcester Royal Infirmary, Worcester*.
ALFRED J. GUNNING, *Contemporary Cardio-Thoracic Surgeon, Oxford*.

The march of events is as follows: The patient experiences vague general malaise. Twenty-four hours later an otherwise unexplained rise of temperature occurs. Pain is felt in the groin and in the medial aspect of the thigh. In a few instances the pain, which varies in severity, is located farther down the leg. During the succeeding 12 hours swelling of the limb appears, but the swelling commences below the knee and spreads to the thigh (*Fig.* 642). Anteriorly it ceases abruptly at the inguinal fold; posteriorly it involves a variable portion of the buttock. It is due to oedema, and pits on pressure. The limb is pale in contradistinction to the condition described below. There is tenderness along the course of the femoral vein and often deep tenderness in the corresponding iliac fossa. The foot feels colder than its fellow. Enlargement of the lymph nodes of the groin is not unusual. The acute phase of this variety lasts 2–6 weeks if untreated. Post-mortem examination of fatal cases of pulmonary embolism arising with this condition often shows that the embolus arose from the clinically silent side so that the *opposite* leg should be examined carefully for signs of phlebothrombosis.

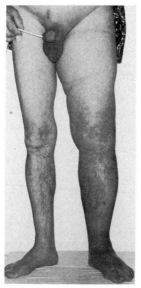

Fig. 642. Phlegmasia alba dolens in a patient with acute retention of urine due to an enlarged prostate.

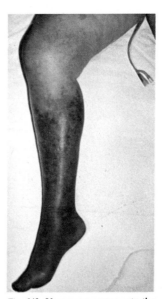

Fig. 643. Venous gangrene; note the massive swelling of the limb.

The acute phase is followed by the chronic phase, which is characterized by a swollen, oedematous limb requiring elastic stocking support, coldness and aching in the limb (venous claudication), and, in a small percentage of cases, the development of a venous ulcer (*see* p. 525).

Phlegmasia Cerulea Dolens is due to massive phlebothrombosis of the iliofemoral vein. It commences with tingling and numbness of the extremity. Suddenly the patient cries out with cramp in the limb (calf or thigh), which soon becomes deeply cyanotic and greatly swollen, especially below the knee.

The pain continues, and is often described as 'bursting' in character. The swollen portion of the limb feels tense, firm yet rubbery, and there is relatively little pitting on pressure. Soon after the iliofemoral vein becomes blocked, shock, proportional to the amount of blood lost to the circulation by being imprisoned in the limb, is always present. The limb cools slowly to room temperature. Gangrene appears to be extensive (*Fig.* 643) but usually the circulation is better than it appears and gangrene of the toes only is the aftermath.

Because he is unable to feel arterial pulsation in the affected limb, often the clinician diagnoses arterial embolism. If he realizes that he cannot feel the pulses in the affected lower limb because the tissues overlying the arteries are bloated and stiff with oedema, absent pulsation in a *greatly swollen limb* suggests that the main vein, and not the main artery, is blocked.

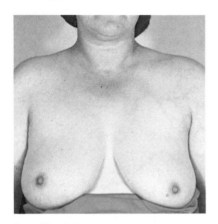

Fig. 644. Enlargement of superficial veins consequent upon spontaneous thrombosis of the axillary vein.

Fig. 645. Swollen arm resulting from spontaneous thrombosis of the axillary vein.

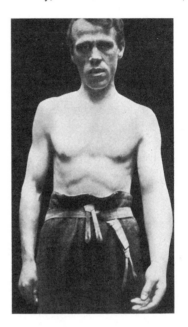

Thrombosis of the Axillary Vein. Although commonly ascribed to trauma many patients have no history of an accident and first notice the abnormality on waking in the morning. On the other hand, in a number of instances the swelling does come on after particularly strenuous use of the arm. Typically the patient is an active young or middle-aged individual, and in 80 per cent of cases male. The temperature and pulse rate are normal. As a rule the swelling involves the whole arm, from the shoulder-girdle to the fingers; not infrequently the lower part of the neck on the affected side shares in the swelling. The superficial veins, especially those running to the superior thoracic inlet, are more prominent than usual (*Fig.* 644). Although pain may be absent, often a dull ache is experienced in the arm and sometimes the axillary vein is palpable as a tender cord. Fatal embolism has not been reported. The swollen arm (*Fig.* 645) is firm, but exhibits slight pitting-on-pressure.

Superficial Thrombophlebitis is, generally speaking, of itself a far less serious condition than deep phlebothrombosis. It can, however, be the only outward and visible sign of grave disease unconnected with the veins or the blood that they transmit.

Superficial Thrombophlebitis of a Varicose Vein (*see Fig.* 73, p. 35). The signs of inflammation are readily apparent and the thrombosed portion of the varix feels like a firm cord. Usually there is no apparent cause; occasionally a leg ulcer is present, from which, presumably, the infection arose.

Two possible complications may supervene: (*a*) Suppuration (a most serious condition because pyaemia threatens), and (*b*) Extension of the thrombus along a perforating vein to the deep veins of the leg, or via the termination of the long saphenous vein to the femoral vein, with all the dangers that attend deep phlebothrombosis. Happily, neither complication is common. Nevertheless it is advisable to mark the upper limit of the inflammation with a skin pen, so that should the inflammation be extending upwards the fact can be noted at the next visit.

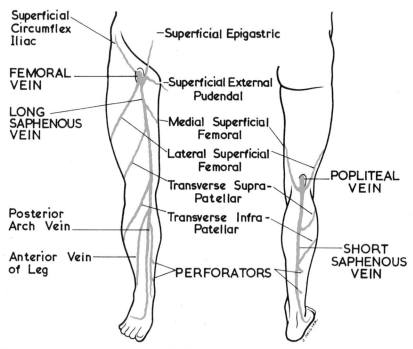

Fig. 646. Showing the possible anatomical distribution of varicose veins and the named intercommunicating veins between the long and the short saphenous veins. A common anomaly of the latter is for it to perforate the deep fascia, more or less in the midline, somewhere below the popliteal fossa. When the long saphenous vein is varicose, blood can pass from it along an intercommunicating vein to the short saphenous vein, and vice versa. The usual ankle perforating veins are also shown, but perforators may be found anywhere in the lower limb notably entering the subsartorial canal above the knee.

Thrombophlebitis Migrans occurs in previously normal veins, and often appears in patients who seem otherwise to be in good health. The thrombophlebitis makes its début spontaneously in almost any superficial vein, and reappears at first here, then there, the intervals between the visitations being days, weeks, or months. On no account regard the condition as a minor malady, and above all do not send the patient on his way rejoicing. Regard it as a sinister sign and one unprecedented, for its presence foretells with almost mathematical precision that one or other of the two following capital diseases is lurking in the background.

a. Visceral Carcinoma (Trousseau's Sign), especially of the pancreas (*see* p.

ARMAND TROUSSEAU, 1801–1867, *Physician, Hotêl-Dieu, Paris, noted the sign as his death warrant, confirming his suspicion of stomach cancer.*

238) or the stomach (*see* p. 228). Therefore, in every case a diligent examination of all the viscera by every means available is imperative.

b. Thrombo-angiitis Obliterans. Wandering superficial thrombophlebitis is one of the diagnostic features of this disease (*see* p. 382).

Mondor's Disease (*Phlébite-en-cordon*; string phlebitis) is a self-limiting thrombophlebitis of veins coursing over the upper chest wall towards the axilla. It is commoner in females, and is, apparently, less rare in France than in Britain. The subcutaneous cord or cords thus produced feel precisely like those that occur in thrombosis of the dorsal vein of the penis (*see* p. 355). In the female a vein overlying the breast may be affected, and has been mistaken for carcinoma. This misdiagnosis has raised the condition from a curiosity to one of real diagnostic importance.

VARICOSE VEINS

Varicose veins are easily the most common of the peripheral vascular diseases. By definition, varicose veins are tortuous, dilated and lengthened, with incompetence of the contained valves. This excludes the visible leg veins of young adult males and athletic females.

Varicosities usually involve either the long or short saphenous vein, or their tributaries (*Fig.* 646). The long saphenous vein (*Fig.* 647) becomes varicose seven times more frequently; sometimes both are implicated.

The Perforating Veins connect the superficial with the deep veins by piercing the deep fascia. They have been described in over 200 varying situations. In the case of the long saphenous vein the main perforators are arranged in three sets—one set in relation to the subsartorial canal, a second set in relation to the calf muscles, and a third set just above the ankle joint. When the valves of the lowest set become incompetent, contractions of the calf muscles (which normally propel the venous blood upwards) cause a reverse flow through the perforating veins and there results a high-pressure reflux which Cockett describes as a 'blow-out', viz.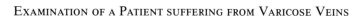

It is this high-pressure reflux that gives rise to the *flare sign* referred to on p. 525.

EXAMINATION OF A PATIENT SUFFERING FROM VARICOSE VEINS

Inspection. With the patient standing, the lower limbs are scrutinized from the umbilicus to the toes remembering to view the back of the legs as well as the front, to avoid overlooking varicosities of the short saphenous vein (*Fig.* 648).

A careful note is made of the anatomical distribution of the varices (*Fig.* 646), particularly of perforating veins.

Inspect the lower abdomen and the pubes. In the male this can be done at this stage; in the female this additional exposure in the standing position is repugnant to the patient, and an abdominal examination with the patient lying down is indicated.

Palpation. The limbs are palpated lightly, particularly over the courses of the short and long saphenous veins. In persons with fat limbs, superficial varicose veins are often palpable when they are not visible. This applies particularly to the areas immediately above an ulcer, and to the proximal portions of both saphenous veins.

HENRI MONDOR, 1885–1962, *Professor of Clinical Surgery, Hôpital Salpêtrière, Paris.*
FRANK B. COCKETT, *Contemporary Surgeon, St. Thomas's Hospital, London.*

At this juncture, especially in cases of bilateral varicosities, it is imperative to ask oneself the question:

Are these Varicose Veins Primary or Secondary? Especially when some of the affected veins do not conform to the usual pattern, e.g. there are varices on the pubis, or there is a lower abdominal operation scar which suggests the possibility of a bygone postoperative thrombosis, secondary varicose veins must be excluded. In practice only the first cause below is at all common.

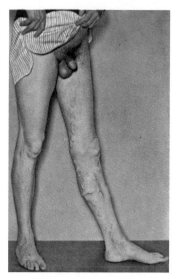

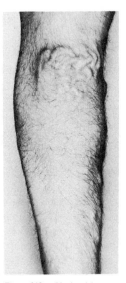

Fig. 647. Varicose veins. Left long saphenous vein mainly affected, but medial perforators are also present.

Fig. 648. Varicosities connected with the short saphenous vein.

1. Pregnancy.

2. An intrapelvic neoplasm (uterus, ovary, rectum) which can obstruct the free deep venous return, and so encourage the development of secondary superficial varicose veins. Usually, however, the presence of such a tumour associated with varicosities is a coincidence.

3. Compensatory varicose veins sometimes are one of the late complications of iliofemoral phlebothrombosis.

4. Superficial varicosities are often present with arteriovenous fistula (*see* p. 398).

Venous Stars are wont to occur in association with elevations of venous pressure. They are common on the dorsum of the foot, as well as on the legs, especially above the knee on the medial aspect of the thigh of patients with varicose veins. They are particularly numerous in persons with obstruction to the vena cava and in pregnant women. Digital pressure easily squeezes blood from the star; upon sudden release, it fills from the centre.

The Cough Impulse Test. When indubitably positive, this test is a clear indication that the valves of the long saphenous vein are incompetent. The fingers are laid on the thigh just below the saphenous opening, in such a way that the pulp of the middle fingers rests upon the vein (*Fig.* 649) or, when not clearly visible, where the vein should be. The patient is asked to cough. A fluid thrill is imparted to the finger if the valve at the saphenofemoral junction is incompetent.

The Percussion (Tap) Sign (Chevrier). With the patient still erect, place the fingers of the left hand just below the saphenous opening. Percuss the main bunch of varicosities once with the right middle finger. When valves within the segment under review are incompetent there will be no barrier to the upward wave of blood, and an impulse will be felt by the fingers overlying the long saphenous vein above. In most instances anatomical charting of the distribution of veins together with the cough and tap signs is sufficient for accurate diagnosis and other tests are relatively infrequently necessary.

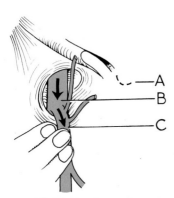

Fig. 649. Eliciting the cough impulse test. **A**, Pubic tubercle; **B**, Femoral vein; **C**, Long saphenous vein.

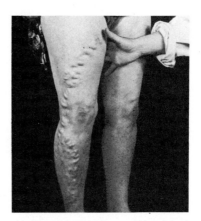

Fig. 650. Varicosity of a very large lateral superficial femoral vein. The Brodie–Trendelenburg test (*see below*) was positive for the whole length of this vein.

The Brodie–Trendelenburg Test. The patient lies down on a couch, and the limb is raised to allow the blood to drain out of the veins (*Fig.* 651 A). The fingers or thumb are placed firmly over the saphenous opening. Keeping firm pressure over this point, lower the limb and instruct the patient to stand (*Fig.* 651 B). The hand is removed suddenly. If the veins fill immediately, it is obvious that the valves in the saphenous vein are incompetent, and the test is positive (*Figs.* 650, 651 C).

Seeking the Sites of Perforators—Fegan's Method. Mark the varicosities with a skin pen while the patient stands; ask her to lie down and raise the affected limb and rest the heel against the examiner's upper chest (*Fig.* 652). Palpate the line of the marked varicosities carefully for gaps in the deep fascia through which the perforating veins pass; they are felt as circular openings with sharp edges and are marked with an X. To confirm that the superficial varicosities fill from the perforators the Brodie–Trendelenburg test can be applied.

Test for Patency of the Deep Veins. It is now realized that deep veins which have been the site of thrombotic occlusion almost invariably recanalize with the passage of time. If the patient complains of persistent 'bursting' pain in the lower leg on standing, the test for deep-vein patency is carried out. While the patient stands, a rubber tourniquet is applied around the thigh, tight enough to occlude the long saphenous vein but not the deep veins. The patient walks for 5 minutes. If the pain

Par L. Chevrier, *Nineteenth century Anatomist, Paris*.
Sir Benjamin Brodie, 1783–1862, *Surgeon, St. George's Hospital, London, described this test most lucidly in 1846*.
Friedrich Trendelenburg, 1844–1924, *Professor of Surgery, Leipzig, popularized the test*.
George Fegan, *Contemporary Emeritus Professor of Surgery, Trinity College, Dublin*.

of which the patient complains is brought on it is proof that the deep veins are still occluded. Additional evidence is that superficial varicosities (if present) become more prominent as their exit (the long saphenous vein) is blocked by the tourniquet.

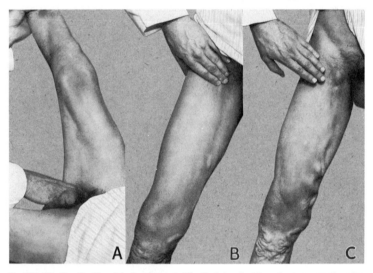

Fig. 651. The Brodie–Trendelenburg test. A, The limb is raised in order to empty the veins of blood, after which a finger (or tourniquet) is placed over the saphenous opening; B, The finger is still kept over the saphenous opening whilst the patient stands upright; C, The pressure over the saphenous opening has just been released, and the vein has filled from above downwards—the test is therefore positive.

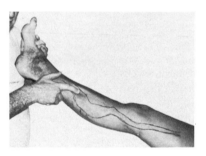

Fig. 652. Fegan's method of palpating for perforating veins after marking the varicosities with a skin pen.

ARTERIOVENOUS FISTULA

Congenital Arteriovenous Fistula. The lower extremity is the most common site, but the upper extremity, the head, or the neck, may be involved in decreasing order of frequency. Presentation in youth is usual. Leading signs are as follows:

1. *Leg Ulcer* (*see* p. 527) is frequently the presenting lesion and is sometimes known as a 'hot ulcer' because the surrounding skin feels warmer than normal. It is due to diversion of blood away from the skin. Often it is extremely painful.

2. *Varicose Veins and Port-wine Discoloration of the Skin* (*Fig.* 653). This combination is always extremely suspicious of arteriovenous fistula.

3. *Local Gigantism.* If, as is frequent, the arteriovenous connections are widespread and the

patient is young, increased length and girth of the limb ensue. It is a mistake to attribute inequality of limb lengths (and the scoliosis that ensues) to shortness of the unaffected leg.

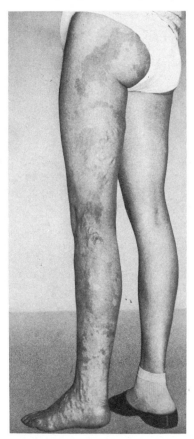

Fig. 653. Varicose veins and port-wine staining due to arteriovenous fistula. The affected leg is shorter than its fellow.

4. *Increased Local Warmth*. The extremity is appreciably warmer, and usually moister than that of the unaffected side.

5. *Collapsing Arterial Pulse* (Corrigan's Pulse). This sign, usually taught on the medical wards, can be demonstrated on the foot pulses.

6. *The Bradycardiac Reaction*. Digital occlusion of the main artery to the limb is followed by slowing of the pulse rate indicating that a considerable volume of blood is being short-circuited.

7. *The 'Machinery' Murmur*. With a stethoscope applied over the fistula a *full-circuit bruit* with systolic accentuation is pathognomonic. The bruit is high pitched and musical.

There are two varieties of congenital arteriovenous fistula—*localized* and *diffuse*. In the diffuse variety, which is relatively common, the arteriovenous communications are deep and clinically indiscernible (probably in the bone). In these (6) and (7) will be absent.

Acquired Arteriovenous Fistula is a result of a wound, usually a stab or through-and-through gunshot wound. Often the superficial situation of the involved vessels enables the clinician to palpate the resultant aneurysm. The sign of an aneurysm (*see* p. 27) may be present. The other signs of arteriovenous fistula described above (except (3)) can be observed, particularly (5), (6) and (7).

This condition is an unusual, but definite, complication of lumbar disc surgery, the communication being between the common iliac artery and vein.

THE LYMPHATICS

SIGNS ASSOCIATED WITH LYMPHATIC OBSTRUCTION

Oedema of the extremities may be due to venous or lymphatic blockage. Persistent swelling of the limb seldom is due to the former unless the inferior vena cava is obstructed (bilateral swelling up to the groin), or a common iliac vein is occluded (unilateral swelling). Look for evidence of venous collateral circulation (*see* pp. 18, 249). Most instances of *long-continued* limb oedema are due to lymphatic disease (lymphoedema) in which the oedema is firm (solid) but will pit to a variable extent (*see* p. 10), particularly in the early stages. Ulceration is rare.

Two varieties of lymphoedema can be distinguished, *secondary* which is commoner by far in practice, and *primary* which is seen more often in vascular clinics. The former follows damage and obstruction to the lymphatic pathways by malignant disease involving the lymph nodes (*Fig.* 654), by filariasis (*see Fig.* 550, p. 337), and by surgical block dissections. Repeated attacks of inflammation (cellulitis) are common in both types and the swelling tends to increase with each attack so that in the course of time the limb reaches massive proportions (*elephantiasis*). The skin becomes hyperkeratotic and fissured so that the limb is pachydermatous in appearance as well as size (*Fig.* 655).

Primary Lymphoedema. Radiological demonstration of the lymphatic pathways (lymphangiography) has clarified the aetiology (Kinmonth). There is a marked female preponderance (75 per cent) although in Milroy's disease the sex distribution is equal.

Aplasia. There is complete absence of subcutaneous lymph trunks. The swelling is present from birth and, if the condition is familial as well as congenital, the term 'Milroy's disease' is correct.

SIR DOMINIC CORRIGAN, 1802–1880, *Physician, Jervis Street Hospital, Dublin, described the collapsing pulse of aortic regurgitation.*
JOHN B. KINMONTH, *Contemporary Professor of Surgery, St. Thomas's Hospital, London.*
WILLIAM F. MILROY, 1855–1942, *Professor of Clinical Medicine, University of Nebraska.*

Hypoplasia is easily the commonest variety. The lymph trunks are fewer and smaller than usual. The oedema commences in childhood or early adult life, usually after an attack of cellulitis (*Fig.* 656).

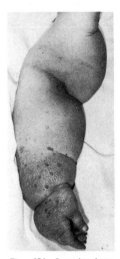

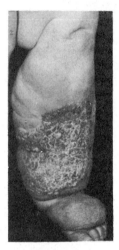

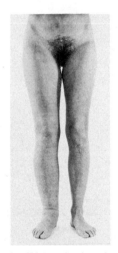

Fig. 654. Lymphoedema-tous arm consequent on axillary lymph-node block-age by secondary breast cancer.

Fig. 655. Pachydermatous skin associated with ele-phantiasis.

Fig. 656. Lymphoedema due to radiologically demon-strated lymphatic hypo-plasia. Onset in early adult life.

Hyperplasia. The lymphatics are enlarged, increased in number and tortuous. This variety is thus analogous with varicose veins. Chyle often runs downwards past incompetent valves and appears on the skin surface as discharging vesicles of milky liquid, a unique sign.

Lymphoedema in the Tropics. Although filariasis is the classical cause, in practice tuberculous lymphadenitis is commoner, with chronic sepsis in second place. The scrotum, which may become enormous, equalling the rest of the body in weight in exceptional cases, the labia (*see Fig.* 550, p. 337), and the lower limbs are notably affected. At first pitting on pressure can be demonstrated, but as the condition becomes chronic the swelling becomes solid.

Chapter 27

THE PERIPHERAL NERVES

The examination of a peripheral nerve lesion consists essentially of three separate parts: (1) General inspection of the injured or otherwise affected limb; (2) Examination of motor defects; (3) Examination of sensation.

GENERAL INSPECTION OF THE INJURED LIMB

a. At times, as the result of a nerve injury the limb, or a portion thereof, takes up an attitude so characteristic as to suggest the diagnosis—for instance, the 'waiter's tip' position of Erb–Duchenne paralysis; the dropped wrist of a radial nerve lesion; the pointing index attitude of median nerve palsy.

b. When a nerve lesion is noted with a *recent* injury bear in mind the following points:

i. A sharp object, e.g. broken glass, has almost certainly severed the nerve. Operative treatment is essential.

ii. Blunt trauma due to a missile may have severed the nerve but rupture of fibres within an intact sheath (*axonotmesis*) is also possible. It is best to explore the nerve at the time of the operation necessary to remove the missile.

iii. A fractured bone or dislocation, when it causes nerve injury, almost always causes axonotmesis, and an expectant attitude can be adopted.

iv. Traction injuries of nerve result in damage (*neurotmesis*) to a long length of the nerve; the outlook for recovery, even with operative repair, is poor.

c. If an *old* wound or scar is present, its position in relationship to underlying structures must be noted. Scars should be examined for tenderness, adherence to deep structures, and bulbous enlargements of divided nerve ends.

d. With a fairly recent complete lesion of a sensory or a mixed nerve, the skin has a pink, or even a rosy appearance, and because of vasodilatation due to severance of the sympathetic nerve fibres, often evidence of desquamation can be seen a few days after the injury. A similar lesion of considerable standing shows dry, mottled blue skin. On the contrary, in the case of an incomplete irritative lesion, the skin may be red, glossy and perspiring (causalgia or Weir Mitchell's skin).

e. The nails should be inspected for curvature, ridging, change in colour and absence of gloss.

Causalgia. * The affected nerves are large, especially the median and tibial, i.e. those supplying the palm and sole; in almost all cases the injured nerve has been divided incompletely. While not uncommon after war injuries, it is exceptional in civil life. It is characterized by pain—persistent, severe and usually described as 'burning' or 'hot'. Many sufferers seek relief by applying cold compresses to the affected part. The threshold for noxious sensory stimuli is lowered—noise, in particular, causes intensification of pain. The *Skin* covering the affected part is tight, thin and glossy. It is *less* sensitive to heat, cold and pin-prick than normal skin, but it is hypersensitive to light touch,

---

* *Causalgia.* Greek, καῦσις = heat + ἄλγος = pain.

Silas Weir Mitchell, 1829–1914, *Neurologist, Jefferson Medical College, Philadelphia.*

and exceedingly tender to pressure. The *Nails* grow rapidly, and are curved due to wasting of the finger pads and are exquisitely tender.

EXAMINATION OF MUSCLES

While the practical clinical methods of ascertaining whether an individual muscle is contracting or not will be described, attention is directed here to a system of grading muscle power* which has earned worldwide approval:

  5. Contraction against powerful resistance (normal power) = 100 per cent.
  4. Contraction against gravity and some resistance = 75 per cent.
  3. Contraction against gravity only = 50 per cent.
  2. Movement only possible with gravity eliminated = 25 per cent.
  1. Flicker of contraction but no movement = 10 per cent.
  0. Complete paralysis = 0 per cent.

The possibility of substitution ('trick') movements are eliminated by adhering to the simple methods described. The hand muscles in particular often have dual innervation (motor overlap).

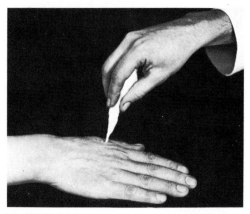

Fig. 657. Testing for touch sensation with a wisp of cotton-wool.

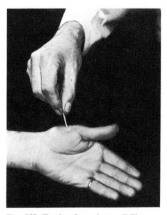

Fig. 658. Testing for pain sensibility.

EXAMINATION OF SENSATION

The patient is placed so that no muscular effort is necessary to maintain the position of the limb. With his eyes closed, he is told to respond as follows:

a. Touch Sensation is tested by stroking the skin with cotton-wool (*Fig.* 657). The patient says 'Yes' when he feels *anything*. This test cannot be relied upon if the skin is clad with hair, e.g. on the dorsum of the hand in men.

b. Pain Sensation. A sharp pin is used (*Fig.* 658), and care must be taken that the patient understands that he is to say 'Sharp' only when he feels the pain of a pin-prick, not when he feels pressure or touch. Unless this precaution is taken, the method is entirely inaccurate.

c. Temperature Sensation. This can be tested readily by filling two test tubes, one with hot and one with cold water, and applying them in turn to the skin of the affected part, at the same time noting

---

* Drawn up by the Medical Research Council, London.

the patient's remarks on whether he feels 'hot' or 'cold'. For practical purposes this test is only of value to the surgeon if syringomyelia is suspected.

In surgical practice a peripheral nerve lesion usually results from trauma (sometimes at operation), and only occasionally from disease (particularly pressure by tumours). Interruption of a nerve trunk can be detected most easily by testing for loss of power of individual muscles, which will be considered for the commoner injuries. The findings for touch and pain sensory loss are not detailed as they are dealt with in neurological and anatomical texts. Neither deep pain sensibility nor tactile localization and discrimination are discussed as they are of purely neurological interest.

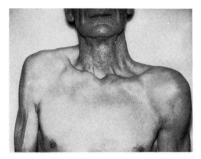

Fig. 659. Paralysis of the accessory nerve. Answer to the request 'Shrug your shoulders'; the shoulder on the side of the lesion fails to shrug.

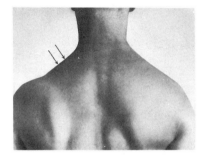

Fig. 660. Characteristic flattening following a lesion of the accessory nerve. Note the winging of the scapula compared with that of the opposite side.

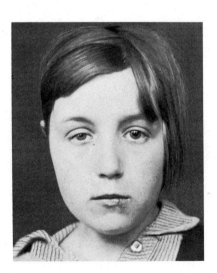

Fig. 661. Paralysis of the right cervical sympathetic. Note the pseudoptosis and myosis.

THE CERVICAL PLEXUS

The Accessory Nerve supplies the sternomastoid and trapezius muscles. Although it is the 11th cranial nerve, and consequently is mentioned in connection with the examination of cranial nerves on p. 60, because it is derived from the cervical plexus, its main consideration has been postponed to this chapter. Paralysis of the above muscles is recognized easily: (1) Ask the patient to shrug his shoulders; that the trapezius is paralysed becomes obvious because the shoulder of the affected side fails to shrug (*Fig.* 659); (2) In cases *of some standing* there is wasting of the trapezius, which causes an alteration in the contour of the lower part of the neck and the adjacent portion of the shoulder of the affected side (*Fig.* 660); (3) There is weakness of the sternomastoid muscle, which is tested as shown in *Fig.* 260, p. 138.

The Cervical Sympathetic Chain. Preganglionic nerve fibres designed for the supply of orbital structures arise in the spinal segments T1 and T2. These fibres traverse the corresponding nerve roots, and, as white rami communicantes, enter the cervical sympathetic chain, lesions of which produce characteristic signs, mainly affecting structures in the orbit.

Horner's Syndrome. In surgical practice this is found most frequently:

1. In Klumpke's paralysis and complete brachial plexus injuries (*see* p. 405).
2. As a complication of a wound in the neck.
3. When the nerve is involved by a cervical (*see* p. 157) or thoracic neoplasm (*see* p. 191).
4. After cervical sympathectomy.

Examine the eyelids. There is pseudoptosis (*Fig.* 661). The upper-lid droops incompletely, for the cervical sympathetic innervates only one-third of the levator palpebrae superioris. The affected pupil is smaller. In this connection a good test is the *spinociliary reflex*: pinch the skin of the neck and the pupil on that side will dilate. In Horner's syndrome no such dilatation occurs. Anhidrosis (absence of sweating) is present on the side of the lesion so that the palm of the hand feels dry.

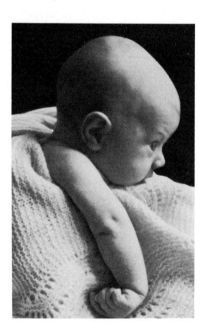

Fig. 662. The arm is held in the 'waiter's tip' position. Erb–Duchenne paralysis.

Johann F. Horner, 1831–1886, *Professor of Ophthalmology, Zürich, Switzerland.*

THE BRACHIAL PLEXUS

Injury of Nerve Roots. There are two types of resulting paralysis, i.e. the upper (Erb–Duchenne paralysis) and the lower (Klumpke's paralysis). Increasingly, with the trauma of modern traffic accidents, complete brachial plexus paralysis is seen; the whole limb shows a flaccid paralysis with loss of pain sensation of the hand, forearm and lower arm. Paralysis of the cervical sympathetic (*see above*) is usual.

Erb–Duchenne Paralysis is due to an injury of C5 and C6 nerve roots, resulting from excessive lateral displacement of the head with forcible depression of the shoulder. Usually it occurs in babies during a difficult confinement, but also later in life from a weight falling upon the shoulder, or an accident producing a similar impact. Diagnosis is easy, for the affected arm lies limply by the side in the characteristic 'waiter's tip' position (*Fig.* 662). Movements dependent upon the integrity of the muscles of the forearm and hand are capable of being carried out, while those of the elbow and shoulder joints are greatly restricted. Thus the successive movements in lifting a drinking glass to the lips are considerably impaired.

Klumpke's Paralysis is due to a lesion of C8 and T1. This is encountered most often as the result of a forceful cephalad pull on the child's arm during birth.

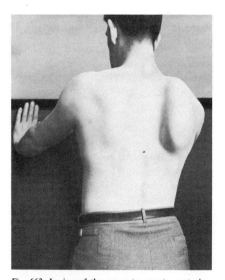

Fig. 663. Lesion of the nerve to serratus anterior. When the patient pushes against a wall with both hands, the scapula on the affected side stands out like a wing.

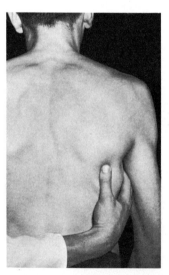

Fig. 664. The normal latissimus dorsi can be felt to contract when the patient coughs.

Less often it is sustained later in life as a result of a dislocation of the shoulder joint or a violent upward pull on the arm, such as might be occasioned by grabbing at a ledge while falling from a height. Paralysis of all the intrinsic muscles of the hand ensues; eventually a true claw-hand results. Loss of sensation along the ulnar side of the arm, forearm and hand also occurs. Finally look for

WILHELM H. ERB, 1840–1921, *Professor of Medicine, Heidelberg.*
GUILLAUME B. A. DUCHENNE, 1806–1875, *Neurologist in Boulogne and Paris. First recognized tabes dorsalis although the cause was unknown.*
MADAME AUGUSTE DÉJERINE KLUMPKE, 1859–1927, *described the syndrome while a medical student in Paris.*

paralysis of the cervical sympathetic (*see* p. 404) because the sympathetic fibres traversing the anterior primary rami of T1 are sometimes implicated indicating that the lesion of T1 is near its exit from the intervertebral foramen, and therefore is in an inaccessible position.

The Axillary Nerve can become torn or compressed in dislocation of the shoulder, in fracture of the neck of the humerus, and occasionally in fracture of the scapula. Palsy results in atrophy of the deltoid muscle (*see Fig.* 721, p. 447) and consequently abduction of the arm is compromised. To avoid 'trick' movement the arm must be parallel to the trunk when testing.

The Musculocutaneous Nerve innervates the biceps, coracobrachialis and brachialis muscles, paralysis of which is detected by asking the patient to stand with his arms outstretched, then to clench his fists and do 'dumb-bell' exercises slowly. The contracted belly of biceps can be seen easily if it is acting.

The Nerve to Serratus Anterior (Nerve of Bell), because of its long straight course, may be traumatized by over-stretching during heavy weight-lifting in certain occupations, for instance that of a furniture remover. It is also liable to be severed during the operation of radical mastectomy. Paralysis is demonstrated by asking the patient to push against a wall with his outstretched hands; the scapula on the affected side becomes *winged* (*Fig.* 663).

The Thoracodorsal Nerve to latissimus dorsi is also sometimes damaged in radical mastectomy. It is remarkable that paralysis of so large a muscle results in but trivial inconvenience, the only movement lost being strong adduction of the shoulder joint. On grasping the muscle belly (*Fig.* 664) its normal contraction can be ascertained by asking the patient to cough deeply.

The three major branches of the brachial plexus provide, in practice, the great majority of nerve lesions. It is not proposed here to enter into more than the minimum details of examination for everyday purposes. Note that the median and ulnar nerves often innervate muscles anomalously due to anastomotic branches.

THE RADIAL NERVE

At the elbow the nerve divides into two terminal branches—*superficial radial*, which is entirely sensory, and *posterior interosseous*, wholly muscular. Paralysis occurs in fractures of the shaft of the humerus, pressure from callus, gunshot wounds of the axilla and arm, and not infrequently from sitting with the arm suspended over the back of a chair or pressure by a crutch (crutch palsy). For radial nerve paralysis to be complete, it must be interrupted in the axilla.

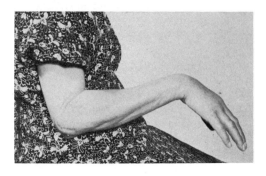

Fig. 665. Wrist-drop due to a lesion of the radial nerve. A 'lipoma' had been excised—note the scar at the elbow—evidently this was a neurofibroma of the radial nerve. The patient is unable to extend her wrist.

SIR CHARLES BELL, 1774–1842, *Surgeon, Middlesex Hospital, London; later Professor of Surgery, Edinburgh.*

Motor Defects. If the injury is situated above the junction of the upper and the middle thirds of the humerus, the action of triceps is lost.

Test for Triceps. Seat the patient with the elbow flexed to a right-angle on a table. This eliminates the force of gravity. If triceps is working the elbow can be straightened easily.

If the lesion is situated at the middle third of the humerus (a frequent site of fracture) the brachioradialis is spared. In all these lesions the characteristic deformity is *wrist-drop*, which is unobtrusive unless the patient flexes the elbow joint with the forearm pronated (*Fig.* 665).

Test for Brachioradialis. Flexion of the elbow is weakened if this muscle is paralysed. When the patient endeavours to flex the elbow joint against resistance, the brachioradialis no longer springs up to bridge the angle between the arm and the forearm as it does normally (*Fig.* 666).

The results of injury of one or other of the terminal branches of the radial nerve are as follows:

The Posterior Interosseous Nerve. Because the extensor carpi radialis longus is not paralysed and the extensor carpi radialis brevis is not always implicated, typical wrist-drop is not present, but the hand is held in radial deviation on attempting extension. Extensor digitorum is paralysed so that the patient is unable to prevent the examiner from flexing the extended fingers easily.

The Superficial Radial Nerve is sometimes severed in operations on the synovial extensor tendon sheaths of the thumb (*see Fig.* 747, p. 462). The sensory loss is depicted in *Fig.* 674. This loss is also found in a higher lesion of the radial nerve.

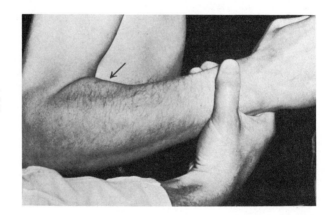

Fig. 666. Contraction of brachio-radialis, absent if the radial nerve is injured in the middle of the arm or above.

THE MEDIAN NERVE

In civilian life the nerve is particularly vulnerable in the cubital fossa, where it is exposed to the risk of damage by misplaced intravenous injections. Another common site of injury—this time by severance—is at the wrist. It controls *coarse* movements of the hand and is the nerve of grasp. In *all* injuries, at whatever level, the patient is *unable to pick up a pin with thumb and index finger*. This is partly due to sensory loss (*see Fig.* 674).

In practice one usually knows the level of the lesion from the position of the injury. In the case of the median nerve a *recent* injury is easily missed on cursory inspection.

RECENT INJURY

The student should recall the following anatomical facts. The nerve gives off no branches until it reaches the elbow. Between the elbow and the middle of the forearm its muscle branches are given off at various levels, to supply the flexors of the wrists and digits and the pronators of the forearm. As some of these muscles have a dual nerve supply, certain movements, which call into action those muscles which are innervated entirely by the median nerve alone, are tested.

Because in the forearm this nerve is so well protected by muscles it is rarely injured here. On this account, an otherwise complex situation is simplified by considering first lesions situated (*a*) in or above the cubital fossa; (*b*) at the wrist.

Lesion in or above the Cubital Fossa. *Loss of the Power to flex the Interphalangeal Joints of the Index Finger*: This can be demonstrated easily by Ochsner's clasping test. Ask the patient to clasp the hands together firmly. If the median nerve has been interrupted above the level where the nerve to flexor digitorum sublimis is given off (crease of the elbow joint) the index finger fails to flex (*Fig.* 667).

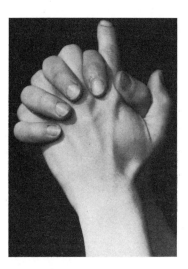

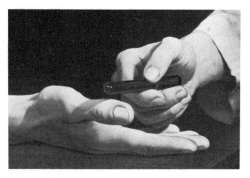

Fig. 668. The pen-touching test. In this case of cut median nerve at the wrist, because of paralysis of the abductor pollicis brevis, the patient can raise the thumb no farther than is shown.

Fig. 667. Ochsner's clasping test in median nerve paralysis. The index finger fails to flex.

Lesion at the Wrist. Below the wrist joint the median nerve usually supplies only the flexor pollicis brevis, the opponens pollicis, and the abductor pollicis brevis. Frequent variations in the nerve supply of the first two dictate that only a non-functioning abductor pollicis brevis can be relied upon.

The Pen-touching Test for Abductor Pollicis Brevis. The patient places his affected hand flat upon a table, palm uppermost. Tell him to keep the thumb straight and rest it upon the table, or as near to the table as possible. The clinician, holding a pen or pencil as shown in *Fig.* 668, rests his hand upon the patient's outstretched fingers (to keep them flat). He is told to touch the pen

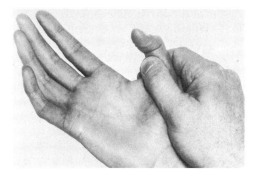

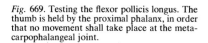

Fig. 669. Testing the flexor pollicis longus. The thumb is held by the proximal phalanx, in order that no movement shall take place at the metacarpophalangeal joint.

with the edge of his thumb. In order to be sure that he understands the instructions clearly it is advisable to touch the lateral aspect of the terminal phalanx and say, 'When I tell you, bring this part of the thumb up to touch my pen.'

Sensory Loss only, by division of the terminal median nerve below the point where the muscular branch to the thenar muscles is given off, is a rare, even theoretical, possibility. *See* again *Fig.* 674.

Lesions in the Forearm involving the Anterior Interosseous Nerve only. This again is unusual.

Loss of Power of the Flexor Pollicis Longus. Can the patient flex the terminal phalanx of his thumb? The thumb is held firmly at the metacarpophalangeal joint so that no movement can take place there; then the patient is instructed to bend his thumb (*Fig.* 669). If he can actively flex the interphalangeal joint the anterior interosseous nerve (and the median nerve above its origin in the cubital fossa) is intact.

LONG-STANDING INJURY. This is comparatively easily detected by the following tests.

Lesion in or above the Cubital Fossa

The Benediction Attitude (*Fig.* 670): When the patient raises his arm with the palm facing the examiner, the outstretched index finger and the serial flexion of the other fingers have been likened to the attitude of the hand of a priest with his arm held aloft.

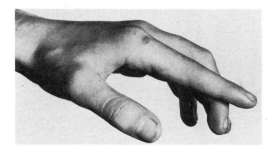

Fig. 670. The pointing index or benediction position of a hand, the seat of long-standing median nerve paralysis due to a lesion at the level of the elbow joint. The pulp of the index finger has atrophied, and the fingernail of the digit is curved like a parrot's beak. Note also the ape-like thumb.

The Ape-like Thumb. The thumb tends to be held in an ape-like position, that is the palmar surface of the thumb lies in the same plane as that of the rest of the palm (simian hand). The reason for this is that the action of the extensor pollicis longus (supplied by the radial nerve) and that of the adductor pollicis (supplied by the ulnar nerve) are unopposed.

Lesion at the Wrist. *Wasting of the Thenar Eminence* (*see Fig.* 4, p. 4) is, in some long-standing cases, so evident that the outline of the first metacarpal bone is visible. It is also present with higher lesions but occasionally is lacking, owing to anomalous innervation of the flexor brevis and opponens pollicis.
Median Nerve Compression in the Carpal Tunnel: see p. 461.

THE ULNAR NERVE

At the level of the elbow joint the nerve is vulnerable (1) from compression by a band (*see* p. 456); (2) from involvement in a fracture of the medial epicondyle or in the resulting callus; (3) from repeated knocks in this part of its course due to cubitus valgus. At the wrist joint the nerve is not infrequently severed, often in combination with the flexor carpi ulnaris (*see Fig.* 743, p. 460), which explains why initially the nerve injury is sometimes overlooked. Again, recent injuries are not so conspicuous as old injuries, but are not so easily missed as is a recent median nerve injury. The ulnar nerve controls the fine movements of the hand, as exemplified in the delicate fingering of the pianist.
RECENT INJURY
Lesion in or above the Cubital Fossa. *Test for Flexor Carpi Ulnaris.* Ask the patient to lay his hand palm upwards flat on a table and, keeping the fingers as straight as possible, to attempt flexion and ulnar deviation of the wrist. If flexor carpi ulnaris is functioning the tendon can be felt, and often seen, in the position shown in *Fig.* 742, p. 460.

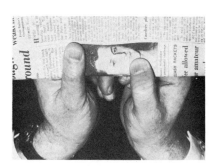

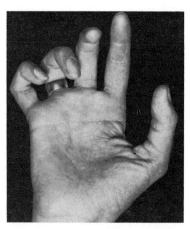

Fig. 671. Froment's sign. A positive result (right side) confirms the diagnosis of ulnar paralysis.

Fig. 672. A claw-like hand resulting from division of the ulnar nerve at the wrist.

Lesion at the Wrist. *Froment's Sign* for demonstrating paralysis of the adductor pollicis is the best test for ulnar nerve injury. The patient is asked to grasp a folded newspaper firmly between the thumb and index fingers of each hand, the thumbs being uppermost, the adductor thus being brought into action (*Fig.* 671). When this muscle is paralysed, the thumb, incapable of adequate adduction, becomes flexed at the interphalangeal joint due to contraction of the flexor pollicis longus (innervated by the median nerve).

JULES FROMENT, 1878–1946, *Professor of Clinical Medicine, Lyons, France.*

Ulnar Claw-hand. The little and the ring fingers are hyperextended at the metacarpophalangeal joints, and are flexed at the interphalangeal joints (*Fig.* 672). The middle and the index fingers are much less affected, owing to the fact that the second and the first lumbrical muscles are supplied by the median nerve. Often, in long-standing cases, the little finger is so crooked that the patient complains that 'it catches in everything'. The ulnar claw-hand is a prerogative of a lesion at the wrist. So it comes about that the *ulnar nerve paradox*—the higher the lesion the less the deformity—beguiles those unfamiliar with the phenomenon. When the nerve is interrupted at or above the elbow joint, the ulnar half of the flexor digitorum profundus muscle is paralysed, and does not act unopposed by the interossei and lumbricals, and so the little and ring fingers are not greatly flexed; consequently there is no 'claw'.

LONG-STANDING INJURY. Some months after interruption of the ulnar nerve it will be noted that, in addition to the above signs:

a. The Little Finger is held in Abduction: The phenomenon, which is more evident when the patient is asked to extend the finger, is due to the unopposed action of the extensor muscles (radial nerve) which also abduct the little finger (*see Fig.* 743, p. 460).

b. Hollowing between the Metacarpal Bones is clearly apparent on the dorsum. Each time the fingers are flexed the intermetacarpal muscular wasting causes the extensor tendons to stand out. The hollowing is due to atrophy of the interossei muscles, and in the case of the interval between the first and second metacarpal bones, to atrophy of the adductor pollicis as well (*Fig.* 673).

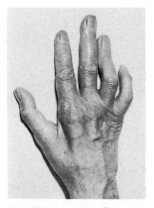

Fig. 673. A long-standing ulnar nerve lesion. Note the abducted little finger and the muscle wasting, particularly between the first and second metacarpals.

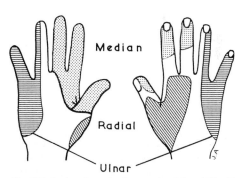

Fig. 674. Average loss of pain sensation (pin-prick) with lesions of the major nerves of the upper limb.

A RAPID METHOD OF ELIMINATING AN INJURY OF A MAJOR NERVE OF THE UPPER LIMB

It is desirable that practitioners acquire a method of examination which will enable quick detection of a nerve lesion. The following routine is virtually completely reliable. If evidence of a lesion is found, more detailed testing as already outlined is necessary.

1. Test for Wrist Drop—Radial Nerve, *see* p. 407.
2. Ochsner's Clasping Test—Median Nerve, *see* p. 408.
3. Froment's Sign—Ulnar Nerve, *see* p. 410.

If fractures of other injuries prevent the above tests being carried out, test pain sensation in the hand. The average loss in lesions of the major nerves is depicted in *Fig.* 674.

CLAW-HAND

A true claw-hand is found in several conditions, most of which have been described in this book.

1. Lesion of both median and ulnar nerves (including leprosy, *see* p. 415).
2. Lesion of the medial cord of the brachial plexus.
3. Klumpke's paralysis.
4. A late and severe Volkmann's ischaemic contracture (*see* p. 479).
5. An end-result of a neglected suppurative tenosynovitis of the ulnar bursa (*see* p. 474).
6. Anterior poliomyelitis.
7. Advanced untreated rheumatoid arthritis.
8. A group of uncommon conditions of neurological interest including syringomyelia, progressive muscular atrophy, polyneuritis and amyotr␣phic lateral sclerosis.

A complete lesion of the ulnar nerve of some standing results in a claw-*like* hand (often called the 'ulnar claw-hand', *see Fig.* 672), but unless the n.␣dian nerve is the seat of a complete lesion also, it cannot be called a true claw-hand.

NERVES OF THE LOWER EXTREMITY

The Femoral Nerve is seldom the seat of a lesion either in peace or war. The disability is great, for the quadriceps femoris, the main extensor and stabilizer of the knee joint, is paralysed. It can be tested by asking the patient to extend the knee with the leg dangling over the edge of the examining couch, i.e. against gravity.

Lateral Cutaneous Nerve of Thigh. *Meralgia Paraesthetica* (*see* p. 501).

The Sciatic Nerve. Morphologically the sciatic nerve consists of two nerves enclosed in a single sheath. Occasionally these two nerves are macroscopically separate throughout their course. Even when, as is usual, a seemingly single sciatic nerve is present, the level of its division (classically at the upper limit of the popliteal space) is inconstant. For these reasons a lesion of the sciatic nerve should be spoken of as a lesion of either the medial or the lateral component of this nerve; if both components are involved, this fact should be recorded.

Lesions of Both Components. In war a gunshot wound is the cause, in peace a fracture-dislocation of the hip joint.

Motor Defects. A complete lesion of the sciatic nerve causes paralysis of all muscles below the knee joint; if the lesion is in the gluteal region, paralysis of some of the hamstrings will occur also, i.e. flexion of the knee is weakened.

Sensory Loss. See Fig. 675.

The Common Peroneal Nerve, the smaller of the two terminal branches, supplies the muscles of the anterior and lateral compartments of the leg below the knee and the short extensors of the toes. In severe injuries of the knee joint due to adduction of the leg on the thigh it is liable to be stretched or, rarely, torn across. *Characteristic Posture or Deformity.* Paralysis causes the foot to assume a position of equinovarus (*see* p. 536), which, by reason of the dropped foot, results in a slapping gait and undue pressure on the outer side of the foot. The toe of the shoe is scuffed.

Motor Defects. The patient can neither extend (dorsiflex) his foot nor extend his toes.

The two terminal branches of the common peroneal nerve are seldom injured alone. When the *superficial peroneal* (musculocutaneous) *nerve* is damaged, on asking the patient to extend the foot it becomes inverted owing to paralysis of the peroneal muscles. In *deep peroneal nerve* lesions a similar request leads to eversion owing to paralysis of tibialis anterior muscle.

Common Peroneal Nerve Entrapment. As the nerve winds round the neck of the fibula deep to the tendinous arch of origin of peroneus longus it is subject to pressure. The first effect is that weakness of the peroneal muscles leads to repeated turning over of the ankle which is liable to be mistaken for an inversion sprain (*see* p. 531). Foot drop is the late result. Burke points out that the lesion can be detected at an early stage by seating the patient with the knees flexed and the heels resting on the floor and requesting him to turn the foot inwards (inversion = deep peroneal nerve) and then outwards (eversion = superficial peroneal nerve) rapidly ⎯⎯⎯⎯⎯⎯⎯⎯⎯⎯⎯⎯⎯⎯⎯⎯⟶
The ability to carry out this action rapidly and repetitively in this position is lost early in this condition.

The Tibial is the larger terminal division of the sciatic nerve. A complete lesion results in paralysis of all the muscles of the gastrocnemius group and all the intrinsic muscles of the sole of the foot.

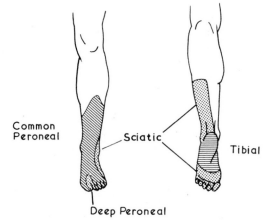

Fig. 675. Average loss of pain sensation (pin-prick) with lesions of the major nerves of the lower limb. A complete sciatic nerve injury causes anaesthesia below the middle of the leg except for an area supplied by the saphenous nerve medially.

Common Peroneal

Sciatic

Tibial

Deep Peroneal

Characteristic Posture or Deformity. The foot is held in calcaneovalgus (*see* p. 538) by the unopposed action of the extensors and evertors. The disability is great, and the patient has a pronounced limp due to difficulty in 'taking off' from the affected foot. He cannot stand on tip-toe. In time the disability in walking becomes less obvious, owing to cicatricial contracture of the calf muscles. The toes become clawed from contracture of their flexors.

DENIS T. BURKE, *Contemporary General Practitioner, Woodville, South Australia.*

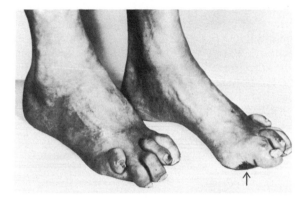

Fig. 676. Typical cock-up deformity of the toes associated with diabetic neuropathy. The arrow points to a gangrenous patch of skin, due to pressure resulting from the deformity.

Motor Defects. The patient cannot fully flex the ankle joint, but a small degree is possible by contraction of the peronei muscles. Inversion against resistance is impossible. Active flexion of the toes is also impossible. The ankle jerk is absent. If the lesion is in the lower third of the leg all the muscular branches are spared, and sensory loss (*Fig.* 675) also is evident.

The loss of sensation of the sole of the foot renders the development of a trophic ulcer or ulcers almost inevitable.

Diabetic Neuropathy of the Tibial Nerve is of particular surgical importance, and although it occurs at all ages, it is more commonly seen in the elderly diabetic. The cock-up deformity of the toes (*Fig.* 676) predisposes to pressure sores over the plantar surface of the heads of the metatarsals, and in diabetics with occlusive peripheral arterial disease it is the chronic infection of such a sore that accounts for the high incidence of infected gangrene in elderly diabetic patients (Oakley). Pressure on the hammer-toe deformity (*see* p. 550) also contributes. In younger patients the anaesthetic sole predisposes to a perforating ulcer in this situation.

A RAPID METHOD OF ELIMINATING AN INJURY OF A MAJOR NERVE OF THE LOWER LIMB

1. Satisfy yourself that the metatarsophalangeal joint is mobile (i.e. that it is not the seat of hallux rigidus). Ask the patient to bend the big toe. If it flexes adequately the tibial nerve is intact.

2. Then request the patient to move his big toe upwards. If strong extension can be performed, the common peroneal nerve is intact.

Fractures and other injuries seldom prevent these simple tests, but in such circumstances test pain sensation in the leg and foot. The average loss is depicted in *Fig.* 675.

NEOPLASM OF A PERIPHERAL NERVE

Neurofibroma of a large or moderate-sized peripheral nerve is not common; all the more reason to be on the lookout for an example, as excision is often disastrous for the patient (*see Fig.* 665). Neurofibroma arises *in* the nerve and cannot be removed without destroying the nerve. Neurilemmoma arises in the sheath and removal is possible with conservation of the nerve. Particular

WILFRID G. OAKLEY, *Contemporary Emeritus Physician, Diabetic Department, King's College Hospital, London.*

diagnostic difficulty arises when a part of the brachial plexus is involved, as the swelling is liable to be mistaken for an enlarged lymph node. The swelling is solitary and, as a rule, fusiform in shape. Its consistency varies; often it is moderately soft, and consequently it is liable to be confused with a lipoma. Pressure upon the lump often gives rise to tingling 'pins and needles', or actual pain down the course of the nerve. These tumours rarely become malignant (with the exception of von Recklinghausen's Disease of Nerve (*see* p. 29) in which individual neurofibromata sometimes become sarcomatous). A similar tumour sometimes occurs at the end of a nerve in an amputation stump (stump neuroma), or in any case where a divided nerve has failed to unite. Any swelling adjacent to a nerve can cause exactly similar signs, e.g. a ganglion.

NERVE COMPRESSION

This denotes a progressive localized pressure on a nerve in an anatomical tunnel, usually near a joint. The commonest examples are as follows:
Carpal Tunnel Syndrome, *see* p. 461.
Elbow Tunnel Syndrome, *see* p. 455.
Cervical Rib Syndrome, *see* p. 146.
Meralgia Paraesthetica, *see* p. 501.
Common Peroneal Nerve Entrapment, *see* p. 413.
Morton's Metatarsalgia, *see* p. 546.
Tarsal Tunnel Syndrome, *see* p. 545.

LEPROSY

Leprosy is being increasingly called Hansen's disease because of the almost universal stigma attached to the term 'leper'. It only occurs in persons with a defect of cellular immunity specific to *Mycobacterium leprae*, who form a very small percentage of any population. Nevertheless there are more than 12 million sufferers in the tropical and subtropical world.

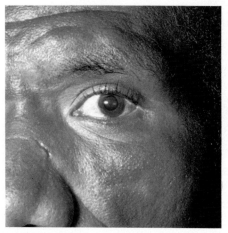

Fig. 677. Loss of the outer half of the eyebrow in leprosy (patient from Papua–New Guinea).

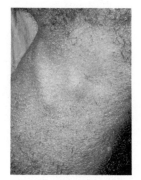

Fig. 678. Thickening of the common peroneal nerve in leprosy.

Lepromatous leprosy is a generalized disease occurring in persons with an absent immune response, with bacillary infiltration of almost the entire skin, and notably of the ears and the nasal

GERHARD H. A. HANSEN, 1841–1912, *Norwegian Physician. Discovered the* Mycobacterium leprae *in 1873.*

mucosa. There is widespread thickening of subcutaneous nerves, but motor and sensory deficit is often of late onset. The deeply lined face (leonine facies), loss of eyebrows, commencing laterally (*Fig.* 677), and nasal collapse due to septal ulceration (c.f. *Fig.* 164, p. 90) are progressively later in appearance, as are testicular atrophy (*see* p. 371) and gynaecomastia (*see* p. 178).

Patients with substantial immunity have a few dry, hairless, anaesthetic, hypopigmented patches. This focal disease is *tuberculoid* leprosy and few nerves will be affected, but because of the intense inflammatory response they may be destroyed. Between these two forms of the disease lies a spectrum of *borderline* forms, identifiable clinically, histologically and immunologically.

Just as there are more skin lesions as the lepromatous pole is approached, more nerves are liable to be affected. Fortunately, thickening does not necessarily mean clinical deficit.

If Hansen's disease is suspected, look for thickening of the following nerves, which may or may not be tender:

Radial nerve at the wrist: very commonly thickened in lepromatous leprosy.
Greater auricular nerve in the posterior triangle below the ear.
Ulnar nerve above the elbow.
Median nerve at the wrist above the flexor retinaculum.
Common peroneal nerve as it approaches the neck of the fibula (*Fig.* 678).
Tibial nerve above the flexor retinaculum, behind the medial malleolus.

Next, test sensory and motor functions of these nerves as described earlier in this chapter.

If there is doubt about the diagnosis of an early case, acid-fast bacilli must be sought in smears of tissue fluid obtained by making tiny slits in the skin, which is held exsanguinated between finger and thumb. Bacilli will also be found in the nasal mucus of lepromatous patients. If not found, or for purposes of exact classification, a skin lesion should be biopsied.

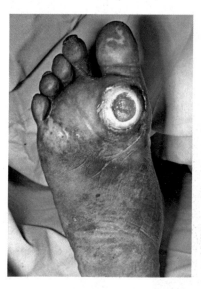

Fig. 679. Plantar ulcer in a leper.

Late Deformities. These are found in communities where there is failure of early case-finding methods, or among patients adequately treated with drugs but who have not been taught to protect anaesthetic areas. Plantar ulcers (*Fig.* 679) are thus common but do not necessarily indicate active leprosy.

Ulnar claw hand (*see Fig.* 672).

Claw foot (*see Fig.* 675).

Progressive absorption of anaesthetic digits due to repeated minor traumata readily occurs. Ultimately, the stumps of hands and feet may suffer similarly.

Chapter 28

BONE

Many bone conditions are described on a regional basis in other parts of this book, particularly tuberculosis (which really involves bone along with joint), and several varieties of osteochondrosis (softening of centres of ossification in certain bones occurring in children and adolescents, i.e during rapid growth).

OSTEOMYELITIS

ACUTE OSTEOMYELITIS

This is mainly a disease of childhood, the bone on the metaphysial side of the epiphysial line being affected (area of richest blood supply). After the age of 12 years there is a decided decrease in incidence, but in 12 per cent the patient is an adult.

Like many surgical infections, the signs are both general and local, and this is a leading example where these two groups of signs must be collected with care, weighed in the diagnostic balance, and then correlated. The younger the patient and the more overwhelming the general infection, the greater the difficulties in arriving at a correct diagnosis. The presenting clinical features are pyrexia (sometimes with rigors denoting septicaemia) 95 per cent, local swelling and tenderness 80 per cent, local erythema and heat 50 per cent, limitation of joint movement 50 per cent, fluctuation 20 per cent and effusion into a nearby joint 10 per cent.

The bone affected is, in order of frequency, a tibia (upper end), femur (lower end), fibula, humerus, calcaneus, radius, ulna. Of the remaining bones of the body, any can be attacked.

Radiography plays such an important part in the diagnosis of bone disease that students, and not a few practitioners, are surprised to learn that radiographs are quite valueless* in the detection of early acute osteomyelitis. This all-important diagnosis—the most urgent connected with bone—must be made by clinical methods. The classic description of the local findings is 'a deep-seated brawny swelling situated near a joint'; but if, before diagnosis, we relied upon the development of this the patient would be robbed of the benefits of early treatment.

The examination should be conducted as follows:

The Pointing Test. If the patient is old enough he will be able to signify which bone is painful (although he may refer the pain to the neighbouring joint).

Inspection. Compare the two sides for minor degrees of swelling. Look for an abrasion or other superficial lesion where organisms might have entered.

---

* In a neonate radiographs, instead of being normal for a period of approximately ten days, show changes in a few days.

417

Test for Localized Heat as described on p. 9. In doing this it may be appreciated that there is exquisite local tenderness.

Pressure over the Bone (*see Fig.* 701, p. 433) is often helpful, especially in early or mild cases. Commence by placing the pulp of the index finger over the bone at a distance from the suspected site of the disease. If pain is not complained of, exercise increasing pressure; sometimes as the pressure increases the patient will cry out quite suddenly. Repeat the manœuvre nearer the suspected epiphysis, proceeding very gently if pain has been caused by more remote pressure. By this means a point of maximum tenderness will be located.

Examine the Suspected Area for Evidence of Superficial Oedema. In cases of some standing, where there is a subperiosteal abscess, overlying oedema is nearly always present. In this connection bear in mind Morison's aphorism concerning cellulitis in children (*see* p. 32).

Examine Neighbouring Joints for Arthritis. It should be noted that in acute osteomyelitis usually a secondary, so-called 'sympathetic', effusion occurs into the nearby joint, e.g. when the upper end of the tibia is infected, there is an effusion into the knee joint.

Palpate the Appropriate Lymph Nodes for example, those of the groin, and compare with those of the opposite side. They are seldom much enlarged.

The diagnosis of acute osteomyelitis in a patient too ill, or too young, to give any information is one of the most difficult tasks in clinical surgery. Pressure over commonly affected bones may reveal that one bone is more tender than others. Signs of septicaemia (*see* p. 44) may be present.

DIFFERENTIAL DIAGNOSIS OF ACUTE OSTEOMYELITIS. Apart from other suppurative processes (acute suppurative arthritis, cellulitis) in which the differential diagnosis for the first 24–48 hours is not of such great importance, as antibiotic treatment must be instituted while awaiting definite signs, the *white blood count* is not greatly raised in the condition mentioned below. In acute osteomyelitis it is generally raised to 20 000 per c mm or more.

Rheumatic Fever. As a rule the pain flits from joint to joint. In a few cases it remains stationary. Although maximum tenderness is situated *at the joint line,* whereas in osteomyelitis it is *near* the joint, in early osteomyelitis good localization of tenderness is uncommon. In rheumatic fever, if tenderness extends beyond the limits of the joint it does so *both above and below.* In acute osteomyelitis it extends *in one direction only.* Cases of acute osteomyelitis especially difficult to differentiate are when the patient has septicaemia and more than one metaphysis is attacked. In both conditions the temperature is raised but in rheumatic fever the heart is affected and the pulse rate is raised relatively higher.

Acute Suppurative Arthritis. As noted, in acute osteomyelitis a 'sympathetic' effusion into the joint nearest the affected epiphysis is not unusual. In primary arthritis the infection is *in* the joint; in osteomyelitis it is the bone *near* the joint. Consequently, when it can be ascertained that one bone only entering into the formation of the joint is tender, the joint signs (effusion) fade into insignificance in the assessment of the signs. Severe pain on attempted movement with distension of the joint capsule and synovial tenderness suggest primary infection of the joint. In the case of sympathetic synovitis, movements of the joint are less painful and the amount of effusion is less.

Cellulitis can present a very difficult problem. Deep cellulitis or a subfascial abscess situated over the region of a metaphysis may be impossible to differentiate from acute osteomyelitis. Again, remember Morison's aphorism.

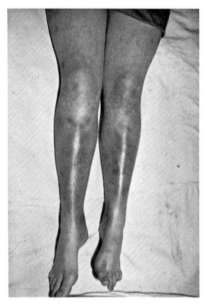

Fig. 680. Erythema nodosum.

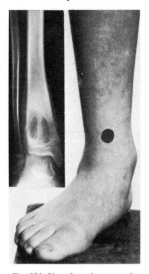

Fig. 681. Site of maximum tenderness over a Brodie's abscess of lower end of tibia. Inset, radiograph displaying intra-osseous abscess.

Erythema Nodosum. The differential diagnosis is less difficult. If the fingers are passed lightly over the plaques (*Fig.* 680), it is evident at once that they are raised above the level of the surrounding skin. Each gives the impression of a miniature Table Mountain. Furthermore, if one of these areas is clasped gently between the finger and thumb, it will be found that it can be made to move on the bone. When this diagnosis is reached remember that some patients with sarcoidosis or ulcerative colitis present with this skin lesion.

Sickle-cell Anaemia (*see* p. 322). Infarction of bone by blockage of a nutrient artery may mimic acute osteomyelitis in susceptible subjects. Secondary infection by *salmonella* may occur so that the condition actually becomes one of osteomyelitis.

Acute Anterior Poliomyelitis. The overall picture is rather similar to that of acute osteomyelitis—an ill child with pain and loss of function of a limb. In anterior poliomyelitis the pain and tenderness are spread throughout the main muscular mass (and often more than one area is involved), whereas in osteomyelitis the tenderness is greatest on direct pressure on the bone. In poliomyelitis, usually the neck is stiff and many of the tendon reflexes are absent.

Malignant Bone Neoplasm is often the greatest problem of all, for sarcoma and subacute osteomyelitis can remain indistinguishable for a considerable time. Radiography may help but often the only certain proof is on biopsy.

Acute Osteomyelitis in Infancy is frequently secondary to umbilical infection. The temperature is often not raised on admission. In an infant, only occasionally does the osteomyelitis manifest itself in the classic manner as regards the general reaction, because at this age the pus is not under pressure; it can readily strip up the periosteum, and soon erodes this veil-like structure. Local oedema comes on much more rapidly, and is much more diffuse than in older patients. In fact, often the whole limb is swollen. Attention is also drawn to acute osteomyelitis of the maxilla (*see* p. 95) caused by pathogens derived from the mother's infected breast. In a breast-fed baby, when acute osteomyelitis of *any* bone is suspected, the mother's breasts should always be examined for inflammatory changes.

DIFFERENTIAL DIAGNOSIS OF ACUTE OSTEOMYELITIS IN INFANCY:

In infancy the particular difficulties in differential diagnosis are:

1. *Acute Infective Arthritis*, especially of the hip joint (*see* p. 496).

2. *Infantile Scurvy*. The diagnosis is often arrived at in the following manner. The mother says that the child (usually between six months and two years of age) is losing weight and its limbs are tender, so tender that the child looks anxious, and screams at your approach; it knows that if its affected limbs are touched it will be hurt. You gently feel the bones; they feel enlarged because of subperiosteal haemorrhage. You now press the gums; they bleed readily*—you diagnose (correctly) scurvy. Slipped epiphysis is a well-recognized complication.

3. *Congenital Syphilis. See* p. 422.

CHRONIC OSTEOMYELITIS

Brodie's Abscess is a localized form of infection of the metaphysis of a long bone, caused by a staphylococcus of low, or of attenuated, virulence. The most frequent sites are the lower end of the tibia, the upper end of the tibia, the lower end of the femur and the upper end of the humerus, in that order.

The patient most often presents during the second decade of life. In a number of instances there is a history of previous attacks of pain and swelling, followed by long periods of freedom from symptoms. As a rule, the pain is typical of bone pain (worse at night), but in some instances it is worse on walking, and relieved by rest. Often the only sign is deep tenderness over the site of the lesion (*Fig.* 681). In cases where the pain comes on after walking, and in all cases during a severe exacerbation, in addition some swelling, pitting oedema and perhaps a cutaneous blush are present. In such cases occasionally the adjacent joint becomes swollen from effusion, but as a rule 'the joint permits of every motion and is apparently normal' (Brodie).

Osteoid-osteoma (Jaffe) is a bone condition of unknown aetiology that closely mimics a Brodie's abscess. As a rule the patient is in the second or third decade of life, males being four times as often affected as females.

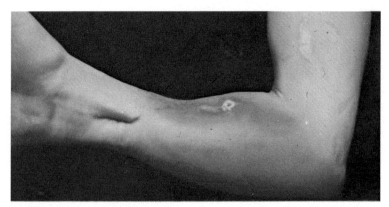

Fig. 682. Chronic osteomyelitis. Recrudescence of infection 16 years after an operation for acute osteomyelitis of the radius.

---

* Only if at least some of the deciduous teeth have erupted.

SIR BENJAMIN BRODIE, 1783–1862, *Surgeon, St.George's Hospital, London*.

HENRY L. JAFFE, *Contemporary Professor of Radiology, University of Southern California School of Medicine, Los Angeles, California*.

Pain is situated in some part of a long bone (often femur or tibia), not necessarily the metaphysial region, as is the case with a Brodie's abscess. At first the pain is intermittent but worse at night; later it becomes continuous, and sometimes very severe. The pain is not relieved by rest in bed, but is sometimes relieved by aspirin.

Tenderness is localized to a comparatively small, circumscribed area, and if the bone is superficial slight enlargement can sometimes be detected.

Superficial Oedema is often present, and slight pitting on pressure can be obtained.

Chronic Osteomyelitis occurring remotely after an Operation for Acute Osteomyelitis

is not, strictly speaking, a Brodie's abscess, because the latter is chronic from the commencement. The interval between the acute attack and the subsequent development of an abscess is a long one, usually over five years. The signs of inflammation and the presence of a scar (*Fig.* 682) adherent to some part of the particular bone that is tender make the diagnosis an easy one.

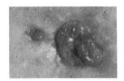

Fig. 683. Sinus following fractured pelvis with extra-peritoneal rupture of the bladder.

Sinus Formation following Osteomyelitis. This, now relatively infrequent, aftermath of an operation for acute osteomyelitis, or of the spontaneous or designed evacuation of pus from a chronic bone abscess, or the supervention of infection on a fracture (*Fig.* 683) is a persistent discharging sinus. The reason for the long-continued, often copious, drainage of pus and the failure of the sinus to close is that necrosis of bone is proceeding in the depths of the sinus; in many instances a sequestrum* is present.

Syphilis of Bone. As a result of early treatment, syphilis of bone has become rare except in parts of the world where medical facilities are poor, but, as of old, it remains the great imitator so that any patient with bone disease (other than obvious acute osteomyelitis) should have a blood test for syphilis carried out. It presents in several guises:

Fleeting Bone Pains. Within three years of untreated or incompletely treated syphilis the patient may suffer from pains in long bones, often worse at night, and boring in character.

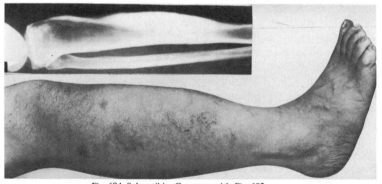

Fig. 684. Sabre tibia. Compare with *Fig.* 692.

---

* *Sequestrum.* Latin, *sequestrum*, deposit = a piece of dead bone that has become separated from the surrounding live bone during the process of necrosis.

Gumma of a Long Bone can simulate, among other conditions, a giant-cell tumour, an eosinophilic granuloma, a Ewing's tumour, and metastatic carcinoma for which the primary growth cannot be discovered. Biopsy will settle the issue if it is felt that the positive blood test may be coincidental.

Syphilitic Osteoperiostitis occurs late in the disease (i.e. after the three-year period referred to above). Usually one bone (less often bilateral symmetrical bones) is attacked, in which event the bone becomes painful, tender, and the seat of a spindle-shaped enlargement. Often the bone gives an illusion of being bent, because new bone is deposited beneath the periosteum of one aspect, for example, *sabre tibia (Fig. 684).*

Syphilitic Metaphysitis is a variety of the above occurring in untreated congenital syphilitics; the swelling and tenderness is at the bone ends.

A SWELLING OF BONE: DIFFERENTIAL DIAGNOSIS

General Considerations. Ascertain by palpation whether the swelling springs from one aspect of the bone, or whether the whole circumference participates in the swelling. In the case of the former try to move the swelling on the bone to make sure that it is intimately attached.

Another basic principle is that when a bone has been examined, movements of related joints should be tested, but first, no matter now insultingly elementary it strikes the reader, the integrity of the bone itself must be tested. Unless it moves in one piece, there is a fracture which may be spontaneous, consequent upon rarefaction due to the swelling; it is also possible that the swelling is composed of excessive callus consequent upon a traumatic fracture or consists of calcification in muscles—*myositis ossificans*.

Having ascertained these points, and bearing in mind the varied nature of swellings of bone, imagine a hypothetical bone with a shaft and two extremities, and consider the principal causes of local enlargement of the bone.

If the swelling envelops the whole circumference and is situated at one end of the bone, so as to further expand the bulbous extremity, viz. ————————————————→ 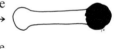 the swelling is likely to be a giant-cell tumour.

If the swelling is situated on one aspect only of the periphery, and located at or very near the epiphysial line, or where the epiphysial line was before growth ceased, viz. ——→ 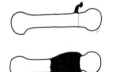 assuredly the swelling is an exostosis.

When the swelling expands the bone, and is situated in the neighbourhood of the metaphysis, viz. ————————————→ 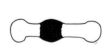 the difficulty of solving the problem increases in complexity. Brodie's abscess, simple bone cyst, and, above all, an osteosarcoma must each be weighed in the diagnostic balance.

When the swelling expands the bone and is situated more nearly midway between the two bone-ends, viz. ——————→ Ewing's sarcoma and eosinophilic granuloma must receive prior consideration.

The physical characteristics of each of these various swellings will be described below. An X-ray is essential but in many instances biopsy is indispensable for completing a diagnosis *which may lead to a decision to amputate the limb.*

The ease or difficulty with which a bone is examined clinically depends, to a large extent, upon whether the bone is superficial. The superficial aspects of the tibia, ulna, patella, clavicle, and skull are readily palpable, but palpation of bones well covered with muscles is extremely difficult. In the latter situations every effort must be made to get the muscles relaxed by attention to the posture.

In answering the all-important question, 'benign or malignant?', the following table may prove helpful:

Benign	Malignant
Swelling often large	Bone not greatly enlarged
Painless	Often painful
Local temperature normal	Warm to touch
Slow growth	Rapid growth or recent enlargement of long-standing swelling

BENIGN NEOPLASMS

Solitary Bone Cyst is the commonest benign neoplasm. It is due to disordered growth at the epiphysis, the swelling appearing in the metaphysis. It is sometimes large enough to be noticed as a swelling but usually presents in childhood as a spontaneous fracture, the fact that a cyst is the cause being noticed on radiology.
Osteoma (Simple exostosis). *See* p. 56.
Solitary Diaphysial Exostosis (Osteochondroma) is also a common skeletal neoplasm, especially in adolescents. It appears only in bones preformed in cartilage, and is most likely to be found on the juxta-epiphysial area of a long bone. It is capped by cartilage, which in turn is sometimes surmounted by an adventitious bursa. Approximately one-half are located at the lower metaphysis of the femur, or the upper metaphysis of the tibia (*Fig.* 685*a*).

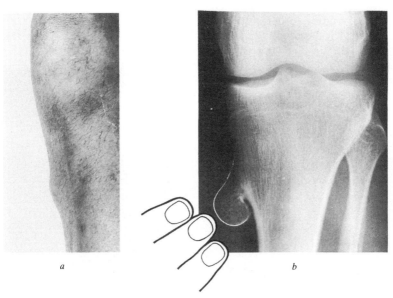

a

b

Fig. 685. *a*, Diaphysial exostosis at the upper end of the tibia. *b*, The sign of diaphysial exostosis. The side farther away from the joint is overhanging (X-ray of the same patient).

The Sign of a Diaphysial Exostosis. Pass the fingers down the side of the bone in such a way as to allow them to ride over the swelling. In the case of a diaphysial exostosis, the side farther away from the joint is overhanging (*Fig.* 685*b*).

Diaphysial Aclasis* (Hereditary Multiple Exostoses) is not rare. About half the offspring of an affected individual manifest the condition. The multiple exostoses, similar to the above, become noticeable during childhood. In addition, during adolescence, not infrequently it becomes apparent that the patient has bowing of one or both forearms with ulnar deviation of the hand. Subjects of this condition are sometimes short of stature.

Aneurysmal Bone Cyst. This expands the bone and the resultant swelling may be confused with giant-cell tumour (*see below*), particularly as the long bones tend to be involved, although the age distribution (most cases are under 20) is slightly different. It can be deemed 'aneurysmal' on three counts, firstly the cause is an arteriovenous aneurysm in the bone (Bissicker), secondly on X-ray the bone is markedly expanded like an aneurysm, and thirdly a few examples are so vascular that they pulsate.

Multiple Enchondromata. *See* p. 428.

MALIGNANT NEOPLASMS

PRIMARY

Multiple Myeloma is not uncommon. Although it can occur at almost any age, as a rule it is found between 50 and 70 years with a male preponderance. The most characteristic early symptom is bone pain of gradual onset often in the back and thoracic cage. It is made worse by movements, coughing or sneezing. Untreated, to intractable bone pain is added the torment of spinal root pain from collapse of a vertebra. Sometimes one of the tumours becomes large enough to be palpable, in which event the swelling feels firm, rubbery, and is rather tender. The location of tumours that can be felt or seen is headed by a rib or the skull (*Fig.* 686); the next in order of frequency is a clavicle or the sternum. Spontaneous (pathological) fracture occurs frequently, more often in a vertebra than elsewhere. In half the cases the urine is loaded with albumin and contains Bence

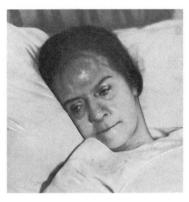

Fig. 686. Multiple myeloma has a predilection for the bones of the trunk. When one of the tumours is situated in a rib or in the skull (as in this case) it may become visible.

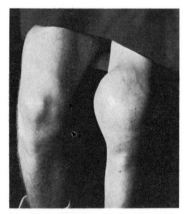

Fig. 687. Advanced giant-cell tumour of the lower end of the left femur causing expansion of the bone.

* *Aclasis.* Greek, ά = not+κλάσις = breaking. Morbid continuity of structures. The outgrowth is structurally similar to tissues from which it springs.

J. L. Bissicker, *Contemporary Fellow in Pathology, Memorial Hospital, New York.*

Jones protein. As the disease advances, general lymphadenopathy, together with enlargement of the liver and spleen, is usual. An invariable finding even in early cases is anaemia. A few patients suffer from a bleeding tendency, and attend first with epistaxis, bleeding gums, haemoptysis, or haematemesis.

Giant-cell Tumour (osteoclastoma) occurs generally between 20 and 40 years, males and females being attacked equally. In 50 per cent of cases the tumour occurs in the region of the knee joint (*Fig.* 687). As a rule the pain is not severe. Increased local heat and dilatation of superficial veins is suggestive of an aggressive tumour. Pulsation and egg-shell crackling are very late signs, and are now seldom seen. This neoplasm is locally malignant, frequently recurs after local removal, and may even metastasize.

Osteosarcoma. Most of these tumours occur in patients between 10 and 20 years of age, and have a male:female ratio of 1·6:1. In elderly subjects osteosarcomata occur in bones the seat of Paget's disease. The lower end of the femur, the upper end of the tibia and the upper end of the humerus are the bones attacked most frequently, in that order. The earliest symptom is pain and this is often present for some time before there is an obvious swelling; like all bone pain, it is worse at night. When a swelling becomes apparent, the limb in the region of the swelling is wont to exhibit increased warmth and this is liable to veer the inexperienced clinician's thoughts to an inflammatory lesion whereas, in this instance, the sign of increased heat should not bias him. Pulmonary metastases occur regularly and comparatively early; they are sometimes present when the patient first attends.

Ewing's Tumour. * Most patients are adolescents, and the tumour is commoner in males. The shafts of the long bones (*Fig.* 688) are the commonest sites. The swelling feels warm but its situation suggests that this is not an ordinary osteomyelitis. In some patients there is pyrexia, in which event the tumour is very malignant. The rapid response to radiotherapy is a therapeutic test.

Eosinophilic Granuloma is a benign bone lesion that simulates a Ewing's sarcoma in some respects, but tends to involve the skull and trunk bones more frequently, and does not cause enlargement of the affected bone to such an extent. A reliable differential diagnosis is only possible with biopsy.

Chondrosarcoma. Many chondrosarcomata have their origin in a pre-existing chondroma. The pelvis is the commonest site, and about 75 per cent of all the tumours are situated in the trunk or the upper end of the femur or humerus. The pain is less severe than in osteosarcoma, and it is often a year before the patient seeks advice. Metastasis occurs comparatively late.

SECONDARY

Before expressing an opinion on a swelling of a bone one must ask the important question, 'Is this swelling primary or secondary?' (*see Fig.* 45, p. 25). Too often this is not heeded; it is taken for granted that the skeletal lesion is a primary tumour. Consequently the general examination of the patient is perfunctory, and it fails to reveal a primary growth, even though the latter might have been discovered easily.

Metastatic Carcinoma is by far the most common malignant bone tumour, particularly after adolescence. Often a metastatic lesion is the presenting complaint, the primary being clinically silent. The breast, the bronchus (*see Fig.* 142, p. 77), the thyroid, the prostate (*Fig.* 689) and the kidney are the organs

---

* A similar tumour often proves to be a secondary deposit from an adrenal neuroblastoma in younger patients or in older patients a lymphoma (reticulum-cell sarcoma) presenting first in bone.

HENRY BENCE JONES, 1814–1873, *Physician, St. George's Hospital, London.*
JAMES EWING, 1866–1943, *Professor of Oncology, Cornell University Medical College.*

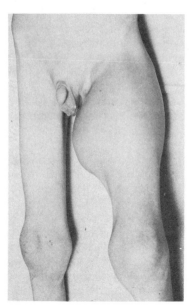

Fig. 688. Ewing's sarcoma.

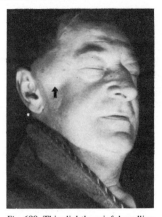

Fig. 689. This slightly painful swelling connected with the zygomatic arch is the patient's only complaint. On examination it is intimately blended with the malar bone, and, although it feels hard, there is an area of softening in the centre. On interrogation he admits to slight dysuria and some increased frequency of micturition. Rectal examination reveals a hard, grossly irregular prostatic enlargement. Diagnosis—secondary carcinoma from the prostate.

upon which to concentrate in the search for a primary growth. A lymphoma not uncommonly is responsible for a localized bone deposit.

GENERALIZED BONE DISEASE

Paget's Disease of Bone (Osteitis Deformans) is, with the lengthening span of life, common. This disease, the cause of which as yet is unknown, presents in two forms: (1) Generalized (*Fig.* 690); (2) Localized to one bone.

1. Generalized Variety. 'Begins in middle life or later, is very slow in progress, and may continue for many years without influence on the general health. It affects most frequently the long bones of the lower extremity and the skull, and is usually symmetrical. Even when the skull is hugely thickened and all its bones extensively altered in structure, the mind remains unaffected.' So wrote Paget. All the leading clinical features are summarized in *Fig.* 691.

As a rule, so very slowly progressive is the disease that although the patient suffers from bone pains, and especially from backache, more often than not these symptoms are attributed to 'rheumatics' or to 'old age coming on'. In a minority of cases the patient complains of headache, deafness, or vertigo, or occasionally failing vision, due respectively to compression of the cerebrum and constriction of cranial nerves at their exits from the skull.

COMPLICATIONS. *Cardiac Failure.* The enlarged bones are very vascular—indeed on occasion they behave as an arteriovenous shunt, and cause cardiac decompensation.

Spontaneous (Pathological) Fracture, especially of the upper femur or upper

SIR JAMES PAGET, 1814–1899, *Surgeon, St. Bartholomew's Hospital, London.*

tibia, is probably the most common complication for, although the bones are thicker than normal, they are very brittle. Typically, the fracture is a transverse one and, although it unites readily, refracture is not unusual.

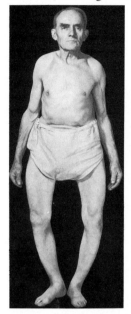

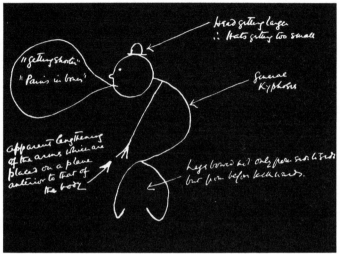

Fig. 690. Paget's disease of bone. Generalized variety.

Fig. 691. Diagram of the essential signs of Paget's disease of bone. This illustration appeared in the first edition of this book and the handwriting is that of Hamilton Bailey.

*Supervention of Sarcoma.** Increased pain with incontestable *recent* enlargement of one bone more than its fellow, together with increased warmth in the overlying skin, makes the diagnosis of bone sarcoma one on which faith can be pinned. This complication is rare (less than 1 per cent of cases).

Spinal Cord or Cauda Equina Compression. Slow progressive narrowing of the vertebral canal by bone proliferation causes neurological signs (*see* p. 221).

2. Monostotic Paget's Disease. A single bone (*Figs.* 692, 693), usually a tibia or femur, but never a fibula, alone is affected—at least for many years. If there is doubt as to the diagnosis, the serum alkaline phosphatase estimation is usually raised (this applies to both varieties of Paget's disease). In 75 per cent of cases eventually the generalized form supervenes.

Osteitis Fibrosa Cystica (von Recklinghausen's Disease of Bone) is a relatively rare manifestation of hyperparathyroidism, recurrent renal calculi being the more usual presentation. Signs and symptoms referable to the skeleton can become manifest at almost any time of life. Often the first symptoms are muscle weakness, gastrointestinal upsets, and muscle pains. The muscle weakness is especially noticeable in the facial muscles, and is often mistaken for myasthenia gravis (*see* p. 91). Cystic degeneration scattered widely throughout the skeleton (but particularly in the mandible) is demonstrable radiographically before it is

---

* Paget's original patient died of this complication 22 years after first being seen.

FRIEDRICH D. VON RECKLINGHAUSEN, 1833–1910, *Professor of Pathology, Strasbourg.*

apparent clinically. Pain in bones, bending of bones, fractures, and possibly localized expansion of one or more bones are the skeletal manifestations.

A suspicion of osteitis fibrosa cystica demands that attention should be directed to the thyroid, which should be palpated thoroughly for the presence of a parathyroid tumour (*see* p. 162), but as a rule the tumour is too small, or too deeply placed, to be palpable. In most instances *the* key to the diagnosis is the finding of an elevated serum calcium level.

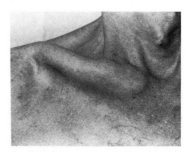

Fig. 693. Monostotic Paget's disease involving the clavicle. The patient had no complaints.

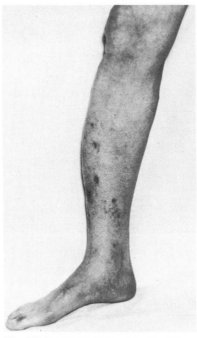

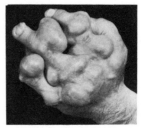

Fig. 694. Multiple enchondromata in a labourer aged 38. Swellings which were present on both hands had been growing slowly larger since early adolescence.

Fig. 692. Paget's disease involving the tibia only. Note that the bone is actually bent; cf. sabre tibia, *Fig.* 684.

Polyostotic Fibrous Dysplasia is similar in as far as the bone and X-ray features are concerned but there is no parathyroid disease or raised serum calcium. A single limb may be affected. The aetiology is not known.

Albright's Syndrome = polyostotic fibrous dysplasia+precocious puberty + *café au lait* skin patches.

Multiple Enchondromata (Dyschondroplasia, Ollier's Disease). Cartilage persists in the shafts of long bones and forms multiple tumours, particularly in the hands (*Fig.* 694). When a major long bone, e.g. femur, is involved the whole limb is shortened and deformed. Almost invariably a single bone is affected.

DWARFISM

Many varieties of generalized bone disease present at birth or arising in infancy and childhood cause stunted growth. Most of these are of interest to paediatricians rather than surgeons, e.g. rickets, or are of great rarity. The following conditions are not so uncommon.

FULLER ALBRIGHT, 1900–1969, *Professor of Medicine, Harvard University, Boston, Mass.*
LOUIS OLLIER, 1830–1900, *Professor of Surgery, Lyons, France.*

Achondroplasia produces the most common variety of dwarfism and is congenital; sometimes it is familial. Achondroplasiacs are seen performing on the stage, screen and in circuses, and they can be observed in the street surprisingly often in some European towns. Subjects have normal intelligence, usually excellent musculature and prominent buttocks due to lordosis. The skull is large with bulging frontal bosses; the nose is flat. The trunk, though somewhat short, is relatively normal compared with the arms and legs. With the arms hanging by the sides, the hands reach only to the level of the upper thighs. In normal individuals the umbilicus is situated above the centre of a line extending from the top of the vertex to the soles of the feet; in achondroplasia alone, due to the relative shortness of the legs, the umbilicus is situated below this centre point (*Fig.* 695).

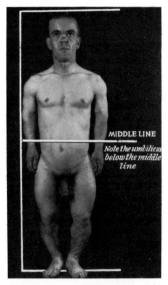

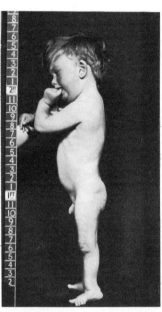

Fiig. 695. Achondroplasia. Normally the umbilicus lies above the middle line of the body. In achondroplasia alone the umbilicus is regularly below the middle line.

Fig. 696. Renal dwarfism. Note the overfull bladder.

Morquio's Disease (Osteochondrodystrophy). The subject has short limbs as has an achondroplasiac, but wedged vertebrae causing kyphosis (*see* p. 203) are additional.

Renal Dwarfism. Rickets caused by deficiency of vitamin D has almost disappeared. Partly for this reason, more attention is being focused on conditions due to renal or intestinal disease (renal or coeliac rickets). Parents seek advice about the child because of (*a*) retardation of growth; (*b*) bone pains; (*c*) mild skeletal deformity, notably genu valgum; and (*d*) hypocalcaemic convulsions. Coeliac disease is of medical importance but renal rickets is of especial surgical interest because not a few are consequent upon congenital urinary obstruction. In this instance the child is found to have an overfull bladder (*Fig.* 696) due to atresia meati, congenital valves of the posterior urethra, or median bar obstruction of the vesical outlet. A larger group of cases is renal in origin so a full examination of the urinary organs is necessary (*see* Chapter 24).

Luis Morquio, 1867–1935, *Uruguayan Physician.*

SOME OTHER CONGENITAL CONDITIONS

There are a large number of syndromes of great rarity, descriptions of which will be found in monographs on bone disease or radiology. The following are of sufficient frequency and exhibit interesting physical signs to concern us here.

Fragilitas Ossium (Osteogenesis Imperfecta) is a congenital, sometimes hereditary, skeletal disease in which the bones are extremely brittle. A particularly arresting feature of the condition is that many of these patients have china-blue sclerotics (*Fig.* 697); indeed, 60 per cent of adult patients with blue sclerotics* suffer from fragilitas ossium. The blueness is due to decreased opacity, which permits the pigment of the deeper coats to show through. Both the fragility of the bones and the relative translucency of the sclera are due to lack of part of their proper matrix.

This disease is encountered in two forms:

a. Becoming manifest in Early Infancy. From birth onwards frequent and often multiple fractures occur. Although the infant has blue sclerotics, this is not such a helpful sign as it is later in life, because normal babies show such a blue tinge. The skull shows parietal prominences and an occipital bulging; the sutures of the cranial bones are late in closing, and soft areas in abnormal situations are not unusual. The lower limbs are stunted. With every bone liable to break on the least provocation, it cannot be wondered at that the chances of survival are seriously curtailed.

b. Becoming manifest in Childhood or Later. The child is normal at birth. The frequency with which fractures occur varies; the longer the occurrence of the first fracture is delayed, the fewer the subsequent episodes. Usually, but not always, the fracture unites readily. An occasional unfavourable feature is that the fracture (usually of the femur) unites with so much callus as to form a palpable, or even a visible, swelling.

Many of these patients have hypermobility of joints, the texture of their skin is fine, their teeth are extremely defective because of imperfect calcification of dental enamel; 25 per cent of them become increasingly deaf from otosclerosis. All are short, due sometimes to kyphoscoliosis (*see* p. 203).

Ochronosis † is easily recognized but rare. Although it can arise from carbolic acid poisoning, all other cases are congenital, and are due to an inborn error of metabolism of tyrosine and phenylalanine. This results in alkaptonuria.

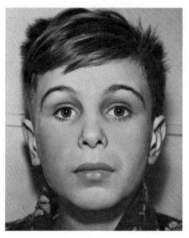

Fig. 697. The blue sclerotics of fragilitas ossium. During the past five years the boy had been admitted to hospital with fractures on many occasions.

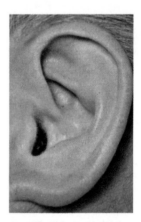

Fig. 698. Ochronosis. Pigmentation of auricular cartilage.

---

* A grossly premature arcus senilis (*see* p. 5) occurs in some patients with blue sclerotics.

† *Ochronosis.* Greek, ὠχρός = yellow, νόσος = disease. When first deposited, the pigment is yellow; later it turns grey-black.

Alkaptonuria should be suspected in infancy because of black discoloration of the diapers. When first voided, the urine is of normal colour, which then passes through slate-blue to brown, and finally to black, on standing.

By the time the patient reaches early middle life, sufficient pigment has been deposited to give rise: (1) to visible bluish discoloration of the auricular cartilages (*Fig.* 698); (2) to circumscribed patches of light brown or slate-blue discoloration of the sclerotics on either side of the corneal limbus; and (3) to discoloration of the skin over bony prominences. Often there is similar discoloration beneath the fingernails and the perspiration is dark brown. The patient suffers from generalized arthritis (ochronotic arthritis) which in 50 per cent of cases becomes severe and is especially evident in the spine. Owing to degeneration of the pigment-laden intervertebral discs, the patient's vertebral column becomes kyphotic and rigid, resulting in a deformity of the spine reminiscent of the curvature produced by ankylosing spondylitis. General osteoporosis also occurs, leading to fractures as a result of minor injuries.

Craniocleidodysostosis. The remarkable feature of this rare hereditary abnormality is the congenital absence of one or both clavicles (*Fig.* 699). Examine for the following additional abnormalities:

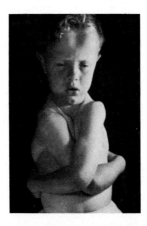

Fig. 699. Craniocleidodysostosis. The shoulders can be almost approximated when the patient hunches the shoulders and crosses the arms.

Skull. Owing to the sagging of the bones of the vault, the cranium presents a flattened appearance. Delayed closure of the fontanelles is usual.

Teeth. The permanent teeth remain unerupted until middle life. The wearing of artificial dentures seems to stimulate eruption, probably from absorption of the overlying bone. Unerupted and incompletely erupted teeth are prone to give rise respectively to cysts or abscesses.

Spine and Pelvis. Frequently accentuation of the normal curves is present, and gives rise to lordosis, kyphosis, or scoliosis.

Lower Extremities. The femoral necks are frequently deformed or absent, and coxa vara is a common abnormality.

Chapter 29

SUSPECTED FRACTURES: EXAMINATION OF JOINTS

FRACTURES

Roentgen's epoch-making discovery was of inestimable value in the diagnosis of fractures and dislocations, but in some situations it is inferior to careful physical examination. Radiographs purporting to reveal an early fracture can be misleading; unless an end of the bone is jutting out through the skin, they fail to signify whether the fracture is closed or open (compound); they may fail to show a fracture of the base of the skull or of the carpal scaphoid (*see* p. 464), a recent march fracture (*see* p. 546), or other stress fracture. In a fractured long bone the crack is sometimes so fine that for a number of days after the injury it cannot be distinguished radiologically from the normal lines of separation of trabeculae. On the other hand, they often reveal a fissured fracture that might be misdiagnosed as a sprain, and also an impacted fracture otherwise overlooked.

Amidst these complexities there has emerged a powerful searchlight focused on the witness-box. In the eyes of the Judiciary the diagnosis of a fracture and an X-ray examination are linked so inseparably that 'No X-ray = negligence!' Thus more than once a practitioner without facilities for radiography at night has sent a patient with an open fracture elsewhere for X-ray examination. Anxious to avoid litigation he has failed to notice that the fracture was compound.

The Diagnosis of a Recent Fracture by Physical Signs. First the injured part must be exposed: severing overlying garments with scissors or slitting a seam with a scalpel is often necessary but with the utmost care and gentleness. Even so, the modicum of movement thus entailed is sometimes sufficient, inadvertently, to call attention to two unfailing signs of complete fracture—*abnormal movement* and *crepitus*—the deliberate elicitation of either of which, for fear of inflicting further damage as well as excruciating pain, is forbidden absolutely.

Three important features of a fracture, *pain, swelling* and *bruising* can be present with lesser injuries. The following signs are only found with a fracture or dislocation.

Loss of Function. Unlike a sprain or a bruise of soft tissues, a fracture usually renders the part almost functionless. To a great extent this is voluntary, for (fractured rib excepted) the patient keeps the fragments strictly at rest. For instance, in the case of a fractured humerus the patient grasps the wrist to prevent movement of the ends of the broken bone, for he has found that such movement causes an exacerbation of exquisite pain.

Deformity (*see* p. 22) is noted. For instance, when an elderly patient falls, and complains of pain in the hip, external rotation of a limb is a characteristic sign leading to a confident diagnosis of fracture of the neck of the femur.

Unless deformity is obvious, time should be spent in comparing the position and contour of the injured part with that of the opposite side of the body, at first by sight, then by palpation, and finally, if necessary, by measurement.

All grades of deformity are encountered. Sometimes it is extravagant, as in the case of a fractured clavicle, the shaft of the humerus (*Fig.* 700) and the middle third of the femur; at others it is slight; often it is absent, as in fractured rib.

WILHELM C. VON ROENTGEN, 1845–1923, *Professor of Physics successively at Strasburg, Giessen, Würzburg and Munich. Discovered X-rays in 1895.*

Having concluded the inspection, the flexor surfaces of the fingers are passed lightly over the entire available area overlying the bone suspected of being fractured. Even with a bone well clothed by muscle, an abrupt angular deformity that was not visible because of swelling of the soft parts sometimes can be felt.

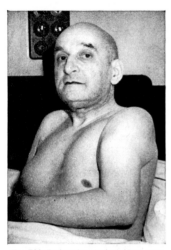

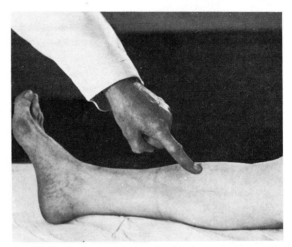

Fig. 700. Deformity produced by a complete fracture at the junction of the upper and middle thirds of the humerus.

Fig. 701. Testing for a point of localized tenderness in the case of a bone with a subcutaneous surface.

Localized Bone Tenderness. Persistent tenderness localized over one part of the bone is an extremely valuable sign; it is the principal sign of impacted and greenstick fractures; usually it is the only sign of a crack fracture. If the bone has a subcutaneous surface or border, the pulp of the index finger is passed along its whole length (*Fig.* 701), exercising moderate pressure, and the patient's face is watched. When the bone in question is placed more deeply, systematic deep palpation is carried out, thus achieving the same objective. A particularly sensitive area is presumptive evidence of a fracture.

Shortening. Details of the method of measuring individual long bones are given on pp. 452 and 491.

Shock is an inconstant finding; it depends largely on the amount of blood lost into the tissues and externally (*see* p. 555).

Inconstant Later Signs

Fracture Blisters. Undiagnosed or treated inadequately, a fracture sometimes proclaims itself by the appearance of cutaneous blebs containing serum or bloodstained serum (*Fig.* 702) which appear 3–5 days after the injury when the skin is unsupported by a pressure dressing. Such blebs are seen most commonly with a fracture of the lower limb below the level of the knee joint. In relevant circumstances they must be distinguished from the blisters of burns or scalds and those of impending gangrene.

Ecchymosis. Cutaneous bruising causes some discoloration at the site of injury within 2 or 3 hours, and within 12 hours the discoloration reaches its zenith. Similar discoloration (depending on the distance the extravasated blood has to travel) coming to the surface 3–10 days after the injury, and possibly some distance from the site of the injury, is strongly suspicious of a fracture.

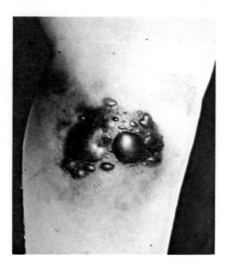

Fig. 702. Fracture blisters.

Swelling due to Callus. Callus takes some time to form. With some greenstick fractures, particularly of a subcutaneous bone, the mother may first bring her child for advice after noticing a swelling (*Fig.* 703) long after the accident.

Atypical Types of Fracture. *Greenstick Fracture* is relatively painless as the fracture is incomplete, no movement between the bone ends taking place. Thus loss of function is not greatly evident. It occurs in children, most commonly in the forearm.

Separated Epiphysis. The injury occurs in an adolescent, before the epiphysis is united to the shaft of the bone. There is nothing to distinguish a separated epiphysis from a fracture clinically except the age of the patient.

Impacted Fracture. The lower end of the radius and the necks of the femur and humerus are the most common sites. The broken ends of the bone being driven into one another, movement between them is impossible. Consequently they are frequently almost painless. Thus the patient who has sustained a Colles's fracture (*see Fig.* 750, p. 464) is likely to dismiss the injury as a sprain. Similarly, a patient with an impacted (abduction) fracture of the neck of the femur can even manage to walk, but usually only after a few days' rest. There is alteration in the contour and length of the limb, the affected bone being shorter. The importance of local tenderness in this type of fracture has been emphasized already.

Spontaneous or Pathological Fracture signifies a fracture from violence that would be insufficient to break a normal bone. The commonest cause is rarefaction of the bone due to a secondary neoplasm. When confronted with a fracture following a trivial injury, do not fail to examine the breasts, the thyroid gland, the kidneys, the testes and the prostate for a primary growth. If these feel normal, think of primary carcinoma of the bronchus. Spontaneous fractures also occur in Paget's disease of bone (*see* p. 426) and in fragilitas ossium (*see* p. 430).

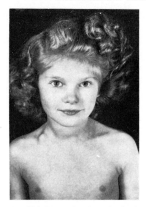

Fig. 703. Excessive deposit of callus around a greenstick fracture
of the right clavicle.

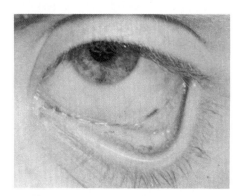

Fig. 704. Subconjunctival petechiae of fat embolism.

Fat Embolism is an uncommon, but most serious, complication of a fracture. Usually the symptoms arise between 36 and 48 hours after the accident. *Second hour—shock, second day—fat embolism, second week—pulmonary embolism* is a wise axiom that warns the clinician of possible impending systemic complications of a closed major fracture.

The signs and symptoms arise suddenly, more commonly after multiple and severe fractures. The patient becomes restless and complains of indefinite pain in the chest. If seen during this fleeting stage, he will be observed to be cyanotic. In a matter of minutes cerebral symptoms supervene. Should the fat globules released into the circulation be large or numerous, their lodgement in the cerebral vessels will cause unconsciousness, with a grave prognosis. More often fewer small fat globules enter the circulation, and drowsiness is produced.

1. *Drowsiness accompanied by Retention of Urine* occurring in a comparatively young patient two or three days after a fracture has been sustained is good presumptive evidence of fat embolism. The pupils are contracted.

2. *Temperature* becomes elevated; in a patient who is going to recover the temperature soon falls, but a second, similar rise the following day is usual. After that only moderate rises occur for several days.

3. *Rash.* A petechial rash is most in evidence on the upper part of the chest, neck, and shoulders 12–96 hours after injury. Occasionally subconjunctival petechiae are present as well (*Fig.* 704).

4. *Thoracic Signs.* There is considerable, slightly purulent expectoration, which is never bloodstained.

5. *Central Nervous System.* In the absence of coma the signs of central nervous involvement are extremely variable, depending upon which part of the brain is mainly involved, and to what extent. In mild cases the signs are few and transitory.

6. *The Sputum and Urine should be examined microscopically for Fat Globules* which, however, are seldom present.

Diagnosis of Dislocations. An X-ray is essential for the reasons mentioned on p. 432, but an accurate diagnosis by clinical means is easily made, as with a fracture. The signs are more or less those of a fracture which may, indeed, be present as well (particularly of the surgical neck of the humerus associated with a dislocated shoulder). There are two points of difference: firstly, the injury is manifestly at the end of a bone; secondly, the bone end may be seen or felt in an abnormal position (dislocated shoulder, *see* p. 447).

Crepitus is not present with a dislocation without fracture and the joint is immobile. For the reasons mentioned above, these points are of no practical importance. The signs can be summarized as follows: *Abnormal Contour, Abnormal Attitude* and *Immobility* (*see Fig.* 738, p. 456).

ROUTINE EXAMINATION OF A JOINT

When a joint becomes inflamed it takes up the position of greatest ease, which is, in fact, the position of greatest capacity for that joint because of the increased amount of synovial fluid secreted. Thus the following are the leading signs of arthritis:

Joint	Position of Greatest Ease	Site of Maximum Swelling
Shoulder	Slight adduction	Under the deltoid, along the tendon of the biceps and in the axilla
Elbow	Flexed at a right-angle; forearm pronated	On either side of triceps tendon
Wrist	Slight flexion	Under extensor and flexor tendons
Hip	Partially flexed, abducted and externally rotated (*Fig*. 705)	Upper part of the femoral triangle
Knee	Semiflexion (*Fig*. 706)	Suprapatellar pouch and either side of patellar tendon
Ankle	Slight plantar flexion and inversion	Anteriorly and on either side of the tendo Achillis

Having studied the position in which the affected joint is held, continue thus:
Compare the Joint with that of the Opposite Side. The joint may be obviously larger than its fellow, but wasting of adjacent musculature can exaggerate the discrepancy. Enlargement may be due to fluid in the joint (fluctuation, *see* p. 12), or to synovial thickening (*see below*), or both.

Wasting of Muscles that move the Joint. Sufficient of the patient's anatomy is displayed to enable a comparison of the limbs with special reference to muscular asymmetry. When a joint is inflamed, wasting of neighbouring muscles occurs, even after a comparatively short time, e.g. a week or ten days. This affects certain groups of muscles in a characteristic distribution; for instance, the quadriceps when the knee joint is involved (*Fig*. 706) and the deltoid in the case

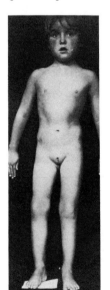

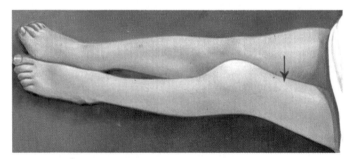

Fig. 706. Wasting of the quadriceps in a case of tuberculosis of the knee joint. This case also demonstrates why bygone clinicians called this condition 'tumor albus' (white swelling).

Fig. 705. Position adopted in early tuberculosis of the right hip joint; the position of greatest ease.

of the shoulder. Minor degrees of muscular wasting can be determined only by taking accurate measurements of the girths of the limbs at identical levels (*see* Fig. 806, p. 492).

The Pointing Test. If pain is a leading symptom, ask the patient to point with one finger to the site of the pain.

Palpation. When a joint has been injured recently, or is acutely inflamed, physical examination must be conducted with great circumspection. In other circumstances, thorough inspection having been concluded, the surface of the joint is palpated and any special points of tenderness noted. In the case of the larger joints (e.g. the knee) attempt to assess whether the capsule is thickened by palpating it between finger and thumb. Synovial thickening gives a boggy sensation as if the capsule consists of sponge rubber. This suggests chronic arthritis.

Movement. The recommendations of the American Academy of Orthopaedic Surgeons contained in the study on 'Measuring and Recording Joint Motion' have been adopted throughout this book. Measurements of joint movement should be recorded in degrees of flexion, extension, abduction and adduction from the Neutral or Zero Starting Position for the Joint. Some joints (hip, shoulder) allow of three-dimensional movement made up of all the above. A goniometer* should be ⟶ utilized for accurate measurement of angles. Needless to say, movements of a joint should be compared with those of its opposite fellow.

Ask the patient to move the joint himself; exhort him to display the full range of movement, first in this, and then in that direction. This is the extent of *active* movement. Then, commencing cautiously, put the joint through as much movement as feasible without causing pain. This is the range of *passive* movement. Limitation of all movements of a joint indicates *arthritis* of that joint. Restriction of certain movements only suggests *an extra-articular lesion* or mechanical block, e.g. by a loose body in the joint. If passive movements exceed active movements paralysis of muscles is likely.

Laxity of Ligaments. If, on testing movements of a major joint, the ligaments are noticed to be unduly slack do not hastily conclude that this is the end result of one of the localized diseases of joints to be described below. Examine the other large joints for similar slackness. Genu recurvatum (*see* p. 521) or recurrent dislocation of the patella (*see* p. 514) suggest that the patient may be suffering from widespread ligamentous laxity. While syringomyelia and tabes dorsalis usually lead to such slackness in the upper and lower limbs respectively, a number of rare syndromes (notably fragilitas ossium, *see* p. 430) are associated with generalized laxity. There are also well-recognized familial and idiopathic varieties in which the laxity occurs as an isolated abnormality. These patients are prone to recurrent joint effusions. Prolonged treatment of a leg fracture by traction leads to looseness of ligaments proximal to the point of traction; in this instance the joint movements (usually the knee) are invariably limited due to disuse while in other varieties the joints are hypermobile.

Joint Crepitus. The significance of this has been discussed on p. 15.

Auscultation of the Joint while passive movement of the joint is in progress, is a means of revealing at a very early stage intra-articular roughness or grating not recognizable by other means. In the earliest stages, fine hair-like crepitations are heard, especially at the end of complete flexion and extension. Sites should be chosen that are as free as possible from hair.

---

* *Goniometer.* Greek, $\gamma\omega\nu\acute{\iota}\alpha$ = angle + $\mu\acute{\epsilon}\tau\rho\sigma\nu$ = a measure.

Methods of examining individual joints are considered in more detail later in this book. At this juncture some points of general diagnostic importance will be considered:

1. *Osteoarthrosis.** In the aggregate, the majority of chronic arthritic joints, particularly after middle age, prove to be due to osteoarthrosis. Hypertrophy of bone, in the form of spurs and osteophytes, is present and may be palpable. There is pain, limitation to a greater or lesser extent of all movements and, during an exacerbation, often an effusion into the joint. In a few instances the lesion is monarticular; in the majority several joints are affected, but, unless the disease is advanced, the main symptoms are confined to one joint, usually a weight-bearing joint (knee, hip, spine). The roughened articular surfaces cause coarse crepitations which can be elicited when a hand is laid over the affected joint which is moved. Sometimes crepitus is loud enough to be heard. As the disease advances movements become more limited and osteophytes sometimes can be felt. One or more osteophytes are liable to become detached and, as free bodies within the joint, cause episodes of locking.

2. *Rheumatoid Arthritis* generally occurs in subjects more youthful than those attacked by osteoarthrosis. Involvement is nearly always bilateral, the metacarpo-phalangeal joints being the joints most frequently first affected. Compared with osteoarthrosis crepitations are relatively fine. The joints are swollen and tender, with movements limited to a lesser or greater extent. An older name is 'arthritis deformans', which signifies that if unarrested, ankylosis with crippling deformities supervenes. Secondary anaemia is found particularly while the disease is active. The typical nodules around the elbow and knee are found in 10 per cent of cases (*see Fig.* 790, p. 491).

3. *Gout* does not always attack the big toe joint (*Fig.* 707). It is easily mistaken for acute bacterial arthritis. In a case of suspected gout look for trophi (*see* p. 82).

4. *Rheumatic Fever* occurs in children and young adults. Characteristically the pain flits from joint to joint, and the arthritis is always multiple and involves the larger joints. Signs of cardiac involvement are usually manifest.

5. *Acute Pyogenic Arthritis* is sometimes difficult to distinguish from acute osteomyelitis; moreover, acute suppurative arthritis is not an uncommon complication of acute osteomyelitis of the upper end of the femur. *See* p. 418.

6. *Tuberculous Arthritis* should be suspected in otherwise unexplained monarticular arthritis particularly in old patients and in the tropics. The somewhat spindle-shaped nature of certain tuberculous joints, with pulpy thickening of the synovial membrane, warmth and the muscular wasting usually present (*see Fig.* 706), serve to distinguish it. The tubercle bacillus can be cultured from fluid aspirated from the joint.

7. *Haemophilia.* A history of a bleeding tendency in a male patient with apparent acute arthritis, not otherwise explained, suggests haemophilia.

8. *Charcot's Joint.* A painless flail joint, often associated with effusion, should bring to mind neuropathy (*Fig.* 708). Test the tendon jerks and the reaction of the pupils. If Argyll Robertson pupils (*see* p. 5) are not present, think of syringomyelia, upper limbs affected (*see* p. 403), leprosy (*see* p. 415) and, particularly if the ankle joints are involved, of diabetic neuropathy (*see* p. 414).

---

* This is a better term than the previously used 'osteoarthritis'; the condition is not inflammatory.

JEAN-MARTIN CHARCOT, 1825–1893, *Physician, Hôpital Salpêtrière, Paris.*

Similar joint changes can follow repeated intra-articular injections of hydrocortisone for rheumatoid arthritis.

9. *Reiter's Syndrome* (non-specific urethritis with arthritis and often conjunctivitis). Multiple arthritis is a usual feature. The joints involved most commonly are the knee, ankle, foot and sacro-iliacs, usually symmetrically. They are hot, swollen, tender and acutely painful; the overlying skin often becomes reddened. This condition is resistant to all antibiotics as yet discovered, which, in the circumstances, often becomes an important sign.

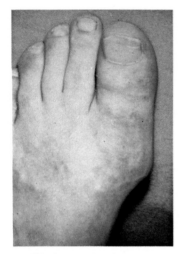

Fig. 707. Gouty arthritis* with an acute exacerbation.

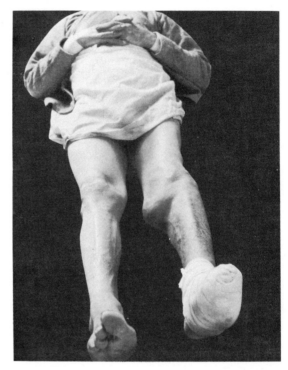

Fig. 708. A case of Charcot's knee. Spontaneous dislocation has occurred. There is also a large perforating ulcer of the foot which is covered by the dressing.

10. *Clutton's Joints,* a manifestation of congenital syphilis, occur usually in childhood. Symptomless, symmetrical synovitis suggests syphilis and baggy fluid distension of both knee joints, accentuated by wasting of the muscles of the thighs, is pathognomonic. This affection commences in *one* joint, and at this stage the local signs are often identical with those of tuberculous arthritis. Often interstitial keratitis is present.

11. *Subacute Arthritis* occasionally complicates bacillary dysentery and brucellosis.

GAIT

Just as observation of the facies may help the clinician, so the scrutiny of the gait as the patient enters the consulting-room occasionally provides a clue to the diagnosis. A limp, particularly a painful limp, can be due to so many causes that

---

* The victim goes to bed in good health. About 2 a.m. he is awakened by pain as though cold water was being poured over the joint; soon afterwards he discovers that the joint is swollen (Sydenham—himself a sufferer).

THOMAS SYDENHAM, 1624–1689, *Physician, London. The Father of English clinical medicine.*
HANS REITER, 1881–1971, *Professor of Hygiene, University of Berlin.*
HENRY CLUTTON, 1850–1909, *Surgeon, St. Thomas's Hospital, London.*

it is unsafe to draw any conclusions as to its origin without a full examination of the lower limbs.

1. The shuffle with everted toes of the extremely flat-footed is characteristic.

2. The waddle of untreated bilateral congenital dislocation of the hip cannot fail to attract attention and the limp in unilateral cases is fairly characteristic, the pelvis on the affected side dipping downwards as weight is placed on that hip.

3. The toddle of a patient with paralysis agitans is hurried as if the centre of gravity is too far forward, and he is trying to keep up with it.

4. A short leg causes a limp that can be recognized easily.

5. A stiff knee causes the affected leg to be swung outwards or else the shoulder to be shrugged. A stiff hip joint causes a bold swing of the limb from the lumbar spine.

6. The patient with hemiplegia has a similar gait to the above; the lower limb is stiff and extended with plantar flexion of the foot so that the limb is circumducted in an arc.

7. The patient with a dropped foot scrapes his toe along the ground, and may adopt a high-stepping gait to enable the foot to clear the ground. An examination of his shoe will reveal that the toe of the sole is worn thin.

8. The tabetic keeps his feet widely apart, lifts them abnormally high, and bang his heels violently on to the ground.

9. The scissors gait of spastic diplegia (Little's disease) is a typical sign. Progression is accomplished by a series of circular steps.

WILLIAM J. LITTLE, 1810–1894, *Physician, The London Hospital.*

Chapter 30

THE SHOULDER JOINT AND SHOULDER GIRDLE

THE SHOULDER JOINT

For an examination of the shoulder joint the patient should strip to the waist.
Bony Landmarks (*Fig.* 709).

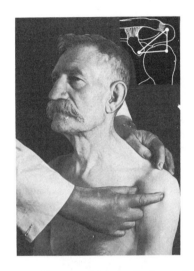

Fig. 709. Three bony points are useful in clinical diagnosis in the neighbourhood of the shoulder joint, a comparison being made with the opposite side. The shoulder triangle: tip of coracoid; tip of acromion; prominence of greater tuberosity.

Testing Movements. These cannot be examined properly from in front; from this aspect it is possible to overlook, and even pass as normal, a completely ankylosed joint. The clinician must stand *behind* the patient, where he can observe any movement of the scapula and, if necessary, fix that bone. It is convenient to grasp the elbow while the various movements are tested, and one should commence by examining the shoulder not complained of, to get an idea of the range of movement to be expected in the particular patient.

Start with the shoulder in the Neutral Position, i.e. with the arms at the sides of the body. Glenohumeral together with scapulothoracic movement is *global*—the arm can normally be placed in any position in any horizontal or vertical plane by a combination of these. In practice it is best to test the following:

Abduction (*Fig.* 710). When scapular and shoulder-joint movements are combined, the normal range is 0–180°. In a normal joint, the scapula commences to move after the first 20–30°; above 90° movement is by scapular rotation; in order to test pure shoulder joint movement, the scapula must be fixed while the arm is at rest by the side. With the scapula so fixed (*Fig.* 710) the patient is told to raise the arm from the side.

Adduction. The normal limit of adduction of the shoulder joint is shown in *Fig.* 711. With the forearm flexed the elbow comes to the midline. Watch, and if necessary fix, the scapula, as in all tests of shoulder movements.

External Rotation is carried out as shown in *Fig.* 712. The flexed forearm should reach a plane almost parallel to the trunk.

Internal Rotation. Ask the patient to place his hand as high as possible on his back (*Fig.* 713).

MOVEMENTS OF THE SHOULDER JOINT

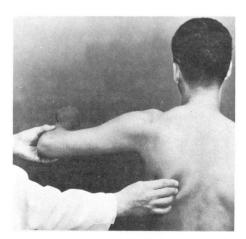

Fig. 710. Abduction.

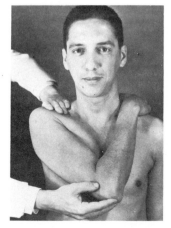

Fig. 711. Adduction.

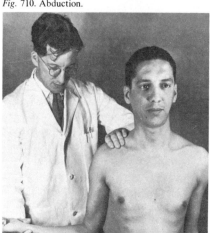

Fig. 712. External rotation.

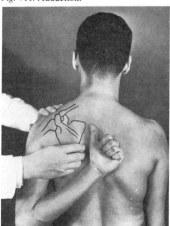

Fig. 713. Internal rotation.

Palpation of the Shoulder Joint. Codman's method. For routine palpation of the shoulder joint and its environs there is no better method than to place the examiner's hands and the patient's limb in the position shown in *Fig.* 714, the hands being reversed when the left shoulder is examined. Note that the pulp of the index finger of the superior hand lies over the supraspinatus tendon near its insertion. When the hands have been positioned correctly, the patient's forearm

ERNEST A. CODMAN, 1869–1940, *Surgeon, Massachusetts General Hospital, Boston, Mass.*

is carried forwards and back again rather slowly and, if necessary, several times. Joint crepitus (*see* p. 15) or crepitus within the subacromial bursa (*Fig.* 715) will be detected by this method, and the forefinger of the uppermost hand is in the optimum position to detect that somewhat elusive, rather common, and extremely important injury—rupture of the supraspinatus tendon.

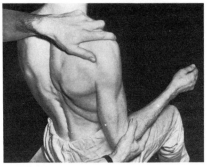

Fig. 714. Codman's method. The thumb lies along the depression below the spine of the scapula; the tip of the forefinger is placed just anterior to the acromion. The other three fingers lie across, and hold, the clavicle. The examiner's lower hand then moves the arm gently back and forth.

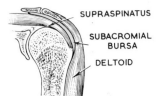

Fig. 715. The subacromial bursa. The tendon of the supraspinatus intervenes between the bursa and the shoulder joint.

Axillary Examination. Routine examination should be completed by passing the fingers, *with the pulps directed laterally*, well up into the axilla. Pulsation of the brachial artery can be felt and in spare individuals the head of the humerus, and in all cases, deep palpation high on the lateral aspect of the axilla brings the fingers against the subglenoid synovial pouch.

ABNORMALITIES OF SHOULDER-JOINT MOVEMENT

Valuable information can be gained by watching a patient *abduct* his arm slowly.

1. If the patient can carry out the movement on the affected side to 90° and then raise the limb perpendicularly above his head (*Fig.* 716), it is proof positive that there cannot be a serious injury to the shoulder joint or to the shoulder girdle.

A quick method of proving that both shoulder joints are normal is to ask the patient to raise both hands above the head and bring the palms together. ⟶

2. If the mid-part of the range (between 60° and 120°) is accompanied by pain, the remainder of the movement being painless, supraspinatus tendinitis, subacromial bursitis or a minor fracture of the greater tuberosity of the humerus is the cause (*painful arc syndrome*).

3. If abduction is possible only to about 40–50° a partial or complete tear of the supraspinatus tendon (*see below*) is likely.

4. If the arm can be raised only very slightly, and, above all, if the patient supports the injured limb with his other hand, then a fracture or dislocation is practically certain. In the absence of bony injury complete rupture of the

supraspinatus, with tearing of the tendinous cuff, is likely, in which case all *passive* movements are full.

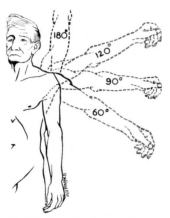

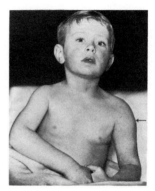

Fig. 716. Observing the patient's per-
formance of abduction gives a great
deal of information.

Fig. 717. Acute pyogenic arthritis
of the left shoulder joint.

5. If pain begins as soon as abduction is commenced and continues throughout the movement, arthritis of one or other form is probable.

Regarding the other movements, over-enthusiastic immobilization in a sling maintains the limb in a position of internal rotation, therefore it is external rotation that suffers most if adhesions ensue.

Effusion into the Joint. Owing to the thick muscular covering of the capsule an effusion is not manifest until it is quite large (*Fig.* 717). The swelling is fluctuant and extends over the whole shoulder and can be palpated by a finger at the apex of the axilla, cf. enlarged subacromial bursa, p. 447.

Chronic Arthritis. All the usual forms of arthritis can attack the shoulder joint. Osteoarthrosis is relatively uncommon as is tuberculosis. 'Frozen shoulder' is now infinitely more common (*see* p. 446).

LESIONS OF SOFT TISSUE OF THIS REGION

Rupture of the Supraspinatus Tendon is a common and important cause of disability of the shoulder joint. The rupture, when extensive, can involve one or more of the structures with which the tendon of the supraspinatus blends before its insertion into the greater tuberosity of the humerus, namely the tendons of the infraspinatus, the subscapularis, the teres minor, and the capsule of the shoulder joint. Together, these constitute the *tendinous cuff*. As the tendon of the supraspinatus forms the roof of the capsule of the shoulder joint and the floor of the subacromial bursa, of necessity, when the tendon ruptures, an open communication results between shoulder joint and bursa.

With advancing age, the tendinous cuff, and especially the tendon of the supraspinatus, undergoes degeneration, rendering it more liable to rupture. Thus this injury can be sustained by lifting a moderate weight.

COMPLETE RUPTURE implies that the whole of the supraspinatus is torn across and that in all probability some other component of the tendinous cuff is implicated as well. Usually the patient is between 55 and 65 years of age. In thin subjects a slight hollowing at the apex of the supraspinous fossa is sometimes visible.

Active Abduction of more than about 50° is impossible. The more the patient struggles (often with puffs and blows) to elevate the limb, the more he shrugs the shoulder. During these efforts often the deltoid can be seen contracting vigorously but the arm cannot be abducted by its action alone (*Fig.* 718).

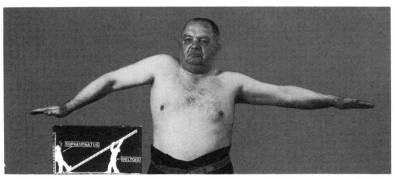

Fig. 718. Complete rupture of the supraspinatus. The more the patient endeavours to lift his arm, the more he shrugs his shoulder. Inset—Showing the fundamental cooperation of the supraspinatus when the deltoid is at work; the supraspinatus must anchor the head of the humerus in the glenoid fossa to enable the deltoid to obtain leverage. If the examiner lifts the arm just above the position shown and then lets go, the arm falls limply to the side.

Passive Abduction is painful but after a lapse of a week or two becomes free and painless. Once the arm has been carried above the head it can be held by the contraction of the deltoid muscle. Before Codman's interpretation the patient was thought to be a malingerer.

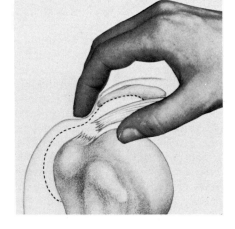

Fig. 719. Seeking a sulcus in rupture of the supraspinatus tendon. (*After Codman.*)

Palpation. The clinician's hands being positioned as shown in *Fig.* 714, as the patient's arm is moved forwards a 'jog', a wince, fine crepitus (*see* p. 15), and a sulcus (*Fig.* 719) make the diagnosis of complete rupture of the tendon of the supraspinatus indisputable (Codman).

PARTIAL RUPTURE. The supraspinatus tendon is partially torn; the remainder of the tendinous cuff is intact. Often the patient is about 45 years of age. The pain is located at the insertion of the deltoid muscle and often radiates down the lateral aspect of the arm, 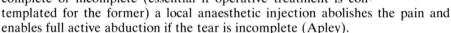 and sometimes along the dorsal aspect of the forearm as far as the wrist.

Active Abduction is limited, as in complete rupture in the acute phase but is regained (unless chronic tendinitis supervenes—*see below*) in a fortnight or so. To find out early whether the tear is complete or incomplete (essential if operative treatment is contemplated for the former) a local anaesthetic injection abolishes the pain and enables full active abduction if the tear is incomplete (Apley).

Passive Abduction also has to be halted because of the pain it produces in the early stages.

Palpation. When elicited as shown in *Fig.* 714, there is unmistakable tenderness just below the acromion process.

Acute Supraspinatus Tendinitis. Calcium salts are deposited rapidly in an area of degeneration of the tendon so that intratendinous pressure rises until liquefied material the consistency of toothpaste bursts through the tendon into the subacromial bursa. An adult of 25–45 years experiences a dull ache in the shoulder which rapidly becomes more severe, until sometimes it is agonizing. All movements of the shoulder joint are limited—abduction especially. There is exquisite tenderness just beneath the tip of the acromion. After two or three days the pain subsides and usually does not return. The calcified material shows on a radiograph.

Chronic Supraspinatus Tendinitis. * The condition probably follows partial rupture of the degenerate supraspinatus tendon. Usually the patient is between 45 and 60 years. The key physical sign is that in mid-abduction (60° to 120°) there is a *painful arc* of movement, as the thickened supraspinatus tendon becomes nipped between the acromion and the greater tuberosity.

Frozen Shoulder. A non-pyogenic inflammatory exudate causes the two layers of the synovia of the shoulder joint to adhere to one another. Usually the patient is 40–60 years of age and more frequently female, but patients with cardiovascular disease, unaccountably, present earlier. The initial symptoms are identical with those of partial rupture of the supraspinatus. The pain, however, increases in severity, occurs at night, and prevents the patient sleeping on the affected side. A time is reached when any movement of the joint causes pain, so the patient keeps the joint still, and stiffness of the shoulder ensues. In a matter of months the 'freezing' process becomes so extensive that the head of the humerus becomes glued to the glenoid cavity, and all movements of the shoulder joint proper are totally restricted. As the process becomes more complete, the pain abates. By this time the muscles around the shoulder show signs of disuse atrophy, but the trapezius is not affected, and a new pain is liable to be located

---

* This is really synonymous with *subacromial bursitis* as the tendon lies in the floor of the bursa.

ALAN G. APLEY, *Contemporary Orthopaedic Surgeon, St. Thomas's Hospital, London.*

in the neck because, with the muscles that activate the shoulder joint proper being *hors de combat*, the accessory muscles that raise the scapula are over-worked. Months later the stiffness gradually lessens. This curious disease recovers spontaneously but the recovery may take up to two years.

Enlarged Subacromial Bursa. Fluid in the bursa presents as a fluctuant swelling in front and to the lateral side of the humeral head and, with large collections, posteriorly as well (*Fig.* 720). The fact that the humeral head can be palpated separately differentiates it from an effusion into the shoulder joint.

BONE AND JOINT INJURIES

Dislocation of the Shoulder follows a fall on the outstretched hand. The usual dislocation is anterior, the head of the humerus coming to lie in the subcoracoid position.

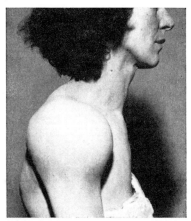

Fig. 720. Fluid in the subacromial bursa.

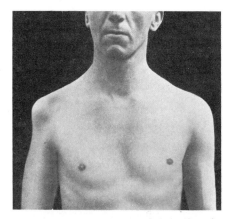

Fig. 721. Right axillary nerve paralysis. Note the wasting of the deltoid muscle.

Inspection. The rounded lateral aspect of the shoulder is lost in favour of a flattened appearance. While flattening of the shoulder is seen typically in dislocation of the joint, it is not an infallible sign. *Fig.* 721 shows a case of paralysis of the axillary nerve with flattening due to wasting of the deltoid muscle. When the shoulder is dislocated, the patient supports the limb with the hand of the opposite side. The arm on the injured side appears longer than its fellow, and the anterior axillary fold lies at a lower level.

Palpation. The cardinal sign of dislocation is the absence of the head of the humerus beneath the tip of the acromion; the fingertips pressed against the upper third of the deltoid muscle, instead of meeting bony resistance, sink in. Conversely, when the fingertips are pressed against the lateral third of the pectoralis muscle, instead of sinking in as they do normally, they meet bony resistance, for here lies the displaced head of the humerus.

Uncommonly the dislocation occurs in a *posterior* direction, and in a thin patient, when the examination is conducted from the posterior aspect, an abnormal prominence below the spine of the scapula near its junction with the acromial process can be seen; this is the head of the humerus.

Because of cursory examination, full reliance being placed on radiography, cases are missed unless movements are carefully tested.

Luxatio erecta, a rarity, can hardly be missed. The arm is held fixed above the head.

Movements. Virtually all active and passive movement is lost with a *recent* dislocation. An *old* missed dislocation usually shows a surprising degree of movement but careful fixation of the scapula as detailed on p. 441, reveals that movements at the shoulder joint have been lost.

Concomitant Injuries. In every case of dislocation of the shoulder the following additional injuries should be sought:

Nerve Injury. The most common is the axillary nerve (*see* p. 406).

Rupture of the Tendon of the Supraspinatus (*see* p. 444). This lesion should be sought early in convalescence after reduction of the dislocation.

Associated Fracture. The neck of the humerus may be fractured at the initial injury. The greater tuberosity of the humerus is sometimes avulsed. Usually radiography is required to detect these fractures.

Blood Vessels. Occasionally the axillary blood vessels are compressed. Always feel the radial pulse both before and after reduction.

Recurrent Dislocation of the Shoulder. After the initial dislocation due to severe trauma, the patient finds that trivial actions, usually involving external rotation, cause frequent episodes of re-dislocation. There are no physical signs but passive external rotation (*see* Fig. 712) causes the patient to become alarmed ('apprehension test') as he knows that the shoulder is about to dislocate.

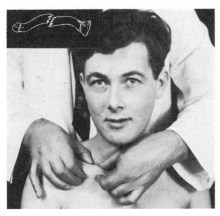
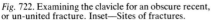
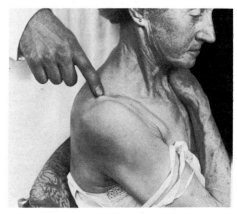

Fig. 722. Examining the clavicle for an obscure recent, or un-united fracture. Inset—Sites of fractures.

Fig. 723. Position to be adopted when the acromioclavicular joint is being examined. This position renders the joint optimally accessible.

Fracture of the Clavicle. The usual situation of this—the most common fracture during the active years of life—is near the bone's centre. As a rule, displacement is considerable. The lateral fragment is pulled downwards by the weight of the arm, while the medial fragment is held up by the cleidomastoid portion of the sternocleidomastoid muscle. Thus, by inspection and, when necessary, by running the finger along the subcutaneous border of the bone, there is no doubt that the bone is broken, for usually the sharp irregular edge of the medial fragment can be felt projecting beneath the skin, and restoration of the normal line of the clavicle is possible only by raising the shoulder above its normal position. On the other hand, under the age of 14 years, greenstick fracture is common, and may require for its diagnosis the method of examination illustrated in *Fig. 722*. An overlooked greenstick fracture with excessive callus formation sometimes proves a less elementary problem (*see* p. 434). A fracture of the lateral or the medial end (*see Fig.* 722, inset) is infrequent, and each is very prone to be overlooked.

Fracture of the Medial End. Impaction is often present causing thickening of this part of the bone, with overlying tenderness. Movements of the arm are limited because of pain.

Fracture of the Lateral End is more elusive, for frequently the lateral fragment is anchored by the acromioclavicular ligament, and consequently there is no displacement and little pain on movement of the arm but there is always some swelling and definite tenderness over the site of the injury. Not infrequently subcutaneous bruising indicates a fracture, but an X-ray is required.

THE ACROMIOCLAVICULAR AND STERNOCLAVICULAR JOINTS

Both joints are readily accessible to the palpating fingers.

The Acromioclavicular Joint. *Subluxation* is not an uncommon injury on the football field and the ice-hockey rink. The extreme outer end of the clavicle can be seen riding above its accustomed level, and light pressure on the prominence imparts to the examining finger a springboard-like sensation, and causes pain; there is also increased costoclavicular spacing. In less obvious cases the patient

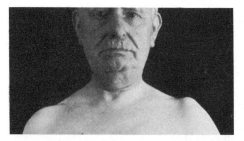

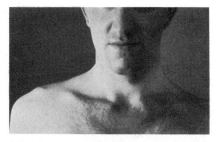

Fig. 724. Osteoarthrosis of the left acromioclavicular joint with effusion.

Fig. 725. Subluxation of the right sternoclavicular joint.

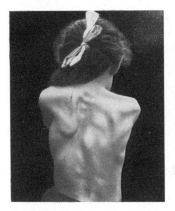

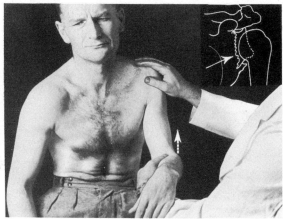

Fig. 726. Sprengel's shoulder. Note the comparatively small, elevated left scapula. Ninety per cent are unilateral.

Fig. 727. Testing for a fractured neck of the scapula.

should adduct the arm by placing the hand of the affected side on the opposite shoulder, and lean slightly forwards. This renders the joint optimally accessible, and enables the area of tenderness (*Fig.* 723) to be pinpointed. In this way this lesion is differentiated easily and certainly from that of a rupture of the tendinous cuff.

Osteoarthrosis of the acromioclavicular joint, commonly post-traumatic, is frequently misdiagnosed as arthritis of the shoulder joint or rupture of the tendinous cuff, for the patient, as a rule, localizes the pain, not on top of the shoulder, but in the shoulder joint. The physical signs usually are quite definite. Sharp pain is experienced when the patient raises his arm *above a right-angle*; this arc contrasts sharply with that of a tendinous cuff lesion. There is tenderness over the joint, and sometimes an obvious swelling in this situation (*Fig.* 724). When the arm is abducted above 90° it is not unusual for crepitus to be elicited over the joint. With upward pressure of the arm carried out in the manner shown in *Fig.* 727, while downward pressure is exerted on the clavicle, the pain of which the patient complains is reproduced at once, due to the joint surfaces grating on one another. **The Sternoclavicular Joint** is very stable and considerable violence is required to dislocate it. Indirect violence causes *forward dislocation*, the most frequent variety. Partial dislocation results in tearing of the intra-articular disc, when a painful clicking occurs in the joint on flexion or circumduction of the arm. In forward dislocation and subluxation (*see Fig.* 725) the deformity is obvious on inspection. Congenital (sometimes familial) forward subluxation is occasionally found. *Backward dislocation* is a rare, but serious, accident due to direct violence, the sternal end being driven backwards, and, unless masked by overlying contusion, there is a hollow in this situation. Often the patient is in considerable distress from dyspnoea and cyanosis and urgent reduction is necessary.

EXAMINATION OF THE SCAPULA

Congenital elevation of the scapula (Sprengel's shoulder) is usually evident on inspection (*Fig.* 726). *Winged scapula* is discussed on p. 406. Bilateral cases must be distinguished from a condition showing a very short neck, and often bilateral webbing of the neck (*Klippel–Feil syndrome*).

A considerable portion of the scapula is readily accessible to the palpating fingers, and, as X-ray examination is sometimes unsatisfactory, clinical methods are all the more important. The spine and acromion are examined by palpating along this bony ridge while the arm is gently hyperabducted. Fractures of the neck of the scapula are particularly liable to be overlooked. Grasp the patient's arm in such a manner that his forearm rests on the examiner's forearm (*Fig.* 727). By this means the whole of the upper extremity can be raised and lowered gently. Provided the clavicle is intact, abnormal mobility and crepitus suggest a fracture of the neck of the scapula.

Otto G. K. Sprengel, 1852–1915, *Surgical Director, Grand-Ducal Hospital, Brunswick, Germany.*
Maurice Klippel, 1858–1942, *French Neurologist.*
André Feil, 1884–1955, *French Physician.*

Chapter 31

THE ARM

THE UPPER ARM

Fracture of the Shaft of the Humerus is common. The arm is rendered useless and is held by the other hand. There may be an obvious angular deformity (*see Fig.* 700, p. 433) and spasms of severe pain (due to muscular contractions) are characteristic. As a rule the diagnosis can be made on inspection alone. If necessary, the fingers on one side and the thumb on the other are run lightly down the medial and lateral surfaces of the upper arm. If X-ray facilities are not available and should there still be doubt, the upper limb is grasped as shown in *Fig.* 728 and the arm is abducted carefully; if a fracture is present, mobility in the length of the bone will become apparent.

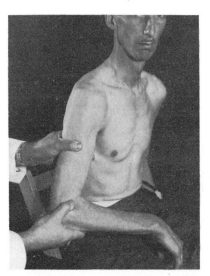

Fig. 728. Testing for fracture of the shaft of the humerus. The forearm is supported, and the arm is abducted carefully.

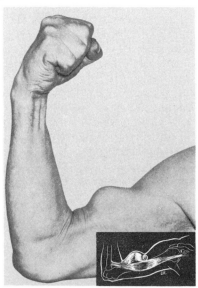

Fig. 729. Rupture of the tendon of the biceps. Inset: the anatomical explanation of the lump.

Test the integrity of the radial nerve (*see* p. 406) in all fractures of the shaft of the humerus, as sometimes it is damaged by the broken ends of the bone where it lies in the spiral groove against the bone. Also feel the radial pulse.

Fracture of the Humerus in a Neonate. The shaft of the humerus is the most common site of any fracture occasioned by difficult delivery.

Fracture of the Neck of the Humerus occurs largely in elderly women, sometimes in children, after a fall on the outstretched hand. There is severe pain, complete loss of function and the arm is supported by the other hand. The region of the shoulder is swollen and ecchymoses are present on the medial aspect of the arm and/or the chest wall. The following tests are advised only in the absence of X-ray facilities:

Sign of Non-rotation of the Head of the Humerus. If the head does not move when the shaft is rotated by very gentle limited circumgyration of the flexed forearm, the diagnosis of fracture of the neck of the humerus is confirmed.

Impacted Fracture. The stumbling-block is that, in the adult, the fracture of the neck of the humerus is frequently impacted, in which event the above sign is null and void. The clinician must resort to *comparative measurement.* The distance between the tip of the acromion and the most prominent portion of the lateral epicondyle is ascertained and recorded on the sound side. This measurement is then repeated on the injured side and the two readings compared.

Fracture of the Greater Tuberosity is commonly associated with dislocated shoulder (*see* p. 447) but occasionally is found as an isolated injury. Palpation reveals tenderness and swelling localized to the tuberosity, and the ability to abduct the shoulder (*see* p. 441) is absent.

Rupture of the Biceps Brachii Muscle. In rupture of the belly of the muscle there are two lumps separated by a gap. In rupture of the tendon there is but one lump. The latter is much commoner and although, as a result of heavy lifting, rupture of a normal tendon can occur, more often the rupture takes place less dramatically, or even spontaneously because the tendon has undergone attrition due to degenerative changes due to advancing age. Therefore always examine the shoulder joint for signs of osteoarthrosis, with which rupture is sometimes associated.

As a rule the signs are unmistakable (*Fig.* 729): when the patient flexes the elbow the belly of the muscle retracts into the lower third of the arm and (accentuated by the hollowing above) stands out in a veritable 'village blacksmith' fashion. When the biceps is wasted and the lump is less conspicuous, flexion of the elbow against resistance causes the swelling to become more evident. In recent cases pain and tenderness along the bicipital groove, with perhaps some ecchymosis below the deltoid muscle, are likely to be present.

Bicipital Tenosynovitis occurs, as a rule, in young adults as the result of excessive use of the biceps while at work or play (e.g. skiing); the pain comes on a day or so after the undue or unaccustomed strain. The patient avoids lifting heavy objects and, unless compelled to do otherwise, keeps his arm by his side and his elbow flexed. Movements of the shoulder are all somewhat limited, abduction being especially painful. He points to the region of the insertion of the pectoralis major as the site of the pain, and in severe cases the pain shoots down the arm.

Yergason's Sign. The elbow is flexed to a right-angle and the forearm is pronated by the patient. The clinician grasps the patient's wrist and then requests him to supinate the forearm against resistance, thus bringing the biceps into action. When pain is localized to the anteromedial aspect of the shoulder, the sign is positive.

THE ELBOW JOINT

Bony Landmarks. Three bony points—the *tip of the olecranon*, the *medial epicondyle* and the *lateral epicondyle*—form an equilateral triangle when the elbow is flexed (*Fig.* 730). When the forearm is extended the tip of the olecranon ascends to bring the three bony points into the same horizontal straight line.

Testing Movements. The normal range is shown in *Fig.* 731. Attention is drawn here to the *carrying angle*, which allows the arm to swing slightly away from the body, and so carry objects more easily. This angle (10° in males and 20° in females) becomes apparent only in full extension of the forearm, and is due to the articular surface of the humerus being set obliquely. The angle may become

ROBERT M. YERGASON, 1885–1949, *Orthopaedic Surgeon, St. Francis Hospital, Hartford, Connecticut.*

altered by fracture of, or injury to the epiphysis of, the lower end of the humerus. If decreased, the condition is known as *cubitus varus*; when increased, as *cubitus valgus*. The importance of the latter is that it causes the ulnar nerve to become stretched or exposed unduly to trauma.

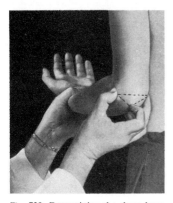

Fig. 730. Determining the three bony points that form the elbow triangle. In full flexion the triangle becomes equilateral.

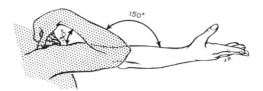

Fig. 731. The normal range of flexion and extension of the elbow joint. Full extension is regarded as the Neutral Position but up to 15° of hyperextension is seen in some normal individuals.

Pronation and supination. *See* p. 458.
Testing the Integrity of the Head of the Radius. This lies more posteriorly than one is apt to think. To find it, rest the tip of the middle finger on the lateral

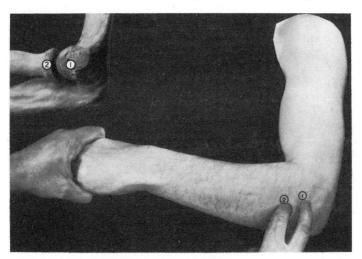

Fig. 732. Testing for the integrity of the head of the radius.

epicondyle (*Fig.* 732), then place the index finger alongside it, the elbow being at a right-angle. The arm is then pronated and supinated and the head of the radius is felt to rotate beneath the index finger.

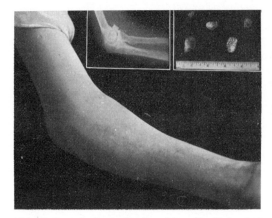

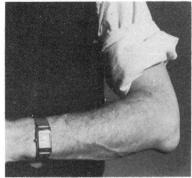

Fig. 733. Loose bodies in the elbow joint with effusion. Left inset, the radiograph. Right inset, the loose bodies removed at operation.

Fig. 734. Effusion into the olecranon bursa. Miner's elbow.

Effusion of the Elbow Joint first manifests itself by filling up of the concavity on each side of the olecranon, because here the synovial cavity is nearest the surface and the posterior ligament is thin and lax. As more fluid accumulates some degree of swelling is also noticeable posterolaterally over the radiohumeral joint. Test for transmitted fluid impulse between this area and the swelling over the medial aspect of the olecranon. This sign distinguishes an effusion into the joint from an enlargement of the bursa beneath the triceps tendon (a rarity). Another point of distinction is that in cases of effusion into the elbow the joint is always held in position of semiflexion—the position of greatest capacity.

Chronic Arthritis. All the usual forms of arthritis can attack the elbow joint. *Tuberculosis* occurs in adults more often than in children, and because of early muscular atrophy the joint assumes a fusiform appearance. When confronted with what appears to be a monarticular *osteoarthrosis* of the elbow joint pause for a moment to consider three other possibilities.

Loose Bodies in the Joint. Especially if there is a history of locking, loose body is a diagnosis that should spring to mind (*Fig.* 733). Occasionally the 'joint mouse' can be palpated.

Osteochondritis Dissecans (*see* p. 513) of the elbow is uncommon compared with that of the knee but the elbow is the second site numerically for the condition. The capitulum is usually involved. Before the stage of loose body in the joint, the only sign is a recurrent effusion.

Charcot's Joint (*see* p. 438).

LESIONS OF THE SOFT TISSUES ABOUT THE ELBOW

Miner's (*syn.* **Student's) Elbow.** The effusion into the bursa over the subcutaneous surface of the olecranon process can hardly be mistaken (*Fig.* 734). This bursa is prone to pyogenic inflammation (olecranon bursitis).

Examination of the Supratrochlear Lymph Node. Quite significant enlargements are missed because a search is made with the arm in the extended position. First flex the arm to a right-angle, in order to relax surrounding structures. When enlarged, the node will be found slipping beneath the finger and thumb on the anterior surface of the medial intermuscular septum a centimetre above the base of the medial epicondyle. Enlargement of this lymph node occurs with some infected lesions of the hand, wrist, and forearm. Bilateral enlargement suggests a generalized disease of lymph nodes and biopsy is necessary for diagnosis; this often applies to unilateral enlargements.

Bicipitoradial Bursitis. There is a bursa beneath the tendon of the biceps, near its insertion. Occasionally this becomes inflamed, especially after repeated throwing of a ball. The inflamed bursa is rarely palpable, but there is pain and tenderness over the insertion of the tendon in front of the elbow joint, and the pain is accentuated by flexion and supination.

Tennis Elbow (Epicondylitis) takes its name from the sprain sometimes sustained by tennis players. Nevertheless, comparatively few of the numerous sufferers play tennis. There is a throbbing ache on the *lateral* aspect of the elbow, or in the region of the origin of the common extensor muscles (a few fibres of which have probably been torn), accentuated by lifting small objects, if that manœuvre entails dorsiflexion of the wrist. To the surprise of all concerned, the patient can carry a bucket of water without any special discomfort. There is no limitation of movement of the elbow joint and no pain on such movement.

Palpation. Usually a point of considerable tenderness will be found over the lateral epicondyle; sometimes this point lies more distally, viz. over the radiohumeral joint or even over the head of the radius.

Cozen's Test. Ask the patient to clench his fist and keep it clenched, and then to extend the wrist. Grasp the lower forearm in the left hand, and while the patient continues to try to keep the wrist extended flex the wrist firmly and steadily (*Fig.* 735). This places considerable tension on the origin of the extensor tendons at the lateral epicondyle, and causes the pain of which the patient complains.

Mills's Manœuvre. With the elbow quite straight and the wrist flexed, pronate the forearm (*Fig.* 736). This brings on the characteristic pain, and does so only in cases of tennis elbow.

Golfer's or **Baseballer's Elbow** is relatively uncommon. The tenderness is situated in the common flexor origin (some fibres of which have probably been torn) from the medial epicondyle.

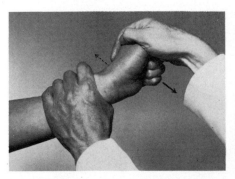
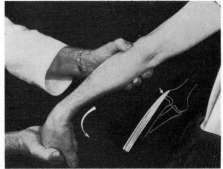

Fig. 735. Cozen's test. Flexion of the wrist against the patient's attempt to keep the wrist extended causes pain in the region of the lateral epicondyle.

Fig. 736. Pronation of the forearm with the arm straight causes pain at the origin of the common extensor muscle (inset). Mills's manœuvre.

The Elbow Tunnel Syndrome is infrequent compared with the carpal tunnel syndrome (*see* p. 461). The pain, which passes down the forearm, is confined to the distribution of the ulnar nerve below the elbow. Muscular wasting affects principally the hypothenar eminence. Compare the carrying angle of the elbow joint with that of the opposite side; if cubitus valgus (*see* p. 453) is present, the cause of the symptoms is explained. Palpate the ulnar nerve in its groove; if

LEWIS N. COZEN, *Contemporary Associate Clinical Professor of Orthopedic Surgery, University of California School of Medicine, Los Angeles.*
GEORGE P. MILLS. 1883–1952, *Surgeon, Royal Cripples' Hospital, Birmingham.*

pressure on the nerve reproduces pain and tingling it suggests that the neuropathy originates here, provided always the signs are limited strictly to those of a lesion of the ulnar nerve at the elbow (*see* p. 408). Signs of osteoarthrosis of the elbow joint are found occasionally. A tight band comprising the fibrous arch of origin joining the two heads of flexor carpi ulnaris compressing the ulnar nerve in, or just below, its groove is found to be the cause when the elbow joint is normal.

FRACTURES AND DISLOCATIONS AROUND THE ELBOW JOINT

The injuries to be described are all accompanied by a greater or lesser degree of traumatic effusion into the joint (*Fig.* 737). The arm is held immobile by the side or supported by the other hand. The diagnosis can be suggested clinically before resorting to X-ray examination which is, however, essential for accurate diagnosis, particularly if multiple fractures are present, as they frequently are with the severe trauma of present-day motorcar accidents.

In particular, dislocated elbow may be associated with any or several of the fractures in this region to be described, and especially the anterior dislocation occasioned by a car driver's elbow protruding from the open window being struck by a passing car ('*side swipe' fracture-dislocation*).

Supracondylar Fracture of the Humerus is a common injury of childhood and adolescence. This fracture, which follows a fall on the outstretched hand, is of exceptional importance because of three threatening complications—two early, and one late—Volkmann's ischaemic contracture (*see* p. 479), injury of the median or, rarely, the radial or ulnar nerves (*see* Chapter 27), and myositis ossificans. Because of the overriding importance of diagnosing the first of these at the very outset, always examine the radial pulse* in every case of a bony

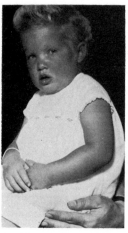

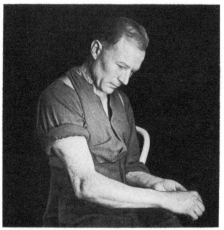

Fig. 737. Traumatic elbow effusion showing the typical posture.

Fig. 738. Characteristic attitude and deformity in backward dislocation of the elbow joint. This illustrates the three characteristic signs of a dislocated joint extremely well: (1) *Abnormal contour*—the olecranon protrudes abnormally; (2) *Abnormal attitude*—the arm is held at 130°; (3) *Immobility*—neither active nor passive movement of the joint is obtainable.

---

* Only rarely is the radial pulse congenitally absent.

injury about the elbow. In most instances posterior displacement of the lower fragment occurs and the elbow, with the forearm, is carried backwards. Therefore, like backward dislocation of the elbow joint, the elbow is unduly prominent, but there is a striking difference: the three bony points are found to be in normal equilateral triangular relationship. With the comparatively uncommon forward displacement of the lower fragment the signs are less striking. This is the fracture above all in which a most careful watch must be kept on the radial pulse *after reduction*.

T-shaped Fracture of the Lower End of the Humerus, in contradistinction to the above, nearly always occurs in an adult, and the fracture is sustained in a different way—the patient falls, striking the elbow. The shaft of the humerus may be driven between the two condyles, giving obvious deformity in the shape of broadening of the elbow. In other circumstances the signs are similar to those of a transverse supracondylar fracture. The bony points cannot be identified on account of swelling, but a haemarthrosis, as evidenced by obvious effusion into the joint (*see* p. 454), leaves little doubt that a serious fracture is present.

Dislocation of the Elbow Joint occurs both in children and in adults as a result of a fall on the outstretched hand (*Fig.* 738). Unlike a supracondylar fracture, when the elbow is dislocated the tip of the olecranon is displaced and the bony triangle (*see* p. 452) is no longer equilateral.

Fracture of the Olecranon Process can occur as the result of direct or indirect violence. There is considerable local swelling, and maximum tenderness is situated in the region of the olecranon. If separation is complete, there is inability to extend the flexed forearm. Wide separation of the fragments due to contraction of the triceps can be detected by palpation when the fracture is complete.

Fracture of the Coronoid Process is much less frequent than the above. This fracture can occur as a complication of backward dislocation of the elbow joint, in which event the dislocation recurs immediately after it has been reduced. Rarely, the fracture occurs in the absence of dislocation, in which case it is unlikely to be diagnosed without the help of radiographs. Tenderness in the front of the elbow joint alone is suggestive.

Fracture of the Head (adults) **or Neck** (children) **of the Radius,** resulting from a fall on the outstretched hand, is a common accident. The three bony points of the elbow are in correct alignment. Flexion and extension are performed somewhat hesitatingly, but to a large degree painlessly. Indeed, up to this stage the possibility of the patient having sustained a fracture often seems remote, but when rotation is attempted tell-tale restriction of movement is most noticeable. Now comes the crux of the examination—there is tenderness, often exquisite, over the head of the radius (*see Fig.* 732, p. 453).

Subluxation of the Head of the Radius ('pulled elbow'). A child's arm is pulled forcibly, either to remove it from danger, or when it indulges in a temper tantrum. As a result the radial head subluxates through the annular ligament. The signs are as above, but a child is much less inclined to allow an efficient examination than an adult.
Fracture of the Lateral Epicondylar Epiphysis. Usually the patient is a child (5–15 years) who, following a fall, has a swollen elbow joint which he will not move. The finger can be run along the back of the upper arm without eliciting tenderness; consequently a supracondylar fracture is most unlikely, but there is tenderness over the lateral side of the joint. An older child can sometimes be coaxed to rotate the forearm proving that the neck of the radius is intact.
Separation of the Medial Epicondylar Epiphysis. Similar signs with tenderness on the medial side in an adolescent are suggestive.

Fracture of the Capitulum. If the effusion is not large it may be appreciated that there is fullness (the displaced fragment) in front of the elbow. Flexion is the movement which is largely lost. This fracture usually occurs in adults.

THE FOREARM

The ulna can be palpated along its subcutaneous border throughout its length. The lower two-thirds of the radius is accessible also.

Testing Movements. The Neutral Position is with the elbow flexed to a right-angle and the thumb upward. Pronation and supination of 90° each is normally possible (*Fig.* 739). If the elbow is extended a further 90° of movement is possible owing to circumduction at the shoulder. Limitation of pronation-supination may indicate a lesion of elbow, forearm, or wrist.

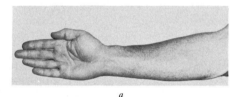

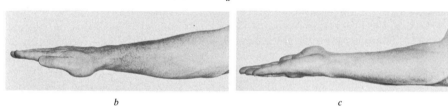

Fig. 739. *a*, The Neutral Position for measuring forearm movement is the thumb-up position with the elbow flexed to a right-angle. *b*, Full pronation. *c*, Full supination.

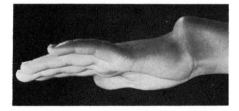

Fig. 740. Madelung's deformity. Female 18 years of age.

Madelung's Deformity. This is a dorsal subluxation of the lower end of the ulna. Usually the patient is an adolescent female who complains of weakness of the wrist, where a very prominent displacement of the lower end of the ulna can be seen (*Fig.* 740). Palpation reveals a grossly unstable inferior radio-ulnar joint. Whether the condition is congenital or acquired is disputed. Many believe that repeated minor injuries delay growth of the radius while the ulna continues to grow, and that this unequal rate of growth forces the lower end of the ulna to subluxate.

Fracture of the Shafts of Both Bones of the Forearm is frequently encountered. In the case of a greenstick fracture both bones are bent but ultra-free mobility in the length of the bones is lacking. When the fractures are complete, there is an angular deformity causing the shape of the forearm to become altered so unmistakably that little more than inspection is required to make the diagnosis. Moreover, the patient supports the forearm and hugs it to the body.

OTTO MADELUNG, 1846–1926, *Professor of Surgery, Strasburg, France.*

Warning. Fracture of a single forearm bone *with displacement* is impossible without dislocation of the head of the radius in the case of the ulna, or of the inferior radio-ulnar joint in the case of the radius. To miss the dislocation is an extremely serious error.

Fracture of the Shaft of the Ulna, which, unlike fractures near the wrist, is due to direct violence, gives rise to comparatively few signs. As the radius splints the broken ulna, there is little displacement of the fragments and the contour of the limb remains normal. For the same reason the patient does not support the injured limb. The diagnosis can be made by drawing the finger along the subcutaneous border of the ulna when the local swelling, tenderness, and possibly other signs of a breach of continuity of the bone will be elicited.

Fracture of the Shaft of the Ulna with Dislocation of the Head of the Radius (*Monteggia fracture-dislocation*). In addition to the signs of a fracture of the shaft of the ulna given above, the fractured bone is bowed, or less commonly the fragments overlap. ————————————————————————→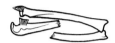

If sought for carefully (and it will be sought only if one is armed with the knowledge of the frequent association of these two lesions) forward displacement of the head of the radius will become evident.

Fracture of the Shaft of the Radius is less common than fracture of the shaft of the ulna. The displacement is variable, but is especially evident when the fracture is associated with dislocation of the lower radio-ulnar joint (*Galeazzi fracture-dislocation*). ————————————→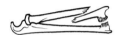

THE WRIST JOINT

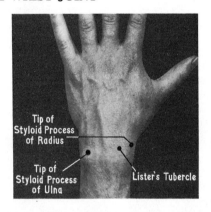

Tip of
Styloid Process
of Radius

Tip of
Styloid Process
of Ulna

Lister's Tubercle

Fig. 741. The bony landmarks on the back of the wrist.

Bony Landmarks (*Fig.* 741). *The Styloid Process of the Ulna*, which lies on the dorsal aspect of the wrist, can be defined at once, for it is completely subcutaneous. *The Styloid Process of the Radius* is truly lateral, projects about 1 cm more distal than the corresponding process of the ulna, but is less obvious than the latter because the tendons forming the radial boundary of the anatomical snuff-box intervene between it and the palpating finger. In spite of this, the styloid process of the radius can be felt beneath and on either side of the tendons in question, and by deep palpation even its tip, which marks the line of the wrist joint, can be discerned. Continuing deep palpation from the base of the styloid process across the anatomical snuff-box towards the ulna, another bony projection will be encountered in a line with the cleft between the index and middle finger, the dorsal tubercle of the radius (*Lister's tubercle*), which marks the lateral boundary of the groove for the tendon of the extensor pollicis longus.

GIOVANNI B. MONTEGGIA, 1762–1815, *Professor of Surgery, Ospedale Maggiore, Milan.*
RICCARDO GALEAZZI, 1866–1952, *Director of the Orthopaedic Clinic, Milan.*
JOSEPH (LORD) LISTER, 1827–1912, *Professor of Surgery, consecutively at Glasgow, Edinburgh, and King's College Hospital, London.*

The Structures in Front of the Wrist, with Special Reference to Flexor Tendons and Nerves. The anterior surface of the wrist is one of the principal finger-posts of the medical and nursing professions. Students of surgery, while sharing the appreciation of the radial pulse, must be familiar with the other structures that can be seen or felt on the volar aspect of the wrist. Usually the most conspicuous of these is the tendon of the palmaris longus. In 10 per cent this is absent on one or both sides. To familiarize yourself with the structures that lie beneath the volar surface of your wrist, proceed as follows: commencing on the ulnar side, locate the pisiform bone. By placing the fingers in the position shown in *Fig.* 742 *a*, the tendon of the flexor carpi ulnaris is rendered tense, and can be traced downwards to its insertion into the pisiform bone. Next, by making a fist, keeping the wrist flexed (*Fig.* 742 *b*), the tendons of the (1) flexor carpi ulnaris, (2) flexor digitorum sublimis to the *ring finger*, (3) palmaris longus, and (4) flexor carpi radialis, can be palpated with certainty (Scheldrup).

At the bottom of the groove between the flexor carpi radialis and the palmaris longus lies the median nerve. Especially if the palmaris longus is absent, in some individuals it is possible to palpate this nerve lying immediately to the ulnar side of the tendon of the flexor carpi radialis muscle. On the radial side of the flexor carpi radialis, lying directly on the bone, is the radial artery.

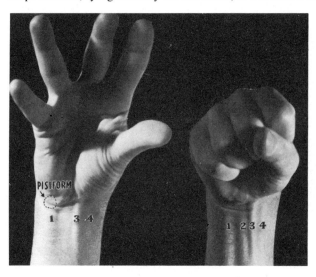

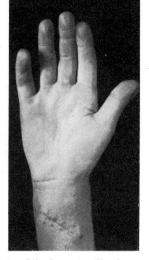

a   b

Fig. 742. 1, Flexor carpi ulnaris; 2, Flexor digitorum sublimis (slip to ring finger); 3, Palmaris longus; 4, Flexor carpi radialis.

Fig. 743. Cut wrist. The flexor carpi ulnaris and the ulnar nerve were found to be severed.

Many opportunities present to apply this knowledge. Take, for example, cut wrist (*Fig.* 743). In this instance the flexor carpi ulnaris tendon and the ulnar nerve were severed—a frequent combination. The state of affairs is shown 3 weeks later. One of the first signs of ulnar paralysis is abduction of the little finger which drifts away from the others (loss of the adductor function of the fourth palmar interosseous), and takes up a position of semiflexion.

EUGENE W. SCHELDRUP, *Contemporary Professor of Medicine, University of Iowa, Iowa City.*

Testing Movements. The Neutral Position is one in which the hand is in line with the forearm. In a young adult the normal range of movement between full extension and full flexion (*Fig.* 744) is 150°. As age advances, especially in those who do not perform manual work or play, this range becomes slightly less. To test radial and ulnar deviation (sum total about 50°) the lower forearm must be held in a fixed position during the test (*Fig.* 745). To test complete mobility of the joint the patient is requested to perform circumduction.

Although it is customary to attribute all these movements to the wrist joint, none can be dissociated from movements of the carpal joints.

Chronic Arthritis produces swelling, tenderness and limitation of movement. *Osteoarthrosis* after injury is fairly common, as is *rheumatoid arthritis*. In Britain, *tuberculosis* of the wrist, in common with tuberculous arthritis of other joints, has become much less frequent and is a disease of the elderly, but this is not the case in many parts of the world (*see Fig.* 5, p. 4). It gives rise to a spindle-shaped swelling of the joint with 'tumor albus' (*see* p. 436), together with palmar flexion. Abscess and sinus formation occur early because the dorsal surface of the joint is superficial.

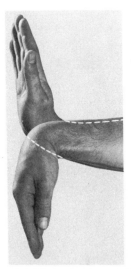

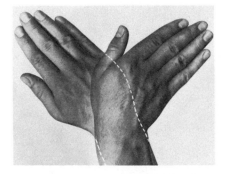

Fig. 744. Normal range of extension (70°) and flexion (80°).

Fig. 745. Normal range of radial (20°) and ulnar (30°) deviation. The latter is slightly greater because of the relative shortness of the styloid process of the ulna.

LESIONS OF SOFT TISSUES ABOUT THE WRIST

The Carpal Tunnel Syndrome* denotes a compression neuropathy of the median nerve as it passes beneath the flexor retinaculum (*Fig.* 746). The majority of patients are women, many of them in the fifth or sixth decade. In more than 50 per cent the symptoms are bilateral, but more in evidence in the dominant hand. The complaint is of progressive weakness or clumsiness, due to impairment of

---

* Ormorod first described the idiopathic variety in 1883.

JOSEPH A. ORMOROD, 1848–1925, *Physician, St. Bartholomew's Hospital, London.*

the finer movements of the hand (e.g. picking up a pin, sewing, knitting), associated with acroparaesthesia, i.e. attacks of pain, tingling and numbness of the affected hand, the ring and little fingers escaping. Often the hand is described as feeling swollen. Characteristically the attacks are nocturnal. Occasionally aching or pain radiates upwards, even as far as the shoulder, but never are there objective sensory changes proximal to the wrist. The syndrome is occasionally secondary to narrowing of the tunnel after a Colles's fracture (*see* p. 464), or in rheumatoid arthritis (*see* p. 483), is seen temporarily in pregnancy, and rarely from other causes, but the great majority are idiopathic.

Wasting of the Thenar Eminence is present only in a few late cases.

Hyperaesthesia is present over the distribution of the median nerve (*see* Fig. 674, p. 411). It can be demonstrated in 96 per cent of cases (Phalen).

The Wrist Flexion Test (Phalen's Sign). The patient is asked to flex both wrists and keep them flexed for 60 seconds. In more than half the patients there is a prompt exacerbation of paraesthesia in one or both hands, and equally prompt lessening of these symptoms when the flexion is discontinued.

The tourniquet test has a similar effect; the cuff is pumped up to the systolic blood pressure for the same time.

If the diagnosis is in doubt studies of the electrical impulses in the median nerve show a delay in motor conduction at the wrist on the affected side.

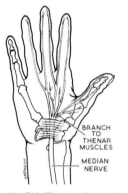

BRANCH
TO
THENAR
MUSCLES

MEDIAN
NERVE

Fig. 746. The carpal tunnel lies between the flexor retinaculum in front and the carpal bones behind. Should the tunnel become narrowed, limitations of space subject the median nerve to compression.

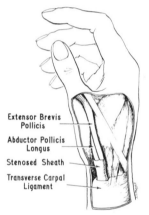

Extensor Brevis
Pollicis

Abductor Pollicis
Longus

Stenosed Sheath

Transverse Carpal
Ligament

Fig. 747. Usual site for stenosing tenosynovitis.

De Quervain's Disease (Stenosing Tenosynovitis), which occurs only in adults, is a painful, disabling condition affecting the common tendon sheath of the abductor pollicis longus and the extensor pollicis brevis which becomes chronically inflamed, and subsequently stenosed at the radial styloid process (*Fig.* 747). The patient, usually female, experiences pain at the site of the affected tendon sheath, and points to this region as the site of pain. In some long-standing cases there is a swelling, likened in size, shape, and consistency to an orange-pip, just proximal to the styloid process. Fine crepitus may be present (*see* p. 15).

GEORGE S. PHALEN, *Contemporary Orthopaedic Surgeon, Dallas, Texas.*
FRITZ DE QUERVAIN, 1868–1940, *Professor of Surgery, Berne, Switzerland.*

Only in man and the gorilla is the extensor pollicis brevis present; it aids in the final movements of the thumb. The addition of this muscle seems to have caused a crowding effect in the tendon sheath, hence this specialized form of tenosynovitis, which occurs as a result of excessive movement of the thumb in certain occupations.

Passive Extension of the Thumb is painless, but active extension brings on the pain complained of.

Localized Tenderness at the site that is illustrated in *Fig.* 747 is always present.

Finkelstein's Test. With the thumb in the palm, the patient is requested to make a fist by superimposing the fingers over the thumb. The hand is then pressed into ulnar deviation (*Fig.* 748). Pain is experienced at the radial styloid process and frequently shoots down to the thumb and/or towards the elbow joint.

Ganglion. A simple ganglion is the result of a myxomatous degeneration occurring in a portion of the connective tissue of the capsule of a joint. The cyst so formed becomes filled with crystal-clear gelatinous fluid. The most common situation for a ganglion is on the dorsal aspect of the wrist over the scaphoid-lunate articulation. The swelling thus produced (*see Fig.* 62, p. 30), is rounded and sessile and becomes tense and prominent when the wrist is flexed, and partially or wholly disappears when the wrist is extended. The second most common site is on the volar surface of the wrist between the tendon of the flexor carpi radialis and the brachioradialis (*Fig.* 749).

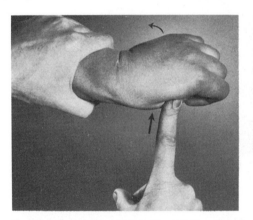

Fig. 748. Finkelstein's test. With the thumb in the palm and the fist clenched, ulnar deviation induces pain in De Quervain's disease.

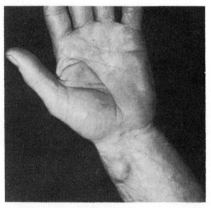

Fig. 749. Ganglion situated between the flexor carpi radialis and the brachioradialis—the second most common situation.

A ganglion giving rise to symptoms is usually between 0·5 and 3 cm in diameter and, more often than not, the swelling is slightly tender to pressure. As a rule it is filled so tightly with gelatinous material that it feels solid. Occasionally fluctuation can be elicited, especially when the swelling lies on the volar aspect of the wrist. When the swelling is large enough to be tested (unusual) it will be found to be translucent.

Ganglion of Finger. See p. 476.
Ganglion of Ankle and Foot. See p. 546.

HARRY FINKELSTEIN, *Died* 1975, *Emeritus Surgeon, Hospital for Joint Diseases, New York.*

BONE LESIONS IN THE VICINITY OF THE WRIST

Colles's Fracture. Although the lower end is the broadest, it is the weakest part of the radius, because except for a thin shell, it is composed of cancellous bone. Thus Colles's fracture—a fracture of the radius within 3 cm of its distal extremity—is the commonest fracture (1 in every 8 fractures). Women of middle age onwards sustain it more frequently than any other type of individual: with few exceptions, the cause is a fall on the palm of the outstretched hand. In about half the styloid process of the ulna also is broken. Impaction of the main fragments is usual. In all cases, whether firmly impacted or not, local tenderness and loss of function of the wrist joint are conspicuous features. The 'dinner-fork' deformity (*Fig.* 750) produced is highly characteristic—the hump is formed by dorsal displacement (*Fig.* 750 inset, right) and by rotation of the lower fragment. An alteration in the normal relationships of the radial and ulnar styloid processes, whereby the former comes to lie at the same level as, or at a higher level than, the latter is a reliable sign.

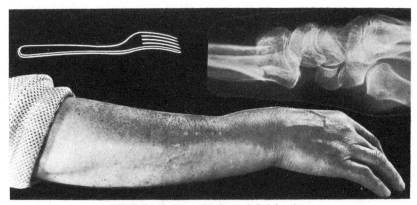

Fig. 750. Colles's fracture. The dinner-fork deformity.

Smith's Fracture (Reversed Colles's Fracture) is similar except that the distal fragment is angulated volarwards, instead of dorsalwards. Smith's fracture, which is much less common, is caused by a sudden force transmitted through the hyperflexed dorsum of the hand, such as would be occasioned by falling and striking the dorsum, and thereby hyperflexing the wrist joint.

Fracture of the Radial Styloid.* This usually occurs in young men. Typically it is caused by forced radial deviation of the wrist on falling. As displacement of the fragment is uncommon the only sign is tenderness on the lateral side of the wrist. **Fracture of the Carpal Scaphoid** is the most common injury to befall the wrist of a working man—the very words *sprained wrist* should arouse immediately a suspicion of a fractured scaphoid. Any accident that imposes violent extension (e.g. a fall on the outstretched hand) is apt to fracture the scaphoid for, willy-nilly, this bone (*Fig.* 751) opposes extension of the wrist, and when the intercarpal joint is excessively extended it breaks.

---

* Formerly known as 'lorry driver's fracture' being due to the kick of a starting handle, now seldom found in a lorry or car except of the 'vintage' variety.

ABRAHAM COLLES, 1773–1843, *Professor of Anatomy and Surgery, Dublin.*
ROBERT W. SMITH, 1807–1873, *Professor of Surgery, Trinity College, Dublin.*

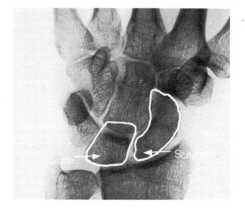

Fig. 751. For practical purposes the scaphoid and the lunate bones are the only carpal bones ever injured and if the clinician orientates them, the subject becomes less difficult.

DIAGNOSIS OF FRACTURE OF THE CARPAL SCAPHOID

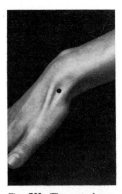

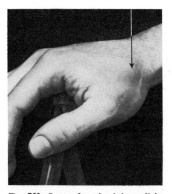

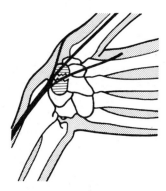

Fig. 752. The carpal scaphoid lies in the floor of the anatomical snuff-box distal to the tip of the radial styloid.

Fig. 753. Soon after the injury slight localized oedema occurs, reducing or obliterating the natural concavity of the anatomical snuff-box.

Fig. 754. In everybody, firm fingertip pressure in the anatomical snuff-box causes some pain, owing to compression of the radial nerve. Therefore test the uninjured side first.

Inspection. The scaphoid lies in the anatomical snuff-box (*Fig.* 752). Oedema appears almost at once (*Fig.* 753) most marked in the snuff-box. The swelling is neither great nor widespread.

Passive Movement. There is pain on attempting to flex or extend the wrist.

Palpation. Grasp the patient's hand in your left hand, and place the tip of your right index finger in the anatomical snuff-box; the scaphoid bone is directly beneath the palpating finger. Now deviate the patient's hand to the ulnar side; this makes the bone more accessible. Palpate again firmly; normally firm pressure at this point causes pain, owing to compression of the radial nerve (*Fig.* 754); therefore do not jump to a conclusion until the same amount of pressure has been applied on the contralateral side. Firm fingertip pressure in the anatomical snuff-box causing pain sufficient to make the patient wince is indicative of fracture. In a recent case these physical signs are often more reliable than an X-ray as the fracture-line may not be visible at first.

Dislocation of the Lunate. There is considerable swelling of the wrist, and usually there are signs of carpal tunnel compression, i.e. the dislocated bone, imprisoned deep to the flexor retinaculum, prevents movements of the flexor tendons causing immobility of the semiflexed fingers and paraesthesiae in the distribution of the median nerve (*see* The Carpal Tunnel Syndrome, p. 461); the signs of a complete median nerve lesion (*see* p. 407) may become apparent. Normally the lunate occupies the hollow that can be felt on the back of the wrist immediately distal to the radius in the line of the middle finger. When the bone is dislocated, this hollow is more concave than usual, and in it lies the site of maximum tenderness. Occasionally the scaphoid is fractured, half of it accompanying the dislocated lunate. This diagnosis cannot be made without X-rays.

Fracture of the Lunate is much less frequent than the foregoing. The site of maximum tenderness is over the lunate (*see Fig.* 751). Extension and flexion of the wrist are greatly reduced. These are the only signs of this fracture. Little wonder that it is overlooked.

Kienböck's Disease of the Lunate is an avascular necrosis probably following repeated minor injury. In a significant proportion of cases the ulna is short in relation to the radius. Persistent tenderness over the lunate and limitation of movement of the wrist joint suggest the diagnosis, which must be confirmed by radiography.

PAIN IN THE UPPER LIMB

This is a common diagnostic riddle. Formerly cervical rib or, in its absence, the scalene syndrome, was blamed frequently and many unnecessary operations performed. The discovery of the common conditions listed below have eliminated this source of error. Having carefully excluded recent injury or angina pectoris as the cause of pain, meticulous examination along the lines suggested will usually enable the clinician to establish the diagnosis, but it should be remembered that some cases are atypical, and X-rays and a therapeutic trial may be necessary before the diagnosis can be regarded as proved.

Consider the following (in approximate order of frequency):

Cervical spondylosis (common), *see* p. 150;
Carpal tunnel syndrome, *see* p. 461;
Supraspinatus tendinitis, *see* p. 446;
Tennis elbow, *see* p. 455;
Secondary malignant disease of bone, *see* p. 425;
Elbow tunnel syndrome, *see* p. 455;
De Quervain's disease, *see* p. 462;
Pancoast's syndrome, *see* p. 191;
Cervical rib syndrome (rare), *see* p. 146.

ROBERT KIENBÖCK, 1871–1953, *Professor of Radiology, Vienna.*

Chapter 32

THE HAND

The findings, particularly in infections and injuries, should be recorded graphically (*see Fig.* 2, p. 3). The fingers should be referred to as index, middle, ring and little, and not by numbers, a practice which is open to misinterpretation with occasionally disastrous results when the incorrect finger is amputated.

ACUTE INFECTIONS OF THE HAND

The prompt diagnosis (and treatment) of acute infections of the hand is extremely important. Without a knowledge of the signs that typify the various lesions, correct treatment is impossible, and unnecessary loss of working time and crippling deformities follow. Observe the inflamed hand:

Posture. When a hand is seriously inflamed it takes up the position of greatest ease, which is, in fact, the position of rest (*Fig.* 755) (Wood Jones).

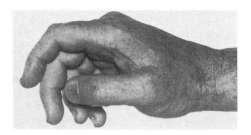

Fig. 755. The position of rest for the hand. The index finger is less flexed than the other fingers.

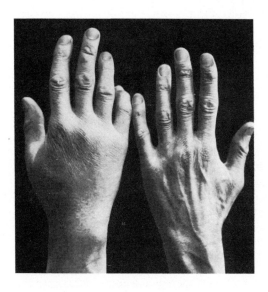

Fig. 756. Oedema of the back of the hand is very common in infections of the palmar aspect. Another example of the value of comparison.

FREDERIC WOOD JONES, 1879–1954, *Professor of Anatomy, Royal College of Surgeons of England.*

Swelling. A fundamental principle is that *the greatest swelling does not necessarily indicate the position of the pus, if such be present.* Oedema is an outstanding feature of all varieties of acute infections of the hand. Because the rich network of lymphatics in the subcutaneous tissues of the dorsum receives efferent vessels from the palm, and because the skin covering the back of the hand is loose and elastic, oedema is often most in evidence on the dorsum (*Fig.* 756), irrespective of the site of the lesion.

The Lymphatic Field of the Hand. After the local examination, always palpate the supratrochlear lymph node (*see* p. 454) and the axillary lymph nodes (*see* p. 174) on the side of the lesion.

POORLY LOCALIZED SUBCUTANEOUS INFECTIONS

Lymphangitis. Organisms gain entrance through an abrasion that may be so minute as to be imperceptible. Within a few hours the adjacent portion of the hand becomes swollen and painful, and there is often considerable elevation of the temperature. Oedema, most in evidence on the back of the hand, comes on early. A little later, red streaks, so characteristic of lymphangitis (*see Fig.* 72, p. 35), can be seen coursing up the arm. Especially in lesions of the ulnar half of the hand, the first lymph node to become enlarged and tender is the supra-trochlear. The lymphatics of the thumb and index finger pass straight to the axillary nodes. Lymphangitis can occur without any other demonstrable manifestation of inflammation, or as an accompaniment of one of the local inflammatory entities to be described.

Cellulitis is the initial lesion of the fascial-space infections to be described. In a proportion of cases, higher in loose subcutaneous than in more confined spaces, the inflammation resolves. In the rest a localized abscess forms. Incision during the stage of cellulitis is highly mischievous. On the other hand, *fluctuation must not be awaited in infection of closed and deep spaces.* In these, swelling, induration and localized tenderness signify that pus is present.

WELL-LOCALIZED INFECTIONS

Intracutaneous and Subcutaneous Abscesses are very common. The volar surface of the hands (including the fingers) of manual workers often is covered with greatly thickened epithelium. Especially in these persons, intracutaneous infections are liable to occur, in which event there may or may not be a history consistent with local implantation of organisms. Signs of local inflammation appear and soon the epithelium is lifted by a collection of pus.

An Intracutaneous Abscess can be situated in the *epidermis*, where it forms an obvious purulent blister (*Fig.* 757 A), or in the *dermis* (i.e. beneath the Malpighian layer of the skin), in which even an obvious dome-shaped elevation is lacking (*Fig.* 757 B), but unless the skin is pigmented or heavily ingrained with dirt, the pus can be seen through the epidermis as an indistinct opacity. The importance of an intraepidermal abscess lies in the fact that it may represent the superficial component of a *collar-stud abscess* (*Fig.* 758), the deeper component of which is commencing to burrow and spread. There is no means of telling if there is a deeper loculus until the superficial component has been uncovered.

A Subcutaneous Abscess (*Fig.* 757 C) does not proclaim its presence so obviously:

MARCELLO MALPIGHI, 1628–1694, *Professor of Physic at Pisa, and later at Messina; is regarded as the Father of Histology.*

the cellulitis, which is its precursor, gives place to a less sharply localized swelling and the formation of pus is surmised from the induration and extreme tenderness.

Fig. 757. Superficial abscesses at various levels. A, Intra-epidermal; B, Intradermal; C, Subcutaneous.

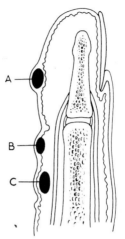

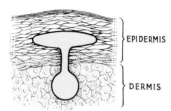

EPIDERMIS

DERMIS

Fig. 758. Epithelial collar-stud abscess, showing the superficial loculus lying between the layers of the epidermis of a horny-handed manual worker.

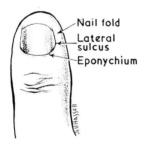

Nail fold
Lateral sulcus
Eponychium

Fig. 759. The parts concerned in paronychia.

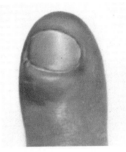

Fig. 760. Paronychia. Often infection occurs as in this case, through a 'hang-nail'.

Paronychia* is the most common infection of the hand (30 per cent). Unlike the others, which occur more frequently in working men, it is encountered in every walk of life, in both sexes, and from infancy to old age. The infection arises from a hang-nail, careless nail paring, or a manicurist's unsterile instrument. The inflammation commences beneath the eponychium (called by manicurists the 'cuticle'). Usually suppuration follows. Confined by the adherence of the eponychium (*Fig.* 759) to the base of the nail, the inflammation advances around the nail fold, even to the contralateral side. In 60 per cent of cases pus burrows beneath the base of the nail (*subungual abscess*).

The diagnosis can be made by inspection alone (*Fig.* 760). If pus is present, light pressure on the inflamed area, or (when pus is present beneath the nail) on the nail itself, evokes exquisite pain.

Apical Space Infection. The infection is confined at first to the space between the distal quarter of the subungual epithelium and the periosteum. Frequently the

---

* *Paronychia.* Greek, παρά = near+ὄνυξ = the nail.

pus bursts through the subungual epithelium to lie beneath the distal portion of the nail (*Fig*. 761). Usually the space becomes infected by running a sharp object under the free edge of the nail into the 'quick'. Although exquisitely painful, there is comparatively little swelling. This not uncommon condition is often confused with terminal pulp-space infection, but unlike the latter, tenderness is greatest at, or just proximal to, the free edge of the nail. Sometimes there is redness extending along one or both of the lateral nail folds, and even prolonged into the eponychium at the base of the nail. In these circumstances, unless the area of greatest tenderness is defined, paronychia is likely to be diagnosed. Pus comes to the surface either just distal to, or just beneath, the free edge of the nail (*Fig*. 761 *b*).

Infection of the Terminal Pulp-space is common and potentially serious. The digital pulps are subjected to more pricks than any other part of the body, index and thumb being affected most often.

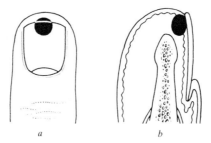

a   *b*

Fig. 761. Location of an apical space abscess. *a*, As seen clinically from in front. *b*, The abscess cavity seen in sagittal section.

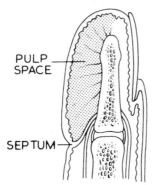

Fig. 762. The confines of the terminal pulp-space. It is separated from the rest of the finger by a fascial septum, at the level of the epiphysial line of the terminal phalanx.

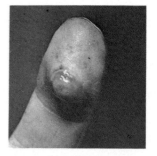

Fig. 763. Exuberant granulation tissue following delayed healing of an incision to drain an infected terminal pulp-space.

The pulp of the distal segment of a digit is closed proximally by fusion of the dermis of the distal flexion crease with the deep fascia, which in turn is attached to the periosteum just distal to the insertion of the long flexor tendon (*Fig*. 762) and is filled with compact fat feebly partitioned by fibrous septa. When infected, tight fixation of the dermis to the fascia, and the fascia to the bone, so interferes with swelling of the parts concerned that the tension within the space becomes extreme. Sometimes not only does necrosis of soft tissue occur, but thrombosis of the vessels traversing the space leads to necrosis of the terminal phalanx.

Dull pain and swelling are the first symptoms. Untreated, by the third day there are severe nocturnal exacerbations of throbbing pain, interfering with sleep. Light pressure over the affected pulp increases the pain. If the pulp is indurated, and has lost its normal resilience, pus is present. Untreated, the abscess tends to point towards the centre of the pulp beneath a patch of devitalized skin. A collar-stud abscess then occurs; still untreated, the abscess bursts. When, following drainage of the space, the wound continues to discharge and becomes filled with exuberant granulation tissue (*Fig.* 763) it is quite certain that necrosis of the terminal phalanx has occurred and this can be confirmed by radiography.

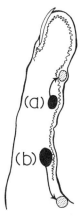

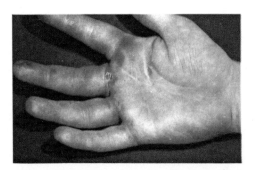

Fig. 764. The direction of spread of an abscess of (a) The middle volar pulp-space; (b) The proximal volar pulp-space.

Fig. 765. Infection of the web space between the index and middle fingers.

Infection of the Middle Volar Pulp-space. In this instance also, the infection follows direct implantation of organisms by a prick, and if the inflammation cannot be controlled, because this, too, is a closed space shut off above and below at the flexion creases, pus under tension causes symptoms and signs similar to those described in connection with the terminal pulp-space. The finger is held in semiflexion: in about one-third of cases an attempt to straighten it is painful. There is tender induration over the space, and while to some extent the terminal and proximal spaces share in the swelling of the digit, palpation over these reveals neither acute tenderness nor induration.

In Early Cases it is difficult to distinguish infection of the middle volar pulp-space from infection of the underlying flexor tendon sheath; however, in the former, some relatively pain-free movement of the finger is possible.

In Late Cases, due to the tracking of pus, frequently a purulent bleb appears in the distal flexion crease (*Fig.* 764 (a)).

Infection of the Proximal Volar Pulp-space (*Fig.* 764 (b)). While this space is well partitioned from the middle space distally, proximally it communicates freely with the web space. Once localization has occurred, infection of this space is comparatively easy to diagnose. There is tender induration in this segment of the digit and frequently a web space becomes involved also (*Fig.* 765).

Web-space Infection. The three interdigital web spaces are filled with loose fat that bulges between the four divisions of the palmar fascia. Infection often results from a purulent blister on the forepart of the palm.

Constitutional symptoms are usually severe; consequently patients with this condition are often seen before localization of the infection has occurred. At this stage there is gross oedema of the back of the hand and although web-space infection can be strongly suspected from the location of the tenderness, it is often difficult to rule out tenosynovitis. Once localization has occurred the involved fingers are separated (*Fig.* 765). In addition to the area of redness shown, there is often a fan-shaped blush on the dorsum extending from the web. The maximum tenderness is found on the volar surface of the web and at the base of one or other of the fingers flanking the affected web. Untreated, pus can track across the volar surface of the base of a finger from one web space into the next web space: also it can track up the side of the proximal volar pulp-space of a related digit.

Carbuncle of the Hand. The dorsal aspect of a proximal segment of a digit and the dorsum of the hand are not uncommon sites, much more frequently in the male because in adult males these areas are often hairy. In either situation the underlying extensor tendon is liable to be involved.

SERIOUS HAND INFECTIONS

These are now infinitely less common than the conditions detailed above. Sometimes they follow a neglected minor infection. When the hand is seriously inflamed it takes up the position of rest (*see Fig.* 755).

Infection of the Thenar Space. This space can be looked upon as a large web space between thumb and index finger. Infection gives rise to the typical 'ballooning' of the thenar eminence, which is quite characteristic (*Fig.* 766). Flexion of the distal phalanx may be pronounced, but it lacks the resistance to extension that is present in tenosynovitis of the flexor pollicis longus.

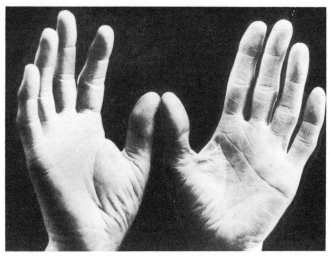

Fig. 766. 'Ballooning' of the thenar eminence (right hand): the sign of an infected thenar fascial space.

Deep Palmar Abscess (Mid-palmar space infection). Pus is situated beneath the thick, strong, resistant palmar fascia. Usually it follows a penetrating injury, but it can result from the bursting of an undrained infected flexor tendon sheath of the index, middle, or ring fingers. Swelling of the back of the hand is extreme. Obliteration of the concavity of the palm with even slight bulging thereof is pathognomonic. By reason of swelling, a very great enlargement of the hand results—it has been likened to a whale's flipper. When the abscess is due to a penetrating wound it decompresses itself along the path of wound infliction and a collar-stud abscess (*Fig.* 767) results, the superficial loculus of which lies beneath the thick fibrocellular layer of the dermis (there is no subcutaneous space in the centre of the palm).

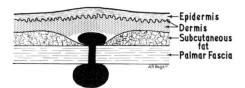

Fig. 767. Deep palmar abscess with an extension along the path of the original puncture resulting in a collar-stud abscess.

Acute Suppurative Tenosynovitis. Infection is usually by the prick of a sharp-pointed object such as a needle, a thorn, or the dorsal fin of a fish, the point of entry being within the territory overlying one of the flexor tendon sheaths (*Figs.* 768, 769). Often the prick is in one of the digital flexion creases—here the sheath is remarkably near the surface. Exceptionally, infection occurs by pus burrowing through the strong proximal septum (*see Fig.* 762) of the terminal pulp-space, or

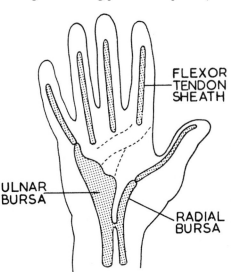

Fig. 768. Showing the relationship of the flexor tendon sheaths to the creases of the fingers and palm. In 11 per cent of cases the sheath of either the index, middle, or ring finger, or combinations of these, communicates with the ulnar bursa (Scheldrup).

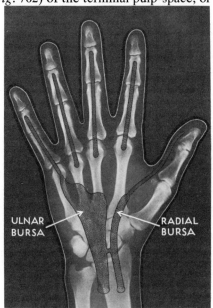

Fig. 769. Showing the relationship of the flexor tendon sheaths to the bones of the hand.

Eugene W. Scheldrup, *Contemporary Professor of Medicine, University of Iowa, Iowa City.*

as a result of an ill-placed incision to give exit to pus previously confined to that space. The whole sheath is rapidly involved. Within a few hours of the injury throbbing pain is felt in the affected digit, and the patient's temperature rises.

Flexion of the Finger. Typically the finger is held in a flexed position. This is an early sign at a stage when diagnosis and treatment are most desirable.

Swelling. There is symmetrical swelling of the whole finger in late cases (*Fig.* 770); soon the back of the hand becomes puffy.

Active Movement. Ask the patient to move the fingers. Note particularly that while the patient with a suppurative tenosynovitis refrains from, and indeed is incapable of, flexing the infected finger, it is not held rigidly immobile. On the contrary, owing to contraction of the lumbrical and interosseous muscles, to-and-fro movement at the carpometacarpal joint occurs which may beguile the clinician, who assumes that such movement excludes a diagnosis of acute tenosynovitis.

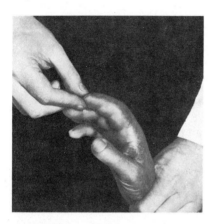

Fig. 770. The '*signe du crochet*'. The affected finger being in semiflexion, any attempt by the examiner to straighten it is resisted, and accompanied immediately by intense pain. A late case seen in the pre-antibiotic era.

Passive Movement. Gently—exceedingly gently—extend the suspected finger. Similarly, test the other digits. Exquisite pain is produced by the slightest attempt at extension (*Fig.* 770) of the infected digit or digits. In infection of the volar pulp-spaces (*see* p. 471) extension may produce pain, but never so severe.

Localized Infected Tenosynovitis is relatively common owing to early antibiotic treatment limiting the infection to a portion of the sheath by adhesions. Swelling and tenderness are confined mainly to one segment of the digit, rendering the differential diagnosis from infection of a middle or proximal volar pulp-space very difficult. Exploration is indicated if the condition does not soon settle completely with antibiotics.

Involvement of the Ulnar or the Radial Bursa, although comparatively rare since the introduction of antibiotics, is always a very serious matter.

Signs of Involvement of the Ulnar Bursa. (1) Flexion of a finger (usually the little finger but, as noted in the caption to *Fig.* 768, the other sheaths may communicate with the ulnar bursa); (2) Fullness of the palm; (3) Fullness immediately proximal to the flexor retinaculum on the ulnar side; (4) A point of maximum tenderness in this position.

Signs of Involvement of the Radial Bursa. (1) Flexion of the thumb; (2) Tenderness over the flexor pollicis longus sheath; (3) Swelling just proximal to the flexor retinaculum on the radial side.

Remember that the radial and ulnar bursae communicate in over 80 per cent of cases. Reference to *Fig.* 768 is again advised. Thus it may be difficult to distinguish infection of one bursa from the other. Sometimes both are infected.

Infection of the Dorsal Space. The frequency with which pitting oedema accompanies pus in the palmar aspect of the hand has resulted in neglect of an appreciation of the dorsal fascial spaces as sites of infection. The most frequent causes of dorsal space infection are a boil of the overlying skin and a penetrating wound. Infection of the dorsal subcutaneous space of the hand is fairly common, as also is that of the corresponding space in the proximal segment of the digits: that of the dorsal subaponeurotic space is rare. If swelling of the dorsum accompanied by tenderness, induration, and perhaps redness is present, a diagnosis of infection of the dorsal space can be made with assurance.

OCCUPATIONAL AFFECTIONS OF THE HAND

For the most part conditions coming into this category are chronic infections.

Chronic Paronychia seldom follows acute paronychia as it is a fungus infection (*Candida albicans*): the onset is insidious with a history dating back months rather than days. The lesions are often multiple. In days gone by washerwomen were especially prone to this condition; today the housewife who does not wear rubber gloves when 'washing up' is the usual sufferer. Another possibility is vascular insufficiency, e.g. Raynaud's disease (*see* p. 382). There is little tenderness. The eponychium is glazed and faintly pink without the redness of acute paronychia or frank pus. The nail itself may be affected, being cross-ridged and sometimes pigmented brown.

Other Common Chronic Affections of Nails (although primarily of dermatological rather than surgical interest) are *psoriasis*, in which the nails are characteristically pitted, and *fungus infection* with *tinea unguium*, in which the involved nails are thickened.

Barber's Pilonidal Sinus.* When clipped, hairs have a cut edge bevelled like the tip of a hypodermic needle and can penetrate the skin, generally in the digital web between the middle and ring fingers of the right hand (*Fig.* 771): the clippings must have penetrated the skin because there are no hair follicles in the web. In the uninflamed state the lesion is characterized by a small black dot (which marks the orifice of the sinus) situated towards the dorsum of the affected cleft. When the skin over the visible lesion is picked up between the examiner's finger and thumb, a nodule can be palpated. In four out of five cases the lesion is multiple. Like its counterpart in the sacrococcygeal region (*see* p. 274), the sinus is the seat of recurrent acute or subacute inflammation. Female hairdressers sometimes develop these lesions in the interdigital clefts of the toes: at work in hot weather they sometimes wear sandals and no stockings.

Grease or Spray Gun Injuries. A worker, with this type of instrument, accidentally injects oil, grease or paint under high pressure into a finger or the hand. Urgent surgical treatment is mandatory if serious loss of function is to be avoided. Immediately after the accident the part feels numb and is pale and swollen (*Fig.* 772). The entry wound is inconspicuous with little or no bleeding. The appearances are suggestive of a space infection if the material is localized in one of the sites described on pp. 472-5 (including tendon sheaths), or of a poorly localized infection if not so localized, but a cardinal sign of inflammation is absent: *the part feels cold.*

Digital Hunterian Chancre. When a painless, elevated indurated sore appears on a finger, especially the right index finger, and the supratrochlear lymph node is considerably enlarged, remember the Hunterian chancre (*see* p. 374). Dental surgeons, doctors and midwives nowadays rarely acquire this infection in the course of their work. 'The primary lesion of syphilis, when it develops on parts of the

---

* In Australia a similar condition is found in sheep-shearers.

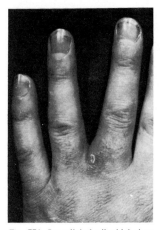

Fig. 771. Interdigital pilonidal sinus in a barber.

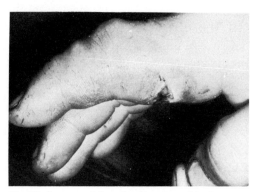

Fig. 772. Grease gun injury; the appearance of the finger soon after the accident.

body other than the genitalia, is protected from recognition by a singularly low threshold of suspicion on the part of clinicians' (Stokes).

Verruca Necrogenica (butcher's wart; pathologist's wart) is due to inoculation with *Mycobacterium tuberculosis* through a breach of continuity of the skin. Formerly milkmaids were prone to this condition, which they acquired from handling tuberculous udders. It commences as a bluish-red patch; later its surface becomes elevated and papillomatous (*Fig.* 773). If squeezed, pus oozes from between the warty projections. It should be suspected if a patient presents with a small warty mass surrounded by pustules, usually on the dorsum of the hand.

Erysipeloid (*see* p. 32).

OTHER LESIONS OF THE SOFT TISSUES OF THE HAND

Syndactyly (webbed fingers) (*Fig.* 774) is congenital and hereditary. Two or more fingers may be involved. Ascertain whether the webbing involves skin only, or whether, in addition, there is fibrous or even bony union.

Implantation Dermoid. Because the digits are pricked frequently—especially the pulps of the fingers—an implantation dermoid cyst is encountered more often in this region than elsewhere. Under the skin there is a painless, soft cyst (*Fig.* 775), which is neither attached to the skin (which is normal) nor to the deeper structures. The inference is that at some previous time a fragment of epidermis was driven beneath the dermis and continued to proliferate.

Compound Palmar Ganglion. This is not a ganglion, as understood by the term at the present time: formerly simple ganglia were thought to arise in tendon sheaths—a hypothesis for which there is no foundation. 'Compound palmar ganglion' is an old term to signify tuberculous tenosynovitis of the ulnar bursa, but at present most are associated with rheumatoid arthritis. In long-standing cases the fingers are partially flexed and there is an hour-glass-shaped swelling bulging above and below the flexor retinaculum. Transmitted fluid impulse can be elicited from one compartment of the swelling to the other (*Fig.* 776), and very characteristic is the soft crepitant sensation derived from the movements of the melon-seed bodies which abound within the bursa.

Ganglion of a Digit is not uncommon on the volar surface beneath a digital

JOHN H. STOKES, *Emeritus Dermatologist and Syphilologist, University of Pennsylvania, Pennsylvania.*

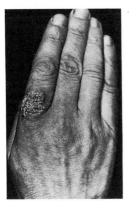

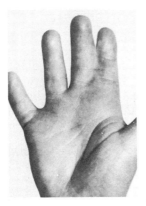

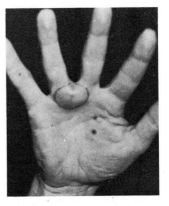

Fig. 773. Verruca necrogenica (butcher's wart).

Fig. 774. Syndactyly.

Fig. 775. Implantation dermoid following a human bite.

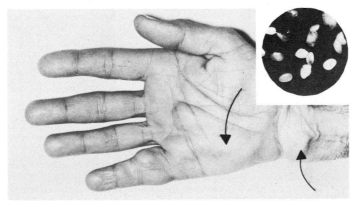

Fig. 776. Compound palmar ganglion. Transmitted fluid impulse accompanied by a peculiar crepitant sensation (due to the movement of melon-seed bodies) could be obtained between the positions marked by the arrows. Also shown are melon-seed bodies found at operation.

flexion crease. The small tense swelling is often mistaken for a sesamoid bone. A giant-cell tumour of the synovial sheath is indistinguishable clinically. More rarely, a ganglion appears on the dorsal surface of a finger in relation to an interphalangeal joint, when it is likely to be confused with a Heberden's node (*see* p. 483).

Glomus Tumour is a small, firm, smooth nodule, rarely more than a few millimetres in diameter. Most examples involve the nail-bed, and present as an exquisitely tender, red or violet-coloured localized area beneath the nail (*Fig.* 777). The tenderness is reduced quite conspicuously by applying a sphygmomanometer cuff and inflating it above the systolic blood pressure (Eastcott). An ordinary haemangioma is, of course, not tender and blanches when pressure is applied. Some cases show disuse atrophy of the digit. The tumour is derived from a glomus body—an arteriovenous anastomosis incorporating muscle and nerve tissue and present mainly in the skin and subcutaneous tissues of the hands and feet, but most numerous in the hands and especially in the nail-beds, which is believed to help in regulating body temperature.

HARRY H. G. EASTCOTT, *Contemporary Surgeon, St. Mary's Hospital, London.*

FLEXION DEFORMITIES OF THE FINGERS

Testing Movements of Fingers and Thumb. The Neutral Position is regarded as that with the fingers straight and the thumb lying next to the index finger. Normally each finger can be flexed so that each joint bends to approximately a right angle (*see Fig.* 788, p. 482). Hyperextension of 45° at the metacarpophalangeal joint is also possible normally. Abduction and adduction of the fingers is measured from the midline of the middle finger ('finger spread') and varies depending on the size of the hand. Compare it with the normal side.

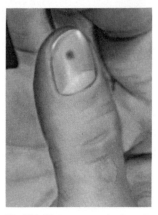

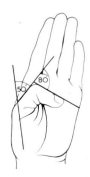

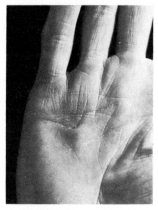

Fig. 777. Glomus tumour in the nail-bed of the thumb.

Fig. 778. Flexion of the thumb. Angles of 80° at the interphalangeal joint, 50° at the metacarpophalangeal joint and 15° at the carpometacarpal joint are normal.

Fig. 779. Early Dupuytren's contracture affecting the slip of palmar fascia of the ring finger.

Thumb movements are more complex. Extension is movement away from the index finger on a flat surface with the hand supine and palm upwards, the angle normally reaching 70°. Normal flexion is shown in *Fig.* 778. The angle of abduction (normal 70°) is that between thumb and index metacarpals with the hand supine, the thumb being raised toward the ceiling (*see Fig.* 668, p. 408).

Dupuytren's Contracture. Occurs usually in males (10:1). The palmar fascia* is obviously thickened and contracted. At an early stage this thickening takes the form of one or more nodules in the palm, and often when the fingers are extended fully a dimple is seen (*Fig.* 779) indicating that the contracted fascia is adherent to the skin. While typically the condition affects the ring finger (*Fig.* 780) and years later the little finger becomes implicated, in about one-third of cases it is the little finger that is affected primarily (Early).

'Congenital' Contracture of the Little Finger develops during early childhood, is frequently bilateral and is the result of contracture of soft tissues (*Fig.* 781) and is similar to Dupuytren's contracture: it is the absence of thickening of the palmar fascia that leaves no doubt as to which is present. Involvement of the ring finger is rare.

Flexor Tendon Adhesions. Should the flexed finger be the aftermath of suppurative tenosynovitis (*see* p. 473), on testing both active and passive movements it will be found that neither extension nor flexion is possible except at the

---

* In about 5 per cent the plantar fascia of one or both feet is affected similarly (*see* p. 538).

BARON GUILLAUME DUPUYTREN, 1777–1835, *Surgeon, Hôtel-Dieu, Paris.*
PETER F. EARLY, *Contemporary Senior Medical Officer (Limb Service), Ministry of Health.*

metacarpophalangeal joint. More than one finger may be affected. Usually there is a clear history of a severe hand infection.

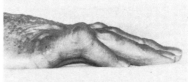

Fig. 781. 'Congenital' contracture of the little finger.

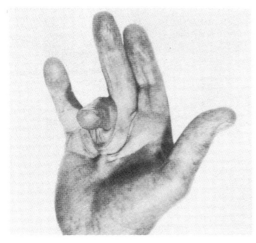

Fig. 780. Dupuytren's contracture of many years' standing.

Volkmann's Ischaemic Contracture is due to vascular injury which results in muscle infarction and muscle-fibre death. Later the lifeless muscle fibres are replaced by fibrous tissue. Obviously, therefore, it is of the highest importance to focus attention on the early signs of muscle ischaemia, so that the clinician can remove the cause while the muscle is still viable.

Stage of Ischaemia. Half the battle is to know the circumstances in which muscle ischaemia is prone to occur. First and foremost, it results from a too-tight plaster cast or, much less frequently, too-tight bandaging. Secondly, it can occur as a result of arterial damage by a fracture. Lastly, it can arise as a result of the intense arterial spasm that follows the accidental injection of certain drugs, notably thiopentone, into an artery in mistake for a vein. *See also* Arterial Trauma, p. 387 *and* March Gangrene, p. 523.

The early signs are *p*ain, *p*allor, *p*uffiness (oedema), *p*ulselessness, and *p*aralysis (Griffiths). As a rule, the first symptom or sign appears within a few hours of injury or the reduction of a fracture. The onset can be delayed for as long as 24 hours, or even more. Pain in the forearm on passive extension of the fingers (*Fig.* 783) is the first serious early sign, as is the assumption of a flexed position. Blue, swollen fingers are by no means invariable: pallor of the hand is not an infrequent early sign. The radial pulse is absent constantly in all severe cases and the skin temperature of the affected hand is reduced.

The Stage of Contracture follows untreated ischaemia, or when effective treatment is commenced too late. In the case of the forearm, the fingers are flexed but they can be, at least partially, extended when the wrist is flexed (*Fig.* 782). This demonstrates that the contracture is in the flexor group of muscles. In extreme cases a complete 'claw-hand' (*see* p. 412) can result.

Burns Contracture. If the history can be elicited, the conclusion that badly treated burns are the cause of contractures becomes obvious.

RICHARD VON VOLKMANN, 1830–1889, *Professor of Surgery, Halle, Germany.*
DAVID L. GRIFFITHS, *Contemporary Director of University Department of Orthopaedic Surgery, Manchester.*

Rupture of the Extensor Tendon of a Digit. Recall the mode of insertion of the extensor digitorum communis (*Fig.* 784). There are two varieties of rupture of the tendon; the first is much the more common.

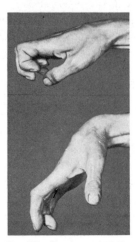

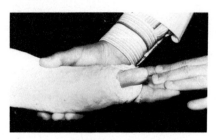

Fig. 783. It should be routine to test for pain on finger extension in all patients with the arm in plaster-of-Paris.

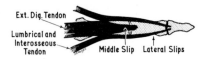

Fig. 782. Showing: *a*, Volkmann's contracture; *b*, That the fingers can be partially extended by flexing the wrist.

Fig. 784. The anatomy of the insertion of extensor digitorum communis.

a. Rupture or Avulsion of the Terminal Lateral Slips occurs as a result of a violent blow on the tip of the finger, as might be occasioned by a cricket-ball. The resulting rupture gives rise to a clinical entity:

Mallet Finger (known in the USA as 'baseball finger') (*Fig.* 785), which is so characteristic that it cannot be mistaken. It can also be due to an avulsion fracture of the base of the terminal phalanx.

b. Button-hole Rupture of the Extensor Tendon at the Proximal Interphalangeal Joint. In this variety of extensor tendon rupture it is the middle slip of the tendon that is torn or avulsed from the base of the middle phalanx. The proximal interphalangeal joint cannot be extended fully (*Fig.* 786), and when it is flexed further sometimes there is a click as the two lateral slips of the extensor expansion jerk sideways over the head of the proximal phalanx. If this click is heard or felt, it must be distinguished from that of a trigger finger proper.

Trigger Finger. A, usually palpable, nodular thickening, not due to trauma or other known cause, develops in the long flexor tendon opposite the head of the metacarpal, most frequently in middle-aged women. The middle or ring finger is usually affected. The 'click' to which it gives rise when the finger springs back into position is often thought by the patient to occur on the extensor aspect, which is not the case. The powerful flexor muscles can pull the bulbous portion of the tendon down the tendon sheath into the palm, but when they relax, the extensor mechanism is unequal to the task of accomplishing the process in the reverse direction (*Fig.* 787). The lump cannot enter the digital sheath without outside assistance, the entrance to the sheath being narrower than the sheath itself. Straightening of the finger is achieved by a momentarily painful snap.

Snapping Thumb is similar. The patient is *usually under 2 years of age*, and the mother is concerned because the infant's thumb becomes fixed in flexion. On the flexor surface over the head of the metacarpal a relatively large orange-pip-like swelling can be felt. Upon gently extending the digit, extension is brought about with a 'click'.

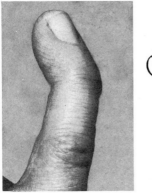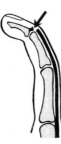

Fig. 785. Mallet finger. The terminal phalanx cannot be extended because the insertion of the extensor tendon has been torn.

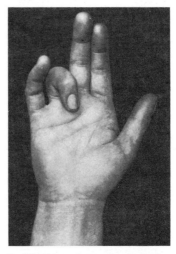

Fig. 787. Trigger finger. After closing her hand the patient was asked to open it, with this result; only when the ring finger was assisted could it be extended: a mere touch towards unflexing and the finger snapped into line with the others.

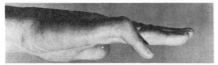

Fig. 786. A button-hole rupture of the middle slip of the extensor tendon of the little finger.

Attrition Rupture of the Extensor Pollicis Longus occurs most often in a middle-aged woman who, while wringing clothes or playing the piano, experiences sudden pain in the base of the thumb, and the thumb falls limply adducted across the palm. The terminal joint is flexed and cannot be extended. It is usually due to rheumatoid arthritis but also occasionally complicates a Colles's fracture. It can occur as early as three weeks (while the wrist is still in plaster), or as late as four months after the injury: the tendon ruptures because it has become frayed in its groove.

INJURIES OF THE TENDONS OF THE HAND

Here we are dealing with a patient with a recent incised or lacerated injury of the wrist or hand, or a person with a defect of finger movement noticed remotely after a wound.

Consider the following two groups:

1. The lesion is, or was, at the wrist, or in the palm, or over the dorsum of the hand; several tendons may have been divided together with, in front of the wrist, the median or ulnar nerve. Diagnosis of the nerve injury is dealt with on pp. 407–11. If only a single tendon is involved, the case falls into the second category discussed on the next page.

Can the Patient flex the Fingers and Thumb fully? If not (and nerve injury and fractures have been excluded), the long flexor tendons to the particular digits have been divided. Remember that the flexor digitorum *sublimis* is *superficial* to

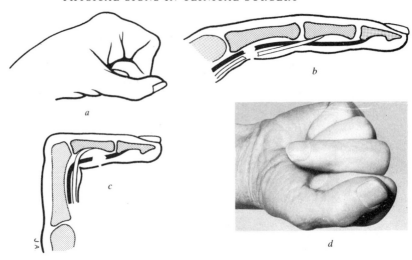

Fig. 788. *a*, Full flexion of a finger is possible if the flexor digitorum sublimis tendon only has been divided. *b*, If both long flexor tendons have been divided flexion is impossible (barring 'trick movement') beyond the point of division. *c*, When flexor digitorum profundus alone has been severed, flexion of the distal interphalangeal joint is lost. *d*, An attempt to flex the middle finger when flexor digitorum profundus alone has been divided.

the profundus from the carpal tunnel to the middle phalanx, and that it alone can be severed in this region without loss of function. As suture in such circumstances is not indicated, it is not important if the diagnosis is missed.

Can the Patient extend the Fingers and Thumb fully? If not, unless another lesion is present causing wrist drop (see p. 407), the relevant extensor tendons have been divided.

In practice the above tests may not be applicable if there has been severe mutilation. Accurate diagnosis must be reached on careful exploration at the necessary operation under a general anaesthetic. On the other hand, with lesser injuries, if tendon damage can be excluded confidently, all that may be necessary is skin suture under local anaesthetic.

2. The lesion is, or was, in a finger, or is, or was, a short incision in the palm, or on the dorsum, which has only involved a single tendon.

Test Flexion and Extension as above. (Also test pain sensation in the affected finger—suture of a severed digital nerve is well worth while.)

If the superficial sublimis tendon to a finger only has been divided, there is no loss of flexion (*Fig.* 788 *a*). Repair is unnecessary.

If both long flexor tendons have been divided, flexion of the finger is lost, commencing at the joint distal to the lesion (*Fig.* 788 *b*).

If the flexor profundus has been severed distal to the proximal interphalangeal joint (*Fig.* 788 *c*) the patient is unable to flex the terminal phalanx.

When the flexor pollicis longus has been divided, the patient is unable to flex the thumb distal to the point of injury.

Division of an extensor tendon is also straightforward—the patient cannot extend the digit at the joint beyond the lesion *with this exception*: division of the middle slip of insertion over the proximal interphalangeal joint gives rise to the typical button-hole deformity (*see Fig.* 786). *See also* Mallet Finger (p. 480).

THE BONES AND JOINTS OF THE HAND

Heberden's Nodes were described by him as 'Little hard knobs, about the size of a small pea, which are frequently seen upon the fingers, particularly a little below the top near the joint'. He also stated that they were not due to gout. The nodes are unsightly rather than inconvenient, and seldom attended by pain. The *terminal* interphalangeal joint of any or all the digits, except the thumbs, usually is involved, the enlargement being sufficient to be seen (*Fig.* 789) and felt as a definite bony ridge across the palmar and dorsal surface of the affected joints. Most cases occur in women about the time of the menopause and do not necessarily herald osteoarthrosis of other joints, as is commonly believed. In males the lesion is nearly always solitary and is the result of bygone trauma, particularly a cricket or baseball injury to the finger, which was of sufficient violence to be remembered by the recipient many years later.

Heberden's nodes are due to osteoarthrosis: they are to be distinguished from the less common spindle-shaped fingers due to swelling of the *proximal* interphalangeal joints which is one of the manifestations of rheumatoid arthritis. **Rheumatoid Arthritis involving the Hand.** Advances in hand surgery have made it possible to remedy the common deformities in selected circumstances. Thus the surgeon should recognize certain conditions due to the disease. Women are affected three times more frequently than men. Any patient with the disease may exhibit a rheumatoid nodule (*Fig.* 790) which is a focal reaction to repeated minor trauma in subcutaneous tissue over bony prominences.

In the first stage hypertrophy of the synovial membrane of joints (*pannus*)* occurs. The most commonly affected are the metacarpophalangeal joints (*Fig.* 791) (index finger most frequently and severely); the proximal interphalangeal joints are next most often involved, and, thirdly, pannus is seen on the dorsum of the wrists. During this stage synovial thickening may also cause trigger finger (*see* p. 480), or the carpal tunnel syndrome (*see* p. 461).

The second stage is characterized by ulnar deviation of the fingers, the angulation occurring at the metacarpophalangeal joints (*Fig.* 792).

Lastly, deformities occur due to dislocations and attrition rupture of tendons. Thus there may be dislocation of a metacarpophalangeal joint or joints. Another typical deformity is 'swan-neck' contracture of a finger (due to hyperextension of the proximal interphalangeal joint and flexion of the distal interphalangeal joint) (*Fig.* 793), the result of fibrosis of the small muscles of the hand. The button-hole deformity is also seen (*Fig.* 793). The commonest tendons to undergo attrition rupture are the long extensors of the fingers and thumb (*see* p. 481).

Dactylitis. † When the phalanges or the metacarpals are inflamed the condition is known as 'dactylitis'. The bone becomes enlarged, spindle-shaped and, in the case of *tuberculous dactylitis* (*Fig.* 794), painful. Within a matter of weeks the skin over the affected bone appears smooth and shiny, then, unless the progress of the disease is checked, red and tender, and frequently an abscess forms. Not

---

* Latin, *pannus* = cloth.
† *Dactylitis.* Greek, δάκτυλος = a finger; inflammation of a finger or toe.

WILLIAM HEBERDEN, 1710–1801, *Physician, who practised in Cambridge and later in London. He was physician to George III and to the illustrious writer Dr. Samuel Johnson.*

ARTHRITIS OF THE HAND

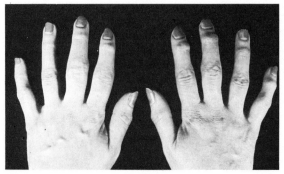

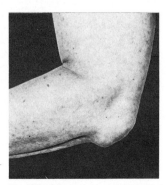

Fig. 789. Heberden's nodes. The distal interphalangeal joints are affected in three-quarters of cases and the proximal in a quarter of cases. The fingers affected are the index, middle, little, and ring fingers in that order of frequency.

Fig. 790. Rheumatoid nodule behind the elbow.

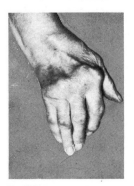

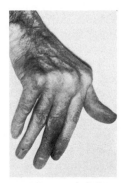

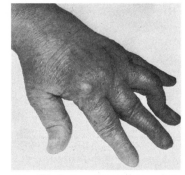

Fig. 791. Pannus in rheumatoid arthritis, most marked over the metacarpophalangeal joints.

Fig. 792. Ulnar deviation.

Fig. 793. 'Swan-neck' contracture of the middle finger and button-hole deformity of the ring finger in rheumatoid arthritis (*see* p. 480).

uncommonly more than one bone of the hand is attacked. In *syphilitic dactylitis* (now rare) a similar *painless* swelling occurs which may also break down. In the tropics *sickle-cell anaemia* (*see* p. 322) causes dactylitis due to infarction of bone resultant on thrombosis of the nutrient artery.

Dactylitis must be distinguished from an **enchondroma**, an example of which is shown in *Fig.* 795.

Sprain of an Interphalangeal Joint also gives rise to spindle-shaped swelling of a digit which is wont to persist for months, and in severe cases is permanent.
Suspected Fracture of a Phalanx or a Metacarpal Bone. All the bones of the fingers and thumb are practically subcutaneous so that when one is fractured completely with displacement (or a dislocation of an interphalangeal joint has occurred), the deformity produced is often obvious. When swelling obscures the

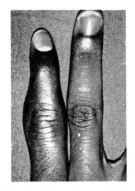

Fig. 794. Tuberculous dactylitis.

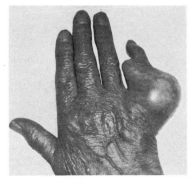

Fig. 795. Enchondroma present in a woman of 75 and growing slowly since adolescence.

displacement, or the bone is incompletely broken, the clinician should run his finger along the dorsum of the relevant phalanx or metacarpal, noting any tenderness or deformity. In the case of a spiral fracture of a metacarpal bone with shortening, *loss of prominence of the relevant knuckle* is a sign of value.

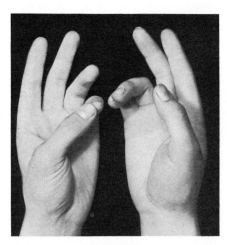

Fig. 796. Bennett's fracture (*right*). The patient cannot approximate the tip of the thumb to the tip of the ring finger. Note the haematoma of the thenar eminence.

Bennett's Fracture is an oblique fracture through the articular surface of the first metacarpal which allows subluxation of the joint. It occurs predominantly through indirect violence—falls or blows against the thumb extended in a parrying gesture, or knocks that strike the distal part of the metacarpal, especially when the hand is clenched, so that it is common in boxers. Directly after the accident restricted movement is evident: not seldom, the thumb is forced into a semiflexed position. Despite every attempt the patient cannot approximate the tips of the thumb and ring finger (*Fig.* 796), let alone the tips of the thumb and the little finger nor can he clench his fist. Soon a large haematoma of the thenar eminence becomes apparent (*Fig.* 796) and the subluxation becomes impalpable.

EDWARD H. BENNETT, 1837–1907, *Professor of Surgery, Trinity College, Dublin.*

Chapter 33

THE HIP JOINT AND THE THIGH

Gait. *See* p. 439.

Preparation of the Patient for the Examination. For a child all clothing is removed. A man only keeps his shirt on. With a female, a nurse sees that the necessary clothing is taken off, and the patient is provided with a pair of bathing triangles to wear during the examination.

Examination Standing. If the patient is ambulatory, inspection is started in the standing posture, first with the patient facing and then with his back towards the clinician.

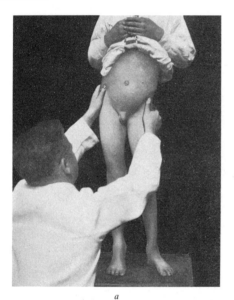 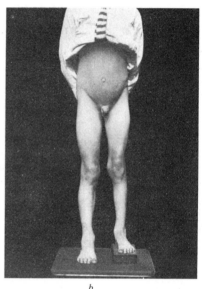

a   *b*

Fig. 797. *a*, Ascertaining if shortening is present. *b*, Measuring the amount of shortening by insinuating blocks beneath the short limb to such a height as to render the pelvis absolutely level. If the trochanters are then level the shortening is below them, if not it is in the head or neck of the femur.

Stance. A patient with arthritis of the hip joint tends to bear most of his weight on the sound leg to lessen weight-bearing. This, in many instances, results in slight flexion of the knee joint on the affected side (*see Fig.* 705, p. 436).

Asymmetry. As seen from the front, the group of muscles most to suffer from disuse atrophy is the adductors. At this juncture ask the patient to turn round for a moment. Flattening of the buttock, due to wasting of the glutei, is often evident with chronic arthritis of the hip joint of some standing.

The presence of scars or sinuses in the immediate neighbourhood is most significant (*see Fig.* 798).

The Pointing Test. Usually pain is experienced in the groin. Less frequently it is felt deeply in the buttock, posterior to the greater trochanter as an increase in tension in the hip joint causes pain and spasm in those muscles with the same nerve supply. Not infrequently pain passes from the hip to the knee. Remember, however, that in some instances the pain is felt *solely in the knee*, although the arthritis is limited to the hip joint of the same side. Branches of the femoral, the sciatic and the obturator nerves all give twigs to both joints. The geniculate branch of the obturator is the main conveyor of pain referred from the hip to the knee joint.

Is there any Tilting of the Pelvis? Concentrate on the anterior superior iliac spines, with a view to ascertaining if they lie on the same horizontal plane. A tilted pelvis usually is the result either of the lower limb being held in an adducted position, or of shortening of one leg, or of surgical arthrodesis in abduction.

If Tilting is present, is the Tilt due to Apparent or to Real Shortening of the Limb? Apparent shortening is due to fixed adduction deformity. Real shortening means that the limb is really short. Both can coexist.

It is of overriding importance to settle at this stage the fundamental question—is tilting due to real shortening of the affected limb? If so, is that shortening situated above the level of the great trochanter? Kneel facing the patient, and place the thumbs on the lowest part of the anterior superior iliac spines and the ring and little fingers behind the greater trochanters, while the

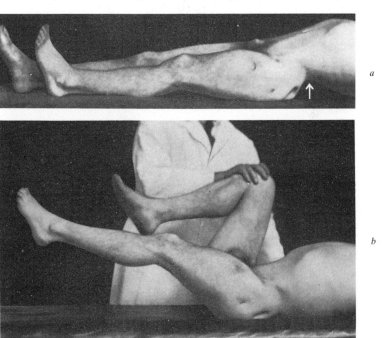

a

b

Fig. 798. Hugh Owen Thomas's sign. Note the result of flexing the normal hip joint of the opposite side. Case of fibrous ankylosis due to tuberculosis. Note the scars of bygone sinuses.

TESTING MOVEMENTS OF THE HIP JOINT

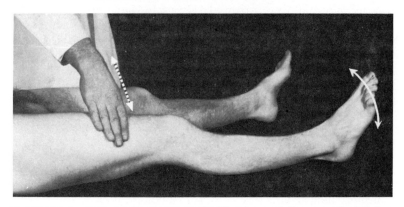

Fig. 799. Rotation. *Method A:* 'Rocking' the hip joint. In this case rotation appeared curtailed on the affected (left) side, and the test is being elicited on the non-affected side. Always compare any restricted joint movement with that of the sound side.

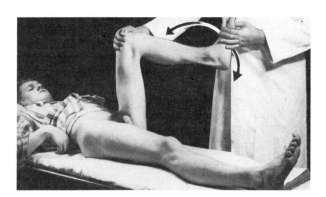

Fig. 800. Rotation. *Method B*. It must be appreciated that *internal rotation* is being tested in this illustration. For *external* rotation the foot is levered inwards.

Fig. 801. The abduction possible in a young child with normal hip joints.

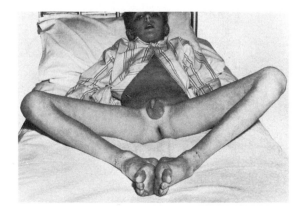

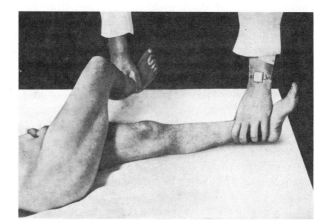

Fig. 802. Adduction. Normally the middle third of the thigh can be crossed.

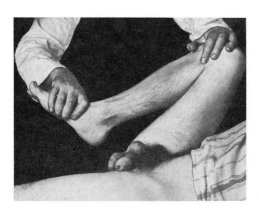

Fig. 803. Flexion.

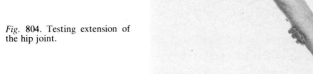

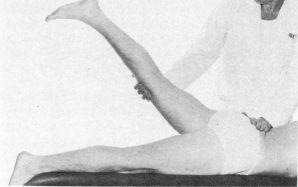

Fig. 804. Testing extension of the hip joint.

middle finger of each hand gropes for, and finds, the tip of each greater trochanter. Slight differences in the height of the trochanters are detected easily in this rapid way (*Fig.* 797 *a*). If the tip of one greater trochanter lies nearer the anterior superior iliac spine than the other, ascertain how much shortening of the limb has resulted:

Build blocks (or books) under the short limb to such a height as to make the pelvis absolutely level (*Fig.* 797 *b*). By measuring the height of the support the amount of real shortening is ascertained with an accuracy unobtainable by any other clinical method. If the patient is ambulatory, undoubtedly this method should be employed.

When the patient is confined to bed, or is too young to cooperate in the rectification of the pelvic tilt just described, careful measurements of the length of each lower limb must be undertaken (*see* p. 491).

Apparent Shortening. If real shortening cannot be demonstrated by these methods it becomes obvious that the shortening *must* be apparent.

Examination of the Patient Lying Supine. After having made certain that the patient is lying without a lateral tilt of the pelvis, seek Thomas's sign, the significance of which must be understood.

Hugh Owen Thomas's Sign. Fixed flexion deformity of the hip joint can be masked by increased normal lordosis. As you look at the patient lying in *Fig.* 798 *a*, you may be deceived, for the whole limb lies flat on the couch. This sign unmasks a possibility that the clinician is being beguiled by the patient's posture and reveals the true position of the affected limb.

Pass the hand (palm upwards) beneath the lumbar spine, and with the other hand flex the *sound* hip until the lumbar vertebrae can be felt hard against the hand. This means that all the lordosis has been corrected. Observe the affected limb. If flexion deformity is present, estimate and record the angle (*Fig.* 798 *b*).

Testing the Movements of the Hip Joint. Make sure that the anterior superior iliac spines are square with the couch and that the pelvis does not move as you proceed:

1. *Rotation.* Lay the flat of the hand upon the thigh, and rock the limb to and fro observing the foot (*Fig.* 799) as an index of the degree of rotation. Performed in this way, this is a delicate test which can be carried out with the utmost gentleness. If it causes pain (e.g. in acute arthritis), the subsequent programme for testing various movements must be curtailed or modified.

Rotation can also be carried out by flexing both the hip and the knee joints to a right-angle, and using the foot to lever the limb round (*Fig.* 800). Common sense dictates that this violent method be employed only in appropriate cases. Its zenith of usefulness is in the early diagnosis of a slipped epiphysis, where limitation of internal rotation is the leading physical sign (*see* p. 498).

2. *Abduction.* Flex the hips to a right-angle and ask the patient to place the soles of the feet together and then to carry the knees outwards as far as they will go (*Fig.* 801). Measure the angle of abduction on both sides. In infants abduction to 80° is possible but this angle is gradually reduced to reach 60° in normal hips in old age. Comparison of the normal (painless) side is often important.

HUGH OWEN THOMAS, 1834–1891, *Orthopaedic Surgeon, Liverpool. He held no hospital appointment.*

3. *Adduction.* Steady the pelvis, and carry the thigh over its fellow. Normally it should cross the middle third (*Fig.* 802). Record in terms of the opposite thigh, i.e. whether the lower, middle, or upper third of the opposite side can be crossed.

4. *Flexion.* Flex the knee on the *affected side* (cf. Thomas's sign, p. 490), and then flex the hip as far as possible, proceeding cautiously (*Fig.* 803).

Up to the present, the examination has been carried out with the patient on his back. Ask him to turn over on to his abdomen, and test:

5. *Extension.* Steady the pelvis. Place the hand behind the knee and lift the limb (*Fig.* 804). Normal extension is only 10° and is limited early in all forms of arthritis.

Telescopic Movement. The pelvis is fixed by an assistant, the thigh is grasped above the knee and the hip joint is flexed to 90°. The thigh is pushed, and then pulled. In congenital dislocation of the hip in a young child and a Charcot's joint (*see* p. 438) the characteristic sensation, which can be likened to that of pulling out a telescope, sometimes can be elicited. Convincing proof is that the greater trochanter and the head of the femur can be felt to move up and down in the buttock.

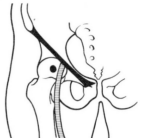

Fig. 805. The black dot represents the spot where tenderness of the hip joint is sought. The thick broken line is that of the femoral artery.

Direct Palpation of the Hip Joint and seeking Joint Crepitus. Lying in its socket, and heavily clothed with muscle, the greater part of the joint is quite inaccessible. The capsule, however, is prolonged down the neck of the femur, and it is here that signs of disease are sought. Place a finger on the anterior superior iliac spine and follow the lower edge of the inguinal ligament medially until the pulsation of the femoral artery can be felt. Just below the inguinal ligament and just lateral to the femoral artery the pulp of the finger will lie directly over that small portion of the head of the bone that is not intra-acetabular (*Fig.* 805). Exert increasing pressure—tenderness suggests arthritis. With the other hand, rotate the hip joint by rocking (*see Fig.* 799)—the head of the bone will be felt to move; joint crepitus may be transmitted to the finger. Absence of the head of the femur signifies that it is dislocated (*see* p. 493).

Mensuration

Girth. Minor degrees of wasting can be revealed by measuring and comparing the girth of the thigh and leg on each side.

    a. From the anterior superior iliac spine, measure off a convenient distance down the thigh. Mark this point. Measure off the same distance on the other thigh, and mark it. At the points marked, measure the girth of the thighs (*Fig.* 806).

    b. From the tibial tuberosity mark off identical points down each leg, and measure the girth of the calves.

Length. The normal limb must be placed in an exactly similar position to the affected limb before the measurements are taken, i.e. if there is an adduction deformity, the normal limb must be adducted a similar amount. Find the tip of the medial malleolus on each side, and mark the point. Define the anterior superior spine on both sides; an error in measurement frequently occurs because an identical point on the spine is not chosen on each side. With one finger palpate the inguinal ligament, and follow this up until the first bony point is reached. If this is done on each side and the first bony part is marked, error from this cause is avoided. Measure the distance (from the anterior superior iliac spine to the tip of the medial malleolus) on each side (*Fig.* 807). Record the measurement of each limb. This is *real* length, not apparent length which is of no importance.

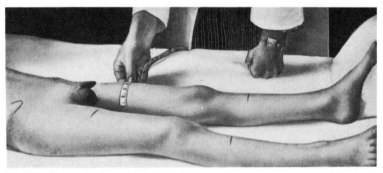

Fig. 806. Mensuration for wasting. Both thighs and both calves are measured at exactly corresponding points.

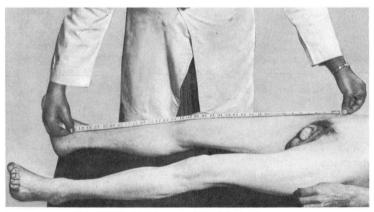

Fig. 807. Measuring the length of the limb. The distance between the anterior superior iliac spine and the tip of the medial malleolus is measured on each side. The tape-measure should lie evenly along the inner border of the patella.

You have discovered real shortening of a lower limb. Where is the shortening? Lie the patient flat with the feet together and the hips and knees flexed. View the patient from the side of the shortening. It is immediately obvious which part of the limb is involved (*Fig.* 808). If the femur is affected proceed as shown in *Fig.* 797 to ascertain whether the shortening is in the head and neck, or in the shaft.

In many instances the examination of the hip joint is complete only when the other major joints, especially the knee joints, have been tested for gross abnormalities.

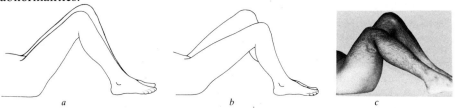

Fig. 808. *a*, Shortening of the femur; *b*, Shortening of the tibia, viewed from the side; *c*, Shortening of the right femur; the aftermath of acute osteomyelitis in childhood. Note the scar on the outer aspect of the lower thigh.

SIGNS IN INDIVIDUAL DISEASES OF THE HIP JOINT

The principal affections of the hip joint encountered at various ages are congenital dislocation (from birth onwards); osteochondritis juvenilis (4–10 years); slipped epiphysis of the head of the femur (10–15 years); osteoarthrosis due to previous disorder of the joint (20–40 years); osteoarthrosis without such a precursor (over 40 years of age). As a rule, tuberculosis of the hip joint commences in early childhood, but there are a number of exceptions.

Congenital Dislocation of the Hip is relatively common, occurring four times more frequently in girls; if the 1 in 3 bilateral cases alone are considered, the female incidence is higher still. There are also racial differences: it is especially common in a belt extending across Southern France, Northern Italy, Austria, Czechoslovakia and Poland, and also in Japan, and particularly rare in Negro and Chinese races who habitually carry their babies on their backs with hips abducted. The earlier the diagnosis, the less difficult is it to remedy, and it is now widely recognized that it should be diagnosed at, or soon after, birth.

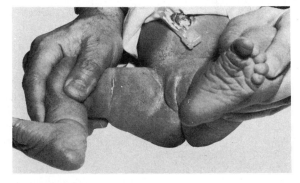

Fig. 809. Limited abduction in flexion of the left hip in congenital dislocation.

SIGNS IN THE NEONATE AND THE INFANT. Before weight-bearing commences, the head of the femur usually is subluxated, but not dislocated. The physical signs during the first six months of life (before the child commences to crawl) are as follows:

Limited Abduction in Flexion of a hip or hips (*Fig.* 809) indicates that actual dislocation is present.

*Barlow's Modification of Ortolani's Test.** The infant is laid on a firm flat surface such as a table. The knees and hips are flexed and semi-abducted. The examiner's fingers over the greater trochanters (*Fig.* 810) push the trochanters forward and medially while the thumbs just below the inguinal ligaments feel for the heads of the femurs which, if subluxated, will slip into the acetabulum on the affected side, or sides, with a palpable jerk. Release of pressure by the fingers leads to another jerk as the subluxation recurs.

Telescopic Movement (see p. 491) often can be obtained.

Other Clinical Findings in Early Life are of academic interest only. Very broad buttocks and undue *widening of the perineum* in bilateral cases, and *extra skin creases* along the adductor aspect of the thigh in unilateral cases (*Fig.* 811) are especially noticeable. Occasionally an observant mother will bring the child because she has noticed that when changing napkins one knee does not spread as far as the other.

Delayed Walking. Although it should now seldom present in this way, unless there is another good reason, any child who is not walking by 18 months should be suspected of having congenital dislocation of the hip.

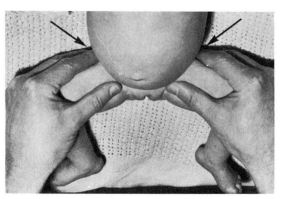

Fig. 810. Method of eliciting Ortolani's 'sign of the jerk'. The arrows indicate the direction of pressure by the fingers over the greater trochanters. The best of all tests for the very early diagnosis of congenital dislocation of the hip joint.

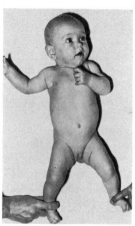

Fig. 811. Additional skin crease on the inner side of the thigh of a patient with congenital dislocation of the left hip joint.

SIGNS IN CHILDHOOD AND IN ADOLESCENT LIFE. After the patient has learned to walk the diagnosis should not present any difficulty:

The Female Contour of the Pelvis. The normal child (male or female) has a male pelvic contour. The child with a unilateral or bilateral dislocated hip has a distinct female pelvic contour (*Fig.* 812). In addition, the buttocks and the abdomen are prominent.

The Trendelenburg Gait. The hip on the affected side lurches up when weight is borne on it. Watch the shoulder, rather than the buttocks. The shoulder dips down on the affected side every time weight is borne on that side. In bilateral cases first one, and then the other, shoulder dips.

---

* As with so many tests and diseases in medicine and surgery this was described long before it was generally recognized: in this instance by Pierre le Darnoy (1870–1963), an orthopaedic surgeon of Rennes, France, in 1912.

THOMAS G. BARLOW, 1915–1975, *Surgeon, Hope Hospital, Manchester.*
MARINO ORTOLANI, *Contemporary Director, Centre for Congenital Subluxation of the Hip, Arcispedale S. Anna, Ferrara, Italy.*
FRIEDRICH TRENDELENBURG, 1844–1924, *Professor of Surgery, Leipzig.*

Trendelenburg's Sign. Normally, each leg bears half the body-weight. When one leg is lifted, as in normal walking, the other takes the entire weight. As a result the trunk has to incline towards the weight-bearing leg, and the pelvis tilts, rising on the side not taking the weight. When this mechanism fails the sign is positive.

The patient stands on the unaffected lower limb first; the buttock on the affected side rises as the pelvis tilts to take the body-weight. Next she stands on the affected side; if it is the seat of a congenital dislocation of the hip joint, the *pelvis on the opposite (normal) side sinks,* as shown by the level of the iliac crests and the gluteal folds. The reason for this is that the head of the femur is out of its socket and the iliotrochanteric muscles are not powerful enough to maintain the horizontal position of the pelvis (*Fig. 813*). Valuable as it is in suggesting the diagnosis of unilateral congenital dislocation, the test is not pathognomonic. It indicates only a defect in the osseomuscular mechanism between the pelvis and the femur. It is also present in poliomyelitis when the glutei are affected, in un-united fracture of the femoral neck, in pathological dislocation, and in coxa vara.*

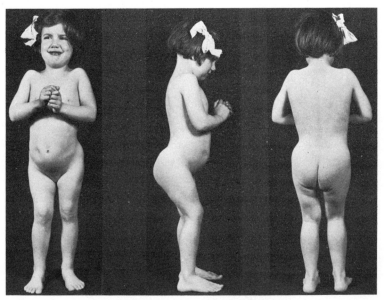

Fig. 812. Bilateral congenital dislocation of the hip.

CONGENITAL DISLOCATION OF THE HIP IN ADULT LIFE. To those features to which the reader's attention has been directed, two more are added: (1) Pain; (2) Joint crepitus, because the patient develops osteoarthrosis in the head of this bone and in the apology for a socket that Nature attempts to provide on the dorsum ilii.

---

* *Coxa vara.* Latin *coxa* = hip joint + *varus* = bent inward. The angle (160° in children, 130° in adults) between the neck and shaft of the femur is decreased, due to a congenital defect, softening of the bone, slipped epiphysis, or malunited fracture.

Pathological Dislocation of the Hip Joint is a complication not only of infected destructive lesions of the hip joint, but also of spastic paralysis, poliomyelitis and spina dysraphism. The signs are those of the causative condition to which are added those of congenital dislocation.

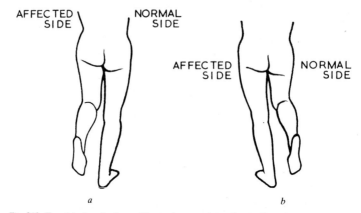

Fig. 813. Trendelenburg's sign. *a*, The patient stands on the unaffected leg. The buttock on the opposite side rises. *b*, The patient stands on the affected leg. The buttock on the other side sinks.

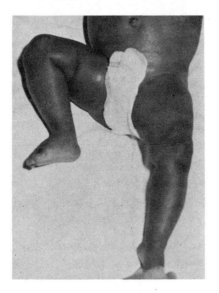

Fig. 814. Acute suppurative arthritis of the right hip joint, showing the 'frog position'.

Acute Suppurative Arthritis of the hip joint is least uncommon in babies, and is nearly always secondary to a more general infection. The diagnosis should be considered in any child who has pyrexia and develops a limp, or refuses to walk. A child of 3 years of age or more is able to locate the site of the pain; otherwise entire reliance must be placed on careful clinical examination. As a result of the effusion, the hip joint takes up a position of flexion, abduction and external rotation—the position of greatest fluid capacity—and in a baby this is so characteristic as to be designated the 'frog position' (*Fig.* 814). Gentle pressure over the capsule of the joint (*see Fig.* 805) causes the child to scream. To confirm the diagnosis, needle aspiration of the hip joint under anaesthesia must be undertaken.

Traumatic (Transient) Synovitis of the hip joint ('irritable hip') is common and impossible to distinguish from the very earliest stages of the following three conditions which may affect the hip joint in childhood; special investigations (X-ray, sedimentation rate) and a period of observation are necessary. The child presents with pain, a limp and a hip in the position of greatest ease (*see Fig.* 705, p. 436), but without the toxaemia or high pyrexia of acute suppurative arthritis. Minor trauma is the presumed cause and the effusion absorbs after a few days' bed-rest, leaving an absolutely normal range of movement.

Tuberculous Arthritis. The hip joint is second only to the vertebral column as the most frequent site of tuberculosis of bones and joints. It has become uncommon except in those primitive communities with poor resistance.

A Limp is the first, and a constant, sign. To commence with, the limp comes on after the patient has walked some distance and is tired; later it is in evidence after resting (e.g. in the early morning) as well.

Pain, more often referred to the thigh or to the knee than experienced locally, is also an early symptom.

Night Cry. Starting pain at night is very important, as it attracts more attention than occasional discomfort during the day (Whitman). Relaxation of protective contraction of muscles allows the inflamed joint surfaces to come in contact with one another and causes the child to utter a sharp cry, usually early in the night. Often he will be found holding the thigh with the hands.

Muscular Wasting. At first revealed only by careful measurement, muscular wasting of the thigh does not linger far behind the above signs—later such wasting, particularly of the buttock, is apparent to the naked eye.

Hugh Owen Thomas's Sign (*see* p. 490) becomes positive at a very early stage, and reveals that the limb is held in concealed flexion. Limitation of extension is also a valuable early sign.

General Signs. Malaise and pallor accompany tuberculous arthritis. The temperature in the early stages is of little diagnostic value.

As the disease progresses (now unusual with adequate treatment) the affected limb passes through three classic successive phases (*Fig.* 815).

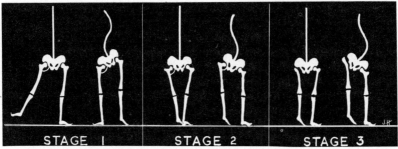

STAGE 1   STAGE 2   STAGE 3

Fig. 815. The stages through which untreated tuberculosis of the hip passes.

Stage 1. The limb is held in slight flexion, slight abduction and lateral rotation (the position of greatest fluid capacity of the joint, which is the seat of effusion). In order to bring the legs parallel

ROYAL WHITMAN, 1857–1946, *Surgeon, Hospital for the Ruptured and Crippled, New York.*

the patients *tilts down* the pelvis on the affected side; to permit this, the lumbar spine becomes curved, the convexity being towards the affected side—the stage of *apparent lengthening*.

Stage 2. As the effusion subsides and spasm of the powerful adductors increases, the position changes to one of flexion, adduction and medial rotation. *Tilting upwards* of the pelvis on the affected side causes *apparent shortening*.

Stage 3. As the head of the bone becomes eroded, *real shortening* supervenes, and increases as dislocation of the head of the bone develops and is supplemented by retardation of growth from the disturbance of the epiphysis.

An Abscess or Abscesses. The longer the disease remains active the greater the liability to cold abscess formation.

Osteochondritis Juvenilis (Legg–Calvé–Perthes Disease). The blood supply of the head of the femur becomes defective, and this part of the bone undergoes very slow, quiet, aseptic necrosis. As a result, the head of the femur collapses and becomes mushroomed. The cause is speculative.

Boys are affected four times more often than girls. The patient remains in good general health and is quite apyrexial (most important facts in differential diagnosis). The most constant early sign is a comparatively painless limp. In the early stages all movements of the hip joint are slightly restricted as there is a traumatic synovitis. Later abduction is found to be considerably diminished, and so is internal rotation. As a rule, other movements are full and painless. Muscular wasting of the limb occurs and moderate flexion and adduction deformity is liable to cause prominence of the greater trochanter. In established cases (after 2 years from the onset of symptoms) a small amount of real shortening is present. Radiography is necessary to confirm the diagnosis, but except in the very early stages a confident clinical diagnosis is possible.

In bilateral cases (10 per cent) the patient develops a characteristic waddling gait, reminiscent of congenital dislocation of the hip. Trendelenburg's sign (*see* p. 495), however, is negative.

Slipped Epiphysis of the Head of the Femur causes limp and pain in the hip during adolescence. The male-to-female ratio is 3:2. Often the child is either obese from hypogonadism (*see* p. 48), or else is tall for his age, thin and growing rapidly. There may be a history of trauma, but usually it was mild. The typical onset is so insidious that the condition is often ignored by the parents and overlooked by the doctor until the deformity is obvious. The earliest symptom is a painful limp with, often, the pain referred to the knee. At this stage ordinary radiographs may be normal, a lateral view of the hip joint being necessary. The cardinal sign is definite painful limitation of internal rotation and abduction of the hip joint. On examination standing the greater trochanter on the affected side feels higher and more posterior than on the normal side. Continued weight bearing leads to more limp, more pain, shortening and external rotation of the femur due to forward and upward displacement of the neck of the femur on its head, so that Trendelenburg's sign becomes positive. A quarter of cases are, or become, bilateral.

Osteoarthrosis is easily the commonest disorder of the hip joint arising in adult life. The triad of pain, stiffness and deformity is found ultimately, irrespective of whether the arthritis is primary or secondary.

Pain is the usual presenting symptom and is of a boring character and mainly localized to the joint concerned, although it may be referred to the knee or the back; shooting pain causing the leg to 'give way' is a variant.

ARTHUR T. LEGG, 1874–1939, *Surgeon, Boston Children's Hospital, Boston, Massachusetts.*
JACQUES CALVÉ, 1875–1954, *Director, La Fondation Franco-Américaine, Berck-sur-Mer, France.*
GEORG PERTHES, 1869–1927, *Professor of Surgery, Tübingen, Germany.*

Stiffness, especially after rest, is common. Rising from a chair is difficult and the patient says it takes him a minute or two to 'get going'. Increasing difficulty in tying the shoelace on the affected side is an important early sign. Stretching the legs apart becomes noticeably restricted early.

Limp. Even in the earliest stages the patient limps, and often this is noticed by friends and not by the patient. The cause is either pain or apparent shortening due to adductor spasm. The limp is increased by weak muscle groups, particularly the glutei of the affected side which may be so weak as to show a positive Trendelenburg's sign.

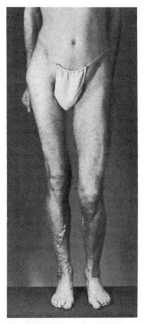

Fig. 816. Male, aged 55 years, with osteoarthrosis of right hip joint. Hip becomes stiff after sitting. Some difficulty in putting on his right shoe. Walks with a stick, and for no farther than half a mile without pain. Five years' history.

Restricted Walking. More and more, walking is restricted, because it induces pain which is inclined to have the characteristics of intermittent claudication, in that the patient must halt to rest at intervals, but the pain is not mainly in the calf or calves. The foot pulses (*see* p. 379) should be palpated carefully.

Stance. The commonest result is adduction of the thigh, eversion of the foot and flexion of the hip joint. As the adduction deformity increases, in order to maintain balance the pelvis is tilted upwards on the affected side (*Fig.* 816). This causes scoliosis, which at first is temporary, when standing or walking. Occasionally adduction is so extreme as to cause a scissors gait. In bilateral cases, in spite of the adduction, scoliosis and pelvic tilt are absent.

Routine Examination of the Hip Joint shows some restriction of all movements, but internal rotation, abduction, and extension are restricted early. Apparent shortening amounts to 2·5–5 cm; real shortening is never great, and occurs (from loss of cartilage and flattening of the head of the femur) only when the disease is fairly advanced.

Swelling of the Joint. As a result of synovial thickening and serous effusion, the joint is swollen. Careful palpation of the joint (*see Fig.* 805) sometimes permits this to be made out when compared with the opposite side.

Joint Crepitus. The irregular surfaces, with or without loose bodies, give rise to coarse grating, which is palpable.

Examine Other Joints. In no other joint condition is this injunction more important. To examine the contralateral hip, knees and the spine is fundamental.

Psoas Bursa. Beneath the inguinal ligament there is a tense swelling (*Fig.* 817) situated in the femoral triangle. Fluctuation is often doubtful because the swelling is so tense and its capsule is so thick. The swelling is too far lateral to be associated with the femoral canal, which excludes an irreducible femoral hernia. The clinician may suspect a psoas abscess, but on deep palpation in the iliac fossa, he fails to find an extension of the swelling so characteristic of an abscess. As a rule a psoas bursa is accompanied by flexion, abduction and external rotation of the limb, an attitude that relieves tension. There is often osteoarthrosis in the corresponding hip joint, for the bursa frequently, but not necessarily, communicates with that joint.

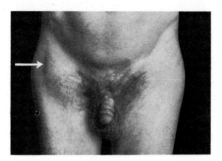

Fig. 817. Psoas bursa. The patient, aged 65, complained of great pain in the groin and difficulty in walking. The latter was due to advanced osteoarthrosis of the hip.

Fibrous or Bony Ankylosis of the Hip Joint? In fibrous ankylosis the patient suffers pain; in bony ankylosis this is absent. Considerable difficulty is experienced in differentiating extensive fibrous ankylosis from bony ankylosis. In the latter there is absolutely no movement at the hip joint; in the former movement may be so slight as to defy detection by routine examination. To detect very slight movement at this joint place one hand over the anterior superior iliac spine and the great trochanter, and rock the thigh from adduction to abduction with the other.

Traumatic Dislocation of the Hip Joint. The commonest variety, *posterior dislocation* (80 per cent), usually results from a traffic accident when the victim's knee hits the dashboard, and the force transmitted up the femur drives the head of the bone out of its socket. Not only is the head of the femur dislocated but, often, the rim of the acetabulum is fractured as well. The patient experiences severe, unremitting pain in the groin and the thigh. The limb lies in a position of adduction, internal rotation and slight flexion (*Fig.* 818): active movement is confined to the foot. The greater trochanter is unduly prominent. The palpating finger over the site of the hip joint (*see Fig.* 805), instead of meeting the usual resistance, sinks in. It may be possible to feel the head of the femur riding the dorsum ilii beneath the gluteal muscles. There is marked shortening. In all varieties of dislocation testing movements is contraindicated for obvious reasons.

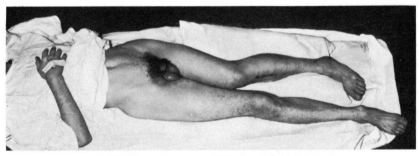

Fig. 818. Traumatic posterior dislocation of the hip joint.

Central Dislocation is infrequent (15 per cent). The limb is abducted but rotation is variable and shortening depends on how far into the pubis the head has been driven.

The above varieties are complicated by injury to the *sciatic nerve* in some 10 per cent of cases (*see* p. 412).

Anterior Dislocation is rare and occurs when the victim falls feet first from a height. It is possible for both joints to be dislocated. Pain and fixation of the joint are present. The limb is abducted, laterally rotated, and slightly flexed. The head of the bone button-holes the Y-shaped ligament of Bigelow, and its neck is held so fast that there is no upward displacement and no shortening.

THE THIGH

Meralgia* Paraesthetica. The lateral cutaneous nerve is compressed as it passes through the inguinal ligament; the result is an area of hyperaesthesia in the lateral thigh and a complaint of a tingling feeling in this region, worse on standing or walking but usually relieved by sitting, as flexion of the hip leads to shortening of the course of the nerve.

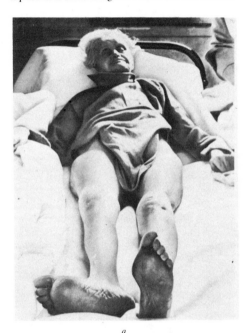

a

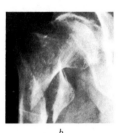

b

Fig. 819. *a*, A typical patient (old lady) with a fractured neck of the femur. Note the 90° of external rotation denoting an extracapsular fracture. *b*, The inset X-ray shows a basal fracture. *c*, The sites of upper femoral fractures. The upper two are intracapsular, the lower two are extracapsular.

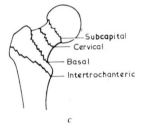

c

Subcapital
Cervical
Basal
Intertrochanteric

Fracture of the Neck of the Femur (*Fig.* 819). Often the patient is an elderly woman, and frequently the accident is trivial—slipping on a polished floor— which suggests that the neck of the femur is the seat of senile osteoporosis (occasionally a bone metastasis). That a fracture of the femur has occurred is usually perfectly obvious on inspection. The leg rotates outwards 90° when the fracture is extracapsular, i.e. a low fracture of the neck. On the other hand an intracapsular fracture (high fracture of the neck) shows only 40° of external rotation, as the capsule prevents further rotation. Patel notes that in extracapsular fractures an additional sign is present—a swelling (haematoma) is found at the inferolateral aspect of the hip joint.

When a fracture of the neck of the femur is impacted (abduction fracture), the patient can lift the heel off the bed; otherwise she is unable to do so.

---

* *Meralgia*. Greek, μηρός = thigh + ἄλγος = pain.

HENRY J. BIGELOW, 1818–1890, *Professor of Surgery, Harvard University, Boston, Mass.*
DINUBHAI PATEL, *Orthopaedic Surgeon, Ahmedabad, India.*

Obscure injuries about the hip joint require careful consideration. Consider the comparatively rare impacted abduction fracture of the neck of the femur; the symptoms are few—the patient may even walk to seek advice. Even the slightest pain on rotation of the hip by *Method A* (*see Fig.* 799) provides sufficient data upon which to order a confirmatory X-ray.

Fractured Greater Trochanter. After a fall on the side there is pain, and bruising (such as might be seen after a fractured neck of femur) is present. Maximum tenderness is over the greater trochanter and full active movements of the hip joint are possible, although painful.

Avulsion Fracture of the Lesser Trochanter is rare but shows a unique sign. It occurs in schoolboys, and is caused by vigorous contraction of the psoas muscles as, for example, when hurdling.

Ludloff's Sign. The sitting patient is unable to flex the affected thigh but all other movements are present. The iliopsoas muscle is an important flexor of the hip joint.

Fracture of the Shaft of the Femur. No other long bone fracture results in so much shock due to the large amount of blood that is extravasated into the thigh. As a rule the limb lies rotated laterally. Often it is obviously deformed, the patient cannot move the limb, and real shortening is present. In this instance the diagnosis presents no difficulty.

Fractures of the Lower End of the Femur are so closely related to the knee joint that they are considered in the next chapter.

KARL LUDLOFF, 1864–1945, *Professor, University Clinic for Orthopaedic Surgery, Frankfurt, Germany.*

Chapter 34

THE KNEE JOINT

For examination the lower limbs should be bare. The patient is examined first in the upright position, both front and back, secondly seated, thirdly supine and finally prone. In the supine position the hip joint should be examined if there is no obvious abnormality in the knee, as pain is sometimes referred from the hip to the knee. When the diagnosis is straightforward the examination may be concluded before the whole of the ritual is complete, but except with localized swellings it is unwise to curtail any part of the routine. In particular, to omit to examine the popliteal space may prove a matter of regret.

Effusion into the Knee Joint. To commence, consider the physical signs of fluid in the joint, irrespective of whether it is the result of a recent injury or not.

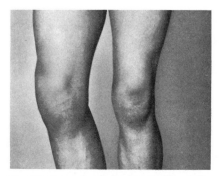

Fig. 820. Traumatic effusion into the knee joint. Note the obliteration of the normal outline of the joint when compared with the other knee.

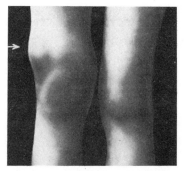

Fig. 821. Large effusion into the knee joint of many weeks' duration. Note the fullness caused by ballooning of the suprapatellar pouch.

Inspection with the Patient Standing. Fluid in the joint can often be seen (*Fig.* 820). Look particularly for a fullness above and on either side of the patella which suggests an effusion into the knee joint. In large effusions, especially in chronic cases, the distended suprapatellar pouch often is outlined as a horseshoe-shaped swelling (*Fig.* 821) because of wasting of the quadriceps femoris muscle.

Testing for the Presence of Fluid in the Knee Joint. The only conditions likely to be confused with an intra-articular effusion are: (*a*) superficial cellulitis; and (*b*) prepatellar bursitis. Fluid *in* the joint is demonstrated in the following ways:

Substantiating Continuity of a Supra- and Infrapatellar Swelling. If the amount of fluid is considerable, transmitted fluid impulse can be elicited from *below* the patella on one or other side of the ligamentum patellae, to that part of the swelling two finger-breadths *above* the upper border of the patella—a point manifestly well clear of a distended prepatellar bursa (*see* p. 517).

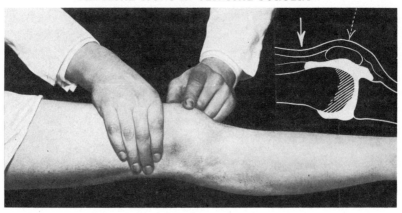

Fig. 822. Testing for a patellar tap.

The Patellar Tap is a pathognomonic sign. In the horizontal position a considerable amount of the excessive synovial fluid gravitates into the suprapatellar pouch. With one hand placed above the patella as shown in *Fig.* 822, exert downward and backward pressure on the suprapatellar pouch, and drive the fluid into the knee joint proper. With the index finger of the other hand, depress the patella with a sharp, jerky movement. Should the characteristic tap be felt, it is proof positive of the existence of excessive fluid in the joint. Too much fluid can prevent the patella being pushed on to the condyles; too little will not lift the patella free from them. There must be a *moderate* amount of fluid for this test to be positive.

Test for a Small Amount of Fluid in the Knee Joint. By compression, displace the fluid from one of the obliterated hollows on either side of the ligamentum patellae into the knee joint proper. In a good light, watch; the hollow refills slowly. Even a small effusion can be confirmed by this test.

Traumatic Synovitis is not a diagnosis; it is a sign of injury (Smillie). There is usually an interval of several hours between the injury and the appearance of the swelling, whereas in acute traumatic haemarthrosis swelling is apparent within half an hour. Varying mixtures of blood and synovial fluid alter this latent period.

Haemarthrosis. In addition to the short interval between the injury and the appearance of the swelling, that the joint is filled mainly with blood, as opposed to synovial fluid, is indicated by the following signs: the knee feels slightly warmer than normal; the swelling is tense and extremely tender; later it feels doughy.

Even more emphatically, haemarthrosis is not a diagnosis but a sign of intra-articular ligamentous tearing, of a torn meniscus, or of a fracture into the joint, each of which must be sought. An X-ray is thus essential, but in addition, in order to elucidate the signs to be described, if no fracture is found, aspiration of the joint with full aseptic precautions and under anaesthesia is necessary.

In cases where the signs point to haemarthrosis, yet the accident was trivial or non-existent, focus attention on the possibility of haemophilia (*see* p. 438).

Examinations of the Movements of a Recently Injured Knee Joint may yield

Ian S. Smillie, *Contemporary Emeritus Professor of Orthopaedic Surgery, University of Dundee, Scotland.*

valuable information, e.g. localized tenderness over the medial collateral ligament; loss of full extension. On the other hand, the examination is often disappointingly uninformative because voluntary muscle spasm of an apprehensive patient makes detailed examination impossible. *In these circumstances any attempt to move the joint must be postponed for a few days*, when the examination is likely to be attended by more satisfactory results.

Testing Flexion and Extension. Should there be free fluid in the joint, full flexion will be curtailed. Likewise full extension is not possible, the fluid preventing the last part of the movement of the leg and thigh into a straight line.

Examination in a Case other than One of Recent Trauma. Needless to say the presence of a scar (or scars) should be noted, and, if present, the patient interrogated.

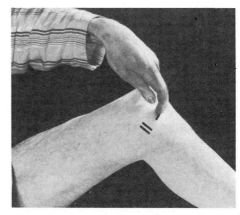

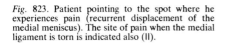
Fig. 823. Patient pointing to the spot where he experiences pain (recurrent displacement of the medial meniscus). The site of pain when the medial ligament is torn is indicated also (ll).

The Pointing Test. If pain is the leading symptom ask the patient to point with one finger to its site. In torn medial meniscus this sign is often particularly valuable (*Fig.* 823). If the patient has felt 'something moving about in the joint', ask him to try to find the 'joint mouse' himself.

Wasting of the Quadriceps. Inspection and comparison with the opposite side will reveal any wasting of the quadriceps muscle; indeed, a better estimation of loss of volume and of tone of this tripartite muscle is obtained by inspection and palpation than by the use of a tape-measure. This is true particularly of a limb which is well covered with subcutaneous fat. The eyes should be directed especially to the vastus medialis, which, in internal derangements of the knee joint of some standing, wastes first and wastes most.

While if the knee joint is insecure the vastus medialis wastes apace, the converse is also true, for when this muscle is paralysed or irreparably injured, an otherwise normal knee joint becomes insecure.

Testing Movements. The Neutral Position is with the knee straight. Ask the patient to bend his knee as fully as possible (maximum flexion = 135°, i.e. until the calf and the back of the thigh are contiguous), and then to straighten it. Measure the degree of flexion and extension attained.

Palpation of the Joint. Acquire the habit of looking upon the knee joint, not as a mere hinge, but as a two-component joint. The patello-femoral component often is neglected in routine examination, yet not infrequently it can provide helpful, and sometimes cardinal, information regarding intra-articular pathology. While the patient is still lying on his back, palpate deeply and systematically beneath the overhanging edges of the patella for tenderness. Next, push the patella medially and laterally. This permits direct palpation of a small portion of the articular surface of the femoral condyles.

Passive Movements. With the left hand laid upon the joint, grasp the ankle with the right; flex and extend the knee joint several times (*see Fig.* 29, p. 16), noting if there is joint crepitus or a click. Crepitus may be felt by moving the patella on the underlying femoral condyles.

Significance of a Click. An intra-articular click is not necessarily due to a torn meniscus. A painless click as the patella moves over the condyle sometimes occurs in a normal joint, especially during childhood. The importance of a click is, 'Is it accompanied by discomfort or pain?'; 'Does the patient associate the sound with the "sickening" sensation that heralds the attack of which he complains?' If not, (*a*) test the lateral mobility of the patella (*see* p. 515); (*b*) test the other knee joint—a click occurring in a normal joint frequently is bilateral.

Differential Diagnosis of a Click. An intra-articular click can in some respects be simulated by the sound of a snapping tendon such as is produced by the semi-tendinosus slipping around and becoming hitched over the medial condyle, or the tendon of biceps over the head of the fibula, or the edge of the iliotibial band over the lateral condyle—or any tendon in the neighbourhood becoming hooked over an exostosis. Provided the phenomenon can be reproduced at the time of the clinical examination, an extra-articular snap should not be confused with an intra-articular click, for the extra-articular sound is a dull thud, often accompanied by a shudder, and the tendon implicated can be seen and felt as a tense sinew.

INTERNAL DERANGEMENTS OF THE KNEE JOINT

This is an old term* which is something of a blunderbuss, and includes such conditions as a tear of a collateral ligament and bruising of the infrapatellar fatpad, neither of which is intra-articular. It is hoped that with increasing experience the reader will use the term less, and with augmented clinical acumen will specify *which* derangement is present. The term covers the conditions which follow, up to but excluding, 'Injuries of the Extensor Apparatus' (p. 513). It is convenient to deal first with lesions of the menisci, the commonest cause by far.

LESIONS OF THE MENISCI

These are very common in males, particularly among footballers and coalminers. With the knee flexed and weight-bearing, a twist occurs with sufficient violence to tear a meniscus. As usually the twist is in a medial direction, and as the medial is longer and more securely attached than the lateral, the medial meniscus

---

* Introduced by William Hey in 1784. Smillie notes that the abbreviation 'I.D.K.' also stands for 'I don't know'. The recent introduction of the arthroscope which enables inspection of the interior of the joint has, in expert hands, helped reduce the number of fruitless surgical explorations of the knee joint.

is injured more often than the lateral meniscus in the ratio of about 5:1 (Smillie). The types of medial meniscal rupture, in order of frequency, are: (1) bucket-handle in which the cartilage can swing laterally to repose in the commodious interior of the joint, and back again to its original position, but it is never anchored; (2) anterior horn tear; (3) posterior horn tear (*Fig.* 824).

In Japan the ratio of medial to lateral is 1:2 (Watanabe) largely due to an increased incidence of discoid meniscus (*see* p. 509).

A meticulous history is almost always a helpmate and usually a co-partner of physical signs, but in this instance the history often assumes the major role—at any rate in the bucket-handle tear of the medial meniscus—for in these cases between the attacks there are often no physical signs whatsoever. So it comes about that the bucket-handle lesion has been called the 'cartilage of symptoms' as opposed to the posterior horn tear, which has been styled the 'cartilage of signs' (Teece) because the history is indefinite and reliance must be placed on physical signs. An injury severe enough to cause a torn cartilage seldom allows of normal activities afterwards (e.g. completion of a game of football).
'Giving Way' or 'Letting Down'. This is a symptom for which the clinician should listen carefully, but not suggest to the patient. While walking or, more frequently, when stepping off a kerb or proceeding down stairs, the affected knee gives way and the patient falls. It occurs particularly with posterior horn tears, but also with old rupture of an anterior cruciate ligament, extreme quadriceps muscle weakness and loose body in the knee, conditions which must be differentiated as described in the sections that follow.

Fig. 824. Tears of the medial meniscus. (1) Bucket-handle. (2) Anterior horn. (3) Posterior horn.

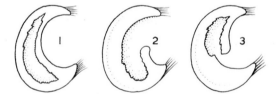

Locking. Only very occasionally is the patient brought with his knee locked. His statement that his knee has previously 'locked' must alwayys be qualified. Ask him to demonstrate the position in which the knee became fixed (10° short of full extension is the position of true locking). Next inquire exactly what he was doing and what he felt at the time of the fixation. Lastly, interrogate him as to how the knee became unlocked. If the locking was true, unlocking occurred with even more dramatic suddenness than the locking. Always listen carefully for the term in the patient's history, but never suggest it to him. Actually the word is unfortunate, because a locked door will not move, whereas a locked knee will flex but not extend. It should be noted that in only 40 per cent of cases of torn meniscus is there a history of locking, and in half of these it occurs at the original accident. In addition to a loose body (*see* p. 512) only a bucket-handle tear and a partially detached tag of anterior cruciate ligament are capable of causing the knee joint to lock. The phenomenon is due to one or other of these three objects becoming rammed between the joint surfaces at the commencement of the screw-home movement of the medial femoral condyle.

MASAKE WATANABE, *Director of Orthopaedic Surgery, Teishin Hospital, Tokyo. Pioneered arthroscopy of the knee joint.*
LENNOX G. TEECE, *Contemporary Orthopaedic Surgeon, Royal Prince Alfred Hospital, Sydney, Australia.*

In recurrent cases the patient learns to unlock the joint by shaking the limb or by performing a rotary motion of the joint.

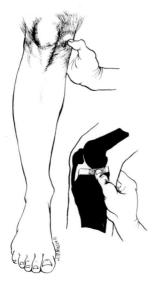

Fig. 825. Method of seeking tenderness over that part of the medial meniscus which lies beneath the medial ligament. Tenderness localized here strongly favours an injury of the medial meniscus.

Clicking is only a subsidiary sign. Of itself, it is not evidence of a tear. In conjunction with other positive features of ruptured meniscus it carries some weight in favour of the diagnosis.

Atrophy of the Quadriceps. At least some wasting and loss of tone of the quadriceps (especially of the vastus medialis muscle) are present in every case of a tear of some duration.

Effusion always follows the original tearing of a meniscus because of the concomitant synovial trauma. Subsequent recurring incidents of locking or 'giving way' of the knee joint are also followed by effusion, but the more frequent the incidents the smaller the consequent outpouring; indeed, a time may come in cases of recurrent displacement where there is no demonstrable effusion at all.

Medial Meniscus. *Tenderness Anterior to the Medial Ligament* becoming apparent as the knee is extended suggests a bucket-handle tear, the cartilage being extruded between the bone ends in this position.

Tenderness Over the Medial Ligament at the level of the joint line (*Fig.* 825): this is the most constant and reliable region of localized tenderness in injuries of the medial meniscus (Smillie). Frequently, tenderness can be elicited here with the knee joint flexed, whereas in the extended position it was indefinite.

Tenderness Posterior to the Medial Ligament suggests a tear of the posterior horn of the medial meniscus.

*Apley's Test.** The patient lies on his face on a couch. He must lie well towards the side of the couch of the affected knee, and the clinician stands on this side. He proceeds to grasp the foot of the affected side with both hands, and then

---

* In the author's opinion this test is easier to interpret and more reliable for the beginner than the classical McMurray's Test which was previously also described.

ALAN G. APLEY, *Contemporary Orthopaedic Surgeon, St. Thomas's Hospital, London.*

flexes the knee to a right-angle. *Lateral* rotation of the foot is performed, and it is noted whether this causes pain or discomfort—normally it should cause no more than slight discomfort. Following this, the clinician places his knee on the patient's ham, so as to fix the femur and without changing the position of his hands he pulls the leg upwards while performing lateral rotation. If, on *distraction*, pain on rotation is produced, a lesion of the medial collateral ligament is diagnosed. The clinician then leans well over the patient, and repeats the test (*Fig.* 826) while his body-weight compresses the tibial plateau onto the condyles of the femur. If lateral rotation with the addition of compression produces increased pain, the *grinding* test is positive and a tear of the medial meniscus is diagnosed.

To test the *lateral* meniscus a reversed test is performed, the foot being rotated *medially* instead of laterally.

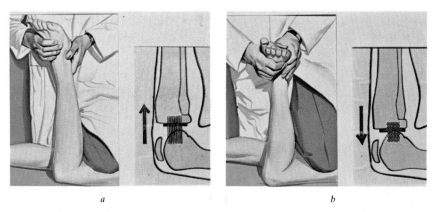

a   b

Fig. 826. *a*, Apley's distraction test. Pain signifies damage to the medial ligament. *b*, Apley's grinding test. Pain signifies damage to the medial cartilage.

Lateral Meniscus. The original accident is seldom definite; sometimes it is so trivial as to have been forgotten. Locking is uncommon, and incidents of this, or of the knee 'giving way', are not necessarily followed by effusion, as injury of the more mobile cartilage causes less synovial reaction. Moreover, to this vague, unhelpful symptomatology must .be added the fact that, for a reason as yet undetermined, *the pain can be referred to the medial aspect of the joint*. However, both tenderness to pressure and pain on manipulation are definitely on the lateral aspect, and coincide with the site of the lesion. Apley's test when modified to try out the lateral meniscus is valuable in confirming the diagnosis.

Combined Lesions of the Menisci. If the history and examination point to lesions of both medial menisci (or less frequently to both lateral menisci), such a diagnosis should be made and appropriate treatment instituted. Similarly, if the data are appropriate, lesions of both menisci of a single knee can be postulated.

Discoid Meniscus is an uncommon atavistic developmental anomaly, almost invariably of the lateral meniscus, in which the cartilage is not only discoid instead of semilunar in shape, but is unattached to the posterior tibial plateau. It is often associated with an unduly high head of the fibula. There is an unmistakable, and often easily audible, 'clunk' when the joint is flexed almost fully, and another 'clunk' when almost fully extended. Usually the patient is in his or her teens. A tear is very liable when the signs and symptoms of this are superadded to the 'clunk'.

LESIONS OF THE LIGAMENTS

Soon after the accident, which must have been considerable to have damaged one or more of the four ligaments of the knee, a haemarthrosis (*see* p. 504) is plainly evident. X-rays are essential for accurate diagnosis and in addition it is often necessary to aspirate the joint under strict aseptic conditions under general anaesthesia in the operating theatre as a diagnostic measure and as a preliminary to definitive treatment.

Rupture of the Anterior Cruciate Ligament comprises approximately 10 per cent of internal derangements of the knee joint. In cases of some standing a leading symptom is instability of the joint, especially on going downstairs.

The Drawer Sign (likened to opening and closing a drawer) is the ability to effect an abnormal amount of movement of the head of the tibia on the condyles of the femur with the knee joint flexed. In order to fix the limb the clinician sits on the patient's foot (*Fig.* 827). Having ascertained the amount of play between the two bones, repeat the manœuvre on the contralateral side for comparison. A positive drawer sign signifies a *dual* lesion, namely that the anterior cruciate and medial ligament (*see below*) have been torn.*

Rupture of the Anterior Cruciate Ligament of Long Standing. In cases of months' or years' duration, the knee joint can be hyperextended.

Rupture of the Posterior Cruciate Ligament is less common than the above. It is most often encountered as a result of the top of the tibia striking the dashboard when a front-seat passenger is thrown forwards—a frequent traffic accident. The signs are similar to those of rupture of the anterior ligament, the leading difference being that the drawer sign is positive backwards, i.e. there is movement of the tibia on the femur when *backward pressure* is exerted.

In a *dislocation of a knee joint*, a rare event, both cruciate ligaments are torn, resulting in a grossly unstable knee joint; common peroneal nerve and popliteal artery injury are common.

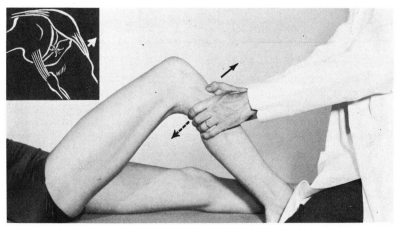

Fig. 827. Testing the knee joint for anteroposterior movement. When the anterior cruciate ligament is ruptured it is the anterior drawer sign that is positive, i.e. there is movement when the leg is *pulled forwards*. Note that the examiner is sitting on the patient's foot.

---

* This has been proved by exploring joints with long-standing injury in which the anterior cruciate ligament is found to be torn and the medial ligament to have healed with lengthening.

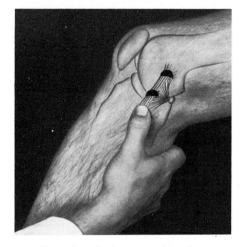

Fig. 828. Method of seeking an area of localized tenderness over the medial ligament. Maximum tenderness over the femoral attachment signifies a tear of this ligament. Maximum tenderness over the joint-line suggests a tear of the medial meniscus.

Traumatic Lesions of the Medial Ligament. Complete lesions are less frequent than lesions of the anterior cruciate ligament. The ligament is not, as is frequently depicted, a rectangular band—its posterior part fans out (*Fig.* 828) so as to make it triangular in shape, the apex of the triangle being attached posteriorly to the medial meniscus. A tear of this ligament is predominantly an injury of ball games and skiing and, because forcible valgus bending of the knee occurs more commonly than varus bending, it is the medial ligament that is ruptured more frequently than its fibular counterpart. Generally the femoral attachment is torn; much less frequently it is the tibial attachment that is implicated; when it comes to the portion of the ligament related to the joint-line, this is so intimately bound to the medial meniscus that, if this part is involved, the meniscus is torn also, and consequently the diagnosis of torn medial meniscus is rightly made.

INCOMPLETE RUPTURE. Although pain is severe at the time, it soon passes off sufficiently for the patient to continue his activities. In a matter of hours a moderate amount of pain returns. Some swelling (rarely ecchymosis) may be discernible over the site of the lesion.

Tenderness is present over the whole of the ligament, but is most acute over the site of the lesion (*Fig.* 828). In incomplete rupture there is *no increased lateral mobility of the joint* (*see below*), but the attempt to invoke such movement causes localized pain in the region of the damaged ligament.

Calcification of the Medial Ligament (Pellegrini–Stieda's Disease). As a rule the patient is a man between 25 and 40 years of age, and following traumatic synovitis (due to incomplete rupture of the medial ligament) with seemingly good progress, but not full recovery, limitation of movement of the knee joint becomes more pronounced. Often the medial aspect of the joint is tender to pressure. As complete extension is painful, the joint is held in slight flexion. The cause is calcification in a ligament. The leading signs are that full extension of the joint is resisted and an attempt to straighten the knee causes pain limited to the femoral attachment of the ligament. In the early stages there is not only tenderness over, but thickening of, this part of the ligament. In 6–18 months a bony prominence can be felt and sometimes seen on the medial aspect of the femoral condyle. By this time the condition is much less disabling. Radiography confirms the diagnosis.

COMPLETE RUPTURE. Haemarthrosis will be present if the capsule of the joint is intact. If not, the blood drains into the periarticular tissues causing a brawny haematoma. All the positive signs of incomplete rupture are present; in addition,

AUGUSTO PELLEGRINI, *Emeritus Chief Surgeon, Ospedale Mellini, Chiari, Brescia, Italy.*
ALFRED STIEDA, 1869–1945, *Professor of Surgery, Königsberg, Germany.*

careful palpation rarely reveals a small, movable particle of bone in the region of the femoral attachment of the ligament. In recent cases lateral mobility of the knee joint is likely to be somewhat increased; later, if this ligament alone is ruptured, muscular spasm makes lateral mobility difficult to elicit, but the attempt to produce lateral rocking evokes pain on the inner side of the knee joint. As noted above *pronounced lateral mobility* of the knee joint occurring recently or remotely after an accident signifies that a *dual* injury occurred— complete rupture of the medial ligament plus rupture of the anterior cruciate ligament.

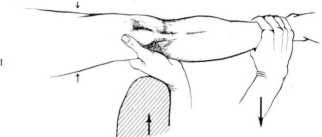

Fig. 829. Method of testing lateral mobility.

Test for Lateral Mobility. With the knee joint extended fully, try to elicit abnormal lateral movement in the manner shown in *Fig.* 829. With the patient seated, the leg is lifted by one of the examiner's hands, holding the back of the knee in such a way as to hook the fingers beneath the upper part of the popliteal space. The free hand is used to grasp the leg above the ankle. The examiner (who is standing) then braces his own knee against the back of his hand supporting the knee while with the other hand he exerts lateral traction on the leg in the direction of the right arrow. Compare the amount of lateral movement with that of the opposite knee joint. Normally there is virtually no lateral play.

Lesions of the Lateral Ligament. This is rounded and cord-like, attached to the lateral condyle of the femur above and to the head of the fibula below, and very strong. On this account, and because adduction injuries are comparatively rare, this ligament is torn much less frequently than its tibial counterpart. The resulting injury is, however, of great importance, because frequently complete rupture is associated with injury of the common peroneal nerve (*see* p. 412).

The ligament is palpated in much the same way as described for the medial ligament, noting that as a rule it is the *lower* (fibular) end of the ligament that is torn, and in cases of complete rupture not infrequently the head of the fibula is avulsed, and can be felt to move and to crepitate.

OTHER CAUSES OF INTERNAL DERANGEMENT

Hoffa's Disease (nipping of infrapatella fat pad or synovial fringes). The fat pads on *both* sides of the ligamentum patellae are tender to pressure ————————→ and forcible extension of the knee may reproduce the pain complained of. Usually the sufferer is obese and the condition is thus commoner in females.

Loose Body. Often the symptoms are not unlike those of a torn medial meniscus (including letting down), but the absence of a history of previous injury to the knee should direct attention to the possibility of a loose body. In the beginning, often the only complaint is vague pain in the joint, made worse by exercise, and attacks of

ALBERT HOFFA, 1859–1908, *Professor of Orthopaedic Surgery, Berlin.*

recurrent effusion that subside rapidly. To these symptoms one day is added locking, which occurs unheralded. Classically the patient volunteers the information that he 'feels something moving about in the joint'; a few declare that they have been able to locate and temporarily imprison a loose body between a finger and thumb.

A completely detached loose body is wont to be located at different positions on successive occasions. Sometimes it remains attached to a pedicle, occupies a more or less constant position, and can be found fairly readily on routine palpation. Request the patient who gives a history of locating a foreign body in a joint to repeat the feat, because for the clinician to fail to catch the 'joint mouse' and then for the patient to succeed, creates a situation best avoided.

In those of advancing years, osteoarthrosis is the most common cause of a loose body or bodies in a joint, in this instance a detached, or partially detached, osteophyte. Routine radiographs, ordinarily normal in internal derangements of the knee joint, are taken in every case to eliminate a loose body or bodies in general, and osteochondritis dissecans in particular.

Osteochondritis Dissecans is the commonest source of loose bodies in young persons, 80 per cent of whom are males. This curious disease is occasionally familial and often bilateral, and is characterized by ischaemic necrosis and partial detachment of a fragment of cartilage with a flake of underlying bone from the articular surface of the medial condyle of the femur, always in exactly the same place, viz. ⎯⎯⎯⎯⎯⎯⎯⎯⎯⎯→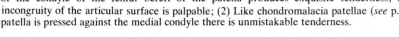
Possibly, it has been conjectured, this phenomenon is due to repeated impingement of the spine of the tibia against the condyle of a joint with a peculiar anatomical configuration.

In addition to letting down and locking, episodes of pain and effusion recur, until the fragment or fragments (rarely more than two) are extruded into the joint. The physical signs are as follows: (1) When the knee joint is flexed, firm pressure over the inferior aspect of the condyle of the femur bereft of the patella produces exquisite tenderness; occasionally incongruity of the articular surface is palpable; (2) Like chondromalacia patellae (*see* p. 515), if the patella is pressed against the medial condyle there is unmistakable tenderness.

INJURIES OF THE EXTENSOR APPARATUS OF THE KNEE

Viewed through morphological spectacles, the patella is a sesamoid bone situated in a tendon of the extensor muscular mechanism as it passes over the knee joint. Lesions due to sudden, violent contraction of the powerful quadriceps muscle (as might be occasioned on stumbling on a stair or catching the foot while walking or running) are considered here. To a remarkable extent, the site of the damage is governed by the patient's age (*Fig.* 830).

Rupture of the Rectus Femoris Muscle occurs at the musculotendinous junction, above the knee joint. The injury can be strongly suspected on inspection, for the knee is held in a semiflexed position and there is a hollow above the patella at the site of the tear. Later the contracted avulsed muscle fibres form a characteristic lump which becomes harder and larger when the patient is requested to brace the muscles of the thigh. Distal to the lump there is a gap into which the fingertips sink and below which the patella can be felt.

Transverse Fracture of the Patella is always accompanied by haemarthrosis. Separation of the fragments, which is frequent, occurs only if the medial and lateral expansions of the quadriceps tendon are torn also. When separation exists the joint is semiflexed, and the patient is unable to extend the knee actively. If there is a great deal of separation a layman knows what has happened. A useful method of examining a doubtful case is to pass the thumb-nail, held nearly horizontal with the surface, over the subcutaneous surface of the patella from above downwards (*Fig.* 831). With even the slightest separation, a sharp crevice is felt.

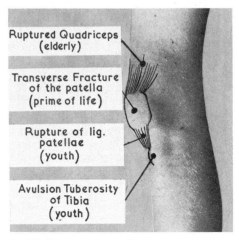

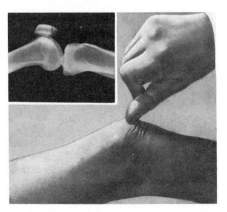

Fig. 830. The principal traumatic lesions of the extensor mechanism of the knee joint tend to vary with the patient's age.

Fig. 831. The thumb-nail test for fractured patella without separation. Inset shows the linear fracture present in this patient.

Rupture of the Ligamentum Patellae. A tender, puffy swelling occurs directly over the ligament. After the tumefaction has subsided somewhat, the breach in continuity of the ligament can be discerned by fingertip palpation. However, the pathognomonic sign of rupture of the infrapatellar ligament is an upward shift of the patella.

Osgood–Schlatter's Disease (Tibial apophysitis*), which is common, is a traction injury of the tuberosity into which the central part of the ligamentum patellae is inserted. Often the history of a specific injury is lacking. A young adolescent complains of pain after exercise in the region of the tuberosity of the tibia, and here a tender, bony lump (*Fig.* 832) is situated. Such signs are present regularly and are pathognomonic. Occasionally the disease is bilateral.

THE PATELLA

Recurrent Dislocation of the Patella. The tendency of females to genu valgum and the relatively small size of their patellae render them much more liable to recurrent dislocation, which occasionally is bilateral. Teenagers are especially prone.

Suddenly the knee gives way, and usually the patient falls to the ground. With recurrent dislocations the attacks are painful, followed by swelling of the joint. With chronicity these unpleasant accompaniments lessen. If the knee is

---

* *Apophysis.* Greek, ἀπό = from + φύσις = growth. A projection of some part, as of a bone.

ROBERT B. OSGOOD, 1873–1956, *Surgeon, Massachusetts General Hospital, Boston, Mass.*
CARL SCHLATTER, 1864–1934, *Professor of Surgery, Zürich.*

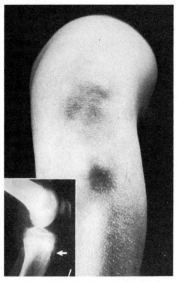

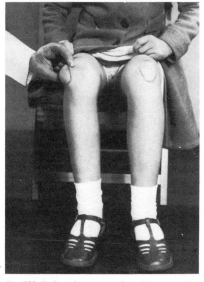

Fig. 832. Osgood–Schlatter's disease. Inset shows the partially avulsed apophysis.

Fig. 833. Referred as a case of possible tear of the medial meniscus, the patella could be manipulated into the position shown when the knee was flexed.

seen while the patella is dislocated the diagnosis cannot be mistaken. Between attacks look for:

1. *Wasting of the Quadriceps.* In cases of some standing the rectus femoris and especially the vastus medialis muscles are wasted.

2. *Excessive Lateral Mobility of the Patella* suggests the possibility of recurrent dislocation which is possible only when the knee joint is flexed while the patella is displaced *laterally* (*Fig.* 833). More usually the patient resists this manœuvre, saying that it brings on the pain ('apprehension test'). So frequently is torn medial meniscus diagnosed that every woman giving a history consistent with that of an internal derangement of the knee joint should be suspected of suffering from recurrent dislocation of the patella until the contrary has been proved.

Chondromalacia Patellae is characterized by fissuring and flaking of the articular surface of the patella, commencing on its medial facet. In some cases there is a history of a direct blow on the patella; in others it is an aftermath of recurrent dislocation of the patella; but in the majority there is no apparent cause. Often the patient is a young adult female, or a male who cycles for sport. Pain is made worse by kneeling or by climbing or descending stairs, when contraction of the quadriceps femoris pulls the patella against the femoral condyles. Examination often reveals a small effusion but after this has subsided, usually movements of the knee joint are full and painless, but sometimes there is a 'catch' when flexing or extending the knee joint. In some instances a tender, irregular, hypertrophied synovial fringe can be felt at the margins of the patellar cartilage. Localized pain on pressing the patella against a condyle, usually on the medial aspect, is present invariably. When the knee joint is moved while keeping a finger on the patella so as to press it against the condyles, unmistakable patellofemoral crepitus becomes apparent. Unless advanced, radiography is of no assistance because the bone is not involved.

In a few patients the disease becomes chronic, when detached or partially detached flakes set up general arthritis of the joint, and eventually the condition becomes indistinguishable from that of osteoarthrosis, which in fact is present.

Stellate Fracture of the Patella arises as a result of a direct blow on the patella. The signs are very similar to those of a transverse fracture, with the obvious difference that the transverse crevice of the latter is not in evidence. Bruising of the skin is much more marked.

ARTHRITIS OF THE KNEE

Acute Pyogenic Arthritis is relatively common in children. The general signs are pronounced. The affected knee joint is swollen and is held in constant, moderate flexion. The overlying skin is sometimes slightly reddened, and is always warm when compared with that of the opposite side. There is exquisite pain on the slightest movement.

It is imperative to exclude osteomyelitis of one of the bones entering into the formation of the joint, particularly the lower end of the femur, for in these cases there is often a 'sympathetic' effusion into the joint, which later sometimes becomes purulent (*see* p. 418).

Tuberculosis of the Knee Joint. The typical case at the present time is a patient, usually between 9 and 30 years of age, complaining of swelling of the joint (*see Fig.*706, p. 436) accompanied by moderate pain of several months' duration. Often there is a history of injury. Usually there is a substantially full range of movement although in the more acute cases slight flexion deformity is present. There may or may not be an effusion, but in the latter event, if the patella is pushed laterally, thickening of the synovia is likely to be discerned. Frequently enlargement of one or more lymph nodes will be discovered in the ipsilateral groin. Examination of the aspirated effusion or synovial biopsy are recommended for absolute diagnosis.

Osteoarthrosis. The knee joint is a more frequent site than any other. Creaking knee joints and difficulty in mounting stairs are one of the penalties of advancing years, and these, particularly common in obese, short, females, require no special comment. Monarticular osteoarthrosis of the knee is much less common than the polyarticular form, and almost always it has a traumatic background. An old bony injury, a long-standing internal derangement (even if eventually remedied by an operation), recurrent dislocation of the patella or genu valgum are all precursors. Crepitus is elicited easily, and it is of the creaking, muffled variety when the articular outgrowths are cartilaginous; later, harsh grating is experienced. Osteophytes should be sought by systematic palpation.

Rheumatoid Arthritis is now relatively common. Other stigmata may be present (*see* p. 483). X-rays, blood tests and, in doubtful cases, a synovial biopsy are necessary to confirm the diagnosis.

THE POPLITEAL SPACE

When the knee is being examined the popliteal space is liable to be overlooked. It is examined best with the patient lying face downwards (*Fig.* 834). Cystic lesions (*see below*) are not uncommon, while the following entities are seldom seen.

Popliteal Aneurysm. Syphilis is now rare but atherosclerotic aneurysms are still encountered and the popliteal space remains the commonest site of a peripheral aneurysm (*Fig.* 835). Consequently in a mature or elderly person always test a centrally placed swelling of the popliteal space for an expansile impulse (*see* p. 27). The condition is frequently bilateral.

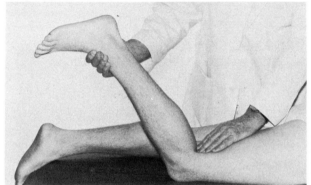

Fig. 834. Palpating the popliteal space.

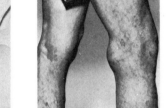

Fig. 835. Popliteal aneurysm.

A Popliteal Abscess is often deep seated; there is but slight fullness of the space. The patient inclines to keep the knee joint somewhat flexed; full extension causes pain. When suspected, the foot and leg must be scrutinized for an infected focus. Commonly the abscess arises from infection of the lymph nodes of the space via lymphatics, from a sore on the heel. In this situation fluctuation occurs late; tender induration should suffice to make the diagnosis.

Nerve Tumours. When a patient presents with what appears to be a typical enlarged bursa in the popliteal space, but it is tender and, when pressed, pain shoots down to the foot, almost certainly the swelling is a tumour of either the tibial or (if in relation to the deep aspect of the biceps tendon) the common peroneal nerve.

CYSTS ABOUT THE KNEE

These swellings are common and no candidate in a surgical examination can expect to pass if he misdiagnoses one of them.

In Front of the Knee. These are the commonest.

Prepatellar Bursitis (Housemaid's Knee) is accounted the most elementary diagnosis in surgery. In this servantless age it is certainly an anachronism to retain its synonym. Today housewives and charwomen rely more on the electric vacuum cleaner than on the brush and dustpan, and coal-miners are those chiefly affected.

The prepatellar bursa is subcutaneous. It covers the lower half of the patella and the upper half of the ligamentum patellae (*Fig.* 836), and the bursa results from friction between the skin and the patella. The distended, uninfected bursa constitutes a most typical circumscribed swelling which permits the sign of fluctuation to be demonstrated in an arresting manner. The bursa is particularly liable to become infected, in which event classic signs of inflammation are found (*see* p. 31).

Infrapatellar Bursitis (Clergyman's Knee) (*Fig.* 837). Again, although the synonym calls attention to kneeling with the trunk upright, and consequent trauma in the region of the tibial tuberosities, as opposed to the patellae (when kneeling 'on all fours'), it is not now representative. Roof-felters, parquet-floor and carpet layers, and those who follow trades in which this type of kneeling is indispensable, are the chief sufferers.

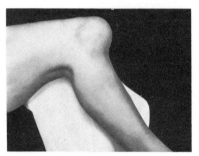

Fig. 836. Prepatellar bursitis.

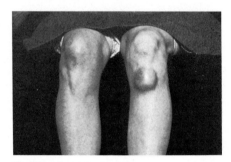

Fig. 837. Infrapatellar bursitis.

At the Back of the Knee. It will be profitable to refresh the mind concerning the relationship of tendons and muscles that are inserted, or arise, in the region of the medial boundaries of the popliteal space (*Fig.* 838).

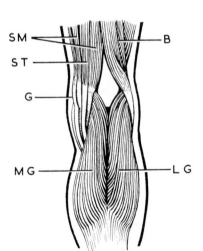

Fig. 838. Tendons and muscles at the back of the knee joint. S M, Semimembranosus; S T, Semitendinosus; G, Gracilis; M G, Medial head of gastrocnemius; B, Biceps femoris; L G, Lateral head of gastrocnemius.

Semimembranosus Bursa is the commonest swelling of the popliteal space. It lies between the medial head of the gastrocnemius and the semimembranosus tendon, slightly more medial and higher than a Baker's cyst and is tense when the knee joint is extended, flaccid when the joint is flexed. If compressed it remains stationary in size—for it does not communicate with the joint. There is

WILLIAM M. BAKER, 1839–1896, *Surgeon, St. Bartholomew's Hospital, London.*

no crepitus on moving the joint, the excursions of which are full unless the cyst is very large. It is found in both sexes from childhood to middle age.

Baker's Cyst. When a swelling in the popliteal space is situated more centrally, and the patient is over 40 years of age, it is likely to be a Baker's cyst, which sometimes is bilateral and is a pressure diverticulum of the synovial membrane through a hiatus in the capsule of the knee joint. It is always located in the midline at or below the level of the joint and stands out when the knee is fully extended but, unless very large, disappears when the joint is even slightly flexed.

Having ascertained that the swelling is cystic, compress it; should the lumen of the stalk be patent, as it is except in cases of long standing, some of the contents of the cyst can be displaced into the knee joint, rendering it more flaccid. Because the communicating channel sometimes is small, the pressure must be exerted for some moments. Next test the joint for signs of osteoarthrosis. As a rule, these and other bursal swellings around the knee are practically painless, and are not tender: also more often than not they are semitranslucent. Unlike bursae situated on the anterior aspect, these swellings seldom become inflamed.

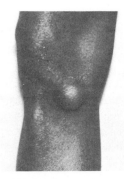

Fig. 839. Enlargement of the bursa anserina.

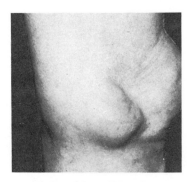

Fig. 840. Cyst of the medial meniscus.

On the Medial Side

*The Bursa Anserina.** Interposed between the tendons of the sartorius, gracilis and semitendinosus (*see Fig.* 838) superficially, and the medial ligament deep to it, lies the bursa anserina, which, when distended, comes to the surface in the position shown in *Fig.* 839.

Cyst of the Medial Meniscus (Fig. 840). If small, the patient is unlikely to be aware of its presence, and complains of a dull pain in the region of the cartilage, accentuated by violent exercise and relieved by rest. As it becomes larger the pain becomes less, and often ceases. A small cyst is situated directly over the line of the joint, but, because an enlarging cyst follows the path of least resistance, as it enlarges it is liable to overlap the line of the joint more in one direction than in another.

While still comparatively small, the cyst is wont to disappear on acute flexion of the joint and to reappear on extension, reaching its maximum dimensions when the knee joint is nearly, but not quite, fully extended. This *disappearing sign* is common (Pisani).

The cyst can protrude through the tibial collateral ligament, or come to the surface in front of, or behind, the ligament. By the time the patient presents, a cyst of the medial meniscus tends to be much larger than a cyst of the lateral meniscus, and is less fixed than its counterpart.

---

* *Anserina.* Latin, *anser* = a goose. Likened to a goose's foot.

ANTHONY J. PISANI, *Clinical Professor of Orthopedic Surgery, Bellevue Hospital, New York.*

On the Lateral Side

Cyst of the Lateral Meniscus. Inexplicably this is encountered much more often. The disappearing sign discussed above is common. The cyst may enlarge in a posterior direction and appear in the lateral part of the popliteal space but most emerge around the posterior border of the lateral ligament (*Fig.* 841). It is not uncommon for a cyst of a *lateral* meniscus to give rise to sufficient pain to cause the patient to seek advice before he has discovered the swelling. When too small to be seen, it feels intensely hard and is tender to pressure. It is completely immobile.

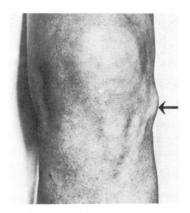

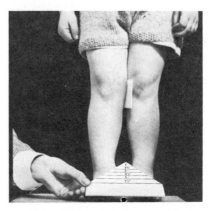

Fig. 841. Cyst of the lateral meniscus.

Fig. 842. Genu valgum. The distance between the malleoli is being measured by a graduated wedge.

DEFORMITIES OF THE KNEE

In assessing the first two conditions mentioned below, the patella must face directly forwards before drawing any conclusions (*see Fig.* 868, p. 540).

Genu Valgum (Knock-knee). There is curvature of the leg with the apex of the convexity disposed medially at the level of the knee, usually bilateral and so common in infancy that it hardly can be regarded as an abnormality. At 3 years 20 per cent of children have knock-knees of 5 cm or more. Over 7 years this percentage is reduced to 1 (Morley). Therefore, in order to ascertain whether the condition is regressing, progressing, or stationary, it is necessary to measure and record the degree of genu valgum present, at intervals. This is done as follows: the inner border of the feet must be parallel, for outward rotation of the feet makes the separation of the knees greater. With his knees braced back, the patient grips a postcard between his condyles. The distance between the medial malleoli is measured (*Fig.* 842). When the deformity is pronounced, the child walks in an unsightly manner; falls are common and synovitis is liable to develop from joint strain.

The common type is *idiopathic*, and consequent upon the somewhat faster growth at the medial compared with the lateral side of the lower epiphysis of the femur. The next common cause of the deformity is *laxity of ligaments* which allows the knee to sag inwards, especially if the child is overweight. When the deformity is unilateral or excessive, an underlying cause of *softening of bones* should be sought.

Genu Varum (Bow-leg) is as a rule bilateral and less common than genu valgum. Up to the age of 2 years it can be regarded as normal. The abnormal convexity

AVISA J. M. MORLEY, *Contemporary, formerly Clinical Assistant, Royal National Orthopaedic Hospital, London.*

is disposed laterally. As a rule it is restricted to the tibia, and is usually the result of a local error of growth of the upper tibial epiphysis but can involve the femur or both bones. The patient walks with the feet separated widely and the toes turned in. In all but minor degrees an obvious waddle is present. In early childhood, while bulky napkins are worn, an apparent bow-leg is usual ('napkin gait').

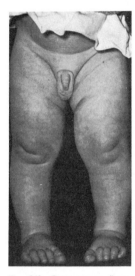

Fig. 843. Genu varum (bow-leg).

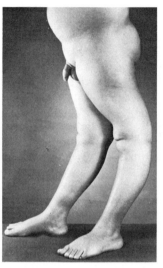

Fig. 844. Genu recurvatum (congenital type).

To measure the degree of bowing the patient should lie supine, the knees extended, the patellae facing the ceiling, and the medial malleoli touching one another. The distance between the knees at the joint line is then measured. Now that rickets is almost extinct, at any rate in developed countries, most examples in childhood (*Fig.* 843) are idiopathic. In jockeys the condition is occupational, and is due to stretched ligaments. Paget's disease of bone (*see* p. 426) is a common cause in the elderly.

Deformity is the only symptom. In well-marked cases persisting into adult life, osteoarthrosis frequently develops eventually.

Genu Recurvatum usually is congenital, and is due to malposition in utero, but the deformity can result from contracture of the quadriceps femoris muscle and from malunion of various fractures about the knee. The joint is hyperextended (*Fig.* 844) and the ability to flex it is very limited, or virtually absent. In the congenital type the patella is small or absent, and in well-marked cases the femoral condyles can be felt in the popliteal space. The hamstring muscles are palpable as tense cords. Osteochondritis dissecans (*see* p. 513) is a frequent complication.

FRACTURES ABOUT AND INTO THE KNEE JOINT

The clinical features only of the common varieties will be considered. X-rays are necessary for the diagnosis of others, and for confirmation of the following:

Supracondylar Fracture of the Femur is confined to adults. There is much swelling above the patella, extreme tenderness and the patient cannot move the limb. As a rule, displacement is not great, but in some instances the lower fragment is rotated backwards by the pull of the gastrocnemius muscle, viz. ⎯⎯⎯⎯⎯⎯⎯⎯⎯→ 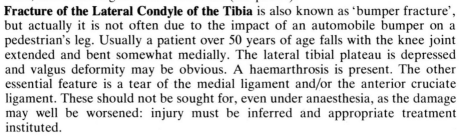 and the shaft overlies it in front. The cardinal importance of this is that the popliteal vessels are liable to compression. Therefore *always palpate the foot pulses* (*see* p. 379) when this fracture is suspected. This applies with the comparable fracture in children (*displacement of the lower femoral epiphysis*).

Femoral Condyle Fractures. One condyle may be driven upwards, or both condyles wedged apart from a T-shaped fracture into the joint. There is obvious widening of the transverse diameter of the knee, and all the signs of haemarthrosis (*see* p. 504).

Fracture of the Lateral Condyle of the Tibia is also known as 'bumper fracture', but actually it is not often due to the impact of an automobile bumper on a pedestrian's leg. Usually a patient over 50 years of age falls with the knee joint extended and bent somewhat medially. The lateral tibial plateau is depressed and valgus deformity may be obvious. A haemarthrosis is present. The other essential feature is a tear of the medial ligament and/or the anterior cruciate ligament. These should not be sought for, even under anaesthesia, as the damage may well be worsened: injury must be inferred and appropriate treatment instituted.

Chapter 35

THE LEG AND ANKLE JOINT

Fracture of the Tibia and Fibula is a common accident in men in the prime of life. This dual fracture is the commonest compound fracture and becomes so as a result of a concomitant laceration of the overlying tissues produced either by a direct injury or by a sharp end of one bone (usually the upper fragment of the tibia) transfixing the skin. Normally the medial side of the great toe, the medial malleolus and the medial side of the patella are in a straight line; this relationship is lost when both the tibia and the fibula are fractured. Frequently the foot is rolled outwards and deformity is obvious, in which event no attempt should be made to palpate or move the leg for fear of inflicting further damage, but the pulsation of the dorsal pedis artery should be sought. As a rule the fibula is broken at a higher level than the tibia.

Fracture of the Shaft of the Tibia alone. *a. A Young Child*, after a fall, although able to stand, refuses to take weight on the injured leg. When recumbent, active movements of the knee are possible and there is little amiss to be made out on inspection, for the fracture is a long spiral one, without displacement. Localized bone tenderness (*see Fig.* 701, p. 433) confirms the necessity for an X-ray.

b. An Adult. A direct blow, such as a kick, is liable to result in a transverse or slightly oblique fracture, and although the skin is often broken the wound is frequently superficial. At first it appears that the fracture is compound, but on examination in the operating theatre this is found not to be so, i.e. the wound does not extend down to the bone.

Fracture of the Shaft of the Fibula alone. A direct blow on the fibula sometimes causes a transverse fracture at the site of impact. This fracture is confined to adults. As a rule the patient is able to stand. Localized bone tenderness is present (*see Fig.* 701, p. 433).

Springing the Fibula. With the patient lying supine on a couch, the clinician stands on the medial aspect of the affected limb and grasps the knee in one hand and the heel in the other. Placing his own knee against the *medial* aspect of the midleg, the limb is pressed against this fulcrum. In this way the crack in the fibula is opened up and pain occurs at the fracture site. Fractures of the lower end of the fibula are so often associated with injuries of the ankle joint that they are best considered with them (*see* p. 530).

Stress Fracture of the Tibia is an incomplete fracture involving only the cortex of the bone. It is confined to athletes,* ballet dancers and soldiers in training and manifests itself insidiously as a dull, gnawing pain in the shin coming on at shorter and shorter intervals after strenuous exercise, lasting for some hours, continuing at night, but rarely severe enough to keep the patient awake for long periods. Eventually it necessitates giving up the exercise that caused the lesion. Physical signs are important, because at first the fracture may be missed on poor-quality radiographs.

Deep Palpation over the Shin reveals a localized area of acute tenderness nearly always along the medial border of the subcutaneous surface of the tibia.

Springing the Tibia. The technique is the same as for springing the fibula (*see above*) but the clinician stands on the lateral aspect of the affected limb and places his own knee against the *lateral* aspect of the midleg. This opens up the crack of the medial cortex, causing pain.

Anterior Tibial Compartment Syndrome (March Gangrene). This more serious lesion occurs after unaccustomed or unusually severe exercise. Soldiers, hikers and footballers are the usual sufferers. Characteristically the first symptom, stiffness followed by pain in the muscular compartment, is delayed for several hours after the exercise has finished; indeed, often until late in the evening. Before morning the anterolateral aspect of the leg has become swollen and extremely tender; it is warmer than the opposite side. By daybreak a blush of the overlying skin can be perceived. So constant is this train of events that, if the condition is known, the diagnosis is simple; if not, usually

---

* Known among athletes as 'sore shin' in Britain and as 'shin splints' in the USA.

phlebothrombosis is diagnosed. Unless the tight fascia is incised promptly, the underlying muscles may become gangrenous (*Fig.* 845).

Dropped Big-toe is an early sign of this condition; extensor hallucis longus becomes paralysed as a result of increased tension in the muscular compartment and the patient cannot extend the toe.

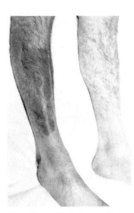

Fig. 845. Gangrene of the muscles in anterior tibial compartment syndrome.

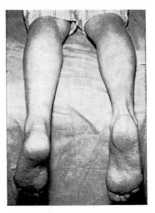

Fig. 846. Rupture of the left tendo Achillis. The patient is attempting plantar flexion of both feet.

THE CALF AND THE TENDO ACHILLIS*

Rupture of the Tendo Achillis. As a rule the patient is a male about 50 years of age. More often than not the rupture is complete and occurs at the narrowest part of the tendon, about 5 cm above its insertion. The injury is not infrequent in tennis, badminton and squash players. There is sudden, agonizing pain, as though the patient had received a direct blow upon the tendon: he is unable even to limp without severe pain. The signs are: when observed in the position shown in *Fig.* 846 the affected foot is held in less equinus than normal. There is a gap into which a finger can be inserted at the site of a complete rupture. The belly of calf muscles appears as a ball-like lump retracted towards the popliteal space. There is an abnormal range of passive movement of the ankle joint as compared with the normal side (absent in partial rupture). If in any doubt, the following test should be applied:

Simmonds's Test. The patient lies prone, the calf is squeezed transversely. If the tendon is intact or incompletely ruptured, the foot, which should project beyond the end of the couch, is seen to plantar flex. If the tendon is completely ruptured, the foot remains still.

Attrition Rupture of the Tendo Achillis. An incomplete rupture of the tendo Achillis is converted into a complete rupture some weeks later. The condition is comparatively painless. The patient falls to the ground, believing that he has been tripped by someone behind him.

A man was walking along the Whitechapel Road, London. He fell down, and rose in anger, hitting the man behind him, who happened to be a policeman! Later, in court, he was discharged when it was explained that he had, in fact, suffered this injury (Robinson).

Tear of the Soleus occurs at the musculotendinous junction. Severe pain and

---

* Achilles, when an infant, was dipped into the river Styx to render him invulnerable. Thenceforth he remained unprotected only in the heel by which he was held. (Greek mythology.)

Franklin A. Simmonds, *Contemporary Orthopaedic Surgeon, Rowley Bristow Hospital, Pyrford, Surrey.*
Walter C. Robinson, *Contemporary Orthopaedic Surgeon, St. Charles's Hospital, London.*

tenderness are experienced half-way up the calf. These are the signs formerly attributed to torn plantaris tendon, a condition which probably does not occur. **Calf Haematoma.** *See* p. 391. **The Heel.** *See* p. 543.

ULCERS OF THE LEG AND THEIR DIFFERENTIAL DIAGNOSIS

The lower leg is the seat of an ulcer many times more often than the whole of the rest of the surface of the body. To be familiar with the diagnosis of the various forms of leg ulcers that are seen the world over is a basic necessity; for those practising in the tropics or subtropics there are other kinds of ulcers that must be recognized in addition.

A Venous Ulcer* arises as a result of increased venous hydrostatic pressure, which causes local oedema, with its low exchange of oxygen and metabolites. Oedematous tissue, especially skin, is more vulnerable to trauma than healthy tissue, and is far less able to combat infection. As a rule, venous ulcers either coexist with incompetent superficial (varicose) veins, or with incompetent perforating veins (i.e. anastomotic veins piercing the deep fascia and linking the superficial with the deep veins) and are accurately termed 'varicose'. A very small percentage of venous ulcers develop without superficial varicosities and are due to deep-vein thrombosis (post-thrombotic ulcer).

A Varicose Ulcer (*see Fig.* 80, p. 38) is shallow, never penetrates the deep fascia, and has irregularly shaped shelving edges, which are often characterized by a thin, blue line of growing epithelium. The base of the ulcer can be formed of (*a*) pink granulations, (*b*) pale granulations, (*c*) slough. The size is variable and in long-standing instances the ulcer may encircle the limb. Often one or more large feeding veins can be seen proceeding towards the edge of the ulcer (*Fig.* 847); when the surrounding skin is scarred, feeding veins are not visible, but can be detected sometimes by digital palpation as a soft furrow in the area of induration. The site of a varicose ulcer is remarkably constant; it is situated on the lower leg, viz. ⟶ 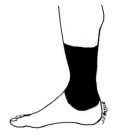 and is more commonly on the medial side (long saphenous vein) than on the lateral aspect of the leg (short saphenous vein); indeed, a considerable proportion lie above and behind the medial malleolus. If the ulcer is *not* situated in the region illustrated above it is improbable that it is venous in origin. Most varicose ulcers are painless but considerable infection and involvement of the saphenous nerve in scar tissue cause pain (Rose).

The precursor of a varicose ulcer is a splay of fine venules that courses from the medial (sometimes the lateral) malleolus, and spreads out to be lost beneath the thick skin of the heel and is known as the 'flare sign'.

Dermatitis is another precursor of ulceration. The commonly used term 'eczema' is incorrect as it is not a sensitivity reaction. The skin is scaly and inflamed with intense itching a subjective feature.

Pigmentation is a sign of venous stasis of long standing in the area in question. It is due to increasing intracapillary pressure, which results in diapedesis of red

---

* So named by John Gay in 1867. An alternative name is *gravitational* ulcer.

JOHN GAY, 1812–1885, *Surgeon, Royal Northern Hospital, London.*
SIDNEY S. ROSE, *Contemporary Surgeon, University Hospital of South Manchester.*

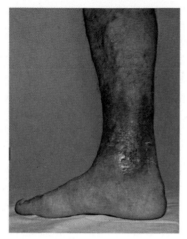

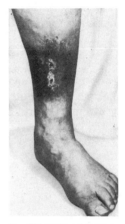

Fig. **847**. Venous ulcer with 'feeding' vein seen above.

Fig. **848**. Profound pigmentation in a case of venous ulcer of many years' duration.

blood corpuscles. Having passed through the walls of the anoxic capillaries, the corpuscles disintegrate and their contained haemoglobin is converted into haemosiderin, which stains tissues brown. Considerable pigmentation can be present in cases of varicose veins without ulceration, but as a rule an ulcer or ulcers (*Fig.* 848) of long standing, or the scar or scars thereof, are present.

Equinus deformity (*see Fig.* 865 *d*, p. 537) is occasionally seen after years of persistent varicose ulceration. It is the result of long-continued walking on the ball of the foot to relieve the pain caused in the region of the ulcer by full dorsiflexion of the ankle joint.

Post-thrombotic Ulcer. In contrast to a varicose ulcer, *pain is a fairly constant accompaniment of a post-thrombotic ulcer.* The common site is similar and, indeed, the ulcer differs in no way from the description given for varicose ulcer. Often there is a clear history of venous thrombosis following childbirth, an abdominal operation, or an accident to the leg, but if not examine the abdomen. Should the abdominal wall, which for this purpose includes the inguinal and the femoral regions, bear a scar, endeavour to obtain evidence of postoperative venous thrombosis. 'Bursting' pain in the limb (*see* p. 397) may be complained of if the deep veins are blocked. Varicose veins are lacking in spite of a very careful search, particularly of the areas where perforating veins are usually found (*see Fig.* 646, p. 394). A sign frequently present in an ulcerated leg, the seat of deep thrombosis, is extensive induration which often extends half-way up the calf, producing a peculiar, but characteristic, shape of the leg, which has been likened to an inverted beer-bottle. ———————————→
The skin is firm and seems to be tethered to underlying structures.

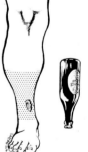

Carcinoma Secondary to a Venous Ulcer.* In a few neglected cases of venous ulcer, or for that matter almost any ulcer of the leg, notably tropical ulcer, carcinoma develops, in which even too often the diagnosis is written on the face of the ulcer (*Fig.* 849). It should be routine to examine the groin for enlarged lymph nodes. It is essential to biopsy any ulcer with a suspicious everted edge in any part of its circumference.

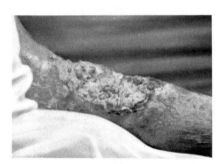

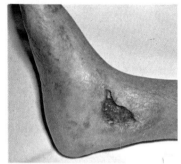

Fig. 849. Carcinoma arising in a venous ulcer of many years' standing.

Fig. 850. Arterial ulcer.

An Arterial Ulcer is rare when compared with venous ulcer. The essential difference is that the former is extremely painful. Varicose veins are likely to be absent, but their presence does not necessarily exclude the diagnosis. Men and women, usually over 60 years of age, are affected equally. The ulcer occurs most commonly in an area exposed to trauma (e.g. the shin; the lateral malleolus) and is deep (*Fig.* 850); not only does it penetrate the deep fascia, but not uncommonly tendons are exposed in its base. The pulsations of the pedal arteries are absent, and the foot is cold. Often there is a history of intermittent claudication and sometimes discoloration of one or more toes is present, in which event the onset of gangrene is imminent.

Congenital Arteriovenous Fistula (*see* p. 398) is a rare cause of an ulcerated leg. As a rule an ulcer consequent upon an arteriovenous fistula appears at an unusually early age.

Ulcer associated with Erythrocyanosis Frigida. This is seen exclusively in women, mostly young, living in cold climes who have plump legs and thick ankles. In even moderately cold weather the skin of the legs is bluish-pink, and in really cold weather blue mottling is strikingly evident. On warming, the skin becomes bright red and painful. When examining the patient on a cold day, before she has had sufficient time to warm up, the skin of the legs feels unduly cold. If there is no evidence of them on the feet or hands, inquiry will disclose that the patient is much troubled by chilblains. Continuing superficial palpation of the legs, often the examiner will encounter small, superficial, painful nodules; these are areas of fat necrosis in the subcutis which are wont to break down to form ulcers (Bazin's disease). Usually such ulcers are small, and multiple (*Fig.* 851). In warm weather the swelling of the ankles becomes a little worse because of superadded oedema.

---

* Marjolin described a carcinomatous ulcer occurring in scar tissue following burns; the term 'Marjolin's ulcer' is inaccurate when applied to this type of ulcer.

JEAN N. MARJOLIN, 1780–1850, *Parisian Surgeon*.
PIERRE A. E. BAZIN, 1807–1878, *Physician, Hôpital St. Louis, Paris*.

An Ulcer occurring on a Paralysed Leg is, in almost every instance, due to erythrocyanosis frigida secondary to the paralysis, the origin of which is frequently anterior poliomyelitis or spinal dysraphism (*see* p. 199). The limb is unduly susceptible to cold, as in the above, but the resulting ulcer (or ulcers) is very indolent.

Leg Ulcer complicating Blood Diseases.

Ulcer of the leg is common in sickle-cell anaemia. It also occurs, too frequently to be coincidental, in acholuric jaundice, Mediterranean anaemia and Felty's syndrome. Therefore examine the spleen for enlargement (*see* p. 236) when the cause of the ulcer is not perfectly clear.

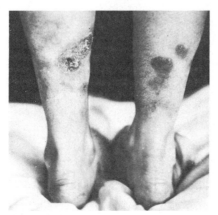

Fig. 851. Ulcers associated with erythrocyanosis frigida. Occasionally there is a single large ulcer low on the back of the calf.

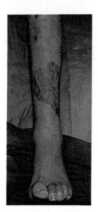

Fig. 852. Ulcer associated with rheumatoid arthritis.

Artefact Ulcer (Factitious Ulcer; Automutilation ulcer). A self-induced ulcer of the leg, which is not exceedingly rare, is encountered either in a highly neurotic individual or in a litigant desirous of obtaining compensation. The mode of production varies. The ulcer is always in an accessible place, often on the anterior or the lateral surface of the leg. Possibly the diagnosis is suggested by the unusual shape or an unusual, or even an artificial, appearance; commonly the ulcerated surface looks so pink, clean and healthy that the clinician is amazed that under treatment it remains stationary, or even increases in dimensions. If the ulcer is covered with a light plaster cast so that the underlying wound cannot be tampered with, a suspicion that the ulcer is factitious can be substantiated, for in these circumstances it will heal with great rapidity. In solving this problem signs that suggest a neurosis (*see* p. 49) can prove extremely valuable.

Gummatous Ulcer. *See* p. 38.

Footballer's Ulcer (Traumatic Ulcer). As its name implies, this occurs directly over the shin in otherwise healthy males. Improperly cared for, it becomes indolent and adherent to the bone. This ulcer follows knocks on the shin from any cause, but is often acquired at football.

Meleney's Ulcer. This was originally described in relation to infected abdominal and thoracic operation wounds which are still its commonest situations (*see* p. 33). However, the infection may occur on the leg (or in the hand) arising either *de novo* (particularly in ulcerative colitis) or, more usually, as a complication of a previously existing ulcer, which, on the law of averages, is usually varicose, at least in temperate climates. The onset is very rapid, and the most important clinical characteristic is burrowing, which may extend 2 cm or even more beneath apparently healthy skin;

the margins therefore are always extensively undermined. The ulcer is painful and tender and shows a tendency to spread ever wider in an alarming fashion.

Leg Ulcer in Rheumatoid Arthritis. This is peculiar to patients with severe, crippling arthritis and *occurs among those* 20 *per cent in whom subcutaneous nodules are plentiful* (Allison). This seems to suggest that it is due to breakdown of a nodule. The ulcer (sometimes multiple) varies in size, is punched-out, shallow (its floor being formed of subcutaneous tissue), and clean. As a rule, it is without surrounding oedema or palpable induration, but is encircled by a dark-red flush, is situated on the lower third of the leg and is painful and slow to heal (*Fig.* 852).

Leg Ulcer associated with Osteitis Deformans. As both Paget's disease of bone (*see* p. 426) and venous ulcer are common conditions, often the ulcer is a coincidental venous ulcer. On the other hand, a small, deep ulcer situated right over the convexity of the anteriorly bowed tibia strongly suggests that the ulcer is an example of this clinical entity. The base of the ulcer is bone, to which the edges are densely adherent. Consequently it is extremely resistant to treatment.

LEG ULCERS IN THE TROPICS

Those best qualified to know recognize three varieties of leg ulcer specific to the tropics and subtropics. To distinguish them with certainty, and thus to cure them, the organisms they harbour must be isolated.

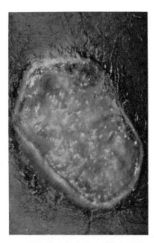

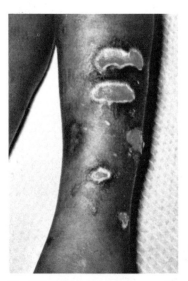

Fig. 853. Tropical ulcer. The patient was an Indian boy of 14 years of age. He sustained a very small puncture wound on the lateral aspect of the left leg two months previously. For one month the resulting ulcer has remained stationary in size, 6×4 cm. Note the raised edge.

Fig. 854. Diphtheritic desert sore. The purulent exudate covering the ulcers was cleaned away before the photograph was taken.

Yaws. The primary sore sometimes is found on the leg or foot (but more often on the buttocks of young children before they walk) as an infected abrasion in which the causative *Treponema pertenue* can be found. It heals in a few weeks. In the tertiary stage multiple deep ulcers, which also contain the spirochaete, are present. They are painless and in the course of healing form tissue-paper-like scars.

Tropical Ulcer (Chronic Phagedenic Ulcer) occurs in the monsoon-ridden humid zone of the tropics, where it is endemic, but breaks out in seasonal epidemics. Sporadic cases occur far out in the subtropics, where the condition is often misdiagnosed, usually as a venous ulcer. The infection develops in a breach of continuity of the skin due to trauma or an insect bite: it occurs practically

JOHN H. ALLISON, *Contemporary Dermatologist, Royal Perth Hospital, Australia.*

exclusively in the lower leg and foot in those who go about bare-legged. The ulcer is due to infection by Vincent's organisms* which, together with many other pyogenic bacteria, are always present in the discharge. It commences as a papulo-pustule which in a matter of hours becomes surrounded by a zone of angry inflammation with induration. Should the patient seek advice at this time, he does so because of the accompanying painful, tender lymphadenitis. In two or three days the pustule bursts and by a process of necrobiosis an ulcer forms and extends rapidly. Its interior is brown, *its edges are undermined*, a zone of skin in the immediate vicinity is infiltrated and raised (*Fig.* 853). There is a copious serosanguineous discharge and considerable pain. In most cases the ulcer remains practically the same size for months, sometimes even for a year or two. In other cases the ulcer assumes phagedenic† characteristics; it can then become of such dimensions with so great a destruction of soft parts of the leg and foot as to call for amputation. In its more usual indolent course it must be distinguished chiefly from yaws. However, at any stage of either course, the profuse serosanguineous discharge, the overpowering vile odour, the unremitting constant pain, the comparatively slight constitutional symptoms and the extreme tenacity of the contained slough should make the diagnosis very easy. On healing, a tropical ulcer leaves a permanent scar which is characteristically circular, parchment-like and faintly pigmented. Occasionally squamous carcinoma supervenes.

Diphtheritic Desert Sore,‡ as its name implies, is peculiar to the hot, parched desert wastes of the world, in all of which it is fairly common. It is due to a true diphtheritic infection by the *Corynebacterium diphtheriae* which commences as a papulo-pustule. Within a few days the top of the papule becomes necrotic, and an ulcer forms. This slowly enlarges, until it attains a diameter of 1–2 cm. Uncommonly the floor of the ulcer is covered by typical *diphtheritic membrane*, which is removed with difficulty. The ulcer (*Fig.* 854) runs a chronic course, and not rarely the patient shows signs of peripheral neuritis due to the toxin produced by the diphtheria bacillus.

THE ANKLE JOINT

Bony Landmarks. The two malleoli are among the most obvious surface markings in the body. The lateral is a little less prominent, and descends lower than the medial malleolus, the tip being 1 cm below and behind the corresponding landmark on the medial side. The line of the ankle joint lies on a plane 1 cm above the tip of the medial malleolus.

Effusion into the Ankle Joint. When the joint becomes distended with fluid the foot takes up a position of inversion and slight dorsiflexion. That an excessive amount of fluid is present is first indicated by a bulging beneath the extensor tendons as they cross the joint-line and a fullness just anterior to the lateral and medial malleolar ligaments. More extensive effusion causes bulging posteriorly, and filling up of the hollow (x) on either side of the tendo Achillis. ───────────────────→ To confirm the presence of fluid, place a finger on either side of the tendon. By digital compression, some of the fluid can be displaced from one side of the tendon to rebound against the watching finger on the contralateral side. For reasons stated on p. 12, it is incorrect to state that this constitutes fluctuation.

Testing Movements of the Ankle Joint. The Neutral Position is with the foot at a right-angle to the leg. The heel is grasped in the left hand, and the midfoot in the right (*Fig.* 855). If the forefoot is held, movement at the subtaloid and midtarsal joints will vitiate the findings.

---

* *Bacteroides fusiformis* and the spirochaete *Borrelia vincentii*.
† *Phagedena*. Greek, φαγεῖν = to eat.
‡ Known in South Africa as 'Veldt sore' and in Australia as 'Barcoo rot'.

HYACINTHE VINCENT, 1862–1950, *Professor of Bacteriology, Val-de-Grâce (Military Hospital), Paris.*

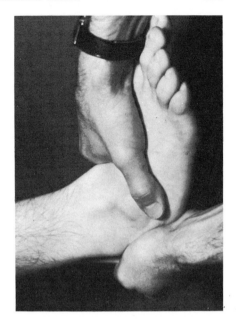

Fig. 855. Method of holding the foot while the movements of the ankle joint are tested. It is of fundamental importance to grasp the *midfoot*, and not the forefoot. Normal extension (dorsiflexion) reaches 20°, flexion (plantarflexion) 50°.

Usually the ankle joint has two movements only—flexion and extension. A few individuals are possessed of a lax lateral malleolar ligament, which allows some lateral movement of the talus within the tibiofibular mortise (Bonnin). The variant is bilateral so that, with painful injury, it can be tested for on the sound side. Patients with hypermobile ankles are prone to recurrent inversion sprains.

Ligamentous Injuries without Fracture. As in other situations, these may be incomplete or complete. 'Sprain' is an ambiguous term, often used to imply that no fracture has been sustained. It should be reserved for tearing of a few fibres of a ligament. If the injury is more severe, it is advisable to employ the terms 'incomplete rupture' or 'complete rupture' of the ligament.

Sprained Ankle is the result of a combined inversion and plantar flexion accident. Pain and tenderness are localized to the front of the ankle towards the fibular side. Directly after the accident a haematoma appears in this situation, but it soon becomes obscured by oedema.

Rupture of the Lateral Ligament. Maximum tenderness is found below the tip of the malleolus, in contrast to a Pott's fracture-dislocation, where the tenderness is over the fibula itself. It is important to be able to distinguish a complete tear of the ligament from an incomplete tear or a sprain. In every relevant case the following test should be carried out, otherwise avulsion of the ligament from the fibula will be overlooked. The ankle is passively inverted—a manipulation which, if carried out slowly, does not cause much pain, but if it does local anaesthetic should be injected before attempting it again. If the ligament is avulsed, an obvious gap appears between the tip of the malleolus and the talus on the anterolateral aspect of the joint. In doubtful cases the findings can be confirmed

JOSIAH G. BONNIN, *Contemporary Emeritus Orthopaedic Surgeon, Central Middlesex Hospital, London.*

by a radiograph taken while the examiner holds the ankle in full inversion (Watson-Jones).

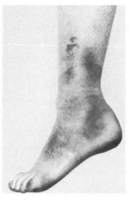

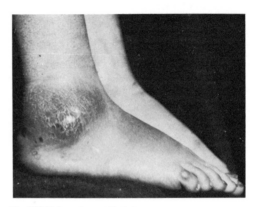

Fig. 856. Third-degree Pott's fracture showing backward displacement of the heel.

Fig. 857. Tuberculous ankle joint.

Rupture of the Medial Ligament. As this is much the strongest ligament of the ankle joint, it is unlikely to be torn unless there is a fracture of the lateral malleolus and a subluxation of the ankle joint (Pott's fracture).

Pott's Fracture-subluxation, easily the most important fracture in the region of the ankle joint, is a break of the lower end of the fibula, usually about 5 cm above the tip of the malleolus with, often, fracture of the tip of the medial malleolus. In almost every case there is some lateral or medial displacement of the talus (*second-degree fracture*), and in many instances there is backward displacement of the talus, too (*third-degree fracture*). For these reasons there is ample justification for designating this fracture a fracture-subluxation*' but the displacement of the talus is insufficient to warrant the term 'dislocation'.

In children and adolescents similar displacements of the lower tibial epiphysis occur.

A patient who has sustained this injury can neither walk nor stand upon that leg; soon the ankle becomes swollen and bruised. On examination it will be found that he cannot move the ankle joint. When compared with that of the opposite side, the distance between the tips of the malleoli is seen to be increased except when there is no bone displacement (*first-degree fracture*). Having ascertained by the principles enunciated in Chapter 29 that a fracture is present in this situation, always observe the heel from the lateral aspect for backward displacement signifying a third-degree fracture (*Fig.* 856). Needless to say, in ordinary circumstances, X-rays are essential for completely accurate diagnosis and reduction of all ankle fractures.

The above is a simple outline for clinical purposes. The student is referred to texts on fractures for details of the subdivision into external rotation, abduction and adduction types.

---

* Subluxation: the joint surfaces are displaced but there is some contact between them.

SIR REGINALD WATSON-JONES, 1902–1972, *Director of the Orthopaedic and Accident Service, The London Hospital.*
PERCIVALL POTT, 1714–1788, *Surgeon, St. Bartholomew's Hospital, London.*

The following two fractures are best regarded as unusual types of Pott's fracture.

Dupuytren's Fracture. When a fracture is sustained by falling from a height on to the feet, the talus is driven upwards and the ligaments which support the inferior tibiofibular joint are torn asunder (*diastasis*). The whole foot is displaced upwards, the width of the ankle between the malleoli being greatly increased, and the distance from the malleoli to the sole shortened.

Maisonneuve's Fracture. A rare variant. If, on X-raying a case of presumed Pott's fracture, *displacement* of the medial malleolus only is found, re-examine the region of the neck of the fibula. Tenderness due to a spiral fracture is probably present, which, together with the malleolar fracture and slight diastasis, constitutes this entity.

Arthritis. In the case of the ankle joint it will be unnecessary to consider all the usual forms of arthritis, for their features in general do not differ sufficiently from those of other major joints to warrant further description. There are, however, a few forms meriting special attention.

Traumatic Arthritis results from repeated minor traumata especially those sustained at football. Should the patient, as is often the case, first be seen with a swollen joint, there may be some difficulty in distinguishing the condition from tuberculosis. In traumatic arthritis there is no radiographic evidence of bone rarefaction, and when the effusion has subsided tiny osteophytes can often be felt in the joint line.

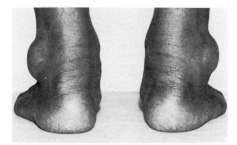

Fig. 858. Tailor's bursae in an Indian 'guru'.

Tuberculosis of the Ankle Joint. Early signs are that the ankle is swollen (*Fig.* 857) and the calf is wasted more than one would expect from disuse atrophy, a useful point in distinguishing from traumatic arthritis. A limp is inevitable, and there is pain in the joint. Soon the patient walks on the forefoot to prevent painful weight-bearing on the heel. A sinus develops in most untreated cases.

Lesions of Soft Tissues peculiar to this Region.

Tailor's Ankle (Tailor's Bursa). Over the subcutaneous area of the lateral surface of the lateral malleolus a sizeable adventitious bursa is wont to appear in old-time tailors or others who work while sitting cross-legged (*Fig.* 858).

Recurrent Dislocation of the Peroneal Tendons from their groove occurs occasionally. One or both tendons slip anteriorly over the lateral malleolus owing to laxity of their restraining ligaments. It occurs on active extension with eversion and is sometimes very painful; at others the patient can demonstrate the dislocation, with an audible click, so that diagnosis is obvious. Otherwise, unless the patient is seen during an attack, it must be surmised from the history.

Chronic Stenosing Tenosynovitis of the Peroneal Tendon Sheath, similar to that found about the wrist (*see* p. 462), occurs rarely. Tenderness and swelling are found in the course of these tendons below and behind the lateral malleolus. Pain occurs only on inversion of the foot.

Swollen Ankle(s). Unilateral or bilateral puffiness around the ankle is a problem which frequently confronts the general practitioner. In bilateral cases it is

BARON GUILLAUME DUPUYTREN, 1777–1835, *Surgeon-in-Chief, Hôtel-Dieu, Paris.*
JULES G. F. MAISONNEUVE, 1809–1897, *French Surgeon.*

essential to exclude a systemic cause—cardiac or renal insufficiency; endocrine disease (*see* p. 11). These having been eliminated, the back as well as the front of the whole of the lower limbs should be inspected and palpated for varicosities. Next, oedema of lymphatic origin (*see* p. 399) must be considered. Foot strain is a cause of slight swelling of the ankles in some heavy individuals.

Unilateral Oedema of the ankles is a frequent accompaniment of a recent bony or ligamentous injury. Not infrequently the swelling persists for months, in which event an original sprain may have been forgotten. Homans stressed that many cases of oedema following a sprain or a fracture are, in fact, instances of phlebothrombosis. Others believe that such swelling is due to Sudeck's atrophy (*see* p. 51) resulting from the injury. It must be conceded that after considering all these possibilities there remain a few cases which defy explanation.

JOHN HOMANS, 1877–1954, *Professor of Clinical Surgery, Harvard University, Boston, Mass.*
PAUL H. M. SUDECK, 1886–1945, *Professor of Surgery, Hamburg.*

Chapter 36

THE FOOT

Examination of the Feet varies widely with the complaint. Thus the examination of talipes equinovarus presenting at birth (*see* p. 536) differs entirely from that of an adult with an ingrowing big toe-nail (*see* p. 549). In all patients other than infants the lower limbs should be exposed at least to the mid-thighs and the gait (*see* p. 439) is observed. If pain is the complaint, unless there is an obvious lesion the patient is asked to point to its site. Comparison of one foot with the other is essential.

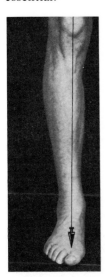

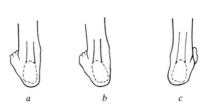

Fig. 860. *a*, The normal heel viewed from the back (left foot). *b*, In talipes equinovarus the calcaneus is tilted outwards. *c*, In marked flat-foot it is tilted inwards.

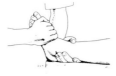

Fig. 861. Inversion.

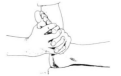

Fig. 862. Eversion.

Fig. 859. Normally a plumb line dropped from the midline of the patella passes to the interval between metatarsals I and II. The heel is aligned with the midline of the tibia posteriorly. These two criteria comprise the Neutral Position of the foot.

The Arches of the Foot. The longitudinal arch (*see* p. 539) and the transverse arch (*see* p. 541) are next scrutinized for evidence of flattening, the patient standing in front of the clinician, preferably on a raised platform, with the feet parallel and slightly apart. In a properly balanced foot, an imaginary plumb line dropped from the middle of the patella should strike the interval between the first and second metatarsal bones (*Fig.* 859).

The Heel. Next, the patient is asked to turn round, with the calves exposed and any shortening of the tendo Achillis or tilting of the calcaneus noted. Normally there is a slight medial tilt (eversion) and in long-standing flat-foot this may be marked (*Fig.* 860 *c*). In uncorrected or partially corrected talipes equinovarus (*see* p. 536) there is a lateral tilt of the calcaneus (inversion) (*Fig.* 860 *b*).

Testing Movements of the Foot. Lastly the patient lies on a couch and, with the knee extended, the foot should be put through its movements (*Figs.* 861, 862). Note that flexion and extension take place mainly at the ankle joint (*see* p. 530).

Further methods of examination are detailed in the rest of this chapter.

Scrutinizing the Patient's Footwear. Unless the patient's shoes are new or have been repaired recently, information can be gleaned therefrom. That part of the sole and/or heel subject to undue pressure in walking is seen to be very worn down. The normal foot tends to wear the outer sides of the heels (*Fig.* 863).

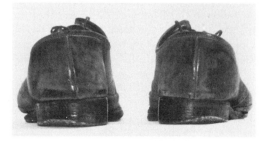

Fig. 863. Wearing down of the outer side of the heels, after some months of use, of shoes by a person with normal feet.

TALIPES* (CLUBFOOT †)

Deformities of the foot are, by convention, named according to the position of the foot. For this purpose the four cardinal positions are called (1) Equinus = flexion; (2) Calcaneus = extension; (3) Varus = inversion; (4) Valgus = eversion. To these are added cavus = an undue hollowing of the instep. These five names, and combinations of any two of them, are all that is necessary to put the deformities illustrated in *Fig.* 865 into words.

Fig. 864. In the newborn infant the little toe can be placed on the shin easily.

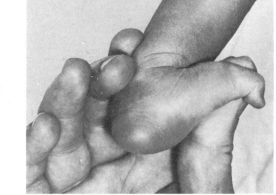

Talipes Equinovarus (*Fig.* 865*b*). By far the most common and important of these deformities is congenital talipes equinovarus which has a strong familial

---

* *Talipes.* Latin, *talus* = ankle + *pes* = a foot. Original meaning: a deformity that causes the patient to walk on the ankle. Present-day meaning: any variety of clubfoot.

† *Clubfoot.* Severe untreated *talipes equinovarus* has a club-like appearance.

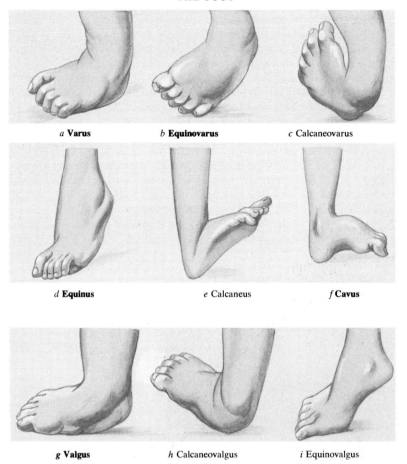

| a Varus | b Equinovarus | c Calcaneovarus |

| d Equinus | e Calcaneus | f Cavus |

| g Valgus | h Calcaneovalgus | i Equinovalgus |

Fig. 865. Varieties of talipes. The commoner varieties are captioned in **bold** type.

incidence (Wynne-Davies). Boys are affected twice as often as girls, and the deformity is bilateral in one-third of cases.

In a normal baby it is not unusual for the feet to repose in an equinovarus position ('in-toeing' or inversion spasm); each foot, however, can be passively extended until the toes touch the anterior aspect of the leg (*Fig.* 864). In talipes equinovarus the deformity strongly resists correction. Furthermore, furrows are formed at the flexures of the foot, the tendo Achillis is short and stands out like a cord when extension is attempted, and the calf muscles are underdeveloped. Calcaneovarus (*Fig.* 865c) is a rare extremely severe degree of equinovarus.

Talipes Equinus* (*Fig.* 865d) is about half as common as talipes equinovarus. It is always an acquired condition, due either to paralysis of the extensors of the foot or to shortening of one leg necessitating continued walking on tip-toe. In women who habitually wear high-heeled shoes a minor degree is often present

---

* *Equinus*. Latin, *equinus* = equine; horse-like. In this instance, like a horse's hoof.

RUTH WYNNE-DAVIES, *Contemporary Senior Lecturer in Orthopaedic Surgery, University of Edinburgh.*

and it is also seen with long-standing varicose ulceration. When examining patients with this condition *the knee should be extended*, as the flexed knee relaxes the tendo Achillis and minimizes the deformity. Callosities may be found beneath the heads of the metatarsal bones.

Metatarsus Varus.* The forefoot is medially deviated but the foot is plantigrade and the heel is normal (*Fig.* 865*a*). This is an occasional congenital anomaly which does not, in later life, cause a serious deformity. If untreated, the person walks with markedly inturned feet ('pigeon toes').

Pes Cavus* (*Fig.* 865*f*) is not uncommon. The toes are clawed and callosities form over the metatarsal heads as in splayfoot (*see* p. 541). Probably the congenital form is due to shortness of plantar fascia but some cases result from brain disease (*Friedreich's ataxia*). The acquired form can be due to paralysis of the small muscles of the foot due to a lesion of the tibial nerve, but where there is no evidence of a nerve lesion pes cavus may be due to:

Contracture of the Plantar Fascia. A small percentage of patients suffering from Dupuytren's contracture (*see* p. 478) have also some degree of contracture of the plantar fascia. As a rule this contracture is unilateral (*Fig.* 866) and asymptomatic.

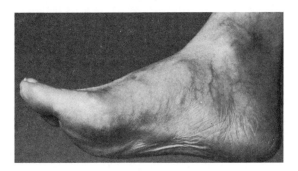

Fig. 866. Contracture of the plantar fascia.

Pes Valgus* is the congenital variety of flat-foot. The foot is plantigrade but the longitudinal arch is defective (*Fig.* 865*g*). The cause of pes valgus is vertical talus (*see* p. 539).

Talipes Calcaneovalgus, with lengthening of the tendo Achillis, is uncommon and congenital (*Fig.* 865*h*). Vertical talus is present and it can be regarded as a more severe form of the foregoing. Sometimes it is associated with dislocated hip or hyperextension of the knee.

Talipes Calcaneus (*Fig.* 865*e*) is an inevitable deformity in cases of isolated paralysis of the gastrocnemius and soleus muscles.

Talipes Equinovalgus (*Fig.* 865*i*) is rare and almost always acquired.

Completing a Diagnosis of Talipes. Having made a diagnosis of talipes, and having decided which variety is present, it is necessary to state whether the deformity is congenital or acquired. Although obviously this is not difficult if the patient is an infant, it is always necessary to look for other congenital deformities, notably one of the varieties of spinal dysraphism (*see* p. 199).

In older children and adults, when the leg is cold, perhaps even livid, and one or more groups of activating muscles are wasted and the patient is unable to

---

* These are usually not classified as talipes as the foot is plantigrade.

Nikolas Friedreich, 1825–1882, *Neurologist, Heidelberg, Germany.*

move the foot and the toes fully, the talipes is certainly paralytic—most commonly a sequel to anterior poliomyelitis.

THE SOLE

FLAT-FOOT

Pes Planus is one of the most common defects of the feet. The causes of the condition are heterogeneous, and in most instances the condition is bilateral. Flattening of the *longitudinal arch* will be considered first (*Fig*. 867).

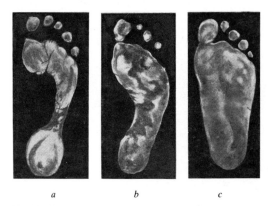

a   *b*   *c*

Fig. 867. Footprints. *a*, Normal; *b*, Early flat-foot; *c*, Advanced flat-foot.

1. *The Pseudo-flat-foot of Infants*. In infants the flat appearance of the feet is normal and it persists for a variable time after the child has commenced to walk. It is due to the normal subcutaneous fat-pad obliterating the arch and may remain up to the age of 3 years.

2. *Congenital Flat-foot due to Talonavicular Dislocation* is rare. The infant is born with the talus dislocated so that its anterior surface is rotated towards the plantar surface (vertical talus), viz. ———→ Usually the dislocation is unilateral. The dislocated head of the bone can be felt beneath the medial and central part of the sole.

3. *Rotation of the Limb*. As a result of either a congenital abnormality or one acquired very early in life, the entire limb is externally rotated (retroversion of the femoral neck); alternatively the rotation is confined to the leg below the knee (tibial torsion). In either the patient stands like Charlie Chaplin (*Fig.* 868), and the line of the body weight, falling too far medially, throws undue strain upon the longitudinal arch, which consequently drops. As the child grows older the deformity is spontaneously corrected.

4. *Genu Valgum* (*see* p. 520) also causes the body weight to be diverted too far medially, with the same result. It is a common cause in children.

Next consider the causes in adolescence or adult life. At an early stage of the examination it is imperative to decide whether the flattening of the longitudinal arch is constantly present (rigid flat-foot) or if the foot assumes an arch when weight-bearing is removed.

Observe the arches with the patient standing and ask him to try to arch the inner border of the foot (*Fig.* 869).
Examination with the Patient Reclining. Put each foot through its movements (*see Figs*. 861, 862) and note whether the arch has returned partially or wholly when the body weight has been taken off it.

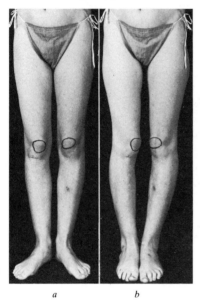

a   *b*   *a*   *b*

Fig. 868. *a*, Flat-foot and 'Charlie Chaplin' stance due to tibial torsion; *b*, When the patient is asked to stand straight the patellae signify that the limbs are rotated medially. Note the apparent bow-leg.

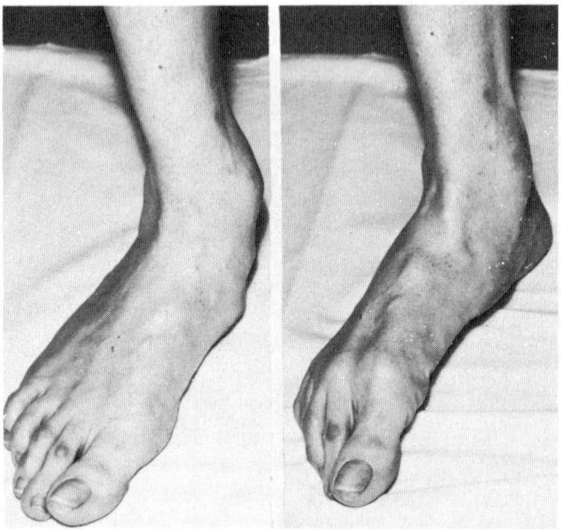

Fig. 869. Rigid flat-foot; *a*, Bearing normal body weight; *b*, Attempted inversion.

Relaxed Flat-foot. A relaxed flat-foot assumes an arch when weight-bearing is removed. This is the most common variety, and it is encountered most frequently in young adults, but it often occurs in middle life, particularly if the patient is called upon to undertake much unaccustomed standing or he or she puts on weight rapidly. Movements are full.

'Foot Strain' is a variety of the above. The patient, often after confinement to bed or unusual exercise, complains of pain over the longitudinal arch (*see Fig.* 878) where there is tenderness, and even oedema on occasion, but not necessarily flattening of the arch.

Rigid Flat-foot is seen principally in middle and late life and is often painless. It is due to fibrous, cartilaginous, or bony ankylosis, most commonly in the talocalcanean or talocuboid joints. Ankylosis can follow a severe or incompletely reduced Pott's fracture-subluxation, an injury involving one or more of the tarsal joints, or it can be the result of acute or chronic arthritis of these joints. All foot movements are limited. In older patients remember to examine the foot pulses (*see* p. 379). Intermittent claudication may present with typical pain in the foot, even in the presence of flat-foot.

Spastic Flat-foot. The peroneal muscles are contracted rigidly. When the condition, which occurs in adolescents (particularly boys), is suspected, the peronei should be palpated early in the course of the examination. *Inversion* alone is limited, because of spasm of the peronei muscles. Often various tarsal bones are fused as shown by a radiograph.

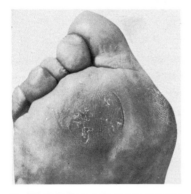

Fig. 870. Callosity over the metatarsal heads which normally do not bear weight (second to fourth) in a patient with transverse flat-foot.

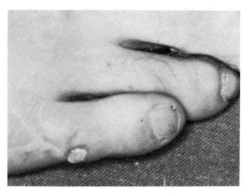

Fig. 871. The most common situation of a hard corn. The central core—a highly distinctive feature—can be seen.

Transverse Flat-foot (Splay Foot), which is common and frequently associated with hallux valgus, is due to flattening of the transverse arch of the forefoot (*Fig.* 870). When the symptoms are due to the fallen arch, as opposed to the hallux valgus, they are those of metatarsalgia (*see* p. 545).

CORNS AND CALLOSITIES AND THEIR DIFFERENTIAL DIAGNOSIS

A Callosity is an area of hard, greatly thickened skin that occurs as a protective measure when intermittent pressure is distributed over a comparatively large area. At the periphery, cornified skin ceases abruptly where it is continuous with normal skin. Callosities appear where the skin is normally thick, most frequently on the soles, beneath the heads of one or more of the metatarsal bones, around the heel and on the inframedial side of the great toe, but never on the dorsum although they may be seen on the outer border of the foot in uncorrected talipes equinovarus.

A Hard Corn. When intermittent pressure occurs over a very limited area, a corn ensues consisting of a conical wedge of highly compressed keratotic epithelial cells which impinges on the nerve endings, hence the pain. It is characterized by a central core of white appearance composed of degenerate cells and cholesterol and is encircled by a narrow area of keratosis, which disappears gradually at the periphery. Palpation reveals the causative bony projection beneath the cutaneous lesion which occurs chiefly where the normal skin is thin, and is found particularly on the fifth toe (*Fig.* 871), and over the dorsal projections of hammertoes.

A Soft Corn is soft because it occurs between the toes, where maceration takes place. The site of election of a soft corn is at the bottom of the cleft between the fourth and fifth toes where opposing prominent bony projections of the bases of the proximal phalanges give rise to pressure and friction. ⎯⎯⎯⟶
The great pressure to which these toes are subjected is shown by their prismatic shape, the apex of the prism being directed towards the intervening cleft. Soft corns are particularly painful and are often mistaken for a wart.

Plantar Wart (*Fig*. 872). As the treatment is completely different from that of a corn or a callosity (*Fig* 873*a*), it is important to be able to diagnose a plantar wart, which presents as a rather dark, obliquely set pearl in the skin, usually

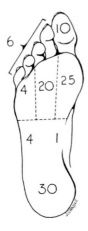

Fig. 872. Percentage distribution of plantar warts averaged from various statistics.

being situated on a weight-bearing portion of the sole or heel so that it soon becomes submerged and surrounded by a collar of cornified skin. Through the cornified skin can be seen red or black spots, which are haemorrhages from attenuated fronds of the submerged papilloma. These spots are recognized more easily through a magnifying glass (*Fig.* 873*b*). A plantar wart is *exquisitely tender* when pressed towards the underlying bone. This is *the* distinguishing feature from a callosity. Mother warts and daughter warts may form a characteristic constellation found with warts in other situations.

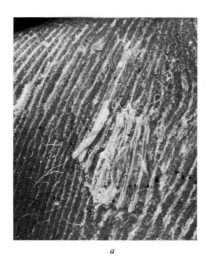
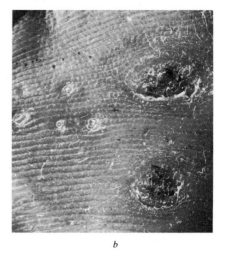

a *b*

Fig. 873. *a*, Callosity; *b*, Plantar wart, each as seen under a magnifying glass (×5).

Perforating (Neurotrophic) Ulcer. The most common situation for a perforating ulcer is beneath one of the metatarsal heads, particularly the first and fifth (*Fig.* 874). The next most common situation is beneath the tips of the terminal phalanges of the toes. Ulcers over the metatarsal heads are always associated with thick callosities. Tabes dorsalis is now an uncommon cause: spinal dysraphism and diabetic neuropathy (*see* p. 414) are frequent, but injury of the spinal cord or sciatic nerve accounts for some cases. The differential diagnosis sign between perforating ulcer (or ulcers) of the toes and a pre-gangrenous appearance of the toes due to occlusive vascular disease is that in the former strong pedal pulses are present.

NEOPLASMS OF THE SOLE OF THE FOOT

Neoplasms of the foot do not differ from those developing elsewhere in skin and bone, but are relatively rare. Two growths, when they occur in the sole, show special characteristics.

Malignant Melanoma. The most frequent site is in the soft skin of the instep (*Fig.* 875). Unfortunately the lesion in its early stage is asymptomatic and unnoticed until ulceration occurs. When suspected the regional lymph nodes (groin) and the liver must be palpated.

Squamous Carcinoma of the Foot. In contradistinction to a melanoma, an epithelioma is almost always confined to the hard skin of the weight-bearing areas of the forefoot (*Fig.* 876). As a result of weight-bearing it soon infiltrates among the tendons and bones so that it is fixed to the deep structures at an early stage.

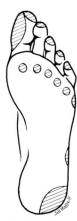

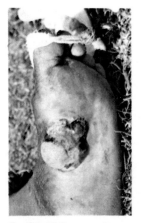

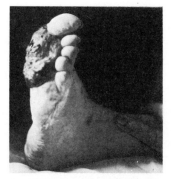

Fig. 874. Distribution of neurotrophic ulcers.

Fig. 875. Malignant melanoma of the foot.

Fig. 876. Carcinoma of the sole of the foot.

THE HEEL

Fracture of the Calcaneus is a common accident in workmen who use ladders or steps. It is due to a fall on to the feet from a height, and is bilateral, and often associated with a *fracture of the vertebral column* as well when the height of the fall is greater than the patient's height.

Signs of Fractured Calcaneus:
1. There is broadening of the heel.
2. Normal hollows below the malleoli are obliterated.
3. Haemorrhage occurs into the sole and a bruise appears on the heel.
4. Maximum tenderness is situated posteriorly near the insertion of the tendo Achillis, rather than upon the plantar aspect.
5. Active and passive movements of the ankle are reduced to about half their normal excursion. In addition, inversion and eversion of the foot (subtaloid joint) are curtailed almost completely because of pain.

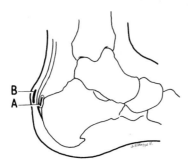

Fig. 877. A, Retrocalcanean bursa; B, Retro-Achillis bursa.

Apophysitis of the Calcaneus (Sever's Disease) occurs most often in boys of 8–12 years of age. Like Osgood–Schlatter's disease (*see* p. 514), the condition is a traction injury of the epiphysial cartilage. The first symptom is a limp, followed by dull pain in the back of the heel. There is tenderness localized to the posterior surface of the calcaneus *below* the insertion of the tendo Achillis; sometimes slight swelling in the region is present.

Retrocalcanean Bursitis. There is a bursa situated between the tendo Achillis and the calcaneus (*Fig.* 877 A). Inflammation of this bursa gives rise to local pain and tenderness. When swelling is present in addition, it is situated *on either side of* the tendon.

Retro-Achillis Bursitis. An adventitious bursa develops between the tendo Achillis just above its insertion and the skin (*Fig.* 877 B). Swelling of the bursa is seen readily: it is situated *over* the tendon, and not on either side of it and is liable to become inflamed from friction of the tendo Achillis against the counter (the stiffener) of ill-fitting footwear particularly in winter. Young women who wear high heels are the chief sufferers, but the condition is met with also in Army recruits.

Calcaneal Exostosis is a not uncommon condition seen in adolescent girls. A bony protuberance is found on the posterior surface of the bone lateral to the insertion of the tendo Achillis.———————————————————————————→ Pain is caused by the shoe rubbing on the lump which is *not* the anatomical lateral tubercle which is situated on the inferior surface.

Achillis Tendinitis. The tendon has no sheath so that pain, tenderness, and swelling are due to rupture of a few fibres of the tendon when the affected part is above the level of the shoe-line although Reiter's syndrome (*see* p. 439) is an occasional cause. On the other hand, with inflammation of one of the above bursae the signs are confined to soft tissues below that line.

Plantar Fasciitis (Policeman's Heel). Any occupation that entails much standing or walking predisposes to this condition, which is common in men of 40–60 years of age. Ossification extending into the posterior insertion of the plantar fascia gives rise to a calcanean spur, which is easily demonstrated by radiography but is impalpable clinically. As the spur is often symptomless, and as 'policeman's heel' is not infrequently encountered in a patient without such a spur, *the finding of a spur on X-ray examination is probably incidental*. The cause is thought to be

JAMES W. SEVER, 1877–1963, *Orthopaedic Surgeon, Children's Hospital, Boston, Massachusetts.*

plantar fasciitis which results in pain in the ball of the heel on walking or standing. There is considerable tenderness in the area, the most acute point being over the medial tubercle of the calcaneus (*Fig.* 878). Reiter's syndrome (*see* p. 439) is sometimes associated.

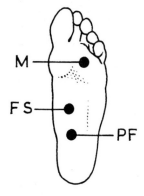

Fig. 878. Sites of plantar pain so typical as to suggest the diagnosis. M, metatarsalgia; FS, foot strain; PF, plantar fasciitis.

THE FOREFOOT

Metatarsalgia. The term implies pain in the metatarsal region without an obvious cause such as a plantar wart. Thus, with greater clinical acumen, less frequent resort to the use of the word is necessary. Examination along the lines already laid down will detect flat-foot (particularly of the transverse variety), plantar wart, soft corn and hallux rigidus, all causes of pain in this region.

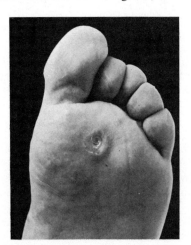

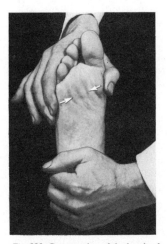

Fig. 879. Plantar corn beneath the second metatarsal head in a case of congenital short first metatarsal.

Fig. 880. Compression of the heads of the metatarsals.

Tarsal Tunnel Syndrome. The cause is similar to that of the carpal tunnel syndrome (*see* p. 461), in this instance the tibial nerve being compressed in the fibro-osseous tunnel deep to the flexor retinaculum behind and below the medial malleolus. However, the condition is very much less frequent and the sex incidence is equal. The patient complains of burning pain and tingling in the toes and the sole of the foot at night. Relief may be attained by hanging the foot out of bed in a dependent position *but the foot pulses are present* (*see* p. 379). As with the carpal tunnel syndrome a sphygmomanometer cuff pumped up to the systolic blood pressure for a minute may reproduce the symptoms.

Congenital Short First Metatarsal is not uncommon. Weight-bearing is transferred from the first metatarsal head with its sesamoid bones on to the second metatarsal head. A corn extending deeply, almost to the bone, develops exactly beneath the second metatarsal head (*Fig.* 879) with localized tenderness. A similar callosity may be found when the foot is involved by rheumatoid arthritis.

Pain in the Ball of the Big Toe. Tenderness strictly confined to this region implies disease of the weight-bearing medial sesamoid. Apley points out that this bone mimics the patella in its pathology. Thus, a fracture (rare), chondromalacia, or osteoarthrosis may cause pain.

If none of the above are present proceed as follows: find the place that is most tender to digital pressure and confirm the exact point accurately by using a blunt object. Next exert transverse pressure across the metatarsal heads, as shown in *Fig.* 880, and observe whether this reproduces the pain. If so, one of the three following conditions is present. The age, occupation and sex give a clue to the exact diagnosis, but radiography is necessary for confirmation.

Morton's Metatarsalgia is due to a neuroma of the medial plantar nerve's contribution to the third cleft (sometimes the second), just before that nerve divides into its two digital branches. This is not a true neoplasm, but a granuloma probably due to intermittent pressure. The neuroma is rarely palpable through the skin. It gives rise to sudden, often extremely severe, pain that shoots *into the toes* supplied by the nerve (*see Fig.* 878) whenever the neuroma is subjected to pressure, as when walking over uneven ground. There is often plantar hyperaesthesia of the third and fourth toes. Females are affected in the ratio of 4:1.

Stress Fracture of a Metatarsal Bone (March Fracture; Fatigue Fracture) occurs in the distal third of one shaft, most often of the second metatarsal of the right foot. This is well known to military surgeons, but occurs also in hikers and even those, like hospital nurses, whose duties entail much standing.

The onset is undramatic. When the boots or shoes are taken off there is a cramp-like pain in the affected forefoot and moderate local oedema appears *on the dorsal aspect.* Move each toe in turn; that of the involved metatarsal causes pain, and when this bone is palpated from the dorsal surface a point of tenderness is found directly over the lesion. *Radiography at this stage is negative,* but the condition is diagnosed correctly by military surgeons without the aid of X-rays. In civil life it is seldom diagnosed for a week or two, when, because of lack of immobilization, there is an excessive deposit of callus (which may be palpable) around the fracture (*Fig.* 881).

Freiberg's Disease (Infraction*) is an affection of the head of the second (uncommonly the third) metatarsal bone that commences in the articular surface as does osteochondritis dissecans (*see* p. 513). It is comparatively rare, with young women much more frequently affected than other persons. In the beginning the condition is extremely painful. At this time there is some local oedema of the dorsum of the forefoot and exquisite tenderness over the affected metatarsal head when even light digital pressure is applied either from the sole or the dorsum. As time goes on, and the metatarsophalangeal joint stiffens, the pain and tenderness become much less, but a bony lump (the thickened metatarsal head) can be palpated.

The Dorsum of the Foot.
The tarsal bones and joints (excluding the calcaneus) are comparatively accessible from the dorsal and medial aspects of the foot.

Ganglion of the Foot
(*Fig.* 882) nearly always arises on the dorsum. It resembles ganglion of the wrist (*see* p. 463), but is much less common.

Köhler's Disease (Osteochondritis of the Navicular Bone) is an uncommon affection commencing in childhood about the fourth year. It causes a pronounced limp and a moderate degree of pain is located in the dorsal aspect of the foot. On palpation of the dorsum of the foot there is an area of tenderness (*Fig.* 883) limited strictly to the navicular bone. The radiographic findings are characteristic: the navicular appears as though it has been crushed.

Tuberculosis of the Tarsus. Pain is an early symptom, but usually it is not so severe as in a case of tuberculosis of the ankle joint. Swelling of the dorsum of the foot is evident, and so is wasting of the corresponding calf muscles. Because of the complexity of the synovial membranes of the region, several tarsal bones become involved. Sinus formation is common.

---

* *Infraction.* Latin, *in* = into+*fractio* = break. Incomplete fracture without displacement.

ALAN G. APLEY, *Contemporary Orthopaedic Surgeon, St. Thomas's Hospital, London.*
THOMAS G. MORTON, 1835–1903, *Surgeon, Pennsylvania Hospital, Philadelphia, Pennsylvania.*
ALBERT H. FREIBERG, 1868–1940, *Orthopaedic Surgeon, The General Hospital, Cincinnati, Ohio.*
ALBAN KÖHLER, 1874–1947, *Radiologist, Wiesbaden, Germany.*

THE TOES

In older patients always examine the foot pulses (*see* p. 379) before advising an operation on the toes. To advise a non-essential surgical procedure on a foot with a deficient arterial circulation is a grave error.

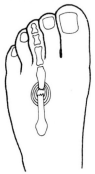

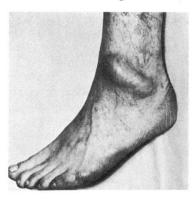

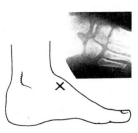

Fig. 881. March fracture. The condition (excessive callus) 3 weeks after the fracture had occurred.

Fig. 882. Ganglion on the foot.

Fig. 883. Site of tenderness in Köhler's disease of the navicular bone. *Inset*: the typical X-ray appearances.

THE GREAT TOE

Hallux* Valgus. This common deformity, which usually is bilateral (*Fig.* 884), can be congenital (rare) or acquired. Especially in the congenital form, the

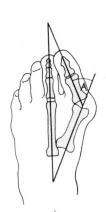

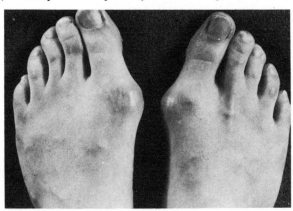

Fig. 884. A fairly early example of bilateral hallux valgus. For accuracy the degree of abduction of the toe on the metatarsal (**A** in diagram) should be measured.

proximal phalanx, in addition to being valgus, is often rotated so that its plantar aspect looks laterally. If so, in all but children, there is likely to be a callosity over the medial aspect of the great toe. Often, in both forms, the second toe comes to overlap or underlap the great toe, or the second toe is a hammer toe.

---

* *Hallux*. Latin = the great toe.

Ask the patient to move the great toe upwards—the extensor tendon stands out as a tight cord. In spite of the deformity the metatarsophalangeal joint has a good range of movement.

Very frequently the deformity, often prominent, is seen when examining the feet for other conditions, the hallux valgus being symptomless. Pain results from one or more of: (*a*) infection of an accompanying bunion (*see Fig.* 68, p. 33); (*b*) an accompanying hammer toe; (*c*) wide splaying of the forefoot giving rise to transverse flat-foot; (*d*) osteoarthrosis of the metatarsophalangeal joint (*see below*). Inspection and seeking a tender place by pressure will quickly reveal which of these is the cause of the pain. Acquired hallus valgus, almost invariably found in women, is one of the the penalties of wearing pointed shoes.

Hallux Rigidus. When, during its period of growth, the great toe is subject to stubbing from a too-short shoe, osteoarthrosis of the metatarsophalangeal joint results, and the joint becomes stiff. A fracture into the joint is also a precursor. Troublesome cases are those in which an unduly long great toe is held rigidly in a position of plantar flexion.

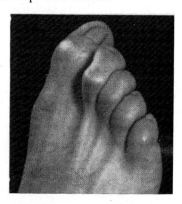

Fig. 885. Hallux rigidus. The patient has been asked to flex his great toe. Only the interphalangeal joint moves.

The great toe is only rarely valgus. Movement in the metatarsophalangeal joint is diminished, extension being especially restricted and painful (*Fig.* 885). In extreme cases all movement is abolished; the condition then becomes relatively asymptomatic. In its more usual, less advanced, state, hallux rigidus, which is seen particularly in young men, gives rise to pain in the metatarsophalangeal joint, especially when walking uphill or over uneven ground. A characteristic sign is palpable irregularity at the joint-line caused by small osteophytic outgrowths on the dorsal articular edge of the metatarsal head (dorsal bunion).

While the following conditions usually are the prerogative of the great toe, on infrequent occasions they may affect one of the other toes.

Gout. In males gout selects the first metatarsophalangeal joint with great frequency. The patient is awakened at night with acute pain. The joint becomes tensely swollen, dusky-red (*see Fig.* 707, p. 439), and exquisitely tender. Pitting on pressure can be obtained in the overlying skin. Suppuration never ensues. As a rule the diagnosis is easy. An inflamed bunion must be eliminated by the absence of hallux valgus (unusual in men), by searching for tophi (*see* p. 82) and if in real doubt by the serum uric acid level.

Ingrowing Toe-nail (Onychocryptosis). There is excessive lateral growth of the nail into the nail-fold, most probably first invoked by cutting off the corners of the nail, viz.————————————————————→ instead of trimming the toe-nails straight across. The sharp lateral edge of the nail digs into, and lacerates, the nail-fold. In the pocket thus formed, chronic infection becomes established and results in a purulent discharge. Recurrent attacks of acute or subacute paronychia punctuate the course of this painful affliction. In cases of some standing, chronic infection of the hidden wound of the nail-fold proclaims itself by protuberant granulation tissue (*Fig.* 886). Nearly always involving the great toe, the lesion is so exquisitely tender that the patient limps with any form of footwear save a sandal.

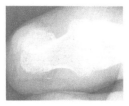

NAIL
SULCUS

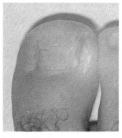

Fig. 886. Ingrown toe-nail with superadded sepsis. A small excrescence of granulation tissue on the *lateral* side is characteristic.

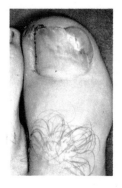

Fig. 887. Subungual exostosis. *Above*: The radiograph of this case.

Subungual Exostosis first makes its appearance beneath the distal half of the nail, which becomes pushed upwards and discoloured. Later the exostosis forces its way through the nail by breaking or distorting it, to reach the surface covered with a mass of granulation tissue (*Fig.* 887). The outgrowth is symptomless until it is traumatized, or becomes infected, when it occasions great pain.

In comparatively early stages, it is confused most often with *onychomycosis*,* a fungus affection causing the nail to become discoloured, much thickened, brittle, and split longitudinally in several places. It may also be mistaken for an ingrown toe-nail. A lateral radiograph renders the diagnosis incontestable.

Subungual Malignant Melanoma. Nearly always early cases are diagnosed incorrectly, being mistaken for a subungual haematoma or a fungus infection, and many months elapse before the correct diagnosis is made. A melanoma occurs as deep pigmentation of the nail bed, or as a pigmented nodule beneath the nail or in the nail groove. Usually in a matter of months, lively proliferation causes the nail to be lifted up, and lost. Then the growth ulcerates, and becomes secondarily infected, but it still retains some of its characteristic brown-black melanin. A similar lesion can occur beneath the thumb-nail.

Onychogryphosis (Ram's Horn Nail) (*see Fig.* 60, p. 30).

Glomus Tumour resembles that occurring beneath the fingernail (*see* p. 477).

---

* *Onychomycosis*. Greek, ὄνυξ= nail+μύκης = *fungus*.

THE SMALLER TOES

Hammer Toe. The proximal phalanx is extended; the middle phalanx is flexed; the distal phalanx can be either flexed or extended, usually the latter. The second toe is involved most frequently. The head of the proximal phalanx is subject to intermittent pressure and a corn, and often in this instance a bursa, too, occurs over the joint, viz.: ⎯⎯⎯⎯⎯⎯⎯⎯⎯⎯⎯⎯⎯⎯⎯⎯⎯⎯⎯→

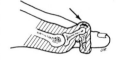

This deformity, which gives rise to much painful disability, is usually bilateral, but often a hammer toe or toes is more advanced on one side. Commonly hallux valgus is associated. The toe deformity in pes cavus (*see* p. 538) is similar but the metatarsophalangeal joint is flexed.

Overlapping Fifth Toe is a common congenital abnormality.

Bunionette. In cases of splay foot (*see* p. 541) the fifth metatarsal bone is displaced away from the fourth, and consequently the head of the fifth metatarsal projects laterally, and is subjected to intermittent pressure from a tight shoe. So it comes about that this bony projection becomes cushioned by an adventitious bursa liable to attacks of inflammation. This is misnamed 'tailor's bursa' which, in fact, is a completely different condition (*see* p. 533).

Ainhum. A painful constricting groove encircles the base of the fifth toe, ultimately causing auto-amputation in an African who habitually walks barefoot (*see Fig.* 63, p. 30).

INFECTIONS OF THE FOOT

Infections of the Sole of the Foot are particularly common among those who walk barefooted and are thus seen mostly in the tropics. Apart from an infected blister (which is also common in those who go about shod) the various infections of the sole are summarized thus:

Infection of a Web Space. These spaces, four in number, extend into the dorsal as well as into the plantar aspects of the foot, and are comparable in every way to those of the hand. Infection is not uncommon in diabetics. There is localized tenderness upon the dorsal, as well as the plantar, aspect of the web.

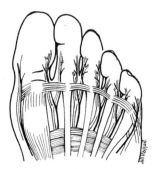

Fig. 888. The four interdigital sub-cutaneous spaces between the five slips of the termination of the plantar fascia.

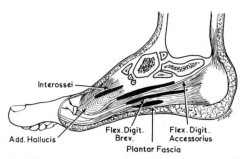

Fig. 889. Sagittal section showing the four compartments of the central plantar space.

Infection of an Interdigital Subcutaneous Space. There are four spaces lying between the digital slips of the central fasciculus of the plantar fascia (*Fig.* 888). Commonly a space is infected by stepping on a thorn or a tack. The patient experiences increasing pain between two metatarsals; soon he is unable to walk. Exquisite tenderness over the infected space proclaims the diagnosis. A collar-stud abscess, with one cavity lying within calloused skin and the other occupying an interdigital space, is present occasionally. When pus decompresses itself into the dorsal subcutaneous space, localization of the abscess is more difficult.

Infection of the Heel Space. The fat pad is intersected by dense fibrous bands extending from the plantar fascia to the skin. The spread of infection from one subdivision to another is therefore slow. Throbbing pain, sufficiently severe to interfere with sleep, is the leading symptom. The patient dare not put his heel to the ground. Swelling of the soft tissues overlying one or both sides of the calcaneus is present. Some oedema around the ankle is usual. Acute tenderness over the space, and, later, fluctuation, leaves no doubt as to the diagnosis.

Infection of the Deep Fascial Spaces of the Sole. There are three deep fascial spaces in the sole—medial, central and lateral. The medial and lateral spaces are of subsidiary importance, for they are comparatively rarely infected. The *central plantar space* is arranged like an apartment house of four storeys (*Fig.* 889). Infection of the various floors of this space becomes increasingly less common as one proceeds from the ground floor upwards. Infection can arise from a penetrating wound, but more frequently it results from extension from an undrained abscess of an interdigital subcutaneous space which spreads along the tunnel that accommodates the digital nerve. As in the hand, the most valuable guides to pus deep in the sole are swelling of the *dorsum* and tenderness of the instep. That the instep is acutely tender serves to distinguish the condition from infection of an interdigital subcutaneous space. In infection of any of these spaces the concavity of the instep is obliterated and in late cases it assumes convexity.

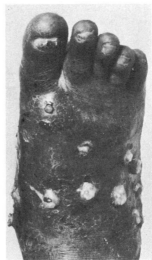

Fig. 890. Madura foot.

Madura Foot* (Mycetoma Pedis), which is endemic in tropical Africa, the Middle East and South-

---

* Due to the *Oöspora madurae* discovered by Hyacinthe Vincent in 1894.

East Asia, is caused by a filamentous fungus that abounds in road dust. In the early stage, especially if the sole is involved, malignant melanoma may be suspected, but later like other invading mycotic infections, sinuses result (*Fig.* 890) giving rise to discharging 'granules' (clumps of the infecting fungus). These may be one of three varieties, known respectively as black, red and yellow mycetoma, because of the colour of the granules. Mycetoma pedis is practically confined to those who go about barefooted, and in the great majority the infection is introduced by a prick, usually by a thorn. The first manifestation is a firm, painless, rather pale nodule, usually on the foot; it increases in size and others appear. In a matter of a week or more, vesicles appear on the surface of the nodules. Soon each vesicle bursts, to reveal the mouth of a sinus, which discharges purulent mucoid fluid containing the characteristic tiny granules. These are sought in the same way as described for actinomycosis (*see* p. 39). *There is no lymphadenitis.* The further course differs according to the variety of mycetoma present. In the black variety the infection spreads mainly subcutaneously. In the red and yellow varieties deep spread occurs early, and muscle and underlying bone become infiltrated, but, unexpectedly, nerve and tendons are highly resistant to invasion, and neurological signs are conspicuous by their absence. Blood-borne dissemination to other parts of the body does not occur. Sooner or later secondary infection supervenes and produces rapid deterioration of the condition. Gross swelling of the foot with obliteration of the concavity of the instep occurs, often with its replacement by a convexity.

The Differential Diagnosis of Multiple Sinuses of the Foot is a common problem in many tropical countries. A veritable host of infections can cause sinuses and basically the diagnosis depends on isolating the causative organism together with a knowledge of local endemic infections. Bear in mind that tuberculosis is common in the tropics and is often long untreated. Kaposi's sarcoma (*see* p. 29), in which the soft nodules often become infected, can resemble Madura foot clinically. Tropical ulcer (*see* p. 529) may occur on the foot.

APPENDIX A

This section has been included to aid the student and newly qualified practitioner confronted with a patient requiring a relatively rapid but efficient routine of examination which will not skimp vital points. It is an attempt to supplement experience which is necessarily lacking. All the methods of examination are to be found earlier in the book, hence the cross-references.

1. THE NEWLY BORN INFANT

In England and Wales infant deaths due to congenital malformations now total approximately 20 per cent of all deaths in infancy (i.e. under 1 year of age). Many of these deaths are of course unavoidable; conversely, the best results for treatment of many congenital anomalies are attained only if the condition is diagnosed early. This applies particularly to neonatal intestinal obstructions (*see* p. 303), talipes (*see* p. 536), congenital dislocation of the hip (*see* p. 493), and spina dysraphism (*see* p. 199). It is advisable therefore for the doctor who has newborn children in his care to apply a scheme of examination for each and every infant.

First, the naked infant should be *inspected*. Some defects which it is essential to remedy are easily seen, e.g. exomphalos (*see* p. 247) and meningomyelocele (*see* p. 199). Birth fractures are usually obvious.

Next the *anus* should be viewed, and in a few instances the little finger passed (imperforate anus, *see* p. 280). This may seem obvious, but, for want of this simple examination, cases of imperforate anus still present after the elapse of several days with advanced intestinal obstruction.

Tracheo-oesophageal fistula will be suspected on inspection if the signs detailed on p. 196 are remembered, particularly that of copious frothy saliva.

Lastly, perform the hip abduction tests (*see* p. 493) to exclude congenital dislocation of the hips, and observe the feet. If there is any suspicion of talipes, test whether the little toes can be placed on the shins (*see* p. 537).

Auscultation of the chest for murmurs, indicating congenital heart disease, is necessary, particularly if the baby is cyanosed, but this is beyond the scope of this work and, indeed, early diagnosis is not so essential.

Conditions to be suspected in the First 12–24 Hours of Life. First and foremost is *neonatal intestinal obstruction* (*see* p. 303).

If very little or no urine is passed, obstruction by a posterior urethral valve is a possibility; examine for a full bladder (*see* p. 337).

Cyanosis on Attempted Feeding. *See* p. 196.

2. EXAMINATION OF THE SEVERELY INJURED PATIENT

Unlike the slightly injured person who will usually indicate the injured part and state what has happened (e.g. a fall on the wrist, a cut finger) the severely injured patient may be unconscious, and the doctor will often have to rely on eye-witnesses or ambulance attendants to relate what has happened.

The first priority in examination is to determine by the methods outlined on p. 42 whether the patient is shocked. In a properly run Trauma Department a nurse will have placed a sphygmomanometer cuff around an upper arm before the doctor reaches the patient. The first blood pressure reading and pulse rate are an important base-line and should be followed by quarter-hourly recording of these data in all serious injuries.

Proceed then to examine the limbs for obvious signs of fracture of a long bone (*see* p. 432) and to question the patient, if possible, regarding pain in the back and elicit signs which might indicate a fractured spine (*see* p. 216). When the possibility of a fractured long bone or spine have been eliminated by clinical means, the nursing staff are asked to undress the patient completely, if necessary cutting the clothes along the seams, to enable a full examination. It is wiser for the doctor himself to supervise this if there is suspicion or certainty of the above injuries.

Reverting to the apparently mildly injured patient, beware the patient who states that there is nothing wrong with him after a serious accident, and examine him most carefully, testing particularly for fractured ribs (*see* p. 181). Numerous instances have been reported, from Coroners' Courts, of patients allowed to leave hospital with multiple fractured ribs (not seen on, perhaps imperfect, X-rays), or with a ruptured spleen, or with cardiac tamponade. Proper application of the compression test will not fail to elicit pain if several fractured ribs are present.

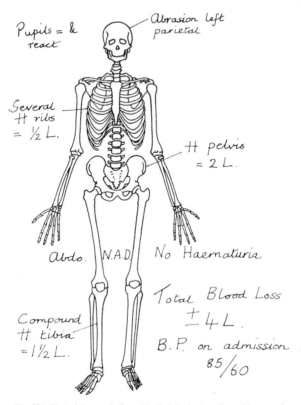

Fig. 891. Pictorial record of a patient's injuries together with a rough calculation of blood loss. The symbol ╫ denotes fracture.

When the patient is completely undressed the examiner should continue in an ordered manner. Apart from obvious fractures, all lacerations and bruises should be noted carefully, even if only for medicolegal purposes. It is useful and expeditious to make a graphic record utilizing a rubber stamp pad of the skeleton (*Fig.* 891). A logical sequence is as follows:

The Head (*see* p. 56). Remember that 60 per cent of accident deaths are due to head injury (Rowbotham).

Fractures of the Facial Skeleton comprise varying combinations of fractures of the zygoma (*see* p. 68), nose (*see* p. 134), maxilla (*see* p. 94), and mandible (*see* p. 96).

The Thorax. Examine for fractured ribs, subcutaneous emphysema (*see* p. 182), pneumothorax, and cardiac tamponade (*see* p. 185). Check that both sides of the chest move equally (*see* p. 192).

The Abdomen. In most cases a rapid palpation of the conscious patient's abdomen satisfies one that there is no intraperitoneal injury.

The Urinary Tract. In relevant instances with trauma to the loins, lower rib cage, or pelvis, the

GEORGE F. ROWBOTHAM, 1899–1975, *Neurosurgeon, Royal Victoria Infirmary, Newcastle upon Tyne.*

patient should be asked to pass urine, which is examined for haematuria (*see* p. 335). Should the patient be unwilling or unable to pass urine the passage of a catheter in the operating theatre under full asepsis is mandatory.

The Limbs. From the point of view of treatment, this is the optimum time to diagnose, or at least suspect, that the major limb artery has been disrupted by the injury. Examine the distal part of the limbs for signs of ischaemia (*see* pp. 385–7).

The Spine (*see* p. 218).

On concluding this detailed examination (and sometimes before), it is often more important to commence treatment for shock immediately, than to send the patient to the X-ray department for an investigation which usually only confirms what is already known.

Diagnosis of the Extent of Blood Loss. The blood loss in the first 24 hours after certain severe injuries is much greater than previously thought. The *average* figures (in adults) for various common *closed* fractures are given below. Compound fractures may show a much greater loss depending on the efficiency of first-aid treatment and the size of divided vessels.

Pelvis   2·0 litres.
Shaft of femur (including basal fractures)   1·0 litre.
Neck of femur   0·5 litre.
Shaft of tibia   0·75 litre.
Ankle fractures   0·5 litre.
Fractures around the knee with effusion   1·0 litre.
Shaft of humerus   0·5 litre.
Fracture-dislocation of elbow   0·5 litre.
Shafts of radius and ulna   0·5 litre.
Colles's fracture   0·25 litre.
3–5 ribs (without haemothorax)   0·5 litre.

In each case reference to a pictorial record as in *Fig.* 891 together with a simple arithmetical calculation will lead to an approximate estimate of the blood loss, often before signs of shock are apparent. It is safer to err on the side of exaggeration of the extent of the haemorrhage in the first place.

The Battered Baby or Child Syndrome (non-accidental injury). The child is said by the parents to fall and break bones frequently. Often there is a stepfather and the mother gives a history inconsistent with the nature of the injury. The child is pale, withdrawn and silent, uncooperative and shrinks away when touched. Diagnosis is frequently rendered more difficult by the mother taking the child to different hospitals with successive incidents, cf Munchausen's Syndrome p. 323.

The Unconscious Patient. Make sure that the airway is unobstructed and insert an endotracheal tube if necessary. The problem of completely accurate diagnosis is much more difficult. In the majority, head injury is the cause of the loss of consciousness. It is important to have the whole scalp shaved as soon as feasible, for a bruise often overlies a fracture.

Even in patients with head injuries, hypoxia may be the factor which precipitates loss of consciousness. Examine carefully therefore for chest lesions and estimate the blood loss due to other injuries. Bleeding into the skull is not an important factor in assessing blood loss, but bleeding from a scalp wound is often quite copious.

Unless the patient is deeply unconscious, an abdominal injury can be detected by the fact that palpation seems to cause pain. Admittedly this is often a most difficult decision to make. Two physical signs are helpful (Lewin). First seek shifting dullness in the flanks (*see* p. 243) and secondly auscultate the abdomen (*see* p. 301). Absent bowel sounds suggest early peritonitis, i.e. that there is an intra-abdominal lesion.

Lastly, bear in mind that coma is due frequently to medical causes, and actually may have caused the accident. Diabetes, a stroke, alcoholic poisoning and barbiturate poisoning are the common causes of coma. In suspected poisoning, a sometimes neglected, common-sense test is to look for a bottle in the patient's pockets. Many people now carry a card detailing their medication (anticoagulants, steroids) or disability (diabetes, haemophilia, etc.).

3. EARLY DETECTION OF CANCER

Although malignant disease is now much more frequent than serious infectious disease in many parts of the world, it is not yet a notifiable condition in Great Britain or any other large country with

WALPOLE S. LEWIN, *Contemporary Neurosurgeon, Addenbrooke's Hospital, Cambridge.*

reasonably developed public health services. Thus any deductions as to the frequency of cancer have to be drawn from the only data available, namely, mortality statistics which are not of extreme reliability. In England and Wales malignant disease causes, at present, approximately one hundred and fifty thousand deaths annually. In *Fig.* 892 is shown the approximate percentage frequency for the most important sites, excluding lymphomata. It is with the early detection of these growths that the student and practitioner are most concerned.

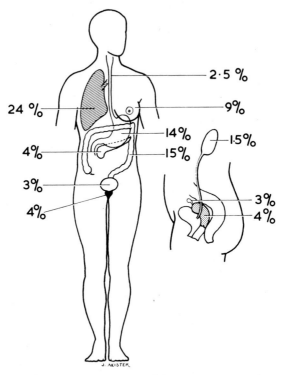

Fig. 892. The frequency of cancer as the cause of death in England and Wales. Colon and rectum are grouped together (15 per cent), as are cervix and body of uterus (4 per cent). Note the comparative rarity of kidney (1·5 per cent) and thyroid and testis (not shown; only 0·4 and 0·2 per cent respectively). All cancers of the upper air passages, mouth and tongue only comprise 2 per cent of the total.

Alteration of Function. It must be stressed that the majority of potentially curable cancers present early with alteration of function and that to wait until physical signs are evident is often to procrastinate until long after a chance of cure has vanished. Thus, one of the following complaints should always be heeded and, in the absence of physical signs, should lead the clinician to request an appropriate X-ray examination and/or arrange to perform an endoscopy.

Indigestion or *loss of appetite* of recent onset, particularly in an older person. Carcinoma of the stomach (*see* p. 228) must be excluded.

Loss of weight is found in the late stages of many malignant conditions (and in many other diseases) but, in the first place, suspect carcinoma of the stomach.

Diarrhoea and/or relative constipation, if of more than 2 or 3 weeks' duration, and in the case of the former not obviously infective in origin, should lead to a suspicion of rectal (*see* p. 275) or colonic carcinoma (*see* p. 240) until proved otherwise.

Hoarseness or loss of voice. Suspect carcinoma of the larynx (*see* p. 133).

Cough. Many smokers cough, and it is a recent alteration in the character of a cough which should induce suspicion and special investigation. Even a few flecks of blood noticed in the sputum is most significant. This is not the place to discuss the early diagnosis of bronchial carcinoma by bronchoscopy and radiology, but it is stressed that this is a highly malignant neoplasm and that presentation with metastases is frequent (*see* p. 190).

Dysphagia. Carcinoma of the oesophagus (*see* p. 197) or of the hypopharynx (*see* p. 132) must be thought of.

Abnormal Bleeding. The presence of blood in the excreta, or in a discharge from any orifice, or in the sputum, must be the signal for the instigation of a vigorous investigation along the lines laid down earlier in this work, namely:

Haematuria see p. 335.

Rectal bleeding. Colonic, rectal and anal neoplasms often bleed.

Vaginal bleeding see p. 286.

Haemoptysis. The importance of this sign has been stressed above in discussing carcinoma of the bronchus.

Haematemesis is unusual as the first sign of carcinoma of the stomach, but this sign must not be neglected lest a serious benign condition requires treatment.

Epistaxis is rarely due to a growth unless oft-repeated, but remember that nasopharyngeal neoplasms are common in some localities (*see* p. 132). Carcinoma of the maxilla (*see* p. 137) may present with nose-bleeding.

Cancer presenting with Physical Signs. The most important are breast cancer (*see* Chapter 15), and ulcerating growths of the skin (*see* p. 33) and mouth. An ovarian cyst (*see* p. 285) must be assumed malignant for there are no physical signs to prove the contrary.

Other important growths which usually can be detected clinically are:

Testicular tumours, *see* p. 369. Penile cancer, *see* p. 354.

Uterine cancer, *see* p. 286. Thyroid cancer, *see* p. 156.

In general, any swelling, unless obviously benign on clinical grounds (e.g. lipoma, ganglion, sebaceous cyst), should be removed and submitted for histology. Unless this is done, the clinician will occasionally commit a serious error of omission.

4. FOLLOW-UP OF CANCER PATIENTS

Following treatment of malignant disease, the conscientious clinician will observe the patient closely for at least 5 years if feasible, a good scheme being to re-examine him every 3 months for 2 years, then every 6 months for 3 years. All neoplasms can recur at any time although the likelihood decreases with the passing of the years. In general it can be said that, after 5 years free of recurrence, cure is probable, but there are exceptions to this rule, notably breast cancers which show a fairly high incidence of late recurrence. In this instance the patient should be seen at yearly intervals after 5 years for the rest of her life if practicable, particularly as the metastases are amenable to treatment.

A few conditions are so highly malignant that it can be said with a fair degree of confidence that, if the patient survives 3 years without evidence of recurrence, they are cured. Into this category fall most neoplasms in infancy and early childhood (nephroblastoma, *see* p. 343; neuroblastoma; and osteosarcoma, *see* p. 425).

The Follow-up Examination

Firstly, carefully scrutinize the *site of the primary growth*. Look particularly for nodules in, or a mass deep to, the operation scar, or for recurrent nodules, or a recurrent mass if treatment has been by radiotherapy.

Next examine the *regional lymph nodes* if these are accessible and have not been removed as part of the operation:

Axilla, *see* p. 174 for primaries in the breast, upper limbs and bronchus.

Cervical, *see* p. 139 for head and neck, breast and bronchus.

Supratrochlear, *see* p. 454 for upper limbs.

Groin, *see* p. 251 for lower limbs, external genitalia, anus and rectum.

Popliteal, *see* Fig. 834, p. 517 for lower limbs.

Supraclavicular, *see* p. 139, particularly for intra-abdominal growths.

Lastly, the *abdomen* must be palpated for enlargement of the liver (*see* Fig. 407, p. 235) and tested for ascites (*see* p. 242).

In appropriate cases vaginal and/or rectal examination is necessary. This applies if the primary growth has been in the uterus or ovaries, or in the left colon, or if deposits of growth in the pelvis are suspected (*see* Blumer's rectal shelf, p. 277 and Krukenberg's tumours, p. 228).

Weighing the Patient. All patients who have suffered from a major cancer (i.e. anything more serious than a rodent ulcer or skin epithelioma) should be weighed at each visit. Loss of weight without dieting (more than 2 kg) indicates that a very careful search must be made for recurrence or metastases. A similar gain in weight should make the clinician suspicious of the development of ascites.

Bone Metastases. Even in cancer patients pain can be caused by non-malignant conditions, e.g. cervical spondylosis, prolapsed lumbar intervetebral disc, and osteoarthrosis of the knee, to mention a few common causes. If such a cause is not apparent, or if ordinary methods of treatment fail, consider a bone metastasis. If accessible, palpate the part carefully for local tenderness. If the metastasis is in a bone anywhere near the surface, the affected area is usually exquisitely tender. A swelling (*see Fig.* 105, p. 55) is exceptional, but a pathological fracture develops in a quarter of long bones which become the seat of a metastasis.

An X-ray is mandatory, but in many cases the first radiograph is normal. In such circumstances a radio-isotope bone scan often demonstrates metastases. Backache, particularly, is suggestive, the vertebrae being the *first* site of half of bone deposits. Paraplegia complicates approximately 10 per cent of these.

Detection of Deeply-seated Metastases. Deposits, initially clinically silent, affect the *lungs* in which metastases have to become remarkably diffuse before the patient becomes short of breath. A pleural effusion, which is probably at least as common, causes dyspnoea earlier. Dullness to percussion and absent breath-sounds are evident on the affected side.

Brain secondaries are commoner than primary brain tumours. Their localization is beyond the scope of this work, but look for changes in personality, paralyses, and cranial nerve palsy (*see* p. 58), particularly in patients who have had carcinoma of the bronchus.

Lymphomata. Examination is directed specifically to all lymph-node areas (*see above*), and to the abdomen for enlargement of liver and spleen. Bone deposits occur in a small proportion (9 per cent).

Further Primary Growths. Any patient who has had a cancer successfully treated is more liable to develop a growth than the average. This may be in the contralateral organ (breast, bronchus, ovary, testis), remnant of the same organ (particularly colon), or in another organ.

5. SURGICAL DIAGNOSIS IN OLD AGE

There is no definition of old age, but it is a truism that a patient considered old by one observer would not be categorized as such by another. A good deal depends on the age of the observer! Be that as it may, the likelihood of the following remarks applying to any given patient is increased *pari passu* with his years and becomes of cardinal importance over the age of 70 years.

Surgical examination in an older person does not differ from that already described in this work but the older the patient the more likely that a given disease process is malignant (i.e. cancerous rather than sarcomatous) in aetiology. This might be termed the first principle of diagnosis in geriatric surgery. The second is that double, or triple, pathology is commoner with increasing longevity. Medical conditions (sometimes multiple) often accompany surgical disease and should be sought by routine methods of examination.

Although the possible combinations of disease are infinite in number, it is convenient to consider the commoner associations on a sexual basis:

In the male, bear the following points in mind in conducting your general examination after examining the part of which the patient complains.

Inguinal hernia (*see* p. 255) is common.

Always inquire regarding frequency of micturition. It is as well to be aware of the degree of risk of acute retention of urine, should an operation prove advisable. If there is any degree of frequency assess the size of the prostate carefully by rectal examination (*see* p. 356).

In the female, be on the lookout for two important unobtrusive conditions:

A small femoral hernia (*see* p. 300) which may, or may not be, the cause of abdominal symptoms.

A painless scirrhous carcinoma of the breast which an old lady is very liable to ignore.

In both sexes, *backache* is often due to secondary carcinoma, originating particularly in the breast or prostate. If these or other primary growths are absent, consider senile osteoporosis (*see* p. 215) as the cause.

APPENDIX B

A list of tropical conditions demonstrating physical signs described in this work has been added for the benefit of students and surgeons in the Tropics.

INDEX

abdomen: acute conditions of, 287–8; conditions
　peculiar to women, 316–19; extra-abdominal
　conditions simulating, 319–20; in the tropics,
　321–2

auscultation of, 217, 301, 312, 555

distension of: by ascites, 242–4; in Hirschsprung's
　disease, (*Fig.* 414) 242; in intestinal
　obstruction, 303; in neonate, 196, 304, 310; in
　paralytic ileus, 311, 312; in peritonitis, 89; in
　potassium deficiency, 46; in pseudo-myxoma
　peritonei, (*Fig.* 419) 244; in retention of
　urine, *see* urine, retention of; in rupture of
　bladder, 331; in spinal cord injury, 219, 220;
　in uraemia, 509; in volvulus of sigmoid colon,
　307; in Wilms's tumour, (*Fig.* 559) 343

fullness of, from fat, fluid, faeces, or fetus, 242–3

increased pressure in, causing hernia, 255

injuries of, 324; detection of, in unconscious
　patient, 555; laceration of mesentery, 326;
　rupture of intestine, 326–7; rupture of liver,
　325–6; rupture of spleen, 324–5

inspection of, (*Figs.* 393–4) 223–4, 227, 240

palpation of, 224–6; beneath bedclothes, for
　infant, (*Fig.* 519) 292, 305; with child's own
　hand, (*Fig.* 509) 242

percussion of, 227; in ascites, 243; in intestinal
　obstruction, 301, 303; in retention of urine,
　(*Fig.* 552) 337

protuberant: in ankylosing spondylitis, (*Fig.* 391)
　214; in congenital dislocation of hip,
　(*Fig.* 812) 494

striae distentiae on, in Cushing's syndrome,
　(*Fig.* 94) 48

'abdominal angina' (mesenteric ischaemia), 229

abdominal aortic catastrophes, 296, 320–1

abdominal crises in medical conditions, 322

abdominal malingerer, 322–3

abdominal reflexes, absent in hemiplegia, 64

abdominal wall:

abscess of, 245–6; in omphalitis, 249

cellulitis of, 33, 245

desmoid tumour in, 28

enlarged veins of, due to portal or vena cava
　obstruction, (*Fig.* 34) 18, 249

infection of, 245

laxity of, in old age, 291

obtaining relaxation of, for palpation of
　abdomen, (*Fig.* 395) 225

oedema of, in meconium peritonitis, 310

passage of extravasated urine up, in subcutaneous
　planes, (*Fig.* 545) 334

rigidity of: involuntary and voluntary, 287; from
　irritation of intercostal nerves by fractured
　ribs, 324

swelling in, (*Fig.* 420) 227, 245, 246

abducent (6th cranial) nerve, injury of, (*Fig.* 109) 59

in Gradenigo's syndrome, 88

in nasopharyngeal carcinoma, 146

abductor pollicis longus: inflammation of sheath of, in
　De Quervain's disease, (*Fig.* 747) 462

abortion:

peritonitis after, 311

vaginal discharge before and after, 283

abscess (*see also* parts affected)

cold, 10, 245

collar-stud, *see* collar-stud abscess

metastatic, 67

possible sites for, in pyrexia after abdominal
　operation, 294

tuberculous, *see* tuberculous abscess

accessory (11th cranial) nerve, injury of, 60, 403

acetabulum, fracture of rim of, 500

achalasia of oesophagus (mega-oesophagus), 197–8

acholuric familial jaundice, 232: ulcer of leg in, 528

achondroplasia, (*Fig.* 695) 429

aclasis, diaphysial (hereditary multiple exostoses), 424

acne rosacea, 5

acoustic (8th cranial) nerve, testing for defect in, 84–5

acrocyanosis (hereditary cold extremities), 382

acromegaly, (*Figs.* 12–13), 7

acromioclavicular joint:

osteoarthrosis of, (*Fig.* 724) 450

subluxation of, (*Fig.* 725) 449–50

acroparaesthesia of hand, in carpal tunnel syndrome,
　462

actinomycosis:

of breast, 174

differentiation of lump due to, from ileitis, 310

of lung, sinus from, (*Fig.* 359) 190

of neck, sinus from, (*Fig.* 83) 39

pus from, (*Fig.* 83) 39

spondylosis due to, 214

adamantinoma, of mandible, 97

Addison's disease, pigmentation of cheek mucosa in,
　126

adductor pollicis, tests for paralysis of:

in median nerve injury, (*Figs.* 668–9) 408–9

in ulnar nerve injury, (*Fig.* 671) 410, 412

adenitis, *see* lymphadenitis

adenocarcinoma:

of Bartholin's gland, 283

of kidney, (*Fig.* 560) 343–4

'adenoid' facies, (*Fig.* 167) 89

adenoids, enlarged:

examination for, (*Fig.* 246) 130–1

snuffles associated with, 134

adenolymphocele: of groin, in onchocerciasis,
　(*Fig.* 442) 253

adenolymphoma, of parotid gland, 104

adenoma:

multiple sebaceous of nose (rhinophyma),
　(*Fig.* 251) 135

pleomorphic salivary, 103

of thyroid gland, (*Figs.* 290, 301) 154, 156, 157,
　161

of thyroid isthmus, 163

of umbilicus, (*Fig.* 433) 250

villous, of rectum, 45

adenomatous polyp, of rectum, (*Fig.* 490) 276

adenomatous polyposis, of intestine, 109–10

adhesions: intestinal, caused by intraperitoneal sepsis,
　40

Adie's syndrome, in head injury, 65

adiposis dolorosa, (*Fig.* 47) 24

adiposogenitalis syndrome, (*Fig.* 95) 48

adolescence, conditions found in (*see also* puberty)

congenital dislocation of hip, 494

imperfectly descended testis, (*Figs.* 599–600) 364

intussusception, 306

kyphosis, 207, 215

recurrent dislocation of patella, 514

slipped epiphysis of femur, 434, 498

cutaneous, in finger-tips in Raynaud's disease, 383
of medial ligament of knee, 511
in multinodular goitre, 161
calculi:
in bladder, 338, 346
in kidney, recurrent, 162, 341, 427
in prostate, 359
in salivary glands: parotid, 102, 105; submandibular, (Figs. 197–8) 105, 106
in ureter, 293, 339, 345; recurrent, 341
in urethra, 338
calf of leg:
crescent sign in haematoma of, (Fig. 641) 391
fibrosarooma of, (Fig. 6)
measurement of girth of, for wasting, (Fig. 806) 491
muscles of: in rupture of tendo Achillis, 524; tenderness in, from phlebothrombosis, (Figs. 639–40) 390–1
pain in: in intermittent claudication, 378; from tear of soleus muscle, 524–5; from thrombosed tibial vein, on dorsiflexion of foot, 390–1
callosities, of foot, (Fig. 873a) 541
callus:
pressure on radial nerve from, 406
at site of fracture, 422; greenstick, (Fig. 703) 434, 449; metatarsal, (Fig. 881) 546
Calve's disease, kyphosis due to, 215
Camper's (Buck's) fascia, 333
cancer (see also carcinoma)
cachexia in, 48–9
early detection of, 555, 556–7
follow-up of treatment of, 557–8
percentages of different sites involved in deaths from, (Fig. 892) 556
cancrum oris, (Fig. 218) 116
Candida infection:
causing chronic paronychia, 475
of mouth, 122
of vagina, 283
canker sore, 111
capillary angioma, (Fig. 49) 27
capillary fragility; excessive, in purpuras, 307
caput medusae, (Fig. 33) 18
in cirrhosis of liver, 239
carbolic acid poisoning, 430
carbuncle, (Fig. 64) 31
of hand, 472
of upper lip, 110
carcinoid facies, (Fig. 171) 91
carcinoma (see also parts affected)
basal-cell, of skin, (Fig. 75) 36
differential diagnosis of lump due to, 310
squamous-cell, of skin, (Fig. 74) 36
of viscera: and supraclavicular lymph nodes, 140; thrombophlebitis migrans as precursor of, 394–5
carcinomatosis:
peritoneal, 244; umbilical hernia in, 248
testing for fluid 'thrill' in, (Fig. 415) 243
carcinomatous ulcer (epithelioma), (Fig. 74) 36
cardiac decompensation:
orthopnoea as sign of, 156
in Paget's disease, 426
in thyrotoxicosis, 156
cardiovascular disease, 'frozen' shoulder in, 446
caries:
of cervical vertebrae, (Fig. 287) 152
dental, 112, 113
Carnett's test, (Fig. 420) 245, 246
carotid artery:
external, displaced by tumour of brachial plexus, 146

internal: fistula between cavernous sinus and, 79; obstruction at origin of, causing hemiplegia, 79; thrombosis of, after trauma, 387
occlusion of, in Takayushu's disease, 385
carotid body, tumour of, (Fig. 274) 144
syncope from pressure on, 144
carpal scaphoid, (Fig. 751) 465
fracture of, (Figs. 752–3) 464–5, 466
palpation of, (Fig. 754) 465
carpal tunnel syndrome, (Fig. 746) 147, 253, 461–2
in dislocation of lunate, 466
due to rheumatoid arthritis, 483
as source of pain in upper arm, 466
carpopedal spasm, 162
carrying angle of elbow, 452–3
in elbow tunnel syndrome, 455
caruncle, urethral, (Fig. 566) 347
castration, gynaecomazia after, 178
cat-scratch disease, 34, 252
cataract:
caused by hypocalcaemia, 162
thrombophlebitis decubiti after operation for, 389
cauda equina:
compression of, in Paget's disease, 427
lesions of, 221–2
tumour of, 202
causalgia, 401–2
cavernous haemangioma, see haemangioma, cavernous
cavernous sinus:
fistula between internal carotid artery and, 79
thrombophlebitis of, (Fig. 123) 70; as complication of carbuncle of upper lip, 110
thrombosis of, after injury, 66
cellulitis, 32
of abdominal wall, 245
from anorectal abscess (Fig. 493) 279
from bulbous periurethral abscess, (Fig. 585) 356
deep, 63; simulating acute osteomyelitic, 419
of face: differentiated from erysipelas, 33; in midline granuloma of nose, (Fig. 252) 135
of hand, 468
from infected bursa, (Fig. 68) 33
of knee, differentiated from effusion into joint, 503–4
in lymphoedema, 399
Morison's aphorism on, 32, 418, 419
of orbit, (Fig. 122) 69–70, 136; infection of cavernous sinus from, 70
of scalp, 52
of scrotum, (Fig. 592) 360
subcutaneous, in lymphangitis, (Fig. 72), 35
cephalhaematoma, 52
cerebellar tonsils, in Arnold–Chiari's malformation, 200
cerebral compression, 61–2
cerebral cortex, localization of various centres in pre-Rolandic area of, (Fig. 115) 62
cerebral irritation, caused by blood in cerebrospinal fluid, 65
cerebral tumour, in pathway of gustatory fibres, causing loss of sense of taste, 98
cerebrospinal fluid:
blood in, 62–3, 65
escape of, from ear, nose, or Eustachian tube, after fracture of skull, 57, 60, 61, 63, 134
cervical lymph nodes:
as lymphatic field: of adenoids, 131; of lips, 112; of maxillary structures, 95
metastases in, (Fig. 276) 140–1, 146; search for primary growth of, 141
palpation of: deep, (Fig. 270) 142; order of, 139–40
stages of breakdown of tuberculous, 142
cervical plexus, injuries to nerves of, (Figs. 659–62) 403–4

arthritis of, 491; acute suppurative, (*Fig.* 814)
496–7; simulated by suppurating deep iliac
lymph nodes, 315, 316; signs of, (*Fig.* 705)
436; tuberculous, (*Fig.* 815) 497–8
dislocation of, congenital, (*Figs.* 809–12) 493–5:
gait in, 216, 440; in infant, (*Figs.* 809–11);
lordosis due to, 203; 'telescopic' movement
of joint in, 491
dislocation of; pathological, 496; traumatic,
(*Fig.* 818) 500
examination of, (*Figs.* 797–808) 486–93
fixed flexion deformity of, (*Fig.* 798) 490
osteoarthrosis of, (*Fig.* 816) 253, 493, 495, 498–9
osteochondritis juvenilis of, 498
pain referred from, 9, 487
palpation of, (*Fig.* 805) 491, 497, 499
stiff, gait due to, 440
traumatic synovitis of, 497, 498
Hippocrates, on head injuries, 57
Hippocratic facies, (*Fig.* 162), 89, 311
Hirschsprung's disease, (*Figs.* 414, 499) 241–2
faeces in, 21
hoarseness, 132, 133
in carcinoma of larynx, 556
from paralysis of laryngeal nerve, in carcinoma of
bronchus, 191, or of thyroid, 157
Hodgkin's disease, (*Figs.* 265, 352) 140, 187
Hoffa's disease, 512
Homan's sign, 390
Hong Kong ear (otitis externa), 83
hordeolum (stye), (*Fig.* 127) 71
interna, 71
Horner's syndrome, (*Fig.* 661) 191, 404
in malignant disease of thyroid, 157
Houston, valve of, 268
Howship–Romberg sign, 266
humerus, fractures of:
capitulum, 458
epicondylar epiphysis, lateral, 457
greater tuberosity, 443, 452
head, causing nerve injury, 456
lower end, T-shaped, 457
neck, 451–2; associated with dislocation of
shoulder, 466
shaft, (*Fig.* 728) 451; causing arterial trauma, 387;
deformity in, (*Fig.* 700) 432; nerve injury
from, 40
supracondylar, 456–7
Hunterian chancre, *see* chancre
Hutchinson's pupils, (*Fig.* 117) 63, 64
Hutchinson's teeth, (*Fig.* 213) 89, 114
Hutchinson's triad, 89
hydatid, Morgagni's, *see* Morgagni's hydatid
hydatid disease, spondylitis due to, 214
hydration, over-
external jugular vein in, 17
hydrocele:
of canal of Nuck, (*Fig.* 451) 259
of femoral hernial sac, (*Fig.* 460) 263
of scrotum; in filarial elephantiasis, 361;
translucent, 363
of spermatic cord, test for, (*Fig.* 450) 259
of tunica vaginalis, (*Fig.* 604.1 and .4) 366:
congenital, 368; fluid from, (*Fig.* 603a), 366;
translucent, (*Figs.* 28, 604.1 and .2) 15, 363,
366, 367
hydrocephalus, (*Fig.* 103) 55
associated with spina bifida, (*Fig.* 368) 200
simulation of, by chronic subdural haematoma, 66
hydromyelia, 199
hydronephrosis, (*Figs.* 25–6) 14
associated with malformation of ear, 343
differentiation of, from enlarged gall bladder, 230
hydropneumothorax, after rupture of oesophagus, 196
hygroma, cystic:

of axilla and groin, 142
of neck, (*Fig.* 271) 142
translucent, 15
hymen, imperforate, 283
in rectovaginal fistula, 281
hyoid bone:
fracture of, 133
greater cornu of, mistaken for hard lymph node,
141–2
hyperadrenocorticism, *see* Cushing's syndrome
hyperaesthesia of skin:
band of, with anaesthesia below, in spinal cord
injury, 219–20
preceding eruption of herpes zoster, 320
saddle-shaped, in lesion of cauda equina, 221
hyperinsulinism, obesity in, 48
hyperkeratosis, senile, (*Fig.* 56) 29
hyperlipidaemia, abdominal pain in, 322
hyperparathyroidism, 162
kidney and ureteric calculi in, 341
osteitis fibrosa cystica in, 427–8
hypertension; causing dissecting aneurysm of aorta,
320
portal, *see* portal hypertension
hyperthyroidism, *see* thyrotoxicosis
hypochondrium: pain in, in cholecystitis, 230
hypogastrium:
swelling in, in rupture of urethra, 331
tenderness in: in aborted ectopic gestation, 316;
in rupture of bladder, 331
hypoglossal (12th cranial) nerve, injury to, 60
tumour of, 146
hypoglycaemic attacks, caused by islet-cell tumour of
pancreas, 239
hypogonadism, obesity in, (*Fig.* 95) 48
hypoparathyroidism, tetany in, 162
hypopharynx, (*Fig.* 244)
carcinoma of, (*Fig.* 266) 132–3, 557
hypospadias, 352–3
perineal, in male pseudohermaphrodite, 353
hypothermia, 159
hypothyroidism, *see* myxoedema
hypoxia, as cause of loss of consciousness, 555
hysteria, urinary retention in, 339

iatrogenic conditions, 46n
icterus neonatorum ('physiological jaundice'), 233
gravis form of, 233
ileitis:
acute terminal, 310
chronic regional, acute episodes in, 310
fistula-in-ano in, 274
ileocaecal valve, (*Fig.* 517) 302
ileostomy, potassium loss from, 45
ileum, obstruction of: dehydration in, 300
signs of, (*Fig.* 517b) 302
ileus:
in acute pancreatitis, 299
gallstone, 307
meconium, (*Fig.* 518) 304
paralytic, 311–12; postoperative, 311; in uraemia,
303, 309
iliac artery, occlusion of, 380
by embolism, 386
by thrombosis, 384
iliac fossa:
left: abscess in, 294; blood in, in ruptured aortic
aneurysm, 320; deep palpation of, (*Fig.* 397)
226; localized peridiverticular abscess in,
295; tenderness in, in diverticulitis of colon,
294

in rupture: of ectopic gestation, 316, 317; of
spleen, 325
in shock, 42
in subdiaphragmatic abscess, 313
in thyrotoxicosis, 155
pulsus paradoxus, in cardiac tamponade, 185
'pump-handle' test, (*Fig.* 384) 210
punctum, in sebaceous cyst, (*Fig.* 39) 23
pupil of eye:
Argyll–Robertson reaction of, (*Fig.* 8) 5, 65, 438
consensual light reflex in, 65n
contraction of, in injury of spinal cord, 219
dilated in shock, 42
in head injury, 57; in neonate, 66
Hutchinson's, (*Fig.* 117) 63, 64
in infection of cavernous sinus, 70
loss of reactions of, 59
myotonic, 65
'pin-point', (*Fig.* 8) 5
purpura:
petechial haemorrhages in, (*Figs.* 521–2) 306
thrombocytopaenic, 306–7
pus:
colour of, 39; 'cayenne-pepper granules' in
actinomycotic, (*Fig.* 83) 39
induration in presence of, 10
odour of, 39–40
sterile, from bubo of cat-scratch disease, 252
pyelonephritis:
as possible cause of postoperative pyrexia, 294
right-sided, simulating acute cholecystitis, 298
pylephlebitis (portal pyaemia), 294, 313, 314–15
pyloric stenosis, 227–8
due to carcinoma, (*Fig.* 394) 224
in infant, (*Figs.* 398–9) 228–9, 305
pyoderma gangrenosum, (*Fig.* 70) 33
pyomyositis, tropical, 246, 316
pyorrhoea alveolaris, (*Figs.* 215–16) 115
in gastric and duodenal cases, 227
pyrexia:
from abscesses, 313, 321
in acute cholecystitis, 298
in acute osteomyelitis, 417
in brain injury, 62; at birth, 66; in cerebral
irritation, 65
causes of, after abdominal operation, 293–4
in fat embolism, 435
in intussusception in infant, 306
in salpingitis, 318
swinging: in pylephlebitis, 314; in
subdiaphragmatic abscess, 314

quadriceps femoris muscle:
paralysis of, 412
rupture of, in old age, (*Fig.* 830) 511
wasting of, (*Fig.* 706) 436, 503, 505, 508, 515
Queyrat's erythroplasia of penis, 354
quinsy, *see* peritonsillar abscess

rachitic . . ., *see* rickets
radial bursa, infection of, 474–5
radial nerve:
injury to, (*Figs.* 665–6) 406–7; in fracture of
humerus, 451, 456
radial pulse, *see under* pulse
radiography, *see* X-rays
radiotherapy, necrosis of tissue due to, 127

radio-ulnar joint, inferior:
dislocation of, in fracture of radius, 459
unstable in Madelung's deformity, 458
radius:
dislocation of head of, in fracture of ulna, 459
dorsal (Lister's) tubercle of, (*Fig.* 741) 459
epicondylar epiphyses of: fracture of lateral, 457;
separation of medial, 457
fractures of: Colles', (*Fig.* 750) 434, 464; of head,
457; of shaft, 459; of shaft, with dislocation
of radio-ulnar joint, 459; of shafts of both
ulna and, 458; Smith's, 464; of styloid
process, 464
styloid process of, (*Fig.* 741) 459
subluxation of head of, in child, 457
test for integrity of head of, (*Fig.* 732) 453
ram's-horn nail (onychogryphosis), (*Fig.* 60)
ranula, (*Fig.* 237) 108, 124–5
rash:
in fat embolism, 435
in septicaemia, (*Fig.* 90) 45
'raspberry tumour' (urethral caruncle), (*Fig.* 566) 347
Raynaud's disease, (*Fig.* 629) 382–3
as cause of gangrene, 388
chronic paronychià in, 383, 475
scleroderma in, (*Figs.* 630–1) 383
Raynaud's phenomenon, in men: 383
rebound tenderness of abdomen, (*Fig.* 504) 288
in aborted ectopic gestation, 316
in appendicitis, 290
in mesenteric vascular occlusion, 308
in obstruction of small intestine, 301
in rupture of small intestine, 326
in salpingitis, 318
recession, sign of, 179
Réclus' disease, 172
records of cases, (*Fig.* 2) 2, 3
of injuries in accidents, (*Fig.* 891) 554–5
of motion of joints, 437
rectal agenesis, (*Fig.* 496) 281
rectal examination (*see also* anorectal examination,
for general principles)
in appendicitis, (*Fig.* 508) 290–1
in ascites, 244
bimanual palpation in, (*Fig.* 473) 267
of bladder, 280, 346
for carcinoma of rectum, (*Fig.* 489) 275–6, or
colon, 280
in congenital megacolon, 242
for metastases from carcinoma of stomach, 228
in neonate and infant, (*Fig.* 499) 280–2, 304
in obstruction of intestine; large, 303; small, 240,
301–2
for pelvic abscess, (*Fig.* 511) 293
of pelvic viscera, 280
in perforated peptic ulcer, 296, 297
of prostate, (*Figs.* 589–90) 357–8, 359–60
revealing loaded bowel, 240, 303
in rupture: of bladder, 331; of urethra, 331
in search for cause of low back pain, 207
rectal shelf of Blumer, (*Fig.* 491) 228, 277–8
rectocele, (*Fig.* 502) 284
recto-urethral fistula, 281
recto-uterine pouch, 285
metastases in, 278
palpable per rectum, 267, 272
rectovaginal fistula, 281
rectovesical pouch:
abscess in, 280
blood in, 280
metastases in, (*Fig.* 491) 228, 277–8
palpation of, (*Fig.* 472) 267–8, 272
tenderness in: in perforated peptic ulcer, 296; in
rupture of bladder, 331
rectum: